OXFORD MEDICAL PUBLICATIONS

Oxford Handbook of
Operative Surgery

Published and forthcoming Oxford Handbooks

Oxford Handbook for the Foundation Programme 4e
Oxford Handbook of Acute Medicine 3e
Oxford Handbook of Anaesthesia 4e
Oxford Handbook of Applied Dental Sciences
Oxford Handbook of Cardiology 2e
Oxford Handbook of Clinical and Healthcare Research
Oxford Handbook of Clinical and Laboratory Investigation 3e
Oxford Handbook of Clinical Dentistry 6e
Oxford Handbook of Clinical Diagnosis 3e
Oxford Handbook of Clinical Examination and Practical Skills 2e
Oxford Handbook of Clinical Haematology 4e
Oxford Handbook of Clinical Immunology and Allergy 3e
Oxford Handbook of Clinical Medicine – Mini Edition 9e
Oxford Handbook of Clinical Medicine 9e
Oxford Handbook of Clinical Pathology
Oxford Handbook of Clinical Pharmacy 3e
Oxford Handbook of Clinical Rehabilitation 2e
Oxford Handbook of Clinical Specialties 9e
Oxford Handbook of Clinical Surgery 4e
Oxford Handbook of Complementary Medicine
Oxford Handbook of Critical Care 3e
Oxford Handbook of Dental Patient Care
Oxford Handbook of Dialysis 4e
Oxford Handbook of Emergency Medicine 4e
Oxford Handbook of Endocrinology and Diabetes 3e
Oxford Handbook of ENT and Head and Neck Surgery 2e
Oxford Handbook of Epidemiology for Clinicians
Oxford Handbook of Expedition and Wilderness Medicine 2e
Oxford Handbook of Forensic Medicine
Oxford Handbook of Gastroenterology & Hepatology 2e
Oxford Handbook of General Practice 4e
Oxford Handbook of Genetics
Oxford Handbook of Genitourinary Medicine, HIV and AIDS 2e
Oxford Handbook of Geriatric Medicine 2e
Oxford Handbook of Infectious Diseases and Microbiology
Oxford Handbook of Key Clinical Evidence
Oxford Handbook of Medical Dermatology 2e
Oxford Handbook of Medical Imaging
Oxford Handbook of Medical Sciences 2e
Oxford Handbook of Medical Statistics
Oxford Handbook of Neonatology
Oxford Handbook of Nephrology and Hypertension 2e
Oxford Handbook of Neurology 2e
Oxford Handbook of Nutrition and Dietetics 2e
Oxford Handbook of Obstetrics and Gynaecology 3e
Oxford Handbook of Occupational Health 2e
Oxford Handbook of Oncology 3e
Oxford Handbook of Operative Surgery 3e
Oxford Handbook of Ophthalmology 3e
Oxford Handbook of Oral and Maxillofacial Surgery
Oxford Handbook of Orthopaedics and Trauma
Oxford Handbook of Paediatrics 2e
Oxford Handbook of Pain Management
Oxford Handbook of Palliative Care 2e
Oxford Handbook of Practical Drug Therapy 2e
Oxford Handbook of Pre-Hospital Care
Oxford Handbook of Psychiatry 3e
Oxford Handbook of Public Health Practice 3e
Oxford Handbook of Reproductive Medicine & Family Planning 2e
Oxford Handbook of Respiratory Medicine 3e
Oxford Handbook of Rheumatology 3e
Oxford Handbook of Sport and Exercise Medicine 2e Handbook of Surgical Consent
Oxford Handbook of Tropical Medicine 4e
Oxford Handbook of Urology 3e

Oxford Handbook of
Operative Surgery

Third edition

Edited by

Anil Agarwal
Consultant General and Colorectal Surgeon,
University Hospital of North Tees,
Stockton on Tees, UK

Neil Borley
Consultant Colorectal Surgeon,
Cheltenham General Hospital, UK

Greg McLatchie
Professor of Surgical Sciences, University of Sunderland;
Consultant Surgeon, Lister Hospital, Stevenage, UK

OXFORD
UNIVERSITY PRESS

OXFORD
UNIVERSITY PRESS

Great Clarendon Street, Oxford, OX2 6DP,
United Kingdom

Oxford University Press is a department of the University of Oxford. It furthers the University's objective of excellence in research, scholarship, and education by publishing worldwide. Oxford is a registered trade mark of Oxford University Press in the UK and in certain other countries

First Edition published in 1996
Second Edition published in 2006
Third Edition published in 2017

Impression: 1

Published in the United States of America by Oxford University Press
198 Madison Avenue, New York, NY 10016, United States of America

British Library Cataloguing in Publication Data

Data available

Library of Congress Control Number: 2016951475

ISBN 978–0–19–960891–1

Printed and bound in China by
C&C Offset Printing Co., Ltd.

Dedication

AKA
For Charu, Mitali, and Kunal

NB
For Alexander, Christopher, and Jennifer

GRM
For Ross, Cameron, Ailidh, Claire, and Calum

Preface to the third edition

'The story always old and always new'
The Ring and the Book

It is twenty years since the first edition of *Operative Surgery* was published. At that time trainees were apprentices in surgery and the emerging consultant was a varied creature in terms of skill and experience, but had the advantage of many hours of exposure to surgical procedures.

By contrast, when the second edition appeared ten years later, the number of training hours had been considerably reduced while training had become more formalized to ensure the standardization of surgical excellence by regular attendance at educational and surgical skills courses. Further, the specialty of general surgery gradually gave way to specialized surgical units including emergency surgery.

As a result this third edition covers the operations listed in the intercollegiate surgical curriculum for each of the ten surgical specialties. It has been extensively updated and rewritten in keeping with the advances of the last ten years.

Trainees in their early years, while sampling a number of surgical specialties, will find in the handbook a detailed description of common operations at which they will assist and ultimately perform. For the specialty-specific intermediate and final stages of training a range of operations that trainees will perform is concisely described. In addition, medical students and housemen will find the descriptions useful during their surgical attachments as will specialist senior nurses and nurse assistants.

A section of 'tips and tricks' is included to add the wisdom of years of experience.

We hope the handbook meets individual needs and will continue to impact on the subsequent production of highly-skilled and well-trained surgeons both now and in the future.

AKA
NB
GRM

Preface to the second edition

The text and increased numbers of contributors reflect the changes that have occurred in general surgery over the past ten years. It is unlikely that in the future we will encounter General Surgical Units. They will be replaced by specialized departments catering for specific areas of surgical expertise. These changes will also fashion future editions of this text in that almost every chapter will become a handbook in itself and the training of surgeons become significantly changed.

GRM
DL
North Tees and Hartlepool NHS Trust
April 2006

Preface to the first edition

This book is a practical guide for the surgeon or surgical trainee about to perform or assist at an operation. The procedures described are those commonly carried out in general, urological, and orthopaedic surgical practice with an introduction on perioperative management and anaesthetics. These should also prove of interest to operating department nurses, assistants, and students of medicine. Indications for, and complications of, procedures are given but more extensive descriptions of these can be found in surgical text books to which the reader should refer.

We emphasize that the book is not for the first-time operator, nor does it embrace the philosophy of 'see one, do one, teach one'. Anyone aspiring to be a surgeon must acquire the basic skills of safe knot-tying and familiarity with surgical instruments. Only by witnessing, assisting at, and then performing many procedures within the structure of a formal surgical training course can the trainee develop the skill, judgement, and the ability to select patients correctly—the recipe for safe surgery.

GRM
Hartlepool
DJL
Stockton on Tees
1996

Contents

Contributors

Anil Agarwal
Chapter 4: Colorectal Surgery
Consultant General and Colorectal Surgeon, University Hospital of North Tees, UK

Reena Agarwal
Chapter 11: Plastic Surgery
Consultant Plastic Surgeon, University Hospitals of Leicester, UK

Andrew Folusho Alalade
Chapter 13: Neurosurgery
Post-CCT Fellow, Victor Horsley Department of Neurosurgery, The National Hospital for Neurology and Neurosurgery, London, UK

James Andrews
Chapter 7: Paediatrics
Specialty Trainee, Paediatric Surgery, Royal Hospital for Sick Children, Glasgow, UK

Sebastian Aspinall
Chapter 6: Endocrine
Consultant Surgeon, Northumbria Healthcare NHS Foundation Trust, UK

Vish Bhattacharya
Chapter 8: Vascular
Consultant General and Vascular Surgeon, Queen Elizabeth Hospital NHS Foundation Trust, Gateshead; Associate Clinical Lecturer, Newcastle University, UK

David Borowski
Chapter 1: General
Specialist Surgeon, Welwitschia Private Hospital, Walvis Bay, Namibia; Honorary Consultant General and Colorectal Surgeon, University Hospital North Tees, UK

Kate Carney
Chapter 1: General
Specialist Registrar in Colorectal Surgery, University Hospital of North Tees, UK

David Chadwick
Chapter 10: Urology
Consultant Urological Surgeon, The James Cook University Hospital, Middlesbrough, UK

Emily Davenport
Chapter 6: Endocrine
Consultant Surgeon, Hawke's Bay DHB, New Zealand

Matei Dordea
Chapter 5: Breast
Consultant Endocrine and Breast Surgeon, North Tees and Hartlepool NHS Foundation Trust, UK

Simon Endersby
Chapter 15: Oral and Maxillofacial Surgery
Consultant Oral and Maxillofacial Surgery, Department of Oral & Maxillofacial Surgery, Sunderland Royal Hospital, UK

Rodrigo Figueiredo
Chapter 8: Vascular
Specialist Registrar in General Surgery, Northern Deanery, UK

Charlie Giddings
Chapter 14: ENT
Locum Consultant Head and Neck Surgeon, Barts Health, UK

Talvinder Gill
Chapter 4: Colorectal Surgery
Consultant Laparoscopic Colorectal Surgeon, University Hospital of North Tees, UK

Morium Howlader
Chapter 15: Oral and Maxillofacial Surgery
General Practitioner, Washington, UK

Richard Jeavons
Chapter 16: Orthopaedics
Consultant Orthopaedic and Trauma Surgeon, North Tees and Hartlepool NHS Trust, UK

Venkatesh Kanakala
Chapter 2: Upper GI, and Chapter 4: Colorectal Surgery
Consultant General/Upper GI and Bariatric Surgery, The James Cook University Hospital, Middleborough, UK

Vijay Kumar Kurup
Chapter 5: Breast
Consultant Surgeon, University Hospital of North Tees, UK

Paul Malone
Chapter 11: Plastic Surgery
Specialist Registrar in Plastic Surgery, East Midlands Deanery, UK

Michael O. Murphy
Chapter 12: Cardiothoracic
Post-CCT Fellow in Cardiac Surgery, Royal Brompton Hospital, London, UK

Robert Nash
Chapter 14: ENT
Specialist Registrar in ENT, Royal National Throat Nose and Ear Hospital; National Hospital for Neurology and Neurosurgery, UK

Jonathan Pollock
Chapter 13: Neurosurgery
Consultant Neurosurgeon, Essex Neurosciences Centre, Queens Hospital, Romford, UK

Peter Radford
Chapter 14: ENT
Specialist Registrar in ENT, Oxford Deanery, Oxford University Hospitals NHS Trust, UK

Amar Rangan
Chapter 16: Orthopaedics
Professor of Orthopaedic Surgery, Faculty of Medical Sciences & NDORMS, University of Oxford; Consultant Orthopaedic Surgeon, The James Cook University Hospital, Middlesbrough, UK

Vedantashankar Sean Sarma
Chapter 15: Oral and Maxillofacial Surgery
Programme Tutor, Master's in Medical Education Programme, Newcastle University, UK

Gourab Sen
Chapter 3: Hepato-pancreato-biliary, and Chapter 9: Transplantation
Consultant Hepatobiliary & Transplant Surgeon, Freeman Hospital, Newcastle upon Tyne, UK

Manoharan Sengamalai
Chapter 7: Paediatrics
Consultant Paediatric Urologist, Regional Paediatric Nephro-Urology Service, Southampton Children's Hospital, UK

Keith Seymour
Chapter 2: Upper GI
Consultant Upper GI and Bariatric Surgeon, Northumbria Healthcare NHS Foundation Trust, UK

Michael Stanton
Chapter 7: Paediatrics
Consultant Paediatric Surgeon, University Hospital Southampton NHS Foundation Trust, UK

Nikhil Vasdev
Chapter 10: Urology
Consultant Urological Surgeon, Lister Hospital, Stevenage; Senior Lecturer in Urology, University of Hertfordshire, UK

Alex Vesey
Chapter 12: Cardiothoracic
Specialist Registrar in Cardiovascular Surgery and Clinical Research Fellow, BHF Department of Cardiovascular Science, The University of Edinburgh, College of Medicine and Veterinary Medicine, Edinburgh, UK

Colin Wilson
Chapter 3: Hepato-pancreato-biliary, and Chapter 9: Transplantation
Consultant HPB and Transplant Surgeon, Institute of Transplantation, The Freeman Hospital, Newcastle-upon-Tyne, UK

Symbols and abbreviations

➲	cross-reference
~	approx.
∴	therefore
↑	increased
↓	decreased
►	important
❶	warning
✍	referral
⚠	warning
🖱	online reference
→	leading to
AAA	abdominal aortic aneurysm
A&E	accident and emergency
ACTH	adrenocorticotropic hormone
AFP	alphafetoprotein
ALT	alanine transaminase
APACHE	acute physiology and chronic ill health score
APD	afferent pupillary defect
APER	abdomino-perineal excision of rectum
ARDS	acute respiratory distress syndrome
ASA	grade American Society of Anaesthesiologists physical status classification system
ASD	atrial septal defects
ASIS	American Society for Information Science
ASIS	anterior superior iliac spine
AST	aspartate transaminase
ATLS	advanced trauma life support
AV	atrio-ventricular
BIPP	bismuth iodoform paraffin paste
BKA	below knee amputation
BMI	body mass index
BNE	bilateral neck exploration
BPD	bilio-pancreatic diversion
BPE	benign prostate enlargement
BPH	benign prostatic hyperplasia
BPPV	benign paroxysmal positional vertigo
BXO	balanitis xerotica obliterans

Ca19.9	carbohydrate antigen 19.9
CABG	coronary artery bypass surgery
CBCT	cone-beam CT
CBD	common bile duct
CEA	carcinoembryonic antigen
CF	cystic fibrosis
CFA	common femoral artery
CIC	clean intermittent catheterization
CNS	central nervous system or coagulase negative staphylococcus
COPD	chronic obstructive pulmonary disease
CPB	cardiopulmonary bypass
CPEX	cardiopulmonary exercise testing
CRPS	complex regional pain syndrome
CSF	cerebrospinal fluid
CT	computed tomography
CVP	central venous pressure
CXR	chest X-ray
DBD	donor after brain-stem death
DBS	deep brain stimulator
DCP	dynamic compression plate
DH	drug history
DHS	dynamic hip screw
DICA	deep circumflex iliac artery
DIPJ	distal interphalangeal joint
DIR	deep inguinal right
DJ	duodenal-jejunal
DPT	deep partial thickness
DRUJ	distal radioulnar joint
dTF	deep temporal fascia
DVT	deep vein thrombosis
EAM	early active mobilization
EBSLN	external branch of the superior laryngeal nerve
ECG	electrocardiogram
eGFR	estimated glomerular filtration rate
EHL	extensor hallucis longus
EMLA	entectic mixture of local anaesthetic
ENT	ear, nose, throat
ERCP	endoscopic retrograde cholangio-pancreatography
ERP	enhanced recovery programmes
ESS	endoscopic sinus surgery

ESWL	extracorporeal shockwave lithotripsy
EUA	examination under anaesthetic
EVD	external ventricular drain
FAP	familial adenomatous polyposis
FBC	full blood count
FCR	flexor carpi radialis
FDP	flexor digitorum profundus
FDS	flexor digitorum superficialis
FEV1	forced expiratory volume (in 1 second)
FFP	fresh frozen plasma
FHL	flexor hallucis longus
FNAC	fine-needle aspiration cytology
FPL	flexor pollicis longus
Fr	French
FT	full thickness
FTSG	full-thickness skin graft
FVC	forced expiratory vital capacity
GA	general anaesthetic
GCS	Glasgow Coma Score
GDA	gastroduodenal artery
GERD	gastrooesophageal reflux disease
GJ	gastro-jejunal
GOJ	gastro-oesophageal junction
GORD	gastro-oesophageal reflux disease
HA	hepatic artery
HCC	hepatocellular carcinoma
HDU	high-dependency unit
HLA	human leucocyte antigen
H-TOF	H-type trachea-oesophageal fistula
IABP	intra-aortic balloon pump
IAN	inferior alveolar nerve
IBD	inflammatory bowel disease
IC	ileo-caecal
ICP	intracranial pressure
ICS	intercostal space
ICU	intensive care unit
IJV	internal jugular vein
IL-1	interleukin 1
ILD	interstitial lung disease
IMF	intermaxillary fixation

INR	international normalized ratio
IPJ	interphalangeal joint
IPMN	intra-pancreatic mucinous neoplasia
ITA	inferior thyroid artery
ITU	intensive-therapy unit
IU	international units
IV	intravenous
IVC	inferior vena cava
LA	local anaesthetic
LABC	lateral antebrachial cutaneous
LAD	left anterior descending artery
LD	latissimus dorsi
LFT	liver function test
LIF	left iliac fossa
LIMA	left internal mammary artery
LMS	left main stem
LMWH	low molecular weight heparin
LOS	lower oesophageal sphincter
LSV	long saphenous vein
LVMR	laparoscopic ventral mesh rectopexy
MCPJ	metacarpophalangeal joint
MDT	multidisciplinary team meeting
MIP	minimally invasive parathyroidectomy
MLB	microlaryngoscopy + bronchoscopy
MR	mitral regurgitation
MRA	magnetic resonance angiography
MRCP	magnetic resonance cholangio-pancreatography
MRI	magnetic resonance imaging
MTPJ	metatarsophalangeal joint
NBM	nil by mouth
NCS	nerve conduction studies
NG	nasogastric
NICE	National Institute for Clinical Excellence
NJ	nasojejunal tube
NPT	negative-pressure therapy
OA	oesophageal atresia
ODS	obstructive defecation syndrome
OGD	oesophago-gastro-duodenoscopy
ORIF	open reduction and internal fixation
OSA	obstructive sleep apnoea

PDA	posterior descending artery
PE	pulmonary embolism
PEG	percutaneous endoscopic gastrostomy
PFA	profunda femoris artery
PICC	peripherally inserted central catheter
PIPJ	proximal interphalangeal joint
PMH	previous medical history
PPPD	pylorus preserving pancreatico-duodenectomy
PPI	proton pump inhibitors
PPV	patent processus vaginalis
PT	prothrombin time
PT	pubic tubercule
PTA	posterior tibial artery
PTC	percutaneous trans-hepatic cholangiographic
PTFE	polytetrafluoroethylene
PTH	parathyroid hormone
PUJ	pelvi-ureteric junction
PUJO	pelvi-ureteric junction obstruction
PV	portal vein
PVC	polyvinylchloride
RA	radial artery
RA	right atrium
RCA	right coronary artery
RFA	radio-frequency ablation of varicose veins
RIMA	right internal mammary artery
RLN	recurrent laryngeal nerve
RSTL	relaxed skin tension line
RUQ	right upper quadrant
RYGB	Roux-en-Y gastric bypass
SAM	systolic anterior motion
SCV	subclavian vein
SFA	superficial femoral artery
SHS	sliding hip screw
SMAS	superficial muscular aponeurotic system
SPA	sphenopalatine artery
SPT	superficial partial thickness
SRP	septorhinoplasty
SSG	split thickness skin graft
SSRIs	selective serotonin reuptake inhibitors
SSI	surgical site infection

SSSI	superficial surgical site infection
STA	superficial temporal artery
STARR	stapled trans-anal rectal resection
STJ	sino-tubular junction
SVC	superior vena cava
TA	transversus abdominis
TAPP	transabdominal preperitoneal
TAT	trans-anastomotic tube
TAVI	trans-catheter aortic valve implantation
TBSA	total body surface area
TCL	transverse carpal ligament
TED	thromboembolic deterrent
TEMS	trans-anal endoscopic microsurgery
TEP	totally extraperitoneal
TIA	transient ischaemic attack
TMD	temporomandibular dysfunction
TME	total mesorectal excision
TNF	tumour necrosis factor
TEO	transoesophageal echocardiography
TOF	tracheo-oesophageal fistula
TPF	temporoparietal fascia
TPN	total parental nutrition
TRAM	tranverse rectus abdominis myocutaneous
TURBT	transurethral resection of bladder tumour
TURP	transurethral resection of prostate
TVT	tension-free vaginal tape
U	units
U&E	urea & electrolytes
ULTRA	Unrelated Live Transplant Regulatory Authority
US	ultrasound
USS	ultrasound scan
UTI	urinary tract infection
VATS	video assisted thoracic surgery
VC	venae comitantes
VF	ventricular fibrillation
VT	ventricular tachycardia
VTE	venous thromboembolism
YAG	yttrium aluminium
ZA	zygomatic arch
ZM	zygomaticomaxillary

Chapter 1

General surgery

Preoperative assessment

Overview

The scope of investigations required preoperatively depends upon the planned operation and the co-morbidities of the patient.

Operations can be classified as minor, intermediate, major, and major plus, depending on the operation undertaken.

- Minor—excision of skin lesion.
- Intermediate—inguinal hernia repair.
- Major—total abdominal hysterectomy.
- Major plus—colonic resection, joint replacement.

A patient's general health may be estimated by their ASA grade:

- Grade 1: normal healthy patient.
- Grade 2: mild systemic disease.
- Grade 3: severe systemic disease that is not a constant threat to life.
- Grade 4: severe systemic disease that is a constant threat to life.
- Grade 5: moribund patient not expected to survive.
- Grade 6: a declared brain-dead patient whose organs are being removed for donor purposes.
- An 'E' may be added to any of the above to denote emergency surgery.

NICE have developed extensive guidance on this topic (for elective surgery) using a simple 'traffic light system' to recommend tests:

- Red: test not recommended.
- Yellow: consider this test.
- Green: test recommended.

Full guidance is available from NICE (1)

This guidance pertains specifically to patients of ASA grades 1–3. Patients with an ASA of 4 will require similar tests to those with an ASA of 3 and may require more in-depth testing, depending on their specific co-morbidities. Patients with an ASA of 5 or 6 are, by definition, unlikely to be 'elective' patients and are, therefore, not covered in this specific guidance.

Cardiopulmonary exercise testing (CPEX)

Patients with cardiorespiratory disease are at higher risk of perioperative complications. CPEX testing allows an objective assessment of the patient's cardiorespiratory reserve and predicts postoperative morbidity and mortality.

Anaerobic threshold (AT) is the onset of anaerobic metabolism during exercise where demand for energy cannot be met by aerobic metabolism alone. It is independent of patient effort. It is an individualized measure of a patient's physiological reserve and, therefore, represents their ability to respond to the metabolic demands of major surgery. This is measured during CPEX testing.

An AT of less than 11ml/min/kg is associated with high rates of perioperative morbidity and mortality.

CPEX testing should be considered in patients planned to undergo major surgery. The evidence for 'routine use' in preoperative assessment in all 'major' case across all surgical specialties is still being gathered—this is exemplified by the common use of CPEX in major vascular cases but the relative lack of use in major colorectal cases.

Mortality and morbidity risk assessment

Accurately assessing patient risk has been shown to enhance subsequent management by aiding clear communication of risk and leading to early critical care involvement/consultant surgical/anaesthetic support.

Commonly used tools for this include the P-POSSUM score. This combines physiological and operative parameters to provide a prediction of operative mortality and morbidity.

An easily accessible calculator is available at:

(http://www.riskprediction.org.uk/pp-index.php).

Preoperative medication review

It is important to review the patient's prescribed medications to understand potential drug interactions and avoid potential complications.

Medications to continue

Cardiovascular system

- *Calcium channel blockers*, *beta blockers*, *nitrates*, and *anti-arrhythmia agents* should continue.
- *Aspirin* should be continued unless major bleeding is expected (cardiac or prostate surgery) or minor bleeding is best avoided (retinal or intra-cranial surgery).

Respiratory system

- *Bronchodilators* should be continued, as withdrawal can precipitate bronchospasm.

Endocrine system

- *Thyroxine/levothyroxine* should continue.
- Steroid intake can cause adrenal suppression. History of steroid intake (10mg prednisolone or more) within the last 3 months requires hydrocortisone supplementation preoperatively.
- Insulin-dependent diabetes—sliding scale/insulin infusion regimes, according to local hospital guidance.

Central nervous system

- *Anti-epileptic medication* should be continued.
- *Parkinson's disease medications* should be continued.
- *Antidepressants: SSRIs (selective serotonin reuptake inhibitors)* can continue but concurrent use with pethidine, tramadol, and pentazocine can precipitate a fatal serotonin syndrome.
- *Antipsychotic drugs* should be continued.
- *Benzodiazepines:* can continue (but may also contribute to respiratory depression/hypotension perioperatively).

Other

- *Anti-reflux medications* should be continued.
- *HIV medications*—a useful website for checking interactions with antiretrovirals is:

(http://www.hiv-druginteractions.org/Interactions.aspx).

Medications to be stopped

Cardiovascular system

- *ACE inhibitors, angiotensin II receptor agonists, and diuretics* should be withheld the day before and the day of surgery, as they may cause severe hypotension perioperatively.
- *Warfarin* should be stopped at least 4 days before surgery. An International Normalized Ratio (INR) of 1.5–2 is acceptable. Reversal agents: vitamin K, fresh frozen plasma, prothrombin complex concentrate—depending on the urgency of reversal required (discuss with haematology).

- *Unfractionated heparin* used as a bridging anticoagulant in patients with a high risk of VTE (venous thromboembolism) should be stopped 6h before surgery and recommenced 12h post-surgery.
- *Clopidogrel* should be stopped 7 days prior to surgery unless cardiac event within 3 months.
- *Factor Xa inhibitors* (*dabigatran, rivoraxiban, apixaban*): stop 2–3 days prior to surgery—note no reversal agent.

Endocrine system

- *Oral hypoglycaemics*: stop on the morning of surgery, usually.
- *Oestrogen-based oral contraceptives/HRT*: increase the risk of thromboembolism; should be stopped 4 weeks prior to surgery (with appropriate counselling, regarding barrier precautions, undertaken); progesterone-only treatments do not need to be stopped.

Central nervous system

- *Antidepressants* (*tri-cyclic antidepressants*): recommend discontinue prior to surgery but will need 1–2 weeks of dose tapering prior to surgery.
- *Monoamine oxidase inhibitors* (*MAOs*): irreversible MAOs should be stopped 2 weeks prior to surgery; reversible MAOs stopped on the day of surgery—can fatally interact with pethidine/ephedrine.
- *Mood stabilizers* (*lithium*): discontinue 24h prior to surgery.

Other

- *Rheumatic disease drugs*: discuss with your surgeon.
- *Methotrexate* may impair wound healing/more infective complications, therefore, some recommend withholding this for 48h preoperatively; similarly with *cyclophosphamide*. Restarting these medications should be discussed with Rheumatology.
- *NSAIDs*: long half-life, discontinue 1 week before surgery; short half-life, discontinue 2–3 days prior to surgery.

Consent

Any decision in healthcare results from a shared discussion between the patient and their healthcare professional.

Doctors must now ensure that patients are aware of any 'material risks' involved in a proposed treatment, and of reasonable alternatives, following the judgement in the case of Montgomery v. Lanarkshire Health Board.

The case: The vaginal delivery of Sam was complicated by shoulder dystocia. The correct manoeuvres to release Sam were performed but during the 12-minute delay Sam was deprived of oxygen and developed cerebral palsy. Mrs Montgomery is diabetic and small in stature; the risk of shoulder dystocia was agreed to be 9–10%. Despite expressing her concerns regarding vaginal delivery, doctors failed to warn Mrs Montgomery of the risk of serious injury from shoulder dystocia or to discuss the possibility of an elective Caesarean section. The court ruled that Mrs Montgomery should had been informed of the risk of shoulder dystocia (material risk) and given the option of a Caesarean section (reasonable alternative).

Test of materiality

Ask yourself: would a reasonable patient think that a particular risk is significant if informed about it? If the answer is yes, it needs to be explored during the consent process.

The patient

To give 'consent' a patient must have 'capacity', which comprises:

- Full understanding of the risks and benefits of having a procedure and the implications of not having the procedure.
- Ability to weigh and retain this information.
- Ability to communicate this decision.

Adults who lack capacity

These patients do not fulfil the above criteria. A good example of this is an otherwise healthy patient with dementia who has a bowel cancer—their dementia takes away their capacity to retain and weigh the information given to them but should not preclude them from consideration of potentially curative surgery. In this situation a '*best interests*' decision must be made.

The decision-maker

The decision-maker must:

- Not make assumptions about a person's wishes based upon their age/appearance/condition or behaviour.
- Consider all the relevant outcomes to taking/not taking a particular course of action at that point.
- Understand the nature of the incapacity. If it is likely to resolve, can the decision be put off until then?
- Involve the patient as much as possible in the decision that is being made on their behalf.

- Consider any wishes or feelings on the subject previously expressed by the patient. Are there any particular religious, cultural, or moral questions to be considered? These may take the documented form of an Advanced Directive or Living Will.
- Consult others: anyone with whom the patient has previously identified as a person to consult in these situations (carer, relative, close friend) or their representative who has Lasting Power of Attorney or a Deputy appointed by the Court of Protection to make their decisions.

Where there are no identifiable patient advocates, an Independent Mental Capacity Advocate (IMCA) should be sought to represent the patient. These are accessible through the safeguarding teams based in all hospitals.

For additional guidance on adults with incapacity please consult: The England and Wales the Mental Health Act (2005) and in Scotland the Adults with Incapacity (Scotland) Act (2000).

Children with capacity

Persons over the age of 16 can give their consent. Those under 16 may also give their consent if they are deemed to have capacity. This is called Gillick Competency. It derives from the case of Gillick v. West Norfolk and Wisbech Area Health Authority (1985) regarding the prescription of contraceptives to children under the age of 16 without parental consent.

If a competent child refuses treatment, those with parental responsibility (except in Scotland) can over-rule the decision, if it is in the child's 'best interests'. If parents refuse treatment that is in the child's 'best interests', this is not legally binding and you may seek a court ruling.

Pregnancy

If the patient is competent, she can refuse treatment for herself and her baby, even if in doing so, she puts her life and the life of the child at risk.

The doctor/healthcare professional

- Must be capable of performing the procedure and understand its steps, risks, and benefits, and the implications of not having the procedure *or* have received specialist training in advising patients regarding the above (delegation of consent).
- *Emergency cases* (adults/children): where consent cannot be obtained—you can provide life-saving treatment.
- Note the existence of Living Wills/Advance Statements.
- Note that *relatives cannot give consent—only the patient involved.*

Which consent form to use?

- *Consent form 1*: used for adults with capacity—patient agreement to treatment/investigation or procedure.
- *Consent form 2*: used for a minor requiring parental/guardian approval for treatment or investigation.
- *Consent form 3*: patient/parental agreement to investigation, treatment, or procedure where consciousness is not impaired (i.e. not for general anaesthetic procedures—use form 2).
- *Consent form 4*: for adults who lack capacity (may be a chronic condition impairing capacity/unconscious).

The key to the consent process is clear communication between doctor and patient.

- Avoid medical jargon.
- Use diagrams/pictures to illustrate your points.
- Check understanding as you go along.
- Get an interpreter if language is a barrier.
- Involve relatives, but remember they cannot give their consent for their loved-one.

For comprehensive guidance, read the GMC's guidance document (2) and the guide from the Department of Health (3).

Prophylaxis

Antibiotics

Surgical site infections (SSIs) are a significant source of morbidity. Specific perioperative antibiotic regimes are available in local formularies designed to counter commensal organisms expected at the surgical site. It is good practice to inform patients that they will receive/have had antibiotics.

NICE recommends antibiotic prophylaxis (<3 doses) in patients undergoing:

- *Clean surgery, with a prosthesis/implant 0–2% SSI risk*, e.g. joint replacement—no breech of the respiratory, gastrointestinal, or genitourinary tract expected.
- *Clean-contaminated surgery 4–10% SSI risk*, e.g. elective sigmoid colectomy—controlled breech of the respiratory, gastrointestinal, or genitourinary tract with minimal contamination.
- *Contaminated surgery >10% SSI risk*, e.g. penetrating trauma with spillage of enteric contents—gross contamination without infection.
- *Dirty surgery*, e.g. perforated viscus, frank pus; compound fracture >4h old—give antibiotic treatment (duration >3doses) in addition to prophylaxis.

Timing of dosage

Consider a single dose of intravenous antibiotics at induction (or 1h before if a tourniquet is being applied). Give a repeat dose of antibiotic if the operation is longer than the half-life of the antibiotic given.

It is not recommended routine use in clean, non-prosthetic, uncomplicated surgery.

Full guidance is available in NICE Clinical guideline 74 (4).

Venous thromboembolism (VTE)

All patients should be given information regarding VTE, its risks and consequences, and the standard local protocols to prevent its occurrence at pre-assessment.

NICE Clinical Guideline 92 (5) offers comprehensive guidance on this topic. Risk factors for VTE are outlined in Box 1.1; the resultant choice of prophylaxis should be weighed against the patient's risk of bleeding, examples of which are shown in Box 1.2.

In general, all surgical patients should have mechanical VTE prophylaxis, unless contraindicated, in the form of one of the following:

- Anti-embolism stockings.
- Foot impulse devices.
- Intermittent pneumatic compression devices.

Do not use mechanical prophylaxis in patients with peripheral vascular disease/previous peripheral arterial bypass grafts/local skin lesions or conditions—limb deformities/heart failure/neuropathy.

Where the risk of bleeding is low, pharmacological prophylaxis should also be added:

- Low molecular weight heparin (unfractionated to be given in those with an estimated glomerular filtration rate (eGFR) <30ml/min/1.73m^2).

Box 1.1 VTE risk

Patient factors

- Age >60 years
- Obesity BMI >30kg/m^2
- Dehydration
- Active cancer/cancer treatment
- HRT/oestrogen-based contraceptive use; pregnancy/post-partum <6 weeks
- Known thrombophilia
- One or more significant co-morbidity factors
- Personal/first-degree relative history of VTE
- Critical care admission
- Varicose veins with phlebitis

Admission factors

- Critical care admission
- Significantly reduced mobility >72h
- Total anaesthetic + surgery time >90min
- Surgery involving the pelvis/lower limb with anaesthetic + surgery time >60min

Box 1.2 Bleeding risk

Patient factors

- Active haemorrhage
- Coagulopathy (acquired—drugs or hepatic failure/innate—haemophillia/von Willebrand's disease)
- Acute stroke
- Thrombocytopenia
- Uncontrolled systolic hypertension 230/120mmHg+

Admission factors

- Neurosurgery/spinal or eye surgery/other procedure with high risk of bleeding
- Lumbar puncture/spinal/epidural—performed in the last 4 hours or expected within the last 12h

- *Duration of treatment*: generally continued until mobility is no longer significantly reduced.
- *Extended treatment*: cancer surgery/major pelvic or abdominal surgery continue treatment for 28 days; elective joint replacements (knee 10–14 days, hip 28–35 days); emergency hip fracture 28–35 days; day surgery patients with reduced mobility 5–7 days.

The WHO surgery checklist

Rationale

WHO estimates of morbidity and mortality following surgery indicates that over *7 million people worldwide will suffer complications following their surgery*. Approximately 1 million will die as a result. Around 50% of these complications are preventable. Haynes et al. (6) demonstrated a reduction of over a third in postoperative morbidity and mortality.

The team brief—at the beginning of the list/session

All members of the team introduce themselves and their role:
- Facilitates communication.
- Breaks down barriers.
- Empowers people to speak up if they see a mistake.

Each case is discussed so all team members know the background and what is planned (patient history/anaesthetic approach/lines/airway equipment/surgical approach/equipment/patient positioning):
- Pre-empts problems: difficult airway/operative equipment.
- The whole team knows what to expect, empowering them to speak up if there is a problem.

Specific considerations discussed:
- ASA grade.
- VTE prophylaxis required.
- Antibiotic prophylaxis.

'Sign in'—before the induction of anaesthesia

- Patient has confirmed identity, site, procedure, and consent.
- Site marked/not applicable.
- Anaesthesia check completed (machine/drugs).
- Ensure the patient has a pulse oximeter attached and that it is working.
- Does the patient have a:
    - Known allergy?
    - Difficult airway/aspiration risk?
    - Risk of >500ml blood loss (7ml/kg in children).

'Time out'—before the skin incision

Team leader should:
- Confirm that all team members have introduced themselves by name and role.
- Confirm the patient's identity, site, and procedure (surgeon, anaesthetist and nurse).
- Ascertain if antibiotics have been given within the last 60min.
- Ascertain if essential imaging is displayed.

The surgeon should confirm:
- Critical or unexpected steps.
- Operative duration.
- Anticipated blood loss.

The anaesthetist should confirm:
- If there are any patient-specific concerns.

The nursing team should confirm:
- The sterility of the equipment.
- If there are any equipment issues or concerns.

'Sign out'—before the patient leaves the operating theatre

Team leader asks:
- Has the name of the procedure been recorded?
- Are the instrument, sponge, and needle counts correct?
- Is the specimen labelled?
- Are there any equipment problems to be addressed?
- What are the key concerns for the recovery of this patient?

The team debrief—at the end of the list/session

Any issues that have been raised during the session are discussed. This is a good opportunity to tell members of the team what they have done well! If a difficult scenario has occurred, this is an important time to make sure all staff members are supported.

A template WHO checklist is provided in Fig. 1.1. This is available as a resource from the WHO site:

(http://www.who.int/patientsafety/safesurgery/ss_checklist/en/).

The WHO actively encourage local adaptations to this template, therefore the actual forms used will differ slightly between individual hospitals.

World Health Organization

Surgical Safety Checklist (First Edition)

Before induction of anaesthesia ▸▸▸▸▸▸▸▸▸ Before skin incision ▸▸▸▸▸▸▸▸▸▸▸▸▸▸ Before patient leaves operating room

SIGN IN

- ☐ **PATIENTS HAS CONFIRMED**
  - IDENTITY
  - SITE
  - PROCEDURE
  - CONSENT
- ☐ **SITE MARKED/NOT APPLICABLE**
- ☐ **ANAESTHESIA SAFETY CHECK COMPLETED**
- ☐ **PULSE OXIMETER ON PATIENT AND FUNCTIONING**

DOES PATIENT HAVE A:

KNOWN ALLERG?
- ☐ NO
- ☐ YES

DIFFICULT AIRWAY/ASPIRATION RISK?
- ☐ NO
- ☐ YES, AND EQUIPMENT/ASSISTANCE AVAILABLE

RISK OF >500ML BLOOD LOSS (7ML/KG IN CHILDREN)?
- ☐ NO
- ☐ YES, AND ADEQUATE INTRAVENOUS ACCESS AND FLUIDS PLANNED

TIME OUT

- ☐ **CONFIRM ALL TEAM MEMBERS HAVE INTRODUCED THEMSELVES BY NAME AND ROLE**
- ☐ **SURGEON, ANAESTHESIA PROFESSIONAL AND NURSE VERBALLY CONFIRM**
  - PATIENT
  - SITE
  - PROCEDURE

ANTICIPATED CRITICAL EVENTS

- ☐ **SURGEON REVIEWS:** WHAT ARE THE CRITICAL OR UNEXPECTED STEPS, OPERATIVE DURATION, ANTICIPATED BLOOD LOSS?
- ☐ **ANAESTHESIA TEAM REVIEWS:** ARE THERE ANY PATIENT-SPECIFIC CONCERNS?
- ☐ **NURSING TEAM REVIEWS:** HAS STERILITY (INCLUDING INDICATOR RESULTS) BEEN CONFIRMED? ARE THERE EQUIPMENT ISSUES OR ANY CONCERNS?

HAS ANTIBIOTIC PROPHYLAXIS BEEN GIVEN WITHIN THE LAST 60 MINUTES?
- ☐ YES
- ☐ NOT APPLICABLE

IS ESSENTIAL IMAGING DISPLAYED?
- ☐ YES
- ☐ NOT APPLICABLE

SIGN OUT

NURSE VERBALLY CONFIRMS WITH THE TEAM:

- ☐ **THE NAME OF THE PROCEDURE RECORDED**
- ☐ **THAT INSTRUMENT, SPONGE AND NEEDLE COUNTS ARE CORRECT** (OR NOT APPLICABLE)
- ☐ **HOW THE SPECIMEN IS LABELLED** (INCLUDING PATIENT NAME)
- ☐ **WHETHER THER ARE ANY EQUIPMENT PROBLEMS TO BE ADDRESSED**
- ☐ **SURGEON, ANAESTHESIA PROFESSIONAL AND NURSE REVIEW THE KEY CONCERNS FOR RECOVERY AND MANAGEMENT OF THIS PATIENT**

THIS CHECKLIST IS NOT INTENDED TO BE COMPREHENSIVE. ADDITIONS AND MODIFICATIONS TO FIT LOCAL PRACTICE ARE ENCOURAGED.

Fig. 1.1 Surgical safety checklist. Reproduced with permission from the World Heatlh Organization.

Skin preparation

Skin preparation

Skin carries commensal organisms and transient bacteria, both of which represent potential sources of SSI. The purpose of skin preparation is to remove transient organisms and to reduce the number of commensal organisms from the surgical field.

Types of skin preparation

Alcohol-based preparations: isopropanol/ethanol

- *Advantages*: fast-acting; minimally toxic; non-staining; non-allergenic; evaporates quickly with good degreasing and cleansing actions; kill most bacteria, viruses, and fungi.
- *Disadvantages*: flammable—fire risk if pooling occurs; repeated use dries skin and can irritate; do not kill bacterial or fungal spores.
- *Not suitable for use near eyes or mucous membranes.*

Chlorhexadine® (cationic bisbiguanide)—aqueous 4% or alcohol-based

- *Advantages*: alcohol-based preparations have been shown to have better bactericidal properties than detergent-based preparations. Persistent antimicrobial action for up to 6h. Low incidence of hypersensitivity and skin irritation.
- *Disadvantages*: little activity against bacterial or fungal spores; emergence of some resistant organisms; stains fabrics; anaphylaxis reported; alcohol-based—fire risk.
- *Not recommended for use on eyes or ears.*

Isophores—iodine-based detergents—(Betadine®, 7.5% povidone-iodine)

- *Advantages*: can be used on skin, mucous membranes, and wounds.
- *Disadvantages*: not sporicidal; can cause staining and irritation of the skin; could theoretically increase circulating iodine (through absorption over a large area) and therefore should be used with caution in patients with hyperthyroidism.
- *Do not use in patients with an iodine allergy.*

Method of skin preparation

Apply using sterile instruments with a non-touch technique, prepping initially over the site of the proposed incision to the periphery. The area should be allowed to dry. Three applications should be sufficient.

Common surgical sutures and needles

Sutures can be classified as *absorbable* or *non-absorbable*, by the origin of their material (synthetic or natural) and their structure (monofilament or braided). *Monofilaments* cause less tissue reaction but require more throws to ensure a secure knot. *Braided* sutures cause more inflammation but require fewer knots. The strength of the suture depends on its size: 0 being the strongest (thickest) to 8/0 the weakest (thinnest). *Cutting needles* are used for skin/tough tissue. *Round-bodied needles* are used when a tissue is more easily pierced and the size of the hole is needed to be consistent and minimized (bowel/vessel).

Absorbable sutures (synthetic: Monocryl®, Vicryl®, PDS®; natural: chromic catgut)

These sutures will be absorbed over a period of time and are generally used inside the body. Table 1.1 shows the time commonly used absorbable sutures take to be fully broken down within the body and the common sites of their use. Suture absorption rates are increased in the presence of fever, infection, or protein deficiency. The tensile strength of the suture reduces, the closer it gets to being absorbed.

Non-absorbable sutures (synthetic: nylon/Ethilon®, Gortex®, Fibrewire®, Ethibond®, Prolene®; natural: silk)

These sutures will not be absorbed. They can be used in skin and subsequently removed. They are used in areas of higher tension where an absorbable suture would be inadequate to allow completion of the healing process. Good examples of this are vascular anastomoses (pulsatile flow exerts pressure) and tendon repairs.

Table 1.1 Absorbable suture time to complete breakdown

Suture name	Complete breakdown time (weeks)	Sites of common usage
Vicryl Rapide™	2	Skin (subcutaneous)
Undyed Monocryl®	3	Skin (subcutaneous)
Dyed Monocryl®	4	Skin closure (stoma formation)/soft tissues
Coated Vicryl®	4.5	Soft tissues
PDS®	9	Soft tissues

Common surgical meshes

Synthetic meshes

- Absorbable: Vicryl®, Dexon®.
- Non-absorbable: Marlex®, Prolene®.
- Composite: polypropylene/expanded polytetrafluoroethylene (ePTFE).

These are widely available and therefore less expensive. However, they are not recommended for use in infected fields and also can potentially erode into adjacent structures (e.g. transvaginal surgery).

Composite meshes are used intra-peritoneally. The upper layer (placed against the abdominal wall) is composed of a standard mesh (polypropylene). The lower layer (exposed to the peritoneal cavity and its contents) is made of biologically inert ePTFE (barrier protecting viscera from adhering to the standard mesh).

Biological meshes

- Collagen-based acellular matrices.
- Cross-linking increases tensile strength.
- Examples include: Permacol®, Alloderm®, Surgisis®.

These implants are more expensive than their equivalent synthetic counterparts, but they can be used in infected fields.

Pore size

The extent of the tissue reaction provoked by the mesh is dependent on the size of its pores. To allow infiltration by macrophages, fibroblasts, blood vessels, and collagen, a mesh must have pores >75μm. Meshes are classified as:

- Type 1 macroporous (pore size >10μm), e.g. polypropylene.
- Type 2 microporous (pore size <10μm), e.g. ePTFE.
- Type 3 composite structure with micro and macroporous components.

Larger pores = more tissue reaction and ingrowth and less 'granuloma bridging' leading to more flexibility. ePTFE is microporous, hence its use in composite meshes as a 'barrier' (no tissue ingrowth, inert).

Weight

The weight of a mesh = weight of the polymer + amount used.

- Heavyweight: thick polymers, small pore sizes, high tensile strength = significant tissue reaction, dense scarring.
- Lightweight mesh = thinner filaments, larger pores (>1mm), reduced tensile strength = less tissue reaction, more elastic and flexible.

Lightweight meshes may hold some advantages over heavyweight meshes in terms of less dense scar formation and hence better elasticity and compliance with the abdominal wall. The available evidence in this area is equivocal.

Strength and elasticity

The composition of the mesh, filament type (monofilament/multifilament), and its pattern (knitted or woven), determines its strength. Knitted mesh can stretch in all directions, whereas woven meshes stretch only in the direction oblique to the 90° intersection of their strands.

When a healthy adult jumps, the maximum intra-abdominal pressure generated is 170mmHg. Any mesh must be able to withstand a pressure of 180mmHg before 'bursting'. All synthetic meshes are designed to withstand this pressure. It is, therefore, not necessary to use heavyweight rather than lightweight mesh for large repairs.

The elasticity of the abdominal wall at 32N/cm is approximately 38%. Lightweight meshes have an elasticity of 20–35% at 16N/cm and heavyweight meshes 4–15%. Reduced elasticity will restrict abdominal distension. It follows that the use of a flexible, lightweight mesh in large repairs would be of benefit (with more elasticity, less restriction on distension).

Principles of enhanced recovery

Overview

Enhanced recovery programmes (ERPs) have revolutionized the management of patients undergoing elective surgery. They have been successfully applied to a range of general surgical specialities, including colorectal, bariatrics, upper GI and ENT surgery. ERPs have also been shown to be of value in the emergency surgical setting.

The aim of ERPs is to expedite recovery after surgery using a targeted, protocol-driven, multidisciplinary team approach in the pre-/peri- and postoperative phases of the surgical journey, involving surgeons, anaesthetists, dieticians, physiotherapists, and specialist nurses. The Association of Surgeons of Great Britain and Ireland (ASGBI) Guidance for implementation of ERPs 2009 is summarized below but can be found in full at:

🔗 (http://www.asgbi.org.uk/en/publications/issues_in_professional_practice.cfm).

Preoperative recommendations

- Preoperative counselling and training.
- A curtailed fast (6h to solids and 2h to clear liquids) and preoperative carbohydrate loading.
- Avoidance of mechanical bowel preparation.
- Deep vein thrombosis prophylaxis using low molecular weight heparin.
- A single dose of prophylactic antibiotics covering both aerobic and anaerobic pathogens.

Perioperative recommendations

- High (80%) inspired oxygen concentration in the perioperative period.
- Prevention of hypothermia.
- Goal-directed intraoperative fluid therapy.
- Preferable use of short and transverse incisions for open surgery.
- Avoidance of postoperative drains and nasogastric tubes.
- Short duration of epidural analgesia and local blocks.

Postoperative recommendations

- Avoidance of opiates and the use of paracetamol and non-steroidal anti-inflammatory drugs (NSAIDS).
- Early commencement of postoperative diet.
- Early and structured postoperative mobilization.
- Administration of restricted amounts of intravenous fluid.
- Regular audit to ensure maintenance of standards and outcomes.

Day surgery

Overview

A patient undergoing 'day surgery' will be admitted, treated, and discharged the same day. A multidisciplinary approach is required to make this work with selection of medically appropriate and motivated patients.

Preoperatively, the patient should be educated regarding the principles of day surgery and receive written information about the process they are going to engage with. The day surgery pathway should be protocol-driven with clear criteria for discharge. Information regarding what to expect in the postoperative period should be provided. Patients should be able to contact the day surgery unit for advice after discharge on an 'as required' basis.

The following should be considered:

Social factors

- Support network—for general anaesthetic procedures, the patient must have a responsible adult to take them home and stay with them for 24h.
- Home environment—must be appropriate for the expected postoperative recovery.

Patient factors

- Patient education—they need to understand the principles of day surgery, consent to the procedure, and commit to the postoperative recovery protocols.
- Fitness for the procedure should be determined by preoperative testing—exclusions should not be made arbitrarily on the basis of ASA/age/obesity.

Surgical factors

- Procedure—should not carry a significant risk of serious complications requiring immediate medical attention (haemorrhage, cardiovascular instability).
- Postoperative symptoms—controllable by oral medication and local anaesthetic techniques.
- Oral intake should be able to be resumed within a few hours.
- Mobilization should not be impaired (ideally).

Anaesthetic factors

- Avoidance of opiates; use of long- and short-acting NSAIDS (as long as not contraindicated).
- Consideration of local/regional blocks.

Energy sources

Electrosurgery: diathermy

This consists of passing a normal electric current through a diathermy machine, creating a high-frequency, alternating current that produces heat to coagulate, cut, and fulgurate tissues. There are two types of diathermy: monopolar (Fig. 1.2) and bipolar (Fig. 1.3).

Potential problems/pitfalls

- Fire risk with flammable skin preparations.
- Patient should not be touching any earthed objects, e.g. the metal edge of the table (this will redirect current flow to this area causing burns).
- Burns under diathermy 'return' pads have been reported.
- Return pads should not be placed over bony prominences, metal implants, scars, hairy areas, or pressure points.
- When not used the active electrode should be placed in an insulated sheath to avoid inadvertent burns to the patient or scrub staff.
- Laparoscopic surgery: non-insulated metal instruments should be kept away from an active electrode to avoid creating an alternative pathway and inadvertent burns.

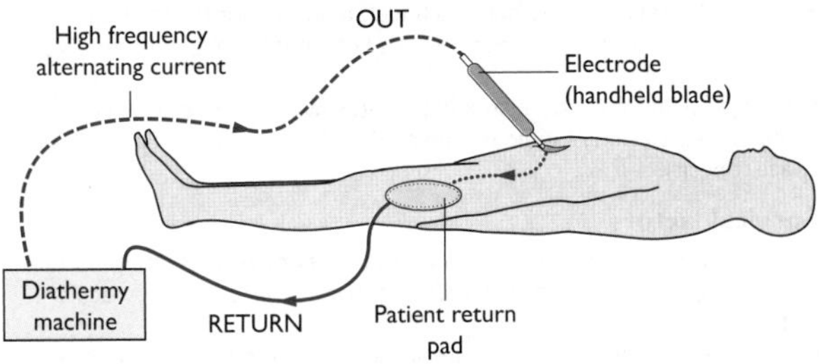
High frequency alternating current
OUT
Electrode (handheld blade)
Diathermy machine
RETURN
Patient return pad

Fig. 1.2 The path of a monopolar current. The circuit is completed through the patient's tissues travelling to a patient return pad.

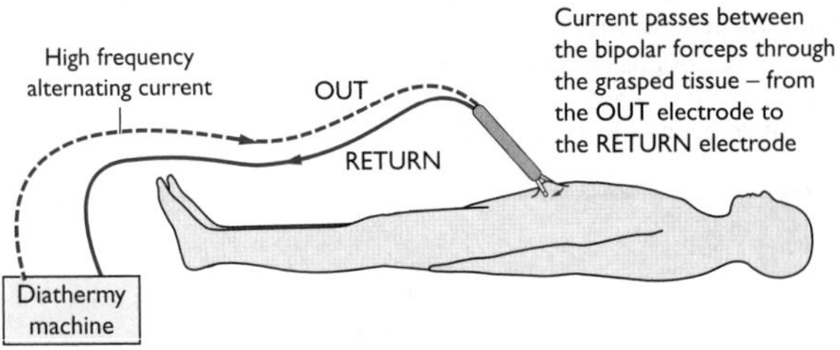
High frequency alternating current
OUT
RETURN
Current passes between the bipolar forceps through the grasped tissue – from the OUT electrode to the RETURN electrode
Diathermy machine

Fig. 1.3 The path of a bipolar current. The circuit is completed through only the tissue grasped between the forceps.

- Pacemakers: use bipolar diathermy, if possible; keep the distance between the electrode and the return pad as short as possible and away from the pacemaker. Implantable defibrillators should be deactivated prior to surgery and a defibrillator should be on hand throughout the operation.

Examples of devices that use bipolar current in common use are the Ligasure® and EnSeal® devices.

Ultrasonic devices

A variety of surgical devices have been developed that use frequencies between 23 and 55kHz to cut, coagulate, desiccate, and vaporize selected tissues. Electrical energy is converted to mechanical energy (vibrations) via the ultrasound generator. Changing the length of the excursion of the oscillating jaw varies the amount of mechanical energy transmitted to the tissue. Fig. 1.4 demonstrates the key components of an ultrasonic device.

The 'Max' setting (large jaw excursion) will result in more rapid cutting but less thermal spread, minimizing haemostasis (coagulation). The 'Min' setting (reduced jaw excursion) will transmit less energy to the tissue, resulting in less efficient cutting but greater thermal transfer of energy, giving better haemostasis.

An example of a device that uses ultrasound in this way is the Harmonic ACE®.

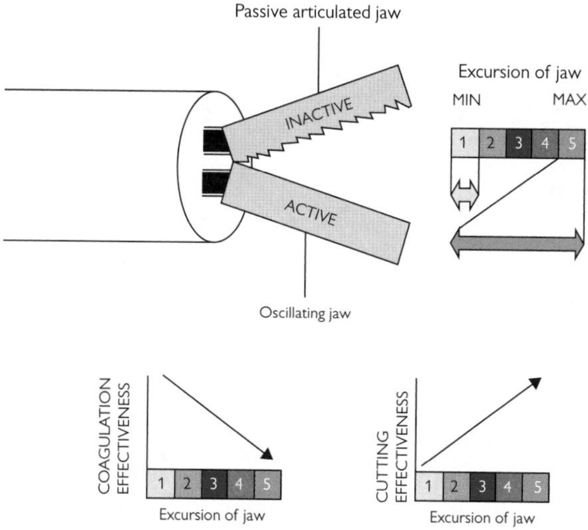
Passive articulated jaw
INACTIVE
ACTIVE
Oscillating jaw
Excursion of jaw
MIN
MAX
1 2 3 4 5
COAGULATION EFFECTIVENESS
1 2 3 4 5
Excursion of jaw
CUTTING EFFECTIVENESS
1 2 3 4 5
Excursion of jaw

Fig. 1.4 An ultrasonic device's key components, settings and effects.

Potential problems/pitfalls

- The active blade tends to retain thermal energy for at least 45s after it has been used—risk of inadvertent injury to adjacent structures (small bowel, ureters).

Lasers

A laser is a concentrated beam of light whose energy is absorbed by tissues and converted to heat, which cuts or coagulates tissue.

Potential problems/pitfalls

- Expensive.
- Fire risk when used near flammable materials.
- Collateral tissue damage around the laser tip.
- Has been associated with air embolism.

Duty of candour

Candour means being open and honest—our duty is to be candid about all aspects of our patients' healthcare, especially when things go wrong. Following the Mid-Staffordshire Public Inquiry, Professor Norman Williams, President of the Royal College of Surgeons, and Sir David Dalton, Chief Executive of Salford Royal Hospital, led a review on how to enhance a culture of candour within the NHS.

When things go wrong

Patients expect to be told:

- Honestly, what went wrong.
- What can be done about any harm caused.
- What can be done to prevent it happening again.

How do we develop this?

- Avoiding a 'blame culture' and 'defensive' behaviour.
- Encouraging incident reporting and reviewing these cases in a structured, objective manner.
- Learning from past mistakes and implementing subsequent change to address these issues.
- Auditing subsequent change in practice to ensure that learning is concrete and sustained.
- Provide support and training for staff in disclosing information about unanticipated events in patient's care and to apologize when appropriate.

The full report, 'Building a culture of candour: a review of the threshold for the duty of candour and of the incentives for care organisations to be candid 2014, D. Dalton and N Williams; Royal College of Surgeons', is available at: (https://www.rcseng.ac.uk/policy/documents/CandourreviewFinal.pdf).

Open and closed midline laparotomy incision

Anatomy

The anterior abdominal wall (Fig. 1.5):

- Muscles: rectus abdominis, external oblique, internal oblique, and transversus abdominis from superficial to deep.
- Linea alba: avascular, midline structure from xiphoid process to symphysis pubis.
- Rectus sheath: above the umbilicus, these form the anterior and posterior rectus sheaths; one-third below umbilicus anterior sheath only.
- Blood supply: superior and inferior epigastric arteries.
- Anterior cutaneous nerves T7–T12 (umbilicus level of T10).

Indications

- Emergency access to the peritoneal cavity and its contents (e.g. widespread faecal peritonitis).
- Elective: if laparoscopic surgery not indicated/possible.
- Incision site is usually midline. Paramedian and oblique approaches are also possible (Fig. 1.5).

Consent

- Procedure-specific consent—will vary with procedure proposed; p-possum scoring of morbidity and mortality.
- Iatrogenic injury to intra-abdominal structures.
- Bleeding, infection, hernia.
- Cardiovascular/respiratory complications.
- Thrombosis.

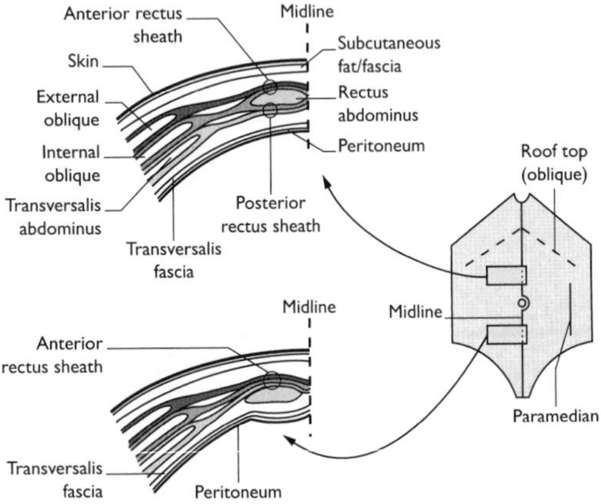
Anterior rectus sheath
Midline
Subcutaneous fat/fascia
Skin
External oblique
Rectus abdominus
Internal oblique
Peritoneum
Roof top (oblique)
Transversalis abdominus
Posterior rectus sheath
Transversalis fascia
Midline
Midline
Anterior rectus sheath
Paramedian
Transversalis fascia
Peritoneum

Fig. 1.5 Anatomy of the abdominal wall and common incisions.

Preoperative preparations

- Resuscitation as per advanced trauma life support (ATLS) guidelines; anaesthetic review; alert emergency theatre team; consider postoperative high-dependency unit (HDU)/intensive-therapy unit (ITU) bed.
- Clear communication to patient and relatives regarding situation and likely outcome.
- Consent—to include procedures as relevant and associated risks, p-possum scoring of mortality and morbidity.
- Mark the surgical site as appropriate, including siting stomas preoperatively.
- Ensure group and save/cross-match, as appropriate.
- Pregnancy test, if applicable.
- Anaesthetic: GA +/– epidural.

Position and theatre set-up

- Patient supine; arms out on boards; legs may need to be in Lloyd–Davies for certain colorectal/gynaecological procedures (supine position of body, hips flexed at 15° with 30° of head-down tilt).
- Patient strapping.
- Gel pads under pressure areas; straps to secure patient.
- Urethral catheterization; nasogastric tube, if GI pathology.
- Hair removal as necessary.
- Patient warmer.
- Consider antibiotic and VTE prophylaxis.
- Display any imaging as relevant.
- Skin preparation from lower chest to groins.
- WHO check (pause). Inform the anaesthetist you are going to start.

Procedure

Midline incision

- Make the skin taut and incise with a blade, in the midline, skirting the umbilicus, as shown in Fig. 1.5.
- Continue incision → subcutaneous fat/fascia → linea alba.
- Incise the linea alba to reveal the peritoneum. Divide any preperitoneal fat to access the peritoneum.
- Grasp the peritoneum between two clips (Fig. 1.6); feel it to ensure no bowel has been picked up.
- Incise the peritoneum. Extend your incision with scissors, lifting the peritoneum away from underlying structures.
- Note: when extending the incision towards the pelvis, take care not to injure the bladder by curving laterally around it.

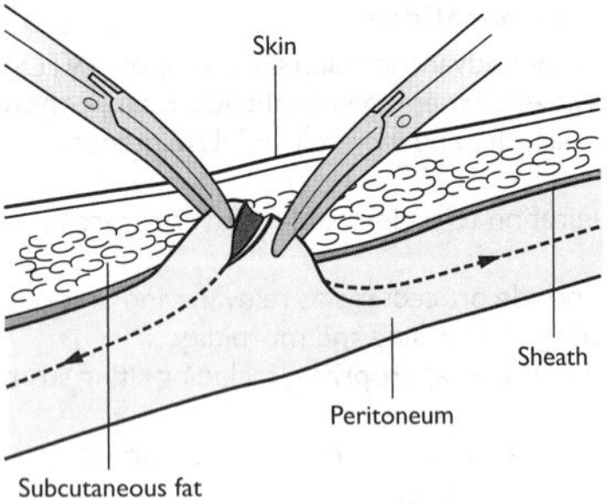
Skin
Sheath
Peritoneum
Subcutaneous fat

Fig. 1.6 Lifting the peritoneum between clips, incise and extend.

Midline closure

- Peritoneum and sheath (mass closure) 0/#1 delayed absorbable (PDS®)/non-absorbable (nylon).
- Suture may be looped (anchors the suture by passing the needle through the tissues then through the loop, i.e. knots itself).
- Blunt needle—lower risk of sharps injury vs. cutting needle—better to use in scar/thick tissue.
- The total length of suture used should be approximately four times the length of the wound. Each bite should be 1cm from the edge of the wound and 1cm from the last bite.
- Tension should be even throughout—undue tension will cause necrosis and impair healing.
- Start from either edge of the wound and meet in the middle.
- Skin continuous (subcuticular) absorbable 3.0 suture (Monocryl®) or staples.

Postoperative care and instructions

Depends upon the type of operation performed, however:

- Analgesia: PCA/epidural—for 24–48h post-op +/− local anaesthetic wound catheters.
- NG tube/catheter—48–72h.
- Continued thromboembolic prophylaxis +/− antibiotics.
- Update patient/ family/relatives of operative findings and current patient status.
- Clips generally removed after 10–14 days.

Complications (specific to a laparotomy incision)

- Wound infection (minor—full dehiscence) 2–30%.
- Incisional hernia 5–30%.

Tips and tricks

- Struggling with access? Extend the wound. This is the first thing your boss will do!
- Pus/ascites on opening—send it for microscopy, culture, and sensitivity or cytology.
- Try to replace the omentum over the intestines before closing to create a barrier between them and the wound.
- Tough sheath using a blunt needle? Mount the needle closer to its tip—it will help get through the tough tissue.
- Use your assistant! They can follow your suture to lift your closure away from any bowel underneath.
- When you are pulling your closure suture tight, place your hand underneath it to ensure no bowel gets caught.
- To efficiently close skin: use a pair of Littlewood's to hold the wound closed at either end. Get your assistant to make the skin taut whilst you clip.

Induction of pneumoperitoneum and diagnostic laparoscopy

Anatomy

The anterior abdominal wall (Fig. 1.5):

- Muscles: rectus abdominis, external oblique, internal oblique, and transversus abdominis from superficial to deep.
- Linea alba: avascular, midline structure from xiphoid process to symphysis pubis.
- Rectus sheath: above the umbilicus, these form the anterior and posterior rectus sheaths; one-third below umbilicus anterior sheath only.
- Blood supply: superior and inferior epigastric arteries—avoid these when placing lateral ports.
- Anterior cutaneous nerves T7–T12 (umbilicus level of T10).
- Important landmark: the vertical fibres of the umbilicus insert into the horizontal fibres of the sheath—where the abdominal wall is thinnest hence easiest point of entry.

Indications

- Emergency: appendicitis, gynaecological pathology, perforated duodenal ulcers, perforated diverticular disease, trauma, or as a precursor to a full laparotomy.
- Elective cases: GI operations, urology, adrenal, gynaecological pathology, staging/biopsies.

Consent

- Procedure-specific consent—will vary with procedure proposed.
- Iatrogenic injury to intra-abdominal structures.
- Bleeding, infection, hernia.
- Cardiovascular/respiratory complications.
- Thrombosis.

Preoperative preparations

- Resuscitation as per ATLS guidelines; anaesthetic review; alert emergency theatre team; consider postoperative HDU/ITU bed.
- Clear communication to patient and relatives regarding situation and likely outcome.
- Consent—to include procedures as relevant and associated risks, p-possum scoring of mortality and morbidity.
- Mark the surgical site as appropriate, including siting stomas preoperatively.
- Ensure group and save/cross-match, as appropriate.
- Pregnancy test, if applicable.
- Anaesthetic: GA +/– epidural.

Position and theatre set-up

A laparoscopy stack generally consists of a monitor, light source, digital capture unit/processor, and gas-delivery system—these are 'stacked' with the monitor at the top. The optimum position of the stack (and ∴ the screen) depends on the procedure; for instance, for a cholecystectomy, the screen should be placed over the patient's right shoulder (i.e. towards the area we are operating in). In some dedicated laparoscopic theatres there will be multiple screens for ease of access.

- Patient supine; legs may need to be in Lloyd–Davies for certain colorectal/gynaecological procedures (supine position of body, hips flexed at 15° with 30° of head-down tilt).
- Patient strapping (across chest)/shoulder supports to avoid falls/slippage.
- Arms may need to be out (anaesthetic access); tucking the arms is to let the surgeon stand close to the patient.
- Gel pads under pressure areas, straps to secure patient.
- Urethral catheterization; NG tube if GI pathology.
- Hair removal as necessary.
- Patient warmer.
- Consider antibiotic and VTE.
- Display any imaging as relevant.
- Skin preparation from lower chest to groins.
- Ensure the camera cable, the gas, and the light leads are not tangled, and are secured to the table prior to starting.
- White-balance the camera; put the light to standby (so it does not set fire to the drapes).
- WHO check (pause). Inform the anaesthetist you are going to start.

Procedure

To establish the pneumoperitoneum:

- Curved, infra-umbilical skin incision ~12mm—make this vertical if a possibility of converting to laparotomy.
- Inside the wound, grasp the umbilicus with a Littlewoods' and lift it vertically.
- Triangulate the wound with two Langenbeck retractors, dissecting until you can clearly see the stalk inserting into the sheath (Fig. 1.7)—note the crossover of the fibres.
- Incise the sheath (10mm) vertically across the umbilicus to the sheath, lifting up away from the abdominal cavity.
- Insert a blunt, curved artery clip, curve upward; gently breach the peritoneum (Fig. 1.8). Insert your port.
- Check your placement (with camera) prior to starting the CO_2 at low flow graduating to high flow with a max. pressure of 12mmHg.
- Decide on working port placement. Infiltrate local anaesthetic and insert under direct vision.

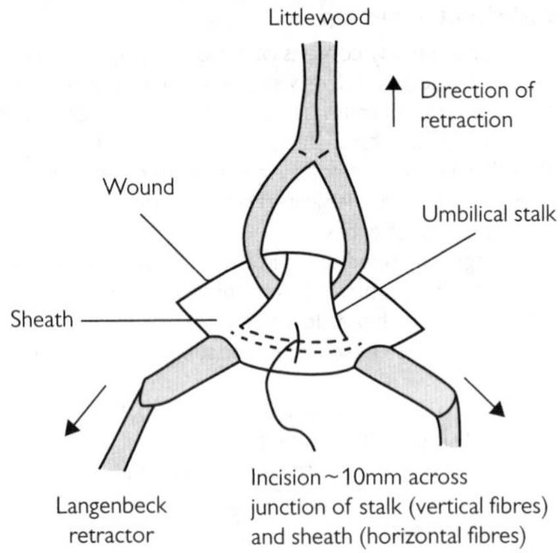
Littlewood
Direction of retraction
Wound
Umbilical stalk
Sheath
Incision ~ 10mm across junction of stalk (vertical fibres) and sheath (horizontal fibres)
Langenbeck retractor

Fig. 1.7 Exposure of the umbilicus and incision of the sheath.

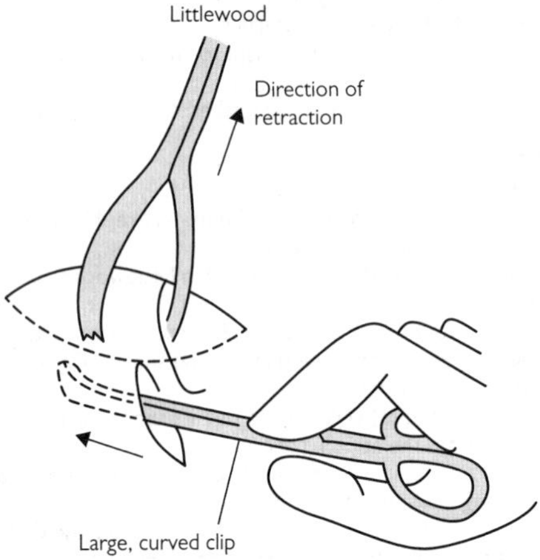
Littlewood
Direction of retraction
Large, curved clip

Fig. 1.8 Insertion of a clip through the peritoneum.

Diagnostic laparoscopy steps

- Head down, right side up: appendix → caecum → ascending colon → transverse colon, also gallbladder, liver, and stomach.
- 'Walk the small bowel'—avoid grasping the small bowel; use your closed instruments where possible; if it is necessary, use an atraumatic grasper under direct vision to ensure no damage is done to the bowel.
- Right side up 'off'/left side up: spleen, descending colon.
- Head down: sigmoid colon, rectum, gynaecological organs.
- Note any free fluid—take a sample for microscopy, culture, and sensitivity.

At the end of the procedure

- Remove all ports under direct vision: check for bleeding.
- Allow complete deflation of the peritoneal cavity.
- All ports 10mm and above require musculo-fascial closure (except in epigastrium).
- The principles of the closure technique outlined below can be applied to all 10mm+ ports.

Umbilical port

- Use your Littlewoods' to lift up the umbilicus.
- Place the blunt end of your forceps under the sheath lifting it up. Take a good bite with your J-stitch. Repeat for the other side (Fig. 1.9).
- Pull up when tying to ensure no bowel is caught in the wound. Check that your closure is satisfactory.

Postoperative care and instructions

- Remove catheter.
- If simply a diagnostic laparoscopy, then patient may eat and drink as tolerated.
- Thromboembolic prophylaxis, consider antibiotic regime.
- Update patient/family/relatives of operative findings and current patient status.

Complications (specific to the procedure of laparoscopy)

- Port site infection <5%.
- Port site herniation <2% if closed.
- Visceral injury during port insertion/basic laparoscopy and assessment <1%.

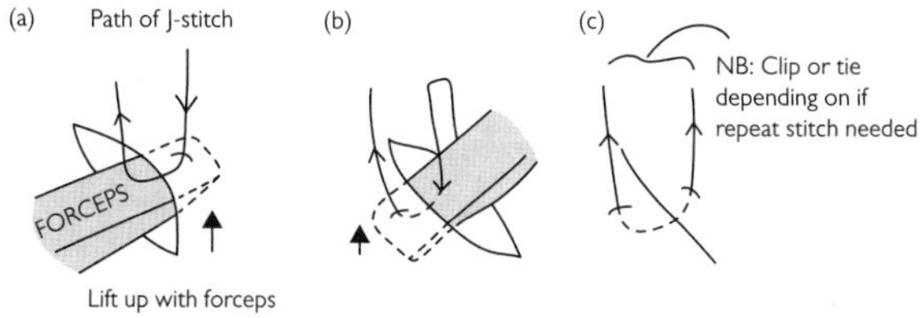
(a)
Path of J-stitch
FORCEPS
Lift up with forceps
(b)
(c)
NB: Clip or tie depending on if repeat stitch needed

Fig. 1.9 Closure of the sheath: follow (a) → (b) → (c) and repeat, as necessary.

Tips and tricks

- Put a purse string suture in the sheath at the start—you can use this to secure your camera port; it allows for efficient closure at the end of the operation (Fig. 1.10).
- Make use of your table—tilt to get best views.
- Use the light on the camera to light up the abdominal wall to see vessels—especially the inferior epigastric artery (in thin people) when inserting ports.
- A supra-umbilical approach in larger people can be easier than an infra-umbilical approach.

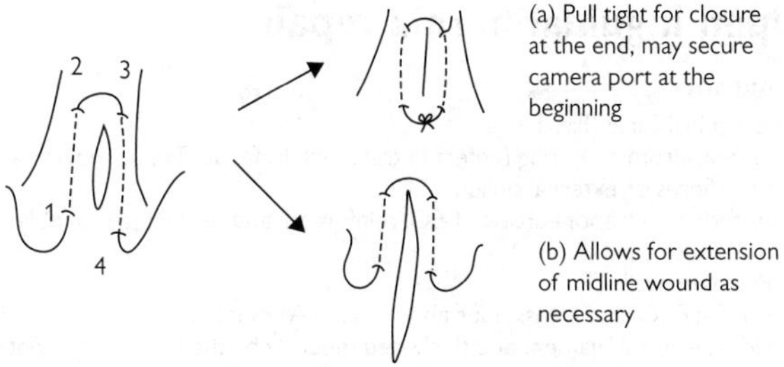
2
3
1
4
(a) Pull tight for closure at the end, may secure camera port at the beginning
(b) Allows for extension of midline wound as necessary

Fig. 1.10 Purse string suture technique—needle entry follows 1–2–3–4, as shown.

Open inguinal hernia repair

Anatomy

The inguinal canal (Fig. 1.11):

- Extends from deep ring (defect in transversalis fascia, TF) to superficial ring (fibres of external oblique, EO).
- Anterior wall: aponeurosis of EO, reinforced laterally by internal oblique (IO) muscle.
- Posterior wall: TF.
- Roof: TF, IO, and transversus abdominis (TA) muscle.
- Floor: inguinal ligament and thickened medially by the lacunar ligament.
- Contents: male—spermatic cord; female—round ligament.
- Nerves: ilioinguinal, iliohypogastric, and genital branch of the genitofemoral nerve—damage to these nerves will result in loss of sensation over the lateral skin of the thigh, the groin, scrotum, or labia.

Indications

- Asymptomatic hernia—majority will develop pain; a number will require emergency repair.
- Symptomatic hernia (elective repair).
- Incarcerated hernia (emergency repair).

Consent

- Bleeding, infection, scar.
- Recurrence.

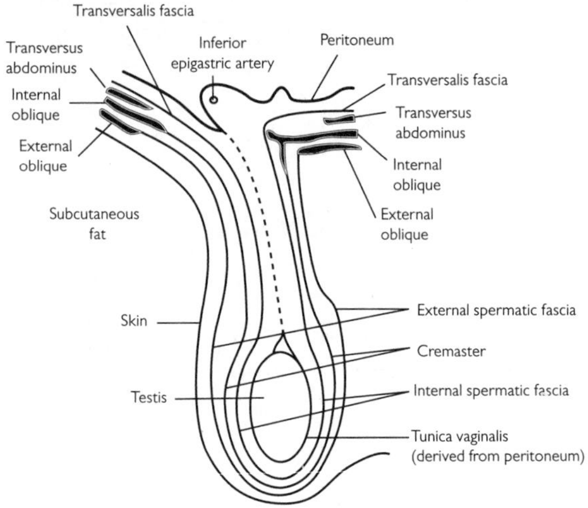
Transversalis fascia
Transversus abdominus
Internal oblique
External oblique
Inferior epigastric artery
Peritoneum
Transversalis fascia
Transversus abdominus
Internal oblique
External oblique
Subcutaneous fat
Skin
Testis
External spermatic fascia
Cremaster
Internal spermatic fascia
Tunica vaginalis
(derived from peritoneum)

Fig. 1.11 The structure of the inguinal canal, the coverings of the testis, and the spermatic cord.

- Chronic pain.
- Testicular ischaemia.
- Emergency: bowel resection +/– anastomosis +/– stoma.
- Cardiovascular/respiratory complications.
- Thrombosis.

Preoperative preparations

- Elective: smoking cessation, weight optimized, medical optimization for respiratory/cardiovascular complaints.
- Emergency: preoperative resuscitation.
- Consent and mark the side of the hernia.
- Group and save.
- Preoperative antibiotic and thromboprophylaxis.
- Anaesthesia: GA/LA/regional—spinal.

Position and theatre set-up

- Supine; knees slightly flexed to reduce tension on the groin.
- Hair removal.
- Patient warmer.
- Skin preparation to include abdomen, groins, and scrotum.
- WHO check (pause). Inform the anaesthetist you are going to start.

Procedure—open repair (Lichtenstein)

- Identify the anterior superior iliac spine (ASIS) and the pubic tubercule (PT). The deep ring: midpoint of these, ~2cm above the inguinal ligament. Skin incision—transverse/curved lateral to the deep ring to just above PT.
- Skin → subcutaneous fat/fascia: ensure haemostasis—tie any sizeable veins 2.0 Vicryl®. Expose external oblique. Note the superficial ring (Fig. 1.12).
- Open external oblique fascia in line with its fibres, as shown Fig. 1.12. Note the ilioinguinal nerve—protect it.
- Clear the leaves of EO fascia superiorly (note IO) and inferiorly (note the inguinal ligament). Indirect sac present?
- Place your index finger on the PT; work around the back of the spermatic cord—protect in hernia ring.

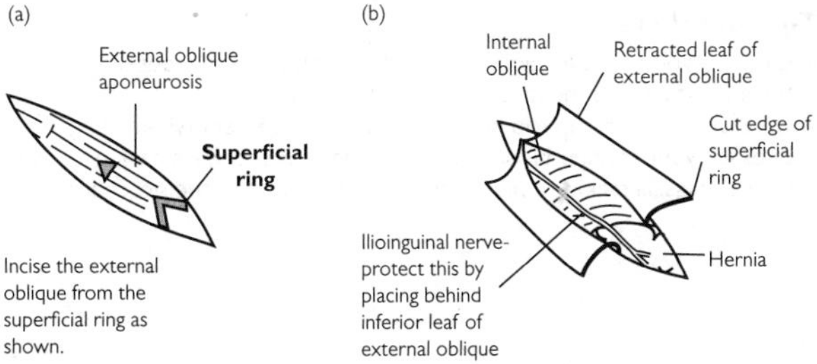
(a)
External oblique aponeurosis
Superficial ring
Incise the external oblique from the superficial ring as shown.
(b)
Internal oblique
Retracted leaf of external oblique
Cut edge of superficial ring
Hernia
Ilioinguinal nerve-protect this by placing behind inferior leaf of external oblique

Fig. 1.12 Exposure of the superficial ring and indirect hernia.

- Divide the cremasteric fibres to expose the indirect hernia sac; hold its edge with a small clip. Dissect it free (Fig. 1.13).
- Open the sac—inspect/reduce contents if viable; insert a finger, twist medially to determine if there is a direct sac.
- Twist the sac to obliterate it; place a transfixion stitch (2.0 Vicryl®) through it; amputate the excess; reduce it.

Direct hernia—inspect the posterior wall (TF)

- The sac may be opened, its contents reduced, and excess sac excised. For small hernia/apparent weakness, the bulge is reduced whilst the posterior wall is reconstructed (Fig. 1.14).
- Use a continuous non-absorbable 2.0 suture, from PT to the level of the deep ring, approximating the TF just above the inguinal ligament to that below the conjoint tendon (Fig. 1.14).
- The resultant deep ring should be snug around the cord.
- Polypropylene mesh: cut, place, and secure it as shown (Fig. 1.15)—continuous 2.0 non-absorbable suture.

Closure

- EO fascia: continuous absorbable (#1).
- Scarpa's fascia: interrupted absorbable sutures (2.0).
- Skin: continuous subcuticular absorbable sutures (3.0).

Postoperative care and instructions

Elective cases (no routine follow up):

- Home same day with routine postoperative care instructions regarding wound care/problems and oral analgesics.
- If a driver—patient to contact their car insurance and DVLA with regard to driving restrictions.
- No heavy lifting/straining for 6–8 weeks.

Complications (specific to the procedure)

- Superficial wound infection <5%.
- Recurrence of hernia 3%.
- Haematoma 2%.
- Chronic pain 1–2%.
- Testicular ischaemia <1%.
- Urinary retention.

Tips and tricks

- Ensure a good hold for your first medial stitch overlying, but not through, the PT as most recurrences are medial
- Careful not to drift up too high on the inguinal ligament when taking the bites for your continuous suture on the mesh as you will steal length from your EO fascia making it harder to close at the end of the procedure!

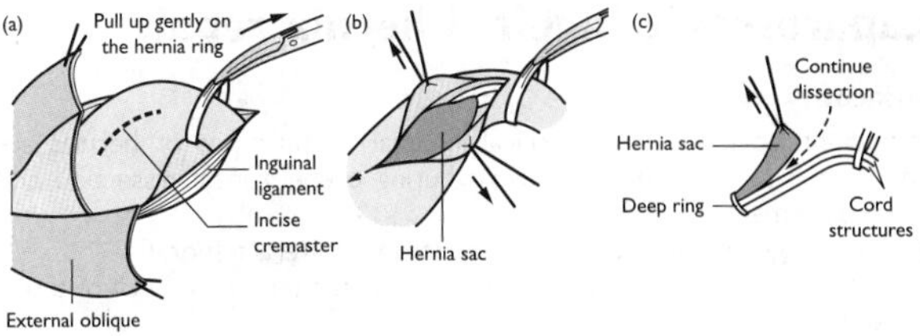
(a)
Pull up gently on the hernia ring
Inguinal ligament
Incise cremaster
External oblique
(b)
Hernia sac
(c)
Continue dissection
Hernia sac
Deep ring
Cord structures

Fig. 1.13 Exposure and clearance of an indirect hernia sac: (a) incise cremaster, (b) identify sac, and (c) protect cord structures and continue dissection of the sac down to the deep ring.

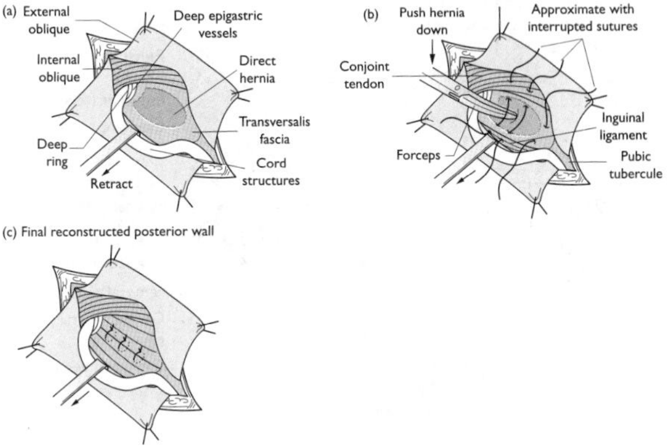
(a) External oblique
Deep epigastric vessels
Internal oblique
Direct hernia
Transversalis fascia
Deep ring
Retract
Cord structures
(b) Push hernia down
Approximate with interrupted sutures
Conjoint tendon
Inguinal ligament
Forceps
Pubic tubercule
(c) Final reconstructed posterior wall

Fig. 1.14 Repairing a direct inguinal hernia (reinforcing a lax posterior wall).

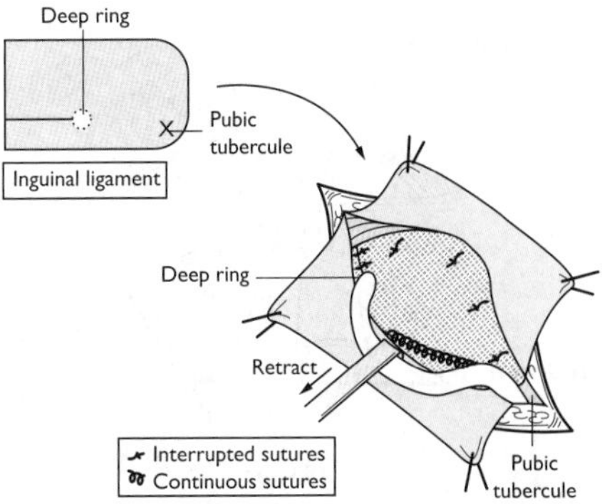
Deep ring
Pubic tubercule
Inguinal ligament
Deep ring
Retract
Interrupted sutures
Continuous sutures
Pubic tubercule

Fig. 1.15 Standard mesh placement in an open inguinal hernia repair.

Laparoscopic inguinal hernia repair

Anatomy

Important laparoscopic anatomical landmarks and types of hernias are shown in Fig. 1.16. Areas to avoid during preperitoneal dissection and mesh placement (Fig. 1.17):

- The triangle of pain—containing the femoral, lateral femoral cutaneous, anterior femoral cutaneous, and the femoral branch of the genitofemoral nerves.
- The triangle of doom—containing the external iliac vein, deep circumflex iliac vein, and the femoral artery.

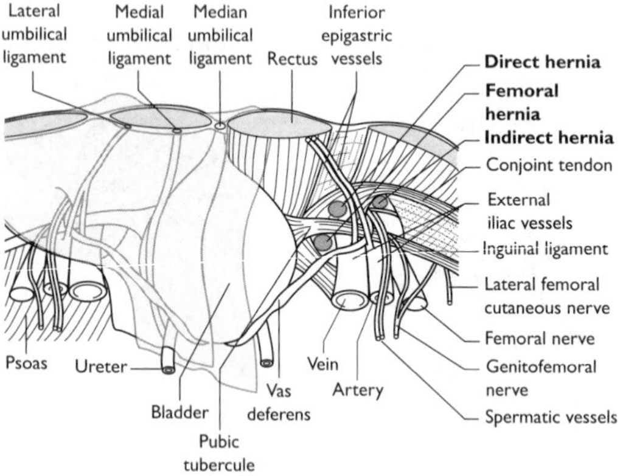
Lateral umbilical ligament
Medial umbilical ligament
Median umbilical ligament
Rectus
Inferior epigastric vessels
Direct hernia
Femoral hernia
Indirect hernia
Conjoint tendon
External iliac vessels
Inguinal ligament
Lateral femoral cutaneous nerve
Femoral nerve
Genitofemoral nerve
Spermatic vessels
Psoas
Ureter
Bladder
Pubic tubercule
Vas deferens
Vein
Artery

Fig. 1.16 Important intra-abdominal anatomical landmarks for laparoscopic hernia repair and areas to avoid.

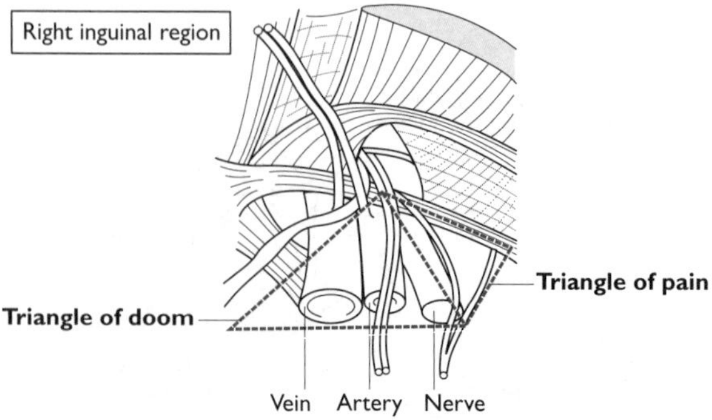
Right inguinal region
Triangle of pain
Triangle of doom
Vein
Artery
Nerve

Fig. 1.17 Areas to avoid in preperitoneal dissection and mesh placement.

Indications

- NICE guidance: can be considered for primary unilateral and bilateral and recurrent herniae.

Consent

- Bleeding, infection, scar.
- Recurrence.
- Chronic pain.
- Testicular ischaemia.
- Iatrogenic injury to intra-abdominal organs.
- Cardiovascular/respiratory complications.
- Thrombosis.

Preoperative preparations

- Elective: smoking cessation, weight optimized, medical optimization for respiratory/cardiovascular complaints.
- Consent and mark the side of the hernia.
- Group and save.
- Preoperative antibiotic and thromboprophylaxis.
- Anaesthesia: GA.

Position and theatre set-up

- Supine, arms tucked.
- Hair removal.
- Stack set up as in Fig. 1.18.
- WHO knife check. Inform the anaesthetist you are going to start

Procedure—transabdominal preperitoneal (TAPP)

- 10mm supra-umbilical port; establish access and pneumoperitoneum using the open Hasson technique.
- 2 × 5mm ports placed under direct vision in the left and right mid-abdomen at the level of the umbilicus (Fig. 1.18).

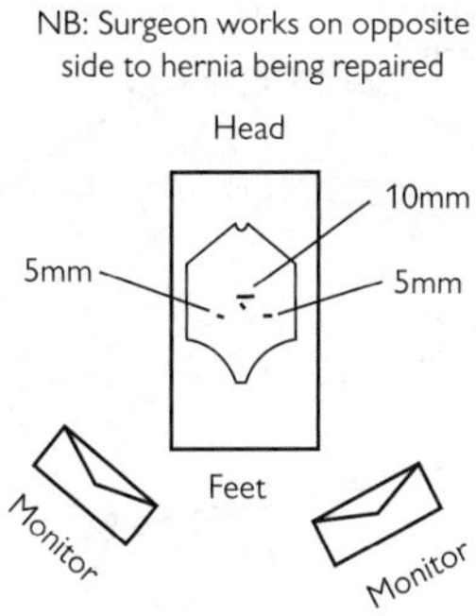
NB: Surgeon works on opposite side to hernia being repaired
Head
10mm
5mm
5mm
Feet
Monitor
Monitor

Fig. 1.18 Theatre set up and port placement in a TAPP hernia repair.

- Perform a diagnostic laparoscopy.
- Create a peritoneal flap from the ASIS laterally to the medial umbilical ligament 2–3 cm above the hernia sac.
- Retract the lower peritoneal flap and use blunt dissection to open the avascular plane between the peritoneum and the transversalis fascia (Fig. 1.19).
- Carefully dissect the indirect hernia sac away from the cord structures.
- It is important to get good medial coverage with the mesh, so ensure you have dissected to the contralateral PT.
- Size the mesh, trim as necessary. Roll it up and place it into the abdominal cavity through the 10mm port or use tip of graspers to hold mesh in centre
- Tap it into the final position, as demonstrated in Fig. 1.20.
- Tack into place medially over the PT and superiorly, avoiding the epigastric vessels.
- Lift the inferior leaf of the peritoneum to check the mesh does not roll. Trim as necessary.
- Either tack or suture the peritoneal leaf back into place to cover the mesh completely.
- Closure—sheath J-PDS® 1, skin 3.0 absorbable.

Procedure—totally extraperitoneal (TEP)

A three-component dissecting balloon should be used to do the initial dissection of the preperitoneal space as outlined (Fig. 1.21).

- 1st port: 2cm incision, lateral and inferior to the umbilicus on the side of the hernia.
- Retract the muscle laterally, exposing the posterior rectus sheath.
- Blunt dissection opens the preperitoneal space. Insert the three-component dissecting balloon into this space through the umbilical incision.

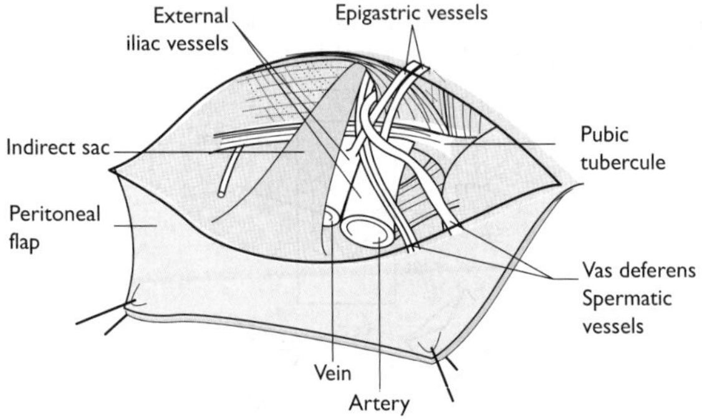
External iliac vessels
Epigastric vessels
Indirect sac
Peritoneal flap
Pubic tubercule
Vas deferens
Spermatic vessels
Vein
Artery

Fig. 1.19 Indirect sac: note this is part of the peritoneum; dissect it carefully off the cord structures to reduce it.

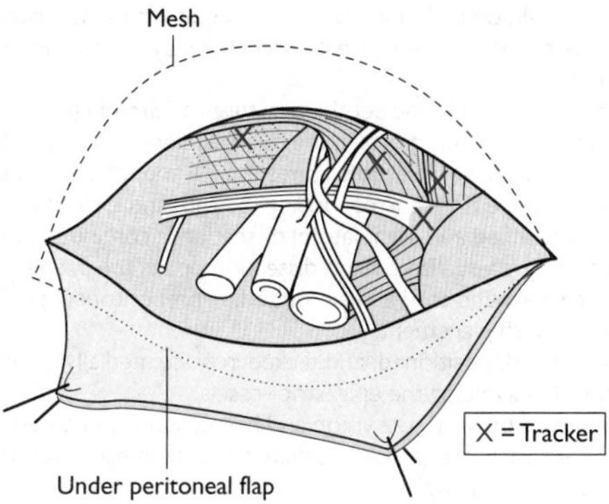
Mesh
X = Tracker
Under peritoneal flap

Fig. 1.20 Placement of the mesh: ensure good medial coverage.

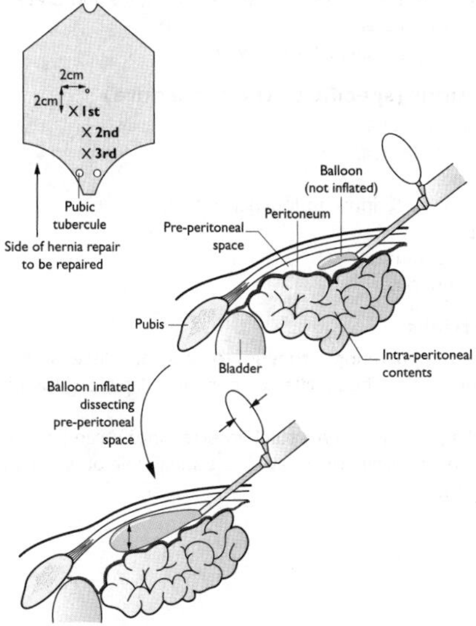
2cm
2cm
X 1st
X 2nd
X 3rd
Pubic tubercule
Side of hernia repair to be repaired
Balloon (not inflated)
Peritoneum
Pre-peritoneal space
Pubis
Bladder
Intra-peritoneal contents
Balloon inflated dissecting pre-peritoneal space

Fig. 1.21 Entry into, and dissection of, the preperitoneal space in a TEP hernia approach.

- Expand the balloon and monitor the dissection with a laparoscope.
- Deflate the balloon and remove it. Insert the stay balloon and inflate it to 40ml of air.
- Attach the CO_2 to this and set the pressure to 15mmHg.
- Insert two further 5mm ports in the midline inferior to the umbilicus (one placed five-finger breadths above the PT and the second two-finger breaths above the PT—corresponding to '2nd' and '3rd' in Fig. 1.21).
- The PT is identified and slight lateral dissection is continued until the obturator vein is visualized. Blunt dissection opens the preperitoneal space, the spermatic cord is skeletonised. A preperitoneal pocket is cleared for mesh placement.
- Mesh is inserted, positioned, and tacked in place medially over the PT and superiorly avoiding the epigastric vessels.
- Ports removed under direct vision and haemostasis is ensured.
- Pneumoperitoneum is gradually deflated and the mesh position is observed on withdrawal.

Postoperative care and instructions

- Home same day with routine postoperative care instructions regarding wound care/problems and oral analgesics.
- If a driver—patient to contact their car insurance and DVLA with regard to driving restrictions.
- No heavy lifting/straining for 6–8 weeks.

Complications (specific to the procedure)

- Superficial wound infection.
- Recurrence of hernia.
- Haematoma.
- Iatrogenic injury to intra-abdominal viscera.
- Chronic pain.
- Testicular ischaemia.
- Urinary retention.

Tips and tricks

- TAPP: use the pneumoperitoneum to help your dissection—once the peritoneum is breached it lifts up your initial flap along the plane of dissection.
- For bleeding: a gauze with a stitch inserted into it can be inserted through the umbilical port (leaving the stitch 'tail' outside) and removed by pulling the 'tail'.

Femoral hernia repair

Anatomy

The femoral canal is ~1.5cm long. The femoral ring is the site of femoral herniation. The boundaries of the femoral ring are:

- Anteriorly: inguinal ligament.
- Posteriorly: pectineal ligament and pectineus muscle.
- Medially: lacunar ligament.
- Laterally: medial border of the femoral vein.

Note that the accessory obturator artery is present in 50% of patients with an aberrant medial course posterior to the lacunar ligament.

Indications

- All femoral hernias should be repaired unless the patient is moribund.

Consent

- Bleeding/infection.
- Recurrence.
- Bowel resection +/– primary anastomosis +/– stoma.
- Proceed to laparotomy.
- Cardiovascular/respiratory complications.
- Thrombosis.

Preoperative preparations

- Elective: smoking cessation, weight optimized, medical optimization for respiratory/cardiovascular complaints.
- Emergency: preoperative resuscitation, NGT, catheter.
- Consent and mark the side of the hernia.
- Preoperative antibiotic and thromboprophylaxis.
- Anaesthesia: GA/regional—spinal.

Positioning and theatre set up

- Supine; knees slightly flexed to reduce tension on the groin.
- NG/catheter if emergency case.
- Hair removal.
- Patient warmer.
- Skin preparation to include abdomen, groins, and scrotum.
- WHO check (pause). Inform the anaesthetist you are going to start.

Procedure

Decide on operative approach (Fig. 1.22):

- Infra-inguinal (Lockwood): over the hernia itself, but no access if bowel resection required; elective repairs.
- Transinguinal (Lothiesen): good access to peritoneal cavity; for inguinal and femoral hernias; predisposes to inguinal hernia if mesh is not used to reconstruct posterior wall.
- Extraperitoneal (modified McEvedy): easy to convert to Pfannenstiel if full laparotomy required. No disruption of inguinal ligament.

Infra-inguinal (Lockwood) approach

- Skin incision below the inguinal ligament, as shown in Fig. 1.22.
- Expose the hernia sac through careful dissection as it emerges below the inguinal ligament lateral to the PT.
- Carefully hold and open the sac inspecting its contents.
- Reduce the contents and ligate the sac as high as possible with a transfixion suture (absorbable 2.0).
- Close the femoral ring (pectineal-inguinal interrupted non-absorbable sutures 2.0 or mesh plug and sutures).
- Close subcutaneous tissue and skin as per inguinal hernia repair.

Transinguinal (Lothiesen) approach

- Skin incision (Fig. 1.22). Expose the inguinal canal as for inguinal hernia repair.
- Incise the TF in an infero-medial direction from the deep ring to PT exposing the peritoneum underneath.
- Clearly identify the femoral vein and the neck of the hernia sac medial to it (Fig. 1.23).
- Open the sac, inspect/reduce its contents if viable and ligate the sac as high as possible (2.0 absorbable).
- Using interrupted non-absorbable 2.0 sutures, close the femoral ring (from pectineal ligament to inguinal ligament) (Fig. 1.23).
- Reconstruct posterior wall: as per direct hernia repair plus consider mesh placement if no contamination.
- Closure. EO fascia: continuous absorbable (#1). Scarpa's fascia: interrupted absorbable sutures (2.0). Skin: continuous subcuticular absorbable sutures (3.0).

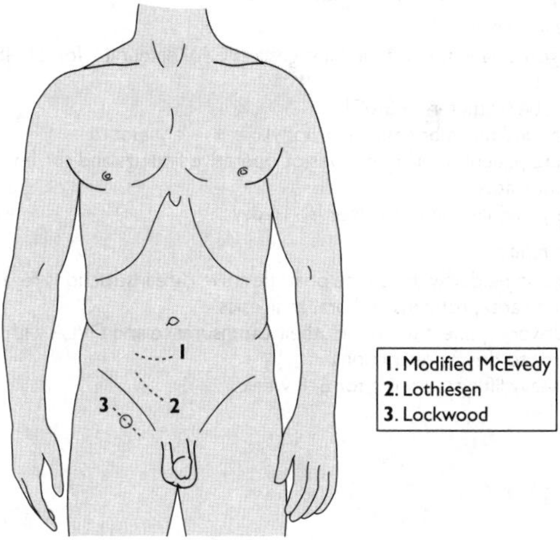
1
2
3
1. Modified McEvedy
2. Lothiesen
3. Lockwood

Fig. 1.22 Operative approaches to a femoral hernia.

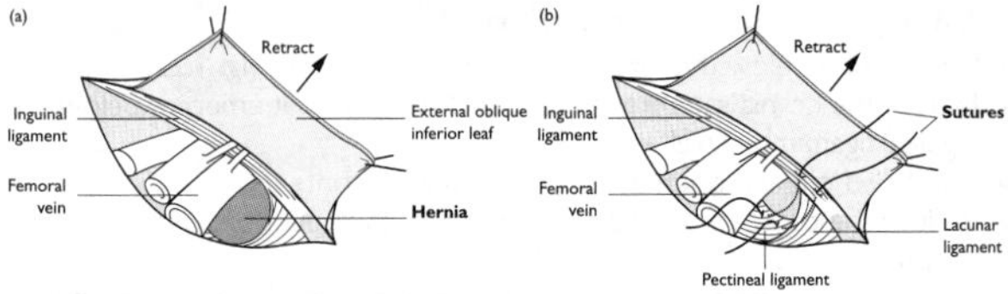
(a)
Retract
Inguinal ligament
External oblique inferior leaf
Femoral vein
Hernia
(b)
Retract
Inguinal ligament
Sutures
Femoral vein
Lacunar ligament
Pectineal ligament

Fig. 1.23 Identifying a femoral hernia sac, open/reduce and repair.

Extraperitoneal (modified McEvedy) approach

- Skin incision, as shown in Fig. 1.22: → subcutaneous fat/fascia → rectus sheath. Insert a self-retaining retractor.
- Incise rectus sheath vertically. Retract rectus abdominis muscle medially. Hold peritoneum between two clips and open vertically.
- Insert retractors to allow you a good view of the internal opening of the femoral canal.
- Insert a finger over the top of the hernia, gently dilating the neck to facilitate its reduction. External pressure/blunt extraperitoneal dissection can help.
- Open the sac, inspect its contents. Replace contents into peritoneal cavity if viable. Ligate with 2.0 Vicryl® and excise the redundant sac.
- Close the femoral ring with interrupted non-absorbable sutures (pectineal to inguinal ligaments).
- Closure: peritoneum 0/#1 Vicryl® continuous, rectus sheath 0/#1 vicryl®/prolene®, Scarpa's 2.0 Vicryl®, Skin 3.0 Monocryl®.

Postoperative care and instructions

Emergency repair

- Analgesia: patient-controlled analgesia (PCA)/epidural—for 24–48h post-op.
- NG tube/catheter—48–72h.
- Continued thromboembolic prophylaxis +/– antibiotics.
- Update patient/family/relatives of operative findings and current patient status.
- Clips generally removed after 10–14 days.

Elective repair

- Home same day with routine postoperative care instructions regarding wound care/problems and oral analgesics.
- If a driver—patient to contact their car insurance and DVLA with regards to driving restrictions.
- No heavy lifting/straining for 6–8 weeks.

Complications (specific to the procedure)

- Injury or narrowing of the femoral vein.
- Injury to the bladder/bowel.
- Superficial wound infection.
- Recurrence of hernia.
- Haematoma.
- Iatrogenic injury to intra-abdominal viscera.
- Chronic pain.
- Urinary retention.

Tips and tricks

- Viability of bowel: pink, peristalsing, mesenteric pulse, shiny. Wrap it in warm soaked gauze and re-assess it.
- Choose the right approach for the right situation.
- If needed, convert to laparotomy.
- Protect vein when taking stitch to close femoral ring and take care not to narrow femoral vein.

Ventral hernia repair

Anatomy

Anterior abdominal wall (Fig. 1.5).

Ventral hernias comprise any hernia of the anterior abdominal wall. They can be spontaneous (epigastric, umbilical, paraumbilical, and spigelian) or acquired (incisional hernias).

Indications

- Symptomatic hernia.
- Prevent strangulation of contents.

Consent

- Bleeding/infection.
- Recurrence.
- Risk of non-viable structures requiring resection.
- Rare: bowel resection +/– primary anastomosis.
- Cardiovascular/respiratory complications.
- Thrombosis.
- Excision of umbilicus.

Preoperative preparations

- Elective: smoking cessation, weight optimized, medical optimization for respiratory/cardiovascular complaints.
- Emergency: preoperative resuscitation, NGT/catheter.
- Consent and mark the extent of the defect.
- Group and save.
- Preoperative antibiotic and thromboprophylaxis.
- Anaesthesia: GA/LA.

Position and theatre set-up

- Supine, with knees flexed to reduce abdominal wall tension. If hernia is not in midline, position with pillows for lateral elevation.
- NG/catheter if emergency case.
- Hair removal.
- Patient warmer.
- Skin preparation to include abdomen, groins, and scrotum.
- WHO knife check. Inform the anaesthetist you are going to start.

Procedure

Open repair—the principle is the same for all types of ventral hernia:

- Incise skin → subcutaneous fat/ fascia over the hernia sac.
- Dissect the sac free, without breeching it, down to its neck at the rectus sheath.
- Open the sac, inspect its contents/reduce if viable.
- Close sac (0/#1 Vicryl®); amputate the excess.
- Create a clear space 360° around the defect between the peritoneum and the sheath (i.e. the preperitoneal space).

If the fascial defect is <2cm diameter:

- Perform a primary suture repair with interrupted non-absorbable 2.0 sutures.

If the fascial defect 2–4cm:

- Close the fascia with a two-layer sutured technique (non-absorbable 0) as shown in Fig. 1.24.
- The upper leaf of fascia is brought down over the lower leaf by mattress sutures and then the free edge is secured with interrupted sutures.

For medium to large defects a mesh repair is preferred:

- Size of mesh: 3–5cm overlap of the defect.
- Siting (Fig. 1.25): preperitoneal onlay, over primarily closed fascial defect or intraperitoneal mesh.
- Intra-peritoneal mesh: dual-sided mesh—non-adherent side (ePTE® surface) to peritoneal cavity, adherent side (Polypropylene®) against the abdominal wall.
- Secure the mesh: non-absorbable 2.0 mattress sutures at 3, 6, 9, and 12 o'clock.
- Closure: fascia: 2.0 non-absorbable sutures, interrupted; Scarpa's fascia 2.0 Vicryl®; Skin 3.0 Monocryl®.

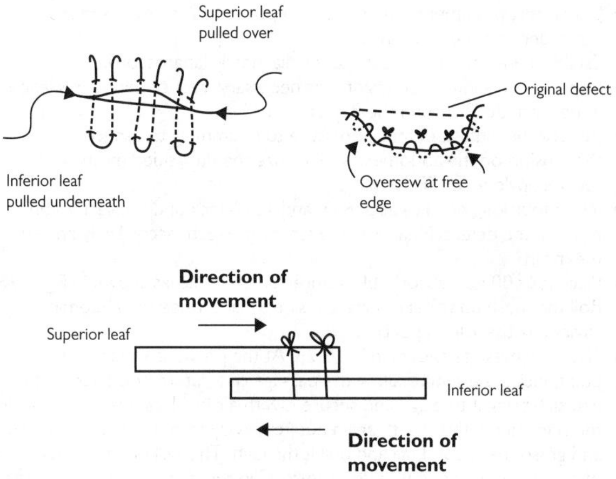
Superior leaf pulled over
Original defect
Inferior leaf pulled underneath
Oversew at free edge
Direction of movement
Superior leaf
Inferior leaf
Direction of movement

Fig. 1.24 Double-breasted primary suture repair.

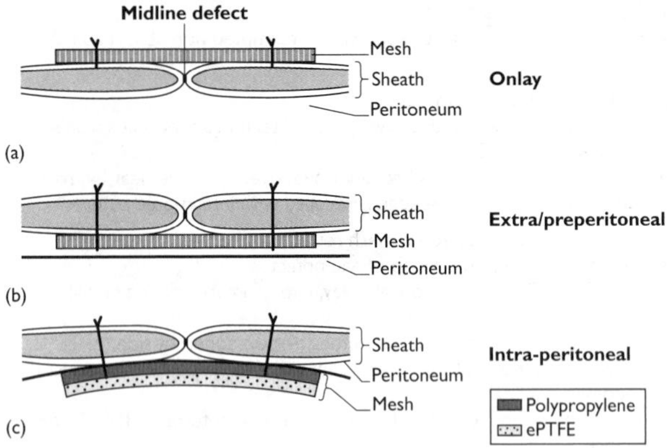

Midline defect
Mesh
Sheath
Peritoneum
Onlay
(a)
Sheath
Mesh
Peritoneum
Extra/preperitoneal
(b)
Sheath
Peritoneum
Mesh
Intra-peritoneal
Polypropylene
ePTFE
(c)

Fig. 1.25 Different sites of mesh placement for incisional hernia repair.

Laparoscopic ventral hernia repair

- Select port placement (10mm camera port and 2 × 5mm ports)—dependent on site of hernia.
- Establish pneumoperitoneum as for diagnostic laparoscopy.
- Inspect hernia; divide adhesions, as necessary; reduce contents; clear a 4–6cm rim 360° around the defect.
- Reduce the intra-abdominal pressure to 6–8mmHg to reduce the tension on the abdominal wall to size the dual-sided mesh (polypropylene/ePTFE).
- Insert four long needles at 3, 6, 9, and 12 o'clock under direct vision to mark the defect. Measure an overlap of 4–6cm accordingly and cut the mesh.
- Place four 00 non-absorbable sutures on the mesh as shown in Fig. 1.26. Roll the mesh up (ePTFE surface inside). Place inside the abdominal cavity (via the 10mm port).
- Place the mesh as shown in Fig. 1.26. At the previously marked skin point, incise the skin to allow the passage of a suture hook. Grasp the first tail, bring it through and secure it with a clip. Using the same hole in the skin, pierce the sheath again but 1cm away from the first entry point and grasp the second tail and pull it through. This will provide a 1cm bite of the sheath when you tie the suture. Clip this pair of tails. Repeat this manoeuvre for the anchoring sutures in positions 3, 6, 9, and 12. Tie.
- Use an endoscopic tacker to seal the perimeter of the repair, each placed 1cm apart.
- Take ports out under direct vision, ensure haemostasis, and close 10mm port site sheath with J-PDS® #1; skin absorbable 3.0.

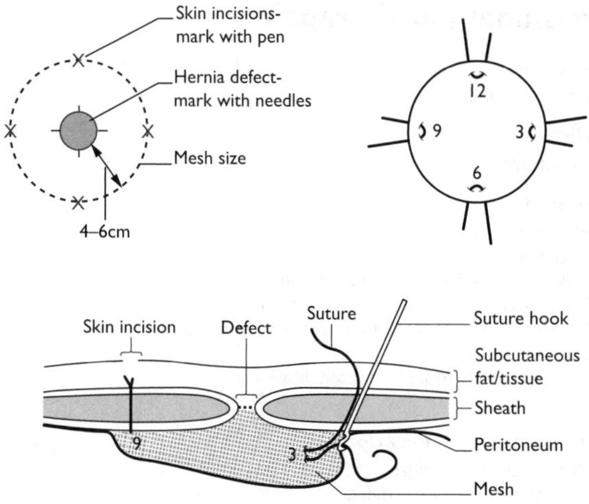
Skin incisions-
mark with pen
Hernia defect-
mark with needles
Mesh size
4–6cm
12
9
3
6
Skin incision
Defect
Suture
Suture hook
Subcutaneous
fat/tissue
Sheath
Peritoneum
Mesh
9
3

Fig. 1.26 Laparoscopic ventral hernia repair technique

Postoperative care and instructions

- Home same day with routine postoperative care instructions regarding wound care/problems and oral analgesics.
- If a driver—patient to contact their car insurance and DVLA with regards to driving restrictions.
- No heavy lifting/straining for 6–8 weeks.

Complications (specific to the procedure)

- Superficial wound infection.
- Recurrence of hernia.
- Haematoma.
- Iatrogenic injury to intra-abdominal viscera.
- Chronic pain.
- Also, excision of the umbilicus/change to its appearance.

Tips and tricks

- For umbilical/paraumbilical hernias—it may be necessary to detach the umbilical stalk from the rectus. Remember to reattach it at the end (2.0 Vicryl®).
- Be vigilant for bowel loops within omentum/hernias!
- Chronic hernias—when opening the sac do not do it right at the top—chronically stuck contents will be fused there, go a little further down either side of the apex, there will be less chance of accidental injury to contents.

Incisional hernia repair

Anatomy

Anterior abdominal wall (Fig. 1.5).

Indications

- Symptomatic hernia.

Consent

- Bleeding/infection.
- Recurrence.
- Risk of non-viable structures requiring resection.
- Rare: bowel resection +/– primary anastomosis.
- Iatrogenic injury to intra-abdominal structures (bladder, bowel, ureters, spleen).
- Cardiovascular/respiratory complications.
- Thrombosis.

Preoperative preparations

- Weight loss to optimize BMI.
- Mark the extent of the defect.
- Elective: smoking cessation, weight optimized, medical optimization for respiratory/cardiovascular complaints.
- Consent and mark the extent of the defect.
- Group and save.
- Preoperative antibiotic and thromboprophylaxis.
- Anaesthesia: GA/LA.

Positioning and theatre set up

- Supine, with knees flexed to reduce abdominal wall tension. If hernia is not in midline, position with pillows for lateral elevation.
- Hair removal.
- Patient warmer.
- Skin preparation to include abdomen, groins, and scrotum.
- Consider urethral catheterization as there may be extensive adhesions and a reasonably long operating time (2+h)
- WHO knife check. Inform the anaesthetist you are going to start.

Procedure

Open repair

- Excise the old scar.
- The skin may be fused to the peritoneum—if so, excise an ellipse of skin to reveal the subcutaneous tissue.
- The incision needs to be deepened down to the rectus sheath and a margin around the defect created (Fig. 1.27).
- Invert the sac—it may need to be opened if narrow necked to reduce the contents. Close the sac if you have opened it.
- For multiple incisional hernias join the defects to give you just one larger defect to address.
- Measure your mesh to ensure an overlap of 3–5cm at the edge of the defect.

Mesh placement

- Onlay: place the mesh anterior to the sheath and defect—you may not have been able to close this defect primarily. Suture it in place as shown in Fig. 1.27.
- Extra-peritoneal: create a pocket (3cm overlap) for the mesh with the peritoneum and posterior rectus sheath below and the rectus muscle above the mesh and suture, as shown in Fig. 1.28.
- Intra-peritoneal: open the hernia sac, divide any adhesions, and clear a 4cm space for the mesh all around the defect. Suture in place as shown in Fig. 1.29.

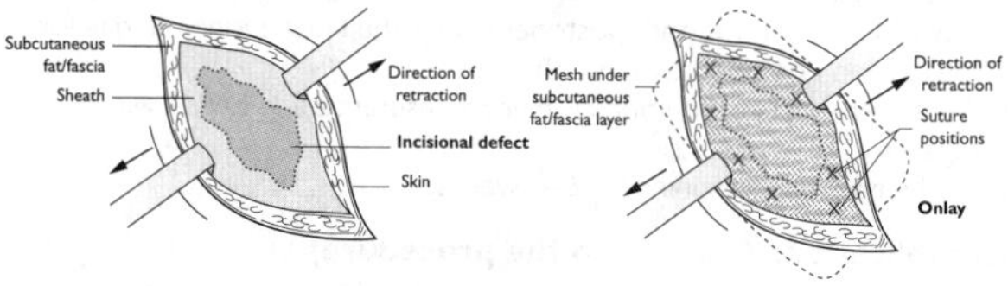
Subcutaneous fat/fascia
Sheath
Direction of retraction
Incisional defect
Skin
Mesh under subcutaneous fat/fascia layer
Direction of retraction
Suture positions
Onlay

Fig. 1.27 Placement of an onlay mesh in an incisional hernia repair.

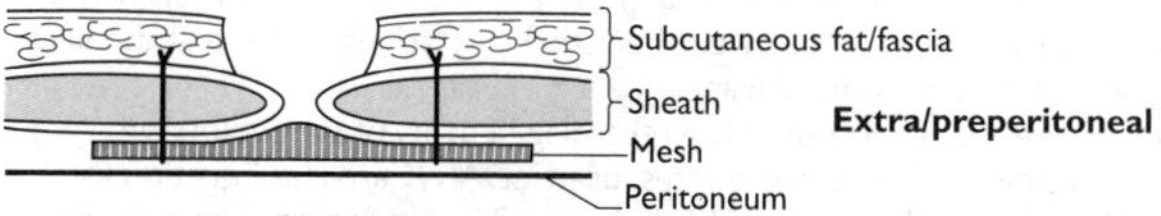
Subcutaneous fat/fascia
Sheath
Mesh
Peritoneum
Extra/preperitoneal

Fig. 1.28 Placement of an extra/preperitoneal mesh for incisional hernia repair.

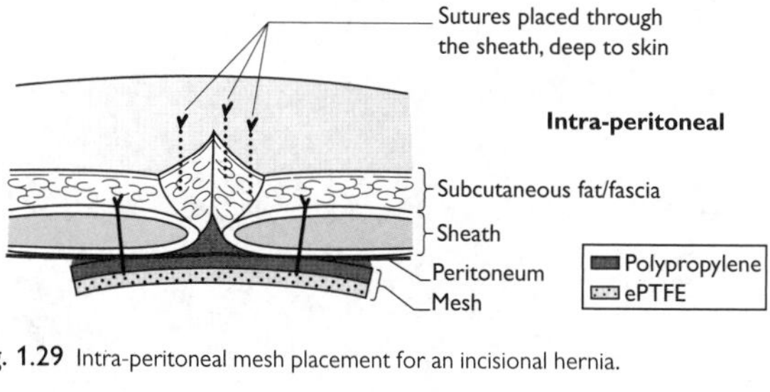
Sutures placed through the sheath, deep to skin
Intra-peritoneal
Subcutaneous fat/fascia
Sheath
Peritoneum
Mesh
Polypropylene
ePTFE

Fig. 1.29 Intra-peritoneal mesh placement for an incisional hernia.

Closure

- Leave one or two Redivac® drains to drain the subcutaneous space.
- Fat/Scarpa's fascia 2.0 Vicryl® interrupted.
- Skin 3.0 Monocryl®.

Laparoscopic repair of incisional hernias would follow the same principles as described for ventral hernias. The size of the defect, however, may preclude this method.

Postoperative care and instructions

- Leave the drains until they are less than 50ml in 24h.
- Abdominal binder—to be sized for the patient through orthotics. To stay on 24/7 for 1 month postoperatively, then just during the day for the second postoperative month.
- If a driver—patient to contact their car insurance and DVLA with regards to driving restrictions.
- No heavy lifting/straining for 6–8 weeks.

Complications (specific to the procedure)

- High recurrence rate 20–40%.
- Persistent seroma requiring aspiration.
- Wound infection.
- Haematoma.
- Injury to viscera intraoperatively.

Tips and tricks

- Consider the use of biological mesh (Permacol®) in infected scenarios.
- Take care to protect bowel when stitching/tacking mesh to abdominal wall in intra-peritoneal plane.
- For preoperative counselling regarding benefits of weight loss on morbidity and recurrence rates, use CeDAR 'Carolinas Equation for Determining Associated Risks' of ventral hernia repairs—free on the App store. Gives the patient some hard facts about the increased morbidity associated with obesity and hernia repairs enabling you to help them set targets preoperatively to hopefully achieve a better long-term outcome.

Excision biopsy of skin lesions

Anatomy

The layers of the skin from superficial to deep:

- Epidermis.
- Dermis.
- Subcutaneous tissues.

Indications

- Benign lump; patient choice to have it excised.
- Suspicious lump. Margins: 4–6mm for squamous cell carcinoma; 2–5mm for basal cell carcinoma; 2mm for pigmented lesion of unknown significance.

Consent

- Bleeding/infection.
- Scar.
- Recurrence.
- Further procedures.

Preoperative preparations

- Consent and mark the site of lesion.
- Consider whether this can be performed under local/general anaesthetic.

Position and theatre set-up

- Ensure good exposure of the lump.
- If under local anaesthetic, set up a screen and have a staff member sit with the patient.
- Shave as necessary.
- WHO check; tell the patient you are ready to start.
- Prepare the area and create a sterile field with your dressings.

Procedure

- Manipulate the skin to evaluate the most cosmetic incision line to take (use Langer's lines).
- Mark the area for excision.
- Proceed to an elliptical incision as demonstrated in Fig. 1.30.
- Excise the lesion. Send it for histological examination. Ensure haemostasis.
- Close with either continuous subcuticular absorbable or interrupted non-absorbable sutures (Fig. 1.30).

Postoperative care and instructions

- Keep the wound clean and dry for 7 days.
- Non-absorbable suture out at 7 days.

Complications (specific to the procedure)

- Wound infection.
- Wound dehiscence.
- Need for re-operation if margins are compromised.

Tips and tricks

- Ensure your incision is perpendicular to the skin to get the best wound edges and resultant scar.
- Use Langer's lines to hide the scar.

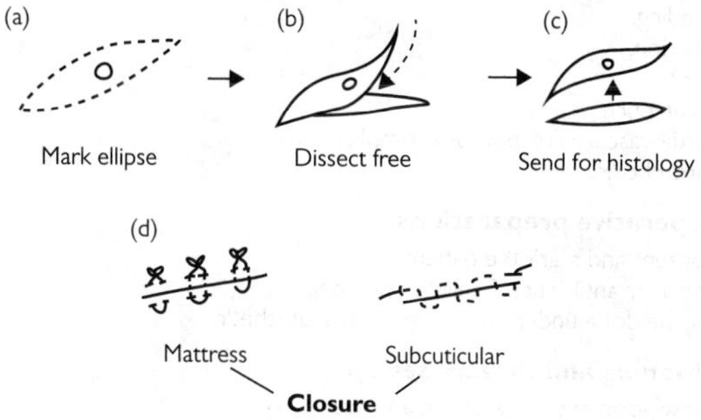
(a)
Mark ellipse
(b)
Dissect free
(c)
Send for histology
(d)
Mattress
Subcuticular
Closure

Fig. 1.30 Excision of a skin lesion, basic steps and options for skin closure.

Abscess incision and drainage

Anatomy

This is dependent upon the abscess site. Specialist areas of abscess drainage are explained in the relevant chapters: please refer to the relevant sections for perianal, pilonidal, axillary, and breast abscesses.

Indications

- All abscesses require incision and drainage in general.

Consent

- Bleeding.
- Infection.
- Scar.
- Recurrence.
- Cardiovascular/respiratory complications.
- Thrombosis.

Preoperative preparations

- Consent and mark the patient.
- Consider antibiotics if cellulitis present.
- May be done under local or general anaesthetic.

Positioning and theatre set up

- Allow good exposure of the abscess.
- Wear eye protection.
- Have access to diathermy if required for haemostasis.
- Apply skin preparation to allow creation of a sterile field and appropriate draping.
- WHO knife check. Inform the anaesthetist you are going to start.

Procedure

- Incise over the most fluctuant point.
- Send a pus swab for microscopy, culture, and sensitivity.
- De-roof the abscess, as shown in Fig. 1.31.

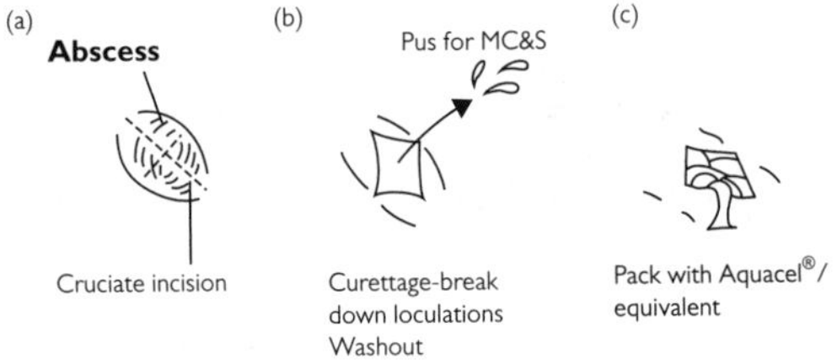
(a)
Abscess
Cruciate incision
(b)
Pus for MC&S
Curettage-break down loculations Washout
(c)
Pack with Aquacel®/ equivalent

Fig. 1.31 Basic steps of incising and draining an abscess.

- Break down any loculations present. Curette the cavity, wash out with normal saline. Ensure haemostasis.
- Pack with Aquacel® or equivalent.
- Dressing gauze +/– surgipad.

Postoperative care and instructions

- Eat and drink, home same day. No routine follow up.
- District nurse/practice nurse to dress the wound until it heals by secondary intention.
- Consider completion course of antibiotics in the presence of cellulitis.

Complications (specific to the procedure)

- Bleeding.
- Infection.
- Residual collection.

Tips and tricks

- Always make a decent incision—not only to allow the pus out, but also to enable the district nurses/practice nurses to pack the wound more easily.
- Eye protection, a must—projectile pus is best avoided!

Surgery for ingrowing toenails

Anatomy

Ingrowing toenails, or onychocryptosis, is a common problem wherein the nail plate punctures the corresponding periungual skin creating a foreign body reaction that can become infected.

Indications

- Failure of conservative therapies.
- Severe pain/recurrent infections.

Consent

- Bleeding/infection.
- Recurrence.

Preoperative preparations

- Consent and mark the patient.
- Performed under local anaesthetic.
- Consider the need for antibiotics if area infected.

Positioning and theatre set up

- Supine with leg at a good height for the surgeon.
- Set up a screen and have a staff member sit with the patient.
- Prepare the whole foot; create a sterile field around this.
- Use plain lignocaine as your local anaesthetic—(adrenaline will cause vasoconstriction in an end arterial system leading to ischaemia).
- WHO knife check. Warn the patient you are about to start and that the local anaesthetic will 'burn and sting' as it is injected.

Procedure

- Infiltrate the local to create a ring block. Check sensation by pinching the skin with toothed forceps.
- Apply a tourniquet around the toe.
- Partial avulsion: elevate the nail from its bed. Split the nail all the way down to its matrix and remove (Fig. 1.32).
- Phenol is applied to the nail bed for 30–60s.
- Total avulsion—the whole nail is removed + phenolization.
- Remove the tourniquet.
- Wrap the toe in a sterile bandage.

Postoperative care and instructions

- Elevate the foot for 1–2 days postoperatively.
- Regular simple oral analgesia.
- Wear soft shoes or open-toed sandals.
- Remove the bandage after 2 days by soaking it.
- Washing the toe in salt water will aid healing.

Complications (specific to the procedure)

- Recurrence 2–3%.
- Infection (rare).

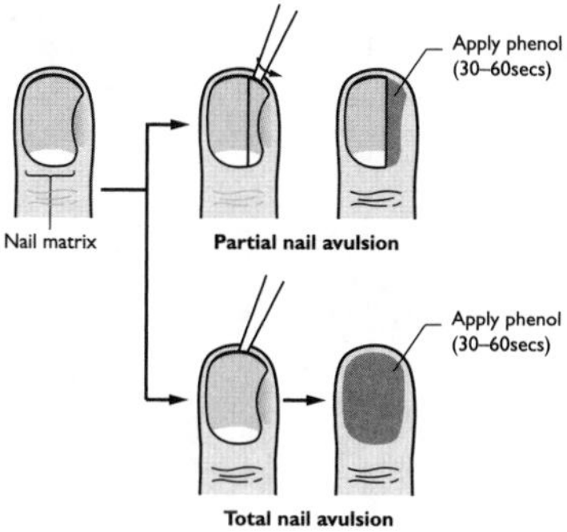
Apply phenol
(30–60secs)
Nail matrix
Partial nail avulsion
Apply phenol
(30–60secs)
Total nail avulsion

Fig. 1.32 Partial and total nail avulsions.

References

1 NICE Guidelines NG45: Routine preoperative tests for elective surgery ☞ (http://www.nice.org.uk/guidance/NG45).
2 GMC. Consent: patients and doctors making decisions together (2008). ☞ (http://www.gmc-uk.org/guidance/ethical_guidance_consent_guidance_index.asp).
3 DoH. Good practice in consent implementation guide (2009). ☞ (https://www.gov.uk/government/uploads/system/uploads/attachment_data/file/138296/dh_103653__1_.pdf).
4 NICE Clinical guideline 74: Surgical site infection: prevention and treatment of surgical site infection (2008). ☞ (https://www.nice.org.uk/guidance/cg74).
5 NICE Clinical Guideline 92: Venous thromboembolism: reducing the risk (2010 updated 2015). ☞ (https://www.nice.org.uk/guidance/qs3).
6 Haynes AB, Weiser TG, Berry WR et al. A surgical safety checklist to reduce morbidity and mortality in a global population. NEJM 2009;360(5):491–99.

Chapter 2

Upper gastrointestinal surgery

Oesophago-gastro-duodenoscopy

Overview

Oesophago-gastro-duodenoscopy (OGD) is a procedure that uses a fibre-optic endoscope (Fig. 2.1), with a light and camera system at the end of a flexible tube, to visualize inside the upper gastrointestinal tract (UGI) tract. The UGI tract includes the oesophagus, stomach, and duodenum. In addition to diagnostic benefit, the endoscope can also be used for therapeutic purposes.

Diagnostic indications

- Investigation of dysphagia with or without weight loss.
- Investigation of upper abdominal pain, dyspepsia, reflux disease.
- Investigation of acute or chronic blood loss.
- Part of investigation of iron-deficiency anaemia.
- Investigation of malabsorption.
- Routine preoperative work-up before upper GI surgery.

Therapeutic indications

- Injection, banding, clips, argon photocoagulation, or diathermy of bleeding vessel from peptic ulcers, varices, or tumours.
- Balloon or bougie dilatation of benign or malignant strictures.
- Stenting for malignant strictures.
- Intra-gastric balloon insertion in super-obese patients.
- Resection of early neoplastic lesions of oesophagus or stomach.
- Retrieval of foreign bodies.
- Endoscopy-guided insertion of fine-bore naso-jejunal feeding tube and percutaneous endoscopic gastrostomy (PEG) for feeding.

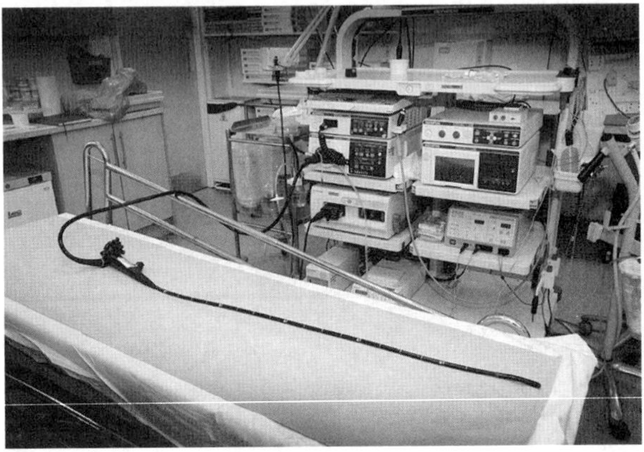

Fig. 2.1 Upper GI endoscopy.

Preparation of patient and positioning

- Informed consent.
- Patient should be fasted for a minimum of 4h.
- Anticoagulation medications can be continued in low-risk diagnostic cases but should be withheld (Clopidogrel for 7 days and Warfarin for 5 days) for therapeutic endoscopy. Occasionally, the anticoagulants are bridged with low molecular weight heparin (CARE: stopping anticoagulants in certain conditions may be unsafe).
- Patient should be consented outside the procedure room.
- The procedure can be done either under topical anaesthesia (lignocaine throat spray) or IV sedation (midazolam).
- During the procedure, patient should be on left lateral position with a mouth guard in place. Heart rate and oxygen saturation are monitored continuously. Nasal O_2 is given to sedated patients.
- Patient is usually fasted for another 1–1½h post-procedure for the sedative to wear off.
- Before starting the procedure:
  - Check that patient is comfortable and in stable condition.
  - Check that nurse assistant is ready.
  - Ensure that the white balance of the scope is done.
  - Lubricate the tip of the scope.
  - Do the final check of the scope for angulation, air insufflation, water irrigation, and the image quality.

Steps of the procedure

- Direct insertion technique is the best and the standard technique.
- Hold the head of endoscope with the left hand and the shaft with the right hand at about the 30cm mark.
- Using the wheels at the head of scope, rehearse the upward and downward movements of the tip, so that correct longitudinal axis can be followed while intubating the scope in pharynx.
- Introduce the scope tip through the mouth guard and over the tongue. Gently angle the tip upwards by rotating the appropriate wheel as it passes over the tongue.
- By looking at the monitor, aim for the scope to be in the midline and advance the scope gently to visualize the epiglottis and cricoarytenoid area.
- Aim for the scope tip to face posteriorly by changing the angle downwards, so that the tip passes inferior to the curve of the cricoarytenoid cartilage.
- Try to pass the scope to one or the other side of the midline and apply gentle pressure. Sometimes it is useful to ask the patient to swallow.
- The instrument should slip into the oesophagus by maintaining gentle inward pressure and insufflating air.
- Throughout this procedure try to be as gentle as possible and do not push the scope against any resistance.
- Once the scope is in the oesophagus, use gentle insufflation of air for thorough examination.
- Measure the gastro-oesophageal junction (GOJ) usually seen at 38–40cm from the incisor teeth. At this junction, the pale pink squamous oesophageal mucosa becomes much darker red gastric mucosa with linear folds.

- After entering into the stomach, rotate the scope towards the left to avoid lesser curvature of stomach. Insufflate air to distend the stomach and aspirate any excessive gastric contents to avoid the risk of aspiration.
- Approach the pylorus after inspecting the stomach. Advance the scope further, keeping the pylorus in centre view.
- Give Buscopan 20mg intravenous if there is excessive spasm and difficulty in intubating the pylorus.
- Once the tip of the scope passes into the duodenal bulb, gently rotate the shaft about 90° to the right and angle up by rotating the wheels. This manoeuvre provides a corkscrew motion at the duodenum and the scope passes into the 2nd part of the duodenum.
- After inspecting the duodenum (give gentle insufflation for good luminal views) withdraw the scope into the stomach. Do the J manoeuvre (retroversion) to inspect the fundus and GOJ.
- Ensure that the scope tip is at the lower part of the stomach. Angle the tip acutely to 180° using the wheels at the scope head. By insufflating more air if needed, and withdrawing the scope gently, view the entire lesser curvature and fundus.
- After retroversion, return the angulation controls into the neutral position for safe extubation.
- Make sure that the stomach and oesophagus is thoroughly decompressed by suctioning the air to avoid post-procedure discomfort.

Risks and complications

- Bleeding is the commonest complication after any therapeutic procedure
- Perforation usually occurs at the cricopharyngeus level of the pharynx or at the lower end of the oesophagus (stricture). The risk of perforation is 1 in 3,000. It is high in elderly patients and following therapeutic procedures (dilatation, stent insertion, or endoscopic mucosal resection). The risk of perforation is high in the presence of anterior cervical osteophytes, Zenker's diverticulum, oesophageal stricture, malignancy, and duodenal diverticula.
- Respiratory depression and arrest due to injudicious use of IV sedation can occur in elderly and frail patients.
- Aspiration and pneumonitis in patients with impaired cough or gag reflex (previous cerebrovascular accident).

Tips and tricks

- Ensure patient is fasted—risk of aspiration.
- Ensure anticoagulants are optimized.
- Do a checklist—it prevents complications.
- Do not push the scope against resistance or blindly, during intubation.

Perforated peptic ulcer closure

Perforated peptic ulcer closure

Overview

The incidence of peptic ulcer perforation is decreasing due to early diagnosis and effective medical management. Around 80% of peptic ulcers are due to *Helicobacter pylori* infections. The remainder are due to consumption of NSAIDS, alcohol, cigarettes, and steroids. A delay in the diagnosis and treatment of >24h is associated with significantly increased morbidity and mortality. Additionally, co-morbidities, shock on admission, age, and frailty are associated with poor outcome.

Indications for surgery

- Generalized peritonitis and typically, but not always, free gas under the diaphragm on erect chest X-ray (CXR).
- Failed conservative management in selected patients. Conservative management can be chosen in patients with a confirmed diagnosis of peptic perforation who are haemodynamically stable and have no, or localized, signs of peritonitis.

Surgical anatomy

Usually perforations occur on the anterior wall of 1st part of the duodenum.

Preoperative preparation

- Resuscitate adequately. Maintain fluid balance. Consider critical care input.
- Pass a nasogastric (NG) tube to decompress the stomach to avoid further contamination of the peritoneal cavity.
- Start 'sepsis six' pathway.

Steps of operation

- Make an upper midline incision extending from the xiphisternum to just below the umbilicus (10–12cm long). Open the peritoneum. You will find a variable quantity of gas and bile-stained fluid. This confirms the diagnosis. Foul-smelling faeculent fluid and gas indicates a large bowel perforation. Use suction. You may encounter fibrinous adhesions between the perforation site and the surrounding structures—liver, stomach, omentum, and colon. Carefully dissect the adhesions to visualize the perforation site. It is commonly just distal to the pylorus.
- If you do not find the perforation, inspect the entire stomach and duodenum carefully. Open the gastrocolic omentum to examine the lesser sac. Visualize the posterior wall of the stomach. Perform a thorough laparotomy if no pathology is found. Remember that multiple perforations can occur. Gastric ulcer perforation may be due to malignancy (3–14%) and may need excision if suitably located.
- Close the perforation by placing two to three parallel 2/0 absorbable sutures about 1cm away from the ulcer margin (Fig. 2.2). Take the sutures along the longitudinal axis of the bowel to avoid narrowing of the lumen of bowel. Deliberately leave the ends of the sutures long. Bring the omentum over the repair and tie the sutures to hold the omentum in place. (Graham patch) (Fig. 2.3). Always make sure that the opposite wall of the duodenum is not incorporated in the sutures to avoid duodenal obstruction.

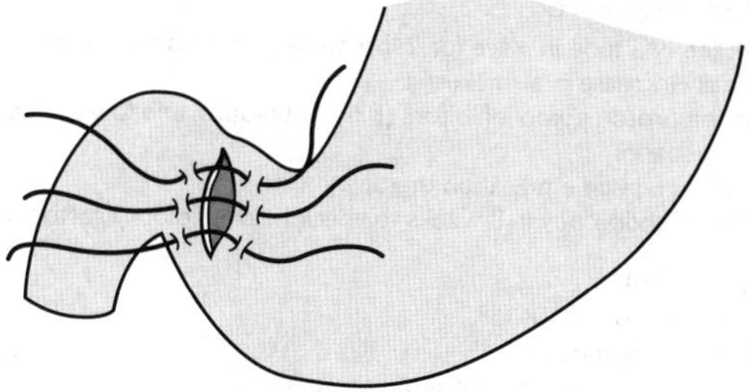

Fig. 2.2 Suture closure of duodenal perforation.

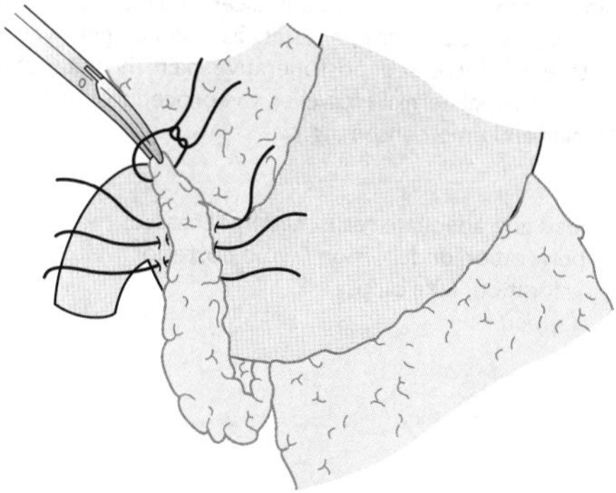

Fig. 2.3 Omental patch technique.

- Some duodenal perforations may be difficult to close. This is because the ulceration is chronic and the margin of the perforation is friable. Attempts at primary closure may cause sutures to cut out or result in duodenal stenosis. These may be managed by the omental plug technique. Place healthy omentum over the perforation to occlude it. Take sutures on the duodenum a distance away from the ulcer margins and tie over the omentum to secure it in position. Rarely, a distal gastrectomy and reconstruction with controlled fistulation of the duodenum is necessary.
- Thoroughly wash the peritoneal cavity with copious amount of warm normal saline (3–4l), until the contents of washout are clear. Leave a drain in the sub-hepatic space selectively.
- Close the laparotomy wound by mass closure using non-absorbable suture.

Postoperative care

- Leave the NG tube in place for 24hrs to decompress the stomach.
- Gradually increase oral intake.
- Prescribe proton pump inhibitors (PPI), antibiotics, and low molecular weight heparin.
- Prescribe *H. pylori* eradication therapy.
- Follow-up endoscopy in 8 weeks to check healing/biopsy gastric ulcer.

Complications

- Mortality is around 10–15%.
- Multi-organ dysfunction.
- Sub-hepatic, sub-phrenic, or pelvic abscess.
- On-going leak and duodenal fistula formation.

Laparoscopic surgery

Consider laparoscopic closure of peptic ulcer in all cases. Advantages of laparoscopic surgery include similar results as open surgery with the additional advantage of decreased postoperative pain, hospital stay, wound infections, and incisional hernia. However, the procedure can be technically more challenging and time-consuming.

Tips and tricks

- Early diagnosis and adequate resuscitation decreases mortality.
- Close the perforation under vision (avoid posterior wall).
- If gastric perforation, take biopsy.
- Eradicate *H. pylori*.

Laparoscopic cholecystectomy

Laparoscopic cholecystectomy is now the treatment of choice for patients with symptomatic gallstone disease. The majority of operations can be performed as day cases.

Indications

- Biliary colic.
- Acute calculous or acalculous cholecystitis.
- Gallstone pancreatitis.
- Symptomatic gall bladder polyp.

Contraindications

- *Absolute*:
  - Cirrhosis with portal hypertension (substantial risk of catastrophic bleeding that is difficult to control).
- *Relative*:
  - Patients with severe cardiorespiratory disease.
  - Pregnancy.
  - Patients with cirrhosis (uncomplicated), coagulopathy.
  - Previous upper abdominal operations.

Surgical anatomy

- The cystic duct arises from the neck of the gall bladder and joins with the common hepatic duct at variable positions.
- Surgically important landmark during laparoscopic cholecystectomy is Calot's triangle. It is formed on the right side by the common hepatic duct, on the left by cystic duct, and the liver surface above.
- The cystic artery derives from the right hepatic artery and supplies the gall bladder. It traverses Calot's triangle; however, there are several anatomical variations. The veins from the gall bladder drain directly into the liver or hepatic veins via the pericholedochal plexus.
- The common bile duct is formed by the union of the common hepatic duct (formed by left and right hepatic ducts outside the porta hepatis) and the cystic duct, and is approximately 8cm in length and 6–8mm in diameter.
- A duct of Luscha can run directly between the liver and gall bladder.

Preoperative preparation

- Perform full blood count, liver function test, coagulation screen, and blood group, and save.
- An ultrasound scan in addition to confirming gallstones can give information about gall bladder wall thickness, oedema of the wall, presence of pericholecystic fluid (acute cholecystitis), and the size of the common bile duct.
- Preoperative magnetic resonance cholangio-pancreatography (MRCP)/ endoscopic retrograde cholangio-pancreatography (ERCP) may be warranted in some cases with deranged liver function tests (LFTs) and/or dilated common bile duct.

- Rule out other causes of right upper quadrant pain and exclude gastritis, peptic ulcer disease, and pancreatitis in patients with atypical symptoms of gallstone disease.
- Ensure preoperative use of TED stockings. Consider prophylactic low molecular weight heparin (LMWH) in high-risk patients.
- Chose a radioluscent operating table for doing perioperative/on table cholangiogram, if necessary.
- Obtain informed consent. Discuss conversion to open cholecystectomy (4–5%), the risk of bleeding, infection, bile leak, and bile duct injury.

Positioning and theatre set-up

- Patient in supine position; consider using table gel mat and strapping to prevent patient sliding.
- Patient's arms can be kept tucked beside body or on arm boards.
- Surgeon and assistant stand on patient's left, monitor on patient's right near head end. Scrub nurse on patient's right side at foot end.

Procedure

- Perform WHO checklist.
- Prepare skin from nipples to suprapubic region.
- Enter the abdomen by the open Hasson technique. Place the trocar directly under vision. In addition to the 10mm umbilical port for a 0° or a 30° camera, insert another 10mm port as a working port about 3–4cm below the xiphisternum. Place a 5mm port at the anterior axillary line on the right side to retract the fundus of the gall bladder and another 5mm port in the midclavicular line on the right side to hold the neck of the gall bladder (Fig. 2.4).

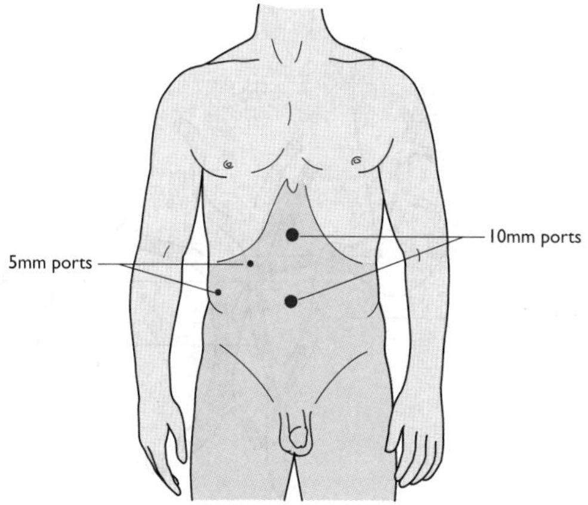
10mm ports
5mm ports

Fig. 2.4 Port sites for laparoscopic cholecystectomy.

- Maintain a pneumoperitoneum of 12mmHg pressure. Tilt the table to reverse Trendelenberg position. Use left side down tilt so that the colon and omentum fall inferiorly.
- Grasp the fundus and lift the gall bladder to display the anatomy.
- Dissect adhesions surrounding the gall bladder to expose Calot's triangle.
- Dissect Calot's triangle by lifting the peritoneal layers on either side of the cystic duct. Use a hook diathermy to incise the peritoneum. Start the dissection by lifting and incising the posterior peritoneal leaf. This will make the gall bladder more mobile. Similarly, dissect the anterior peritoneal leaf starting from Hartmann's pouch moving towards the fundus. This is particularly important in acute cholecystitis as the anatomical landmarks can be difficult to find. Use a dissector or Peterlin forceps to isolate the cystic duct and artery, and to create the so-called critical window (Fig. 2.5). This is the space between the cystic duct and the artery and the liver at the base of the gall bladder fossa. Clear all tissues around the cystic duct and artery to make sure that these two structures are definitely entering the gall bladder. Do this to avoid inadvertent injury to the right hepatic duct, artery, and common bile duct.
- Using a clip applicator, apply two titanium clips proximally and one distally to both the cystic duct and the artery. Divide the structures between the clips.
- Retract the gall bladder upwards to find the plane between gall bladder and liver. Free the gall bladder from the liver using a hook diathermy.

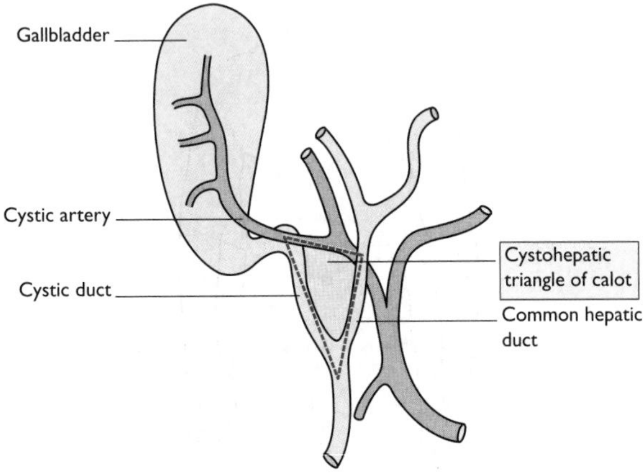
Gallbladder
Cystic artery
Cystic duct
Cystohepatic triangle of calot
Common hepatic duct

Fig. 2.5 Calot's triangle (critical window).

- Before disconnecting the gall bladder inspect the hepatic bed and cystic duct and the artery stumps for bleeding. Control minor bleeding from the liver bed by gentle pressure.
- Deliver the gall bladder via either the umbilical or epigastric port. Use an endobag to avoid spillage of bile or stones from the gall bladder. If necessary stretch the port site using a straight blunt artery forceps while extracting the gall bladder. Extend the incision if the stone in the gall bladder is larger than the port site.
- Do not use a drain if the field is dry.
- Remove ports under vision. Inspect the sites for bleeding. Do a final inspection before deflating the abdomen.
- Close the rectus sheath at the umbilical port under vision. Hold the umbilical tube with a Littlewoods' forceps and use the Langenbeck retractor to expose the cut ends of the fascial sheath. Using a J-shaped PDS(polydiaxanone) or Ethibond (braided, polyester) take interrupted sutures under vision to approximate the fascial sheath.
- Close the skin using subcuticular sutures.
- Infiltrate local anaesthetic.

Postoperative care

- Postoperative observations as per day unit protocol.
- Check for blood or bile in the drainage bag.
- Most patients are discharged on the same day.

Complications

- Bleeding.
- Visceral injury—may present after 24–48h.
- Bile leak.
- Major bile duct injury.
- Intra-abdominal infection—higher risk if spilled stones.
- Wound infection.
- Post-cholecystectomy pain syndrome.
- Port site incisional hernia.
- Retained stones.

Tips and tricks

- Expose the critical window and clearly identify the cystic duct gall bladder junction before clipping or dividing any tubular structure.
- Seek senior advice if difficulty with identification of the critical view. Consider performing cholangiogram or converting to open procedure.
- Aspirate pus/mucus/bile in tense distended gall bladder before proceeding to dissect Calot's triangle.
- Use locking clips or ligature in dilated cystic duct.
- If there is severe chronic inflammatory change at Calot's triangle, do a 'fundus-first' method. Separate the gall bladder from the liver at the fundus and work towards the cystic artery and duct.
- Clip and divide the cystic artery before the cystic duct to avoid traction injury and bleeding.

Open cholecystectomy

Only the operative steps are discussed in this section. See 'Laparoscopic cholecystectomy' (p. 74) for indications, contraindications, preoperative preparation, and positioning of the patient.

Procedure

- The preferred method to access the gall bladder is by an oblique subcostal muscle cutting incision (Kocher's). Make an incision approximately 20cm long, two-finger breadths below the right costal margin. Divide the muscle with diathermy in the line of skin incision. Open the peritoneum in the same line.
- Place two packs, one on the hepatic flexure of the colon and one on the duodenum to get a clear view of gall bladder and Calot's triangle. These packs may be retracted using either the hand of the assistant or a Kelly's retractor. Have the second assistant retract the liver using a Deaver retractor. Place gauze in between to prevent injuring the liver.
- Apply an artery forceps or a sponge-holding forceps to Hartmann's pouch and retract downwards to stretch Calot's triangle. Commence dissection by dividing the peritoneal layer working from the cystic duct towards the cystic artery and liver.
- If there are severe chronic inflammatory changes at Calot's triangle, do a 'fundus-first' method. Separate the gall bladder from liver at the fundus and work towards the cystic artery and duct.
- If the gall bladder is very distended, aspirate it before commencing the dissection to avoid perforation and spillage of bile. Also, handling of the gall bladder is easier when it is empty.
- Expose the cystic duct and artery by dissecting the fatty tissue in Calot's triangle. Isolate the cystic duct and clearly ascertain its position. Then dissect the cystic artery and trace it to the gall bladder to avoid injury to the right hepatic artery. Once the critical window is developed, divide the cystic artery and then the cystic duct between two ligatures in continuity. The cystic artery is tied first to avoid traction injury. Also, dividing the cystic artery first will straighten the cystic duct.
- Retract the gall bladder away from the liver and dissect it off using diathermy.
- Close the peritoneum with absorbable suture and the rectus sheath and muscle with continuous 2.0 Prolene®/PDS suture. Close the skin with subcuticular Monocryl® or with staples.

Surgery for bleeding peptic ulcer

Overview

Bleeding from a peptic ulcer can be life-threatening. NICE recommend using risk-stratification tools like Blatchford and Rockall scoring in triaging patients for urgent endoscopy. Urgent endoscopy is performed to identify the site and cause of bleeding, and also to institute appropriate therapeutic intervention. Early endoscopy within 24h of admission has been shown to reduce blood transfusion and length of hospital stay. Most, but not all, bleeding is controlled in this way. Urgent surgical intervention is occasionally required.

Indications

- Failure of endoscopic control.
- Re-bleeding after successful endoscopic therapy.
- Elderly and unfit patients may not cope with bleeding—consider early surgery.
- Patients with ongoing blood transfusion requirements.

Preoperative preparation

- Resuscitation in critical care is ideal.
- Clotting abnormalities must be corrected and cross-matched blood should be available.
- Supine position.

Procedure

- Make an upper midline incision.
- A bleeding ulcer in the duodenum is found on the posterior wall, typically eroding the gastroduodenal artery. Kocherization of the duodenum may be necessary. Perform a longitudinal duodenotomy between two long-stay sutures. Suction the clots and blood for visual inspection. If bleeding is profuse, occlude the gastroduodenal artery using a pledget in a forceps. Put two sutures on either side of the bleeding site to tie off the artery (see Fig. 2.6).
- Extend the incision proximally to inspect the stomach if no cause for bleeding is found in the duodenum.
- Close the duodenotomy transversely to avoid narrowing of the duodenum (Heineke–Mikulicz pyloroplasty). If a transverse closure is not possible due to long duodenotomy, carry out a longitudinal closure and perform Roux-en-Y gastroenterostomy. An alternative is a Finney pyloroplasty, an inverted U-shaped anastomosis between the stomach and the duodenum.
- With giant ulcers the first part of the duodenum may completely disintegrate and, once opened, prove difficult to close. Manage this situation with an antrectomy and Roux-en-Y reconstruction. Close the duodenal stump primarily with a linear stapler or suture. Alternatively, suture the margins to the fibrous ulcer cavity overlying the pancreas (Nissen technique). To prevent duodenal stump leak, drain the duodenum with a Foley catheter inserted through the closure line or preferably by a T-tube in the healthy lateral wall of the second part of the duodenum.

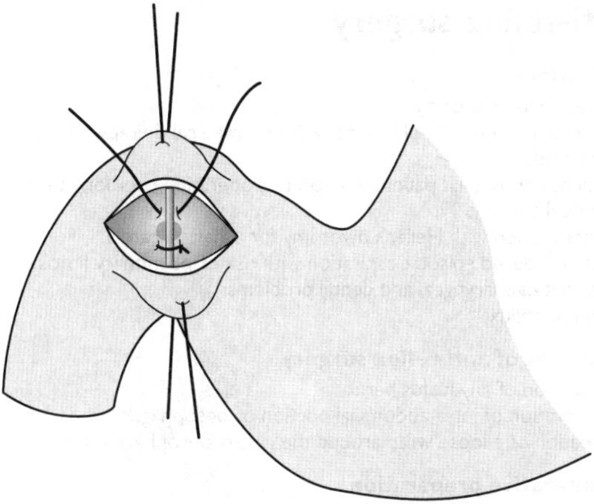

Fig. 2.6 Duodenotomy and ligation of gastroduodenal artery.

Postoperative care
- Monitor closely and observe for further evidence of bleeding.
- Allow clear fluids after 24h. NG tube can be taken out after 48h followed by soft diet.
- Give *H. pylori* eradication therapy when oral feed commenced.
- Do OGD after 6–8 weeks.

Complications
- Recurrent bleeding.
- Duodenal fistula.
- Duodenal stenosis.
- Obstructive jaundice (injury to common bile duct).

Tips and tricks
- Exclude other sources of bleeding.
- Keep endoscopy equipment in theatre.
- If duodenotomy cannot be closed consider controlled fistula.

Anti-reflux surgery

Indications

- Failed medical therapy.
- Development of complications whilst on medical therapy (ulcer, stricture).
- Patient's choice. Fit patient who prefers operation over long-term medical therapy.
- In association with Heller's myotomy for achalasia cardia.
- Reflux-induced episodic aspiration with risk of pulmonary fibrosis, associated pharyngeal and dental problems.
- Volume reflux.

Principles of anti-reflux surgery

- Reduction of any hiatus hernia.
- Restoration of intra-abdominal portion of oesophagus.
- Creation of a loose wrap around the gastro-oesophageal junction.

Preoperative preparation

- Endoscopy to identify erosive oesophagitis, strictures, and other gastro-oesophageal pathology.
- 24h pH study to estimate the severity of acid reflux.
- Manometry to rule out motility disorder.
- Contrast swallow to delineate anatomical details of gastro-oesophageal junction (GOJ) and associated para-oesophageal hernia.

Surgical approaches

- Trans-thoracic.
- Transabdominal.
- Open method.
- Laparoscopic method.

Types of surgery

A range of different anti-reflux operations are practiced worldwide. Some are historical. Three common types of procedures performed are:

- Nissen fundoplication (360° wrap)—Fig. 2.7.
- Anterior partial fundoplication (Dor fundoplication)—Fig. 2.8.
- Posterior partial fundoplication (Toupet)—Fig. 2.9.

Nissen fundoplication (360° wrap)

This procedure involves mobilization of oesophagus from hiatus and reducing stomach and hiatus hernia sac into the abdominal cavity. A hiatal repair is performed and the fundus of the stomach is wrapped around the intra-abdominal oesophagus.

Anterior or Dor fundoplication

This is an anterior hemifundoplication, which provides a good mucosal protection after a cardiomyotomy. The stomach is brought forward and sutured on either side of the oesophagus.

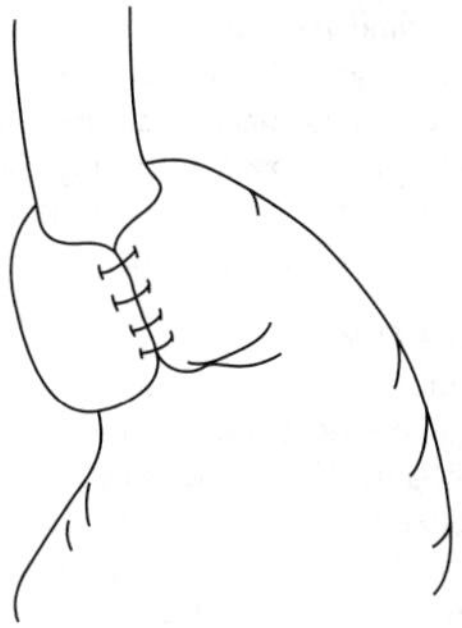

Fig. 2.7 Nissen fundoplication.

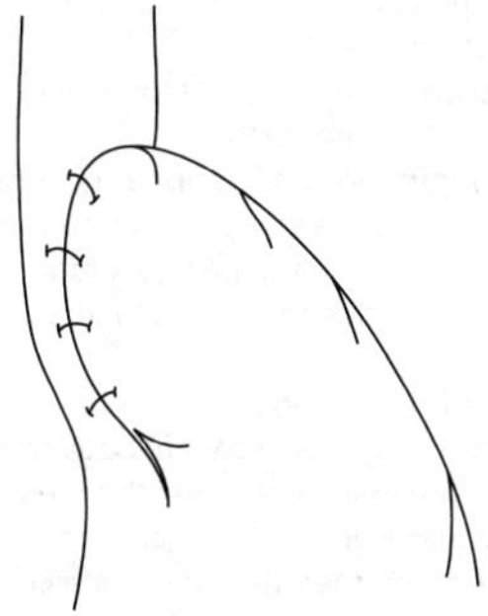

Fig. 2.8 Dor fundoplication.

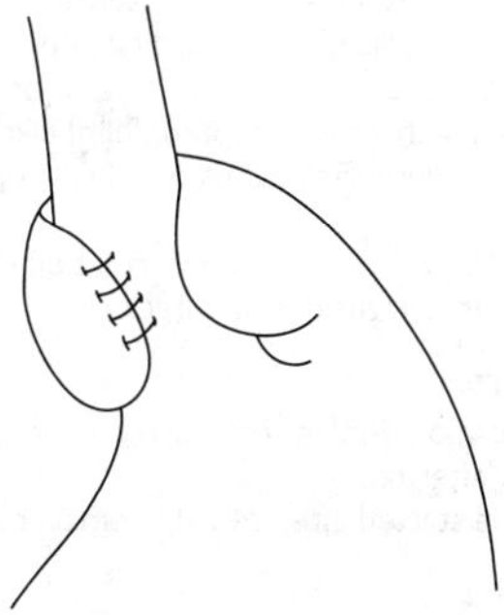

Fig. 2.9 Toupet fundoplication.

Posterior partial or Toupet fundoplication

The difference in this procedure is that an incomplete wrap of stomach is made posteriorly, where the stomach is sutured to the oesophagus side leaving a strip of oesophagus exposed anteriorly. Although a low incidence of dysphagia is noted with this procedure, it is associated with higher incidence of failure to control reflux symptoms.

Position and theatre set-up

- Patient in supine position.
- The surgeon stands on the right side and the assistant stands on the left side. Alternatively, a modified lithotomy position can be given with knees partially flexed. The surgeon stands between the patient's legs. With a 20–30° reverse Trendelenberg (head-up) position, the abdominal viscera can move downwards exposing the hiatus.

Procedure

- With the advent of minimal invasive surgery and availability of suitable retractors to use in the upper abdomen, anti-reflux procedures are usually done laparoscopically.
- Create a pneumoperitoneum using Hasson's open technique with a sub-umbilical incision. Insert 11mm port.
- Under vision insert 11mm port in left upper quadrant in mid-clavicular line. Insert a 5mm port in the same position on the right side. Insert a 5mm port 5cm lateral to the left upper quadrant port. Put a 5mm port in the epigastrium and use this to insert a Nathanson self-retaining liver retractor.
- Use the retractor to lift the left lobe of liver.
- Divide the gastrohepatic ligament/pars flaccida using harmonic diathermy. Following the white line along the medial edge of the right crus, develop a plane between the crus and the oesophagus. Do the same dissection on the other side. Safeguarding both vagus nerves, mobilize the distal oesophagus. Use a nylon sling to retract the oesophagus.
- Repair the hiatal defect with non-absorbable sutures. Ensure that the oesophagus is not angulated and the approximation is not too tight.
- The gastric fundus is mobilized and pulled behind the oesophagus using the 'shoe-shine' technique.
- Secure the wrap taking three interrupted, full-thickness sutures on the stomach and seromuscular sutures on the oesophagus using 2-0 Ethibond.
- In order to ensure the wrap is floppy, insert a bougie or balloon or endoscope in the oesophagus during surgery.

Postoperative care

- These operations can be done as day-case procedures.
- Allow liquids orally after 6h.
- A sloppy diet can be started after 24h. To remain on sloppy diet for 3–4 weeks.

Postoperative complications

- *Nausea and vomiting*: about 50–60% patients experience this symptom. This is usually transient. Further investigations are required if conservative measures fail.
- *Dysphagia* (3–8%): usually transient after Nissen fundoplication and should settle within a few days. If symptoms persist, endoscopy to assess the luminal patency is needed. Endoscopic dilatation, if the hiatal closure is tight or the wrap is tight, may resolve the situation. Some cases may require re-operation to release the wrap. Occasionally the Nissen wrap is converted to a partial wrap.
- *Wrap migration*: herniation of the fundoplication wrap into the chest through hiatus is a recognized complication. Migration is usually due to inadequate hiatal closure, failure to recognize shortened oesophagus, early return to strenuous exercises, or postoperative vomiting. Due to risk of strangulation, this needs urgent surgical attention.
- *Pnemothorax/pneumomediastinum/surgical emphysema*: these are common due to mobilization of the oesophagus. Usually resolves conservatively.
- *Gas bloat syndrome and increase in flatulence*: inability to vent the air from the stomach is noted in 70% of cases. Occurs due to altered GOJ or injury to vagus nerve causing delayed emptying and relaxation of the pylorus.
- *Oesophageal perforation*: more common during re-do fundoplication. Use bougie or endoscope during the operation to delineate anatomy.
- *Splenic injury*: occurs during mobilization of the fundus and/or division of short gastric vessels.
- *Recurrent symptoms*.

Surgical outcome

Anti-reflux surgery is successful in 85–90% of patients. The overall postoperative mortality is <1 in 1,000 (0.1%). Perioperative complications comprise of pneumothorax, splenic injury, and oesophageal perforation in <1%. Late complications can occur in 10–15%. These include gas bloat syndrome, temporary dysphagia, and increased flatulence.

Tips and tricks

- Exclude achalasia or motility disorders before offering anti-reflux procedure.
- Address patient's expectations during preoperative counselling.
- Requires meticulous handling of oesophagus.
- Type of anti-reflux procedure is tailor-made to patient and experience of the operator.
- Use bougie or endoscope in revision procedures.

Gastrectomy

Surgical anatomy

The stomach is divided into the fundus, body, and pyloric regions. The fundus is the most proximal part of the stomach, separated from the oesophagus by the cardiac notch and is attached to the diaphragm by the gastro-phrenic ligament. The pyloric region consists of the antrum and pylorus. The thickened circular muscle fibres form the pyloric sphincter.

The stomach has a rich blood supply from the coeliac axis. On the lesser curve, the left gastric artery forms an anastomotic arcade with the right gastric artery, which arises from the common hepatic artery. The gastroduodenal artery, which is a branch of the hepatic artery, divides into the superior pancreaticoduodenal artery and the right gastroepiploic artery. The right gastroepiploic artery runs along the greater curvature and forms anastomosis with the left gastroepiploic artery, which is a branch of the splenic artery. The fundus of the stomach is supplied by short gastric vessels arising from the splenic artery. The veins along the lesser curve drain into the portal vein and on the greater curve into the splenic vein.

Understanding the lymphatic drainage of the stomach is paramount in the surgery of gastric cancer. The lymph nodes concerned in the drainage of the stomach are divided into hepatic, subpyloric, suprapyloric, perigastric, and pancreaticolienal groups. Due to the complexity of lymph node stations, the Japanese Gastric Cancer Association (JGCA) has mapped out these stations to 23 major stations (Table 2.1). These consist of six perigastric and 17 extra-gastric lymph node stations.

Preparation for gastric surgery

All patients require thorough fitness assessment (cardiac, respiratory, nutritional). CT/PET CT, endoscopic ultrasound, and staging laparoscopy to assess the liver and the hiatus are used in combination for accurate staging.

Extent of gastric resection

The objective of gastric cancer surgery is to completely excise the disease with clear margins. The stomach is resected to obtain a 5cm clear margin, both longitudinal and circumferential. In addition, an en-block regional lymphadenenectomy is performed. This is also used for staging purposes.

Anatomically, the stomach can be divided into thirds (lower—L, middle—M, upper—U). Distal-third (L) tumours require subtotal gastrectomy (~80% of the stomach) with preservation of the fundus and short gastric arterial supply. Middle-third (M), proximal-third (U), and whole-stomach tumours (LMU) require total gastrectomy. Tumours at the cardia require total gastrectomy with excision of 5cm of distal oesophagus. The GI continuity is established through Roux-en-Y anastomosis.

Lymphadenectomy

Gastric cancer with lymph node metastases may remain a loco-regional disease and radical excision with lymphadenectomy can be justified on the following grounds:

- Optimal pathological disease staging and estimate of prognosis.
- Improved loco-regional control.
- Prolonged survival and possible cure.

Table 2.1 Classification of regional lymph nodes of the stomach

Perigastric lymph node stations		Extra-perigastric lymph node stations	
Station	Location	Station	Location
1	Right paracardial	7	Along the trunk of left gastric artery
2	Left paracardial	8a	Anteriosuperior nodes along common hepatic artery
3a	Lesser curvature, along the branches of left gastric artery	8p	Posterior nodes along the common hepatic artery
3b	Lesser curvature, along the 2nd branch and distal part of right gastric artery	9	Around coeliac artery
4sa	Along short gastric vessels (perigastric area)	10	Splenic hilar lymph nodes
4sb	left gastroepiploic vessels (perigastric area)	11p	Along proximal splenic artery
4d	Right gastroepiploic vessels	11d	Along distal splenic artery
5	Suprapyloric, along the 1st branch and proximal part of right gastric artery	12a	Hepatoduodenal ligament nodes along the proper hepatic artery
6	Infrapyloric, along the first branch and proximal part of the right gastroepiploic artery down to the confluence of the right gastroepiploic vein and the anterior superior pancreatoduodenal vein	12b	Hepatoduodenal ligament nodes along the bile duct
		12p	Hepatoduodenal ligament nodes behind the portal vein
		13	Posterior to pancreatic head
		14v	Along superior mesenteric vein
		14a	Along superior mesenteric artery
		15	Along middle colic vessels
		16a1	Para aortic nodes in the aortic hiatus
		16a2	Around abdominal aorta(from coeliac trunk till left renal vein)
		16b1	Around abdominal aorta (from left renal vein till inferior mesenteric artery)

(Continued)

Table 2.1 (*Contd.*)

Perigastric lymph node stations		Extra-perigastric lymph node stations	
Station	Location	Station	Location
		16b2	Around abdominal aorta (from inferior mesenteric artery till bifurcation of aorta)
		17	Anterior surface of pancreatic head
		18	Along the Inferior margin of the pancreas
		19	Infradiaphragmatic nodes along the subphrenic artery
		20	In the oesophageal hiatus of the diaphragm
		110	Paraoesophageal (lower thorax)
		111	Supradiaphragmatic nodes separate from the oesophagus
		112	Posterior mediastinal nodes separate from the oesophagus and he hiatus

Japanese Gastric Cancer Association Classification: 3rdeEdition. Gastric Cancer (2011) 14:101–2.

The pattern of lymphatic spread has been carefully documented in relation to the primary tumour and divided into three tiers based on the relative incidence of nodal disease:

- N1 (perigastric tier).
- N2 (nodes along main arterial supply to the stomach).
- N3 (distant nodal stations away from the stomach).

The amount of nodal dissection performed is represented as D1, D2, or D3, depending on how many tiers are removed.

Procedure

Total gastrectomy

- Patient in supine position.
- Obtain access via upper midline incision. It is sometimes necessary to excise the xiphoid process.
- Use a self-retaining retractor like Omnitract or Octopus to expose the hiatus and retract the left lobe of liver.
- Carry out a thorough inspection to exclude ascites, peritoneal deposits, and to assess resectability before commencing the operation (preoperative understaging in 15–20% is quoted in the literature).

- Commence dissection by mobilizing the greater omentum from the transverse colon and mesocolon. Continue dissection until reaching the lower border of the pancreas, safeguarding the middle colic and marginal vessels.
- Commence the dissection at 1st part of duodenum by releasing any retrogastric adhesions. Expose and doubly ligate the right gastroepiploic vessel at its origin, where it separates from gastroduodenal artery.
- Pull the stomach downwards to stretch the gastrohepatic ligament and continue dissection by dividing the ligament. Continue dissection caudally to expose right gastric vessels. Ligate them and divide in continuity
- Divide the short gastric vessels.
- Divide the 1st part of duodenum using a surgical stapler. Over-sew with absorbabale sutures (surgeon's choice). Take down the hepatic, suprapyloric, and subpyloric nodes.
- Continue the dissection to clear the lymph nodes along the left gastric artery and divide it flush at its origin. Dissect the lymph nodes along the superior border of the pancreas, splenic artery, and hilum. This dissection completely mobilizes the stomach.
- Apply stay sutures on the oesophagus. Divide the oesophagus with adequate margins after applying a purse-string applicator.
- Using a circular stapler, perform an end-to-side anastomosis between the distal oesophagus and the afferent jejunal limb.
- Maintain gastrointestinal continuity by creating Roux loop.

Subtotal gastrectomy

- This procedure is performed for tumours confined to the distal stomach; it is unnecessary to remove the whole stomach.
- The steps are the same as for total gastrectomy, except that the upper-third of the stomach is left behind with the blood supply from the short gastric vessels.
- The anastomosis of the proximal stomach to the jejunum is either hand sewn or a stapling device is used.
- A Roux-en-Y gastroenterostomy is almost always preferred as it is associated with the lowest degree of bile reflux.

Billroth 1 (gastroduodenal anastomosis) reconstruction after subtotal gastrectomy produces bile reflux into the gastric remnant. Billroth II/Polya (retro-colic loop gastro-jejunostomy) reconstructions were frequently carried out for benign peptic ulcer surgery. It also produces bile reflux and in symptomatic patients required revision to a Roux-en-Y configuration. Loop gastro-jejunostomy continues to be employed for palliative bypasses. It may be combined with a division of the stomach above the site of the malignant obstruction to prevent future in-growth into the anastomosis as a 'divine exclusion'.

Roux-en-Y reconstruction

The Roux-en Y reconstruction configuration proceeds as follows:

- *Total gastrectomy*: the anastomosis is performed between the jejunum (50cm from DJ flexure) to the oesophagus using hand sewn or circular stapler (Fig. 2.10).
- *Subtotal gastrectomy*: the anastomosis is performed between the jejunum (50cm from DJ flexure) to the most dependent part of the stomach using hand sewn or linear stapler (Fig. 2.11).

Most surgeons perform the anastomosis through the retro-colic route:

- Divide the proximal jejunum 50cm away from the DJ flexure (minimum of 50cm to avoid bile reflux).
- Divide the mesenteric vessels to provide a mobile well-vascularized distal jejunal segment.
- Create a retro-colic window in an avascular part of the transverse mesocolon.
- After total gastrectomy, perform a stapled oesophago-jejunal anastomosis. Place 2/0 Prolene® purse-string sutures at the cut end of the oesophagus, securing the anvil (head of the stapler gun) of the appropriately sized circular stapler (usually 25–28mm size).

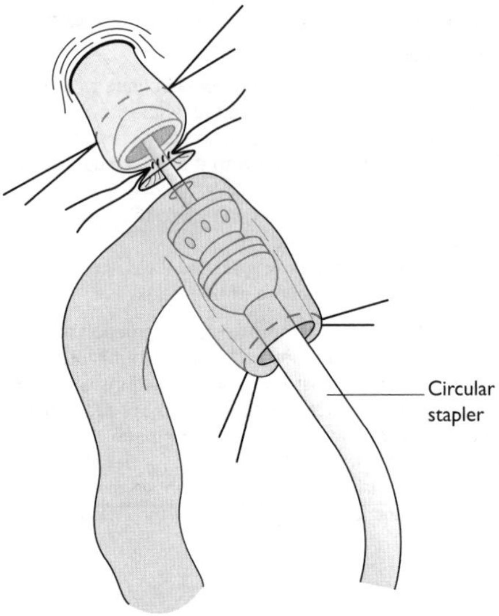
Circular
stapler

Fig. 2.10 Jejuno-oesophageal anastomosis using circular stapler.

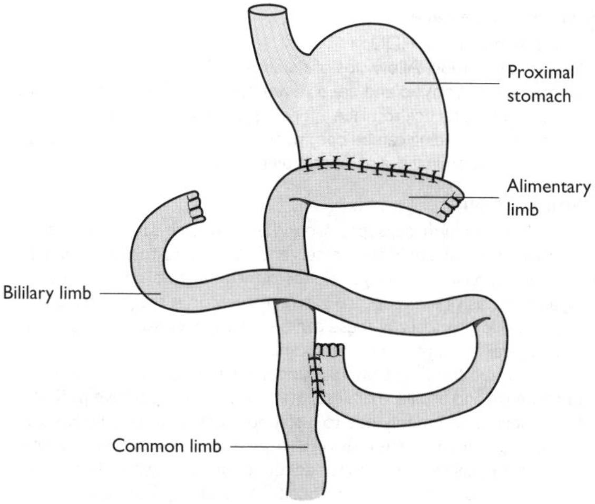
Proximal
stomach
Alimentary
limb
Bilitary limb
Common limb

Fig. 2.11 Subtotal gastrectomy with Roux-en-Y anastomosis.

- Insert the staple gun into the open end of the Roux loop from the left-hand side of the patient and create an end-side oesophago-jejunal anastomosis, taking care not to twist the mesentery or catch additional tissue in the anastomosis.
- Keep the blind end of the jejunum as short as possible. Close with a linear stapler. Over-sew with 2/0 Vicryl®.
- After subtotal gastrectomy, employ a hand-sewn, continuous two-layer anastomosis after subtotal gastrectomy between the lowest part of the gastric remnant and the Roux loop, using 2/0 PDS or Vicryl®. An end–side anastomosis is usually too narrow and a side–side anastomosis is preferred.
- Close the blind end of the Roux loop with a linear stapler and oversew it. In constructing the anastomosis this blind end is positioned on the patient's right-hand side (in contrast to total gastrectomy) so that there is dependent drainage from the stomach.
- After completing the gastro-jejunostomy, secure it beneath the colon and incorporate closure of the window in the transverse mesocolon.
- Perform the distal Roux anastomosis 40–50cm distally as a side-to-end jejuno-jejunostomy, using one or two layers of 2/0 PDS or Vicryl®.

Loop gastro-jejunostomy

- Identify a mobile proximal jejunal segment. The retro-colic route is the shortest and is associated with the best position for drainage.
- Perform the anastomosis along the lower greater curve in two layers with 2/0 Vicryl® or PDS with 5–10 cm of iso-peristaltic jejunum. Then secure the gastro-jejunostomy below the transverse mesocolon.

Postoperative care

- Close monitoring in HDU.
- Keep the NG tube. Allow sips of fluids after 48h.
- Continue chest physio and deep vein thrombosis (DVT) prophylaxis.
- It is common practice to place a feeding jejunostomy after a total gastrectomy. Feeding can be commenced from 1st postoperative day.
- Leave the abdominal drains till soft diet is commenced.

Complications

- *Secondary haemorrhage*: sepsis around the stomach can erode the sutures on important blood vessels and can lead to torrential bleeding.
- *Anastomotic leak*: oesophago-jejunostomy (after total gastrectomy), GJ anastomosis (after subtotal gastrectomy), or at the jejunojejunal anastomotic site. Usually these can be managed conservatively with radiological drainage of any significant collection.
- *Duodenal stump leak or blowout*: duodenal stump blowout is very uncommon and usually manifests in the early postoperative period. Stump leak is commonly due to distal obstruction where the Roux limb was created due to a stenosis or kink. A stump blowout will require prompt surgical intervention for adequate drainage with a large-bore catheter to convert it to a controlled fistula. Stump leaks can be managed by conservative methods and adequate radiological drainage.
- *Dumping syndrome*: group of symptoms noticed in post-gastrectomy patients consisting of abdominal cramps/pain, sweating, flushing, light headedness, diarrhoea, and palpitations.
  - Early dumping:
    —Occurs 20–30min after ingestion of food. Hyperosmolar food is emptied too quickly into small bowel causing fluid shift from intestine into lumen to make it isotonic. Results in luminal distention, which induces autonomic response. Patient education about eating small quantities of food frequently and avoiding a high-sugar diet should resolve the symptoms.
  - Late dumping:
    —Occurs 2–3h after a meal and is less common than early dumping. In addition to rapid emptying of food into small bowel, the carbohydrate-rich food gets absorbed in to the bloodstream. This results in release of large amounts of insulin. The insulin causes reactive hypoglycaemia, which in turn stimulates the adrenal gland to release catecholamines, resulting in the symptoms described.
- *Recurrence of disease*.
- *Nutritional deficiencies*: severity of these symptoms is related to the extent of gastric resection. Most common deficiencies are iron & vitamin B12.

Tips and tricks

- Adequate preoperative assessment is key in patient selection and resectability of the tumour.
- Radical nodal dissection (D2) is unnecessary if the surgery is palliative.
- Awareness of complications and timely management is vital for best outcomes.

Oesophagectomy

Due to the complexity of this particular operation and variations in access and techniques, this procedure is discussed as different approaches.

Indications

- Malignancy.
- End-stage benign disease (very late presentation of achalasia).
- Occasionally emergency resection required for corrosive injury/perforation or spontaneous rupture.

Assess fitness for surgery

- Full blood count/electrolytes/LFTs.
- Pulmonary function tests.
- Arterial blood gases.
- Exercise test.
- ECG.
- Cardiological/respiratory consultation.
- Nutritional assessment and hyperalimentation.
- Anaesthetic assessment—single lung anaesthesia/thoracic epidural.

Preparation for surgery

- Stop smoking.
- Thrombo-embolic prophylaxis.
- Intravenous broad-spectrum antibiotic cover.
- Cross-match four units of blood.
- Intensive care/high-dependency bed availability.
- Colon preparation if required for a conduit.
- Psychological preparation and counselling.

Rationale for radical surgery and lymphadenectomy

- Optimal staging.
- Improved loco-regional control.
- Improved cure rate.

Left thoracic subtotal oesophagectomy

Some thoracic surgeons favour a left thoraco-laparotomy (Fig. 2.12) for lower and middle-third oesophageal tumours. It is contraindicated for malignancy above the aortic arch for which a right-sided three-phase approach is required. The theoretical advantage is that tumour operability is assessed as the initial part of the procedure, although with modern imaging, inoperability in the chest is rare. Disadvantages include poor access to the abdomen (poor nodal clearance) and insufficient mediastinal access to nodal tissue and the thoracic duct.

Position of patient

- Right lateral decubitus position with left arm flexed at 90° and placed on arm-rest.

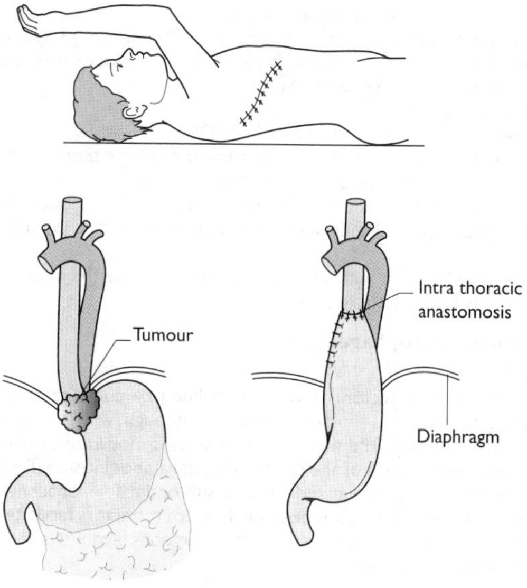
Tumour
Intra thoracic anastomosis
Diaphragm

Fig. 2.12 Thoraco-abdominal approach for lower third oesophageal carcinoma.

Steps of operation

- Make an oblique incision from the left hypochondrium over the costal margin along the 6th, 7th, and 8th ribs to its posterior angle till erector spinae muscle. Divide the thoracic wall muscles with diathermy and open the pleural space at the upper border of the 7th rib.
- Collapse the lung (single lung ventilation).
- Divide the costal margin and detach the diaphragm from the ribs peripherally, avoiding damage to phrenic nerve.
- Open the peritoneum along the upper midline incision from rectus sheath to costal margin and exclude distant/unresectable disease.
- Mobilize the oesophagus and adjacent tissue from the hiatus upwards.
- Preserve the left recurrent laryngeal nerve as the oesophagus is freed by blunt dissection around the aortic arch.
- Pass a tape around the oesophagus at this point to aid retraction and dissect into root of the neck, identified by the 1st rib.
- Mobilize the stomach in a similar fashion to that described for the abdominal Lewis–Tanner approach.
- Divide the gastrosplenic, gastrocolic, and gastrohepatic ligaments with preservation of the right gastric and gastroepiploic vessels.
- Ligate and divide the left gastric vessels.
- Carry out a pyloroplasty.

- Kocherize the duodenum to gain length.
- Divide the oesophagus above the aortic arch after applying stay sutures
- Divide the stomach with a linear stapler across the lesser curve towards the fundus to create a gastric tube.
- Deliver the specimen.
- Over-sew the gastrotomy line with 2/0 PDS.
- Pass the high point of the fundus up to the apex of the thorax and anastomose it to the oesophageal stump.
- Repair the diaphragm and costal margin with continuous 1 nylon suture.
- Insert apical and basal underwater seal chest drains and re-expand the lung.
- Approximate the ribs with interrupted 0 Vicryl®. Close the muscle in layers with 1 PDS. Clips to skin.

Trans-hiatal oesophagectomy

Rationale

Trans-hiatal oesophagectomy has fewer pulmonary complications when compared to the trans-thoracic approach, although with no significant reduction in mortality. The thoracic oesophagus is mobilized by blunt dissection with anastomosis of the conduit through a neck incision (Fig. 2.13). Major blood loss can occur and there is sub-optimal lymphadenectomy producing a higher local recurrence rate. Modern retractors facilitate more dissection under direct vision. Many thoracic surgeons favour this approach, particularly for benign disease.

Abdominal phase

- Patient in supine position.
- Make a midline incision.
- Exclude distant or unresectable disease.

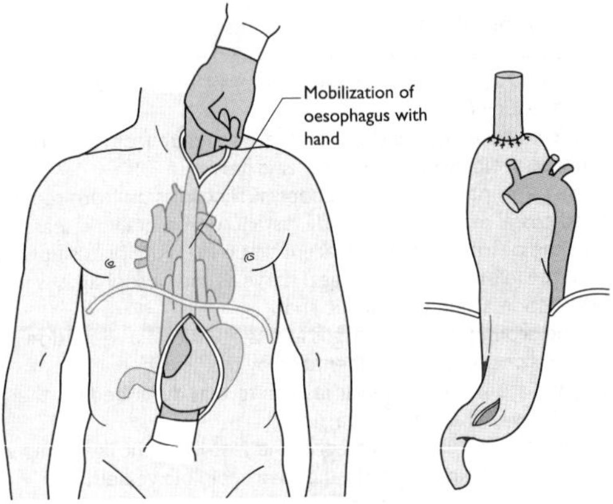
Mobilization of oesophagus with hand

Fig. 2.13 Trans-hiatal mobilization of oesophagus.

- Carry out routine gastric or colonic mobilization to allow tension-free passage up to the neck.
- Divide the phreno-oesophageal ligament.
- Mobilize the lower 5–10cm of oesophagus and tumour checking that there is no fixation to the aorta or tracheo-bronchial tree.
- Perform a pyloroplasty.

Cervical phase

- Patient's neck is extended, supported by head-ring and turned to the right.
- Make a 5cm oblique left cervical incision parallel to the sterno-cleidomastoid centred at the level of the cricoid cartilage.
- Divide the platysma and omohyoid.
- Ligate the inferior thyroid artery and divide it.
- Retract the carotid sheath laterally and the larynx and trachea medially, avoiding damage to the recurrent laryngeal nerve in the tracheo-oesophageal groove.
- Mobilize the oesophagus posteriorly by blunt dissection from the pre-vertebral fascia into the superior mediastinum. Dissect the oesophagus free by sharp dissection from the trachea avoiding damage to the posterior membranous aspect. Once encircled with a sling, the cervical and upper thoracic oesophagus can be mobilized to the level of the carina by further blunt dissection.

Mediastinal phase

- Now pass a hand through the hiatus and free the oesophagus by blunt finger dissection. Carry out sequential division of the posterior attachment to the aorta and the anterior connection to the tracheo-bronchial tree. Finally mobilize the oesophagus from its lateral pleural adhesions. Much of this can be achieved under direct vision with adequate retraction and synchronous dissection from the neck.
- If there is uncontrollable blood loss pack the area and convert to an open thoracotomy.
- Penetration of either pleural space necessitates chest drain.
- Divide the proximal oesophagus in the neck and suture a drain to the distal cut end and bring this out in the abdomen. Then excise the specimen and prepare the colonic or gastric conduit, suturing it to the drain and passing it up into the neck. Anchor the conduit to the pre-vertebral fascia in the neck.
- Insert a feeding jejunostomy and close the abdomen with 1 PDS and clips to skin.

Anastomosis

- Fashion an end-to-end oesophago-gastric or oesophago-colic anastomosis with interrupted 2/0 PDS.
- Insert a 24Fr Wallace–Robinson drain adjacent to the anastomosis and close the wound in layers with 2/0 Vicryl® and subcutaneous 3/0 Monocryl® to skin.

Abdominal and right thoracic subtotal oesophagectomy (Ivor Lewis)

This is the Ivor Lewis or Lewis–Tanner procedure, commonly used for middle and lower third oesophageal tumours. Reconstruction is usually carried out with a gastric pull-up anastomosed at the apex of the thorax (Fig. 2.14).

Abdominal phase

Steps of operation

- Patient is supine position.
- Exclude distant and unresectable disease via an upper midline incision.
- Use modern fixed retracting devices (omnitract/octopus) to enhance gastric and hiatal exposure.
- Mobilize the stomach as previously with preservation of the right gastric and gastro-epiploic vessels (Fig. 2.14). Carry out a lymphadenectomy. Drains are usually not required. Consider a feeding jejunostomy. Close the abdomen with mass closure with 1 PDS and clips to skin.

Thoracic phase

Steps of operation

- Patient is put in left lateral position.
- Perform a postero-lateral thoracotomy with diathermy. Retract the inferior aspect of the scapula upwards and enter the thorax through the 5th or 6th intercostal spaces (the 2nd rib is at the apex of the sub-scapula space). Divide the intercostal muscles above the rib.
- Collapse the lung (single lung ventilation).
- Excise the neck of the lower rib to allow a controlled fracture and better exposure.
- Ligate the intercostal vessels and destroy the nerve to decrease postoperative pain.
- Exclude distant or unresectable disease.
- Divide the right pulmonary ligament up to the inferior pulmonary vein. Ligate the arch of the azygous vein and divide it in continuity with 2/0 Vicryl®.
- Develop the plane between the azygos vein and the aorta with en bloc excision of the thoracic duct and para-aortic nodes.
- Ligate oesophageal aortic branches with 3/0 Vicryl® and skeletonize the antero-lateral descending thoracic aorta. Dissect the oesophagus medially from the lung hilum and pericardium taking all nodes en bloc.
- Pass a tape around the oesophagus to aid retraction.
- Expose proximally the right and left main bronchi with en bloc excision of carinal, bronchial, and para-tracheal nodes, avoiding damage to the posterior membranous aspect of the tracheo-bronchial tree.
- Ligate the thoracic duct just above the diaphragm to prevent chylothorax.
- Excise para-oesophageal tissue en bloc with mediastinal pleura posteriorly and inferiorly, exposing the left lung.
- Continue oesophageal mobilization to meet the trans-abdominal dissection.

- Divide the final pleural attachments to allow entry of the stomach into the thorax.
- Withdraw the NG tube. Apply oesophageal stay 2/0 Vicryl® sutures and transect the oesophagus at the apex of the thorax.
- Divide the proximal stomach along the lesser curve with associated abdominal nodes and fashion a gastric tube.
- Carry out a gastro-oesophageal anastomosis, as shown in Figs 2.15–2.17.
- Insert apical and basal underwater seal drains. Approximate the ribs and close the wound with interrupted 0 Vicryl®. Close the muscle in two layers with 1 PDS and apply clips to skin.

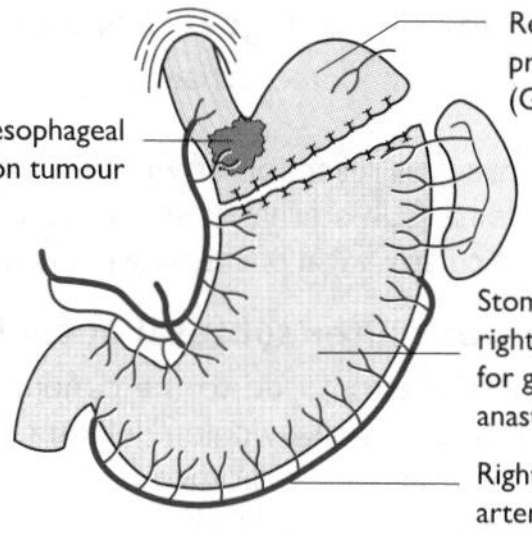
Resected part of proximal stomach (GOJ cancer)
Gastro-oesophageal junction tumour
Stomach tube with intact right gastroepiploic artery for gastro-oesophageal anastomosis in chest
Right gastroepiploic artery

Fig. 2.14 Gastric resection for two-stage oesophagectomy.

Three-stage oesophagectomy (McKeown)

Overview

Some surgeons prefer to expose/divide and anastomose the oesophagus in the neck. The additional resection of the oesophagus is not much more than that achieved by the Ivor Lewis technique, although this technique is required for proximal tumours so that an adequate proximal resection margin can be achieved. The procedure is commonly referred to as a 'McKeown' oesophagectomy. It involves the same initial approach as an Ivor Lewis oesophagectomy but with complete dissection of the thoracic oesophagus up to the thoracic inlet. The addition of a left or right neck approach is then carried out for the additional resection.

Colonic interposition for oesophageal replacement

- When the stomach is absent, rendered ischaemic, or damaged by caustic injury.
- Where tumour extent requires resection of whole stomach.
- For extra-anatomical bypass (sub-sternal or subcutaneous routes).
- Surgical preference (particularly vagal preserving procedures).

Oesophageal anastomosis after subtotal oesophagectomy

The oesophageal remnant is anastomosed to the conduit used for reconstruction, usually stomach or occasionally colon. Jejunum is rarely used for replacement except as free graft after pharyngo-laryngo-oesophagectomy for hypo-pharyngeal and proximal cervical tumours.

Oesophago-gastric or oesophago-colic anastomoses are hand sewn or stapled in the neck or upper thorax. The outcome is similar and surgical preference/approach dictates the selection of anastomotic technique. Cervical anastomoses have a higher leak rate, although a neck leak may not produce as severe clinical consequences as an intra-thoracic leak. Circular stapled anastomoses produce a higher stricture rate than sutured anastomoses, particularly if using guns smaller than 25mm. Irrespective of technique, anastomoses should be tension-free and have a good blood supply with close application of epithelial margins. Trauma from non-crushing clamps should be avoided.

Stapled oesophageal anastomosis

- Prepare the oesophageal remnant by NG tube withdrawal, aspiration, and insertion of a 2/0 Prolene® purse-string. Pass a double-ended straight needle suture through a purse-string clamp applied across the oesophagus before transection. Divide the oesophagus close to the margin of the clamp. Alternatively, use a small round-bodied needle to place the Prolene® purse-string by hand at 5–7mm intervals with 5mm bites circumferentially, the oesophagus being held open by multiple full thickness 2/0 Vicryl® stay sutures (Fig. 2.15). Insert the head of the staple gun and secure the purse-string around its neck (Fig. 2.16).

- If a gastric tube is used, insert the staple gun through the proximal resection margin and site the anastomosis posteriorly at the high point of the stomach, away from the gastrotomy line so as not to compromise the blood supply. Pass the spike through and secure the gastric wall with a 2/0 Vicryl® purse-string suture around the neck of the gun. After firing the gun, inspect the completeness of the donuts. Advance the NG tube and close the gastrotomy line with a linear stapler and over-sew it with 2/0 PDS. Variations of this approach can be used to produce end-to-end or end-to-side oesophago-colic anastomoses in the thorax or neck.

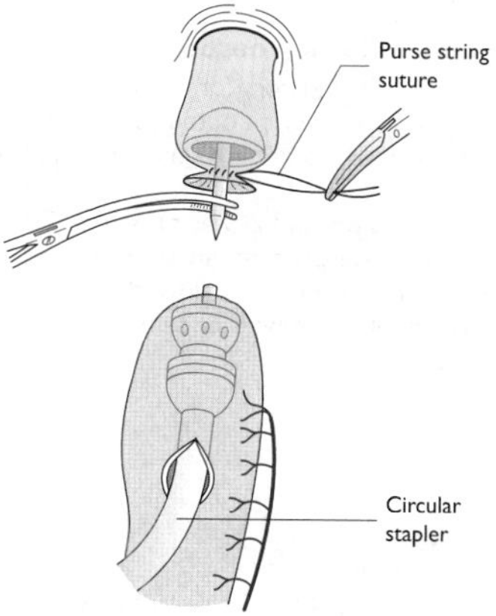
Purse string
suture
Circular
stapler

Fig. 2.15 Purse-string suture placed to secure the anvil of circular stapler.

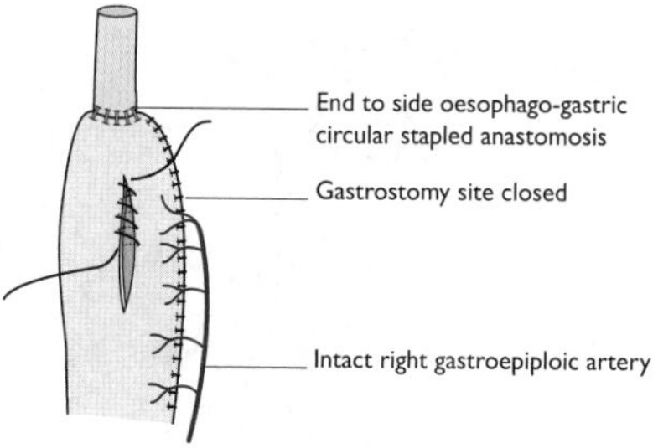
End to side oesophago-gastric
circular stapled anastomosis
Gastrostomy site closed
Intact right gastroepiploic artery

Fig. 2.16 After circular stapled anastomosis, the gastrostomy is closed with continuous sutures.

Sutured oesophageal anastomosis

(See Fig. 2.17)

- The simplest approach is a single layer of interrupted full-thickness 2/0 Vicryl® or PDS sutures.
- First form the gastric tube completely and make a 2cm incision at the site where a stapled anastomosis would be fashioned. Place lateral stay sutures and suture the posterior wall initially with the knots internally. In the thorax the whole row is placed first and then the oesophagus parachuted down with sequential ligation of the sutures. Then complete the anterior row with knots externally and avoid redundant tissue from size discrepancy. A similar technique can be used to fashion end-to-end oesophago-colic anastomoses.

Postoperative care following oesophagectomy

- HDU/ITU monitoring is mandatory for the first few days after surgery (hourly observations of vitals, urine output, and chest drains).
- Blood pressure maintained systolic >100mmHg. Humidified oxygen is supplied.
- Non-invasive continuous positive airway pressure (CPAP) ventilation is avoided, as the gastro-oesophageal anastomosis can fall apart due to over distention of stomach due to swallowed air.
- Continuous aspiration of NG tube is done to decompress the stomach tube

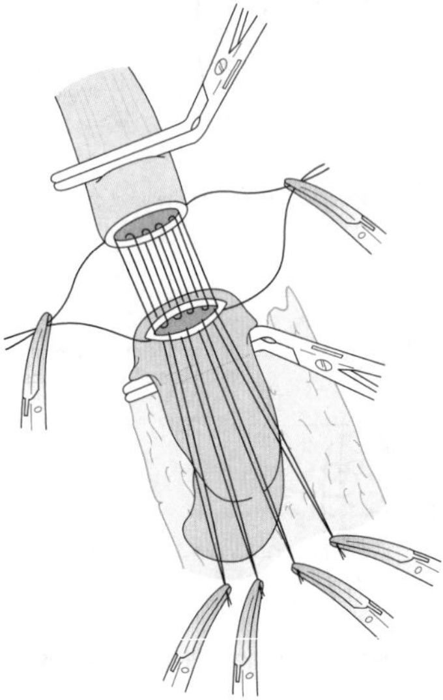

Fig. 2.17 Sutured oesophago-gastric anastomosis.

- It is debatable whether to do contrast study after 48h to check the anastomosis, before commencing oral fluids (surgeon's choice).
- Once the chest drains cease to drain, they should be removed and chest assessed by series of CXR.
- Oral diet is usually commenced from day 5 and all the drains are removed if no visceral contents are spilling through the drains.

Complications following oesophagectomy

Early complications

- Haemorrhage.
- Pneumonia/acute respiratory distress syndrome (ARDS).
- Pneumothorax/pleural effusion.
- Thromboembolic complications.
- Anastomotic leak.
- Chylothorax.
- Recurrent laryngeal nerve palsy.
- Gastric outlet obstruction (if no pyloroplasty performed).
- Mortality (5–10%).

Late complications

- Anastomotic stricture (particularly for stapled anastomoses).
- Post-thoracotomy pain.
- Dumping.
- Post-vagotomy diarrhoea.
- Reflux.
- Cancer recurrence (loco-regional and/or metastatic).

Oesophageal cardiomyotomy (Heller's) for achalasia

Achalasia is characterized by a hypertensive non-relaxing lower oesophageal sphincter (LOS). It is associated with non-coordinated spastic oesophageal peristalsis due to loss of ganglion cells in Auerbach's plexus. Pneumatic balloon dilatation of the LOS and cardiomyotomy has similar results.

Preoperative investigations

- Clinical history: classical triad of symptoms of dysphagia, recurrent chest infections, and weight loss.
- Endoscopy: food residue in oesophagus with tight cardia.
- Barium swallow: 'bird's beak sign', absent air bubble in stomach.
- Oesophageal manometry: hypertensive lower oesophageal sphincter (LOS), aperistalsis of oesophageal body, and raised resting pressure.

Cardiomyotomy

Although this procedure was traditionally done by open transabdominal or trans-thoracic routes, the minimally invasive route is now most common. The aim of this procedure is to weaken the LOS sufficient enough to allow food and avoid gastro-oesophageal reflux simultaneously. It is recommended that myotomy is not carried more than 2cm on to the stomach and to add an anti-reflux procedure (Dor fundoplication is recommended).

Laparoscopic cardiomyotomy

Position and preoperative preparation

- Though some surgeons prefer to operate standing on patient's left side, commonly the patient is positioned in lithotomy position with the operator standing between the legs. Reverse Trendelenburg position is preferred to expose the hiatus and upper abdominal structures.
- Apply intermittent pneumatic compression stockings to reduce DVT risk.
- Undertake preoperative endoscopy.

Steps of operation

- Insert the first port 5–10cm above the umbilicus. Create a pneumoperitoneum (10mm port and 12–14mmHg pressure).
- Use a 30° laparoscope.
- Insert a 5mm port just below the xiphisternum. Put a Nathanson retractor through the port. Elevate the left lobe of the liver to visualize gastro-oesophageal junction.
- Insert two further 5–10mm left and right subcostal ports for the hiatal dissection and subsequent suturing. Insert an additional 5mm left upper quadrant port for gastric retraction using an atraumatic Babcock.
- Divide the proximal gastrohepatic ligament using the harmonic scalpel, preserving the hepatic branch of the vagus and exposing the right crus. These vagal fibres supply the gall bladder and division can result in cholestasis and cholelithiasis in the long term. However, they can be divided if it interferes with access.
- Divide the phreno-oesophageal ligament around its antero-lateral aspect. Mobilize the dilated oesophagus by blunt mediastinal dissection, preserving the anterior vagus. Then free the oesophagus from the left crus and retract at least 5–6cm into the abdomen. If an anterior fundoplication is planned, then a large retro-oesophageal window in front of the crura is not required. A crural repair is not carried out unless the hiatus is widened.
- Create a 6cm myotomy over the right antero-lateral aspect of the oesophagus using bipolar scissors or the harmonic scalpel to divide the longitudinal and circular muscle fibres (preserve the anterior vagus). Continue the myotomy over 2cm of the cardia.
- Suture a Dor partial anterior fundoplication intra-corporeally as described in anti-reflux surgery (Fig. 2.8).
- Check for haemostasis and perforation.
- Drains are not usually required.
- Bleeding from the divided muscle fibres is usually self-limiting and excessive diathermy is avoided to prevent mucosal damage.
- Immediate laparoscopic repair is recommended if any mucosal injury is detected. Water-soluble contrast study may be done selectively before commencing oral intake.
- Close the umbilical port as described in laparoscopic cholecystectomy (Fig. 1.9).

Postoperative care

- These operations can be done as day-case procedures.
- Allow liquids orally after 6h.
- A sloppy diet can be started after 24hs. To remain on sloppy diet for 4–6 weeks.

Complications

- Perforation (7–15%), risk is increased in patients who had previous dilatation or Botox injections (submucosal fibrosis).
- Recurrent dysphagia due to inadequate myotomy or too tight fundoplication.
- Gastro-oesophageal reflux.
- Diverticulum formation.
- Malignant change (surveillance endoscopy is indicated).

Tips and tricks

- Exclude malignancy preoperatively.
- Consider primary repair if oesophageal mucosa is breached.
- Submucosal fibrosis is expected in patients already treated with Botox injections.
- Add anti-reflux procedure with cardiomyotomy

Obesity surgery

Overview

People with a body mass index (BMI) equal to or exceeding 40kg/m^2, or between 35 and 40kg/m^2 with significant co-morbid conditions satisfy the criteria as having morbid obesity. In UK the prevalence of obesity has tripled in females between 1980 and 2004 (from 8% to 23%) and quadrupled in men (from 6% to 23%). Currently it is estimated that nearly 2.55% of the adult population in the UK are obese with a BMI >40.

Surgery is recommended as a management alternative for morbidly obese people, provided the following criteria are met:

- They should have been receiving multidisciplinary intensive management in a specialist weight-management clinic.
- There should be no specific clinical or psychological contraindications.
- They should be aged 18 years or over.
- They should demonstrate that all appropriate non-surgical measures have been sufficiently tried and failed.
- They should be fit for anaesthesia and surgery.
- They should be self-motivated and understand the need for long-term follow-up.
- In addition, NICE 2014 guidelines recommend surgery in the following group of patients:
  - BMI 30–34.9 with recent onset of diabetes.
  - Consider waist circumference as an assessment tool and set low BMI target compared to others in patients of Asian origin with recent onset diabetes.

Preoperative preparation

- Comprehensive multidisciplinary assessment involving various professionals, such as an endocrinologist, dietician, physiotherapist, upper GI surgeon, clinical psychologist, and anaesthetist, is necessary.
- Diabetes, hypertension and hypoventilation syndrome are common conditions in obese patients. These conditions must be optimized preoperatively. Patients with obstructive sleep apnoea (OSA) need sleep capnography.
- Patients are encouraged to stop smoking at least 6 weeks before surgery. Use of NSAIDS during the operation and postoperatively is contraindicated to prevent marginal ulcers.
- Some surgeons prefer to do preoperative upper GI endoscopy to rule out co-existing pathology and to exclude *H. pylori* infection.
- Preoperative blood tests (FBC, U&E, LFT, vitamin levels, thyroid and parathyroid levels).

Positioning of patient and access

- Patient in supine, modified lithotomy position with knees partially flexed. The surgeon stands between the patient's legs. With a 20–30° reverse Trendelenberg (head-up) position, the abdominal viscera moves downwards exposing the hiatus to commence the operation.
- Adequate measures are taken to secure the patient to the table.

- Most of the bariatric procedures are done laparoscopically. Insert the first port by using Veress needle or Visiport technique using 0° scope and then changing to 30° scope (12mm port). Place this port one-hand's breadth (10–15 cm) below the left costal margin about 2cm to the left of midline.
- Place two 12mm ports in left and right upper quadrants (working ports). Insert two 5mm ports, one in the epigastrium (Nathanson retractor for liver) the other in anterior axillary line parallel to previous 12mm port in LUQ region.

Types of surgical procedures

Purely restrictive operations

- Laparoscopic gastric banding.
- Sleeve gastrectomy.

Combined restrictive and malabsorptive procedure

- Roux-en-Y gastric bypass.
- Loop or 'mini' gastric bypass or one anastomosis gastric bypass (OAGB).

Predominantly malabsorptive procedures

- Bilio-pancreatic diversion (BPD).
- BPD+ duodenal switch (DS).

Laparoscopic adjustable gastric banding (LAGB)

An adjustable band is used to create a small pouch at the fundus with an adjustable outlet. The adjustable band is made of silicon with an inflatable balloon that is in contact with the stomach. It has a buckling mechanism to fix it at the desired level. This band is connected to a port via the tube; this port is used to adjust the band size. It is thought the mechanism of action is to increase vagal stimulation by pressure when food bolus passes. It works by neuro-modulation rather than true restriction.

- For this procedure one of the ports should be 15mm size (instead of 12mm) to introduce the band device into the peritoneal cavity.
- Identify the angle of His and expose the left crus. Divide the gastrohepatic ligament to expose right crus. Incise the overlying peritoneal layer to enter the areolar plane.
- Insert a blunt instrument in this plane. It should reach the angle of His area without any resistance.
- Draw the band behind the stomach. Position and secure it.
- To stop slippage, suture the stomach fundus over the band to the pouch created using interrupted non-absorbable sutures (2-0 Ethibond).
- Bring the connection tubing system through the 15mm port. Connect it to the port that is secured to the rectus sheath. At this stage the port is completely empty.

Postoperative care

- Patients are allowed liquid diet from the same day and are usually discharged.
- Band adjustments usually commenced in 6–8weeks (ensure Huber needles are used to fill the port).
- Where early or late complications are suspected, always ensure the band is completely empty of fluid.

Complications

- Slippage causing large pouch or necrosis of stomach.
- Erosion into stomach.
- Oesophageal dilatation.
- Infection at the port site.

Sleeve gastrectomy (LSG)

In this procedure the stomach is reduced to a narrow tube by removing four-fifths of it (Fig. 2.18).

- Position of patient and the ports are similar to LAGB.
- Commence dissection from greater curvature of stomach. Divide the gastroepiploic vessels and continue dissection to the crus by dividing short gastric vessels.
- Using the pylorus as a land mark, commence stapling, leaving 4–5cm of antrum (use 60mm green cartridge) staying close to the bougie (32–36Fr), which is pressed against lesser curvature of stomach.
- Continue dividing the stomach to the angle of His.
- Secure haemostasis; apply liga clips for bleeding from staple line.
- Extract the excised stomach via 15mm port.
- Perform a methylene blue dye test to check the integrity of staple line.

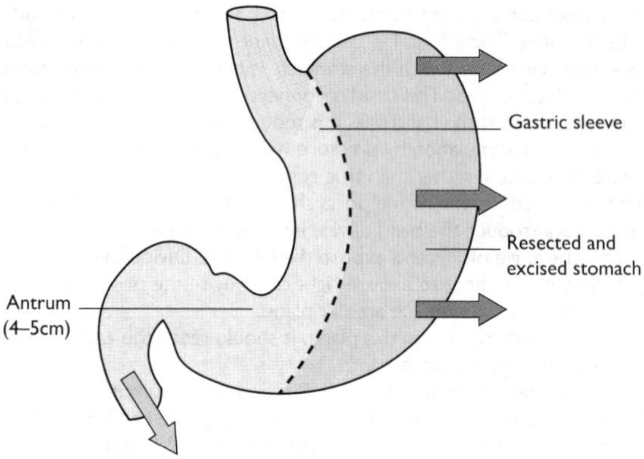
Gastric sleeve
Resected and excised stomach
Antrum (4–5cm)

Fig. 2.18 Sleeve gastrectomy.

Postoperative instructions
- Commence clear fluids same day and soft diet on 2nd day. Discharge patient following this.
- DVT prophylaxis.
- Vitamin supplements and B12 replacement.

Complications
- Bleeding from the staple site.
- Leak from staple line (especially where two staple lines cross over or at angle of His).
- Sleeve dilatation and gain in weight.
- Severe acid reflux.
- Kink or obstruction of sleeve is reported, but rare.

Roux-en-Y gastric bypass (RYGB)

RYGB (Fig. 2.19) is the commonest bariatric operation performed across the world for morbid obesity. The intention of this procedure is to restrict the capacity of the stomach by reducing its size to 40–50ml and to create a Roux pattern small bowel continuity. This procedure has combined restrictive and malabsorptive effects.
- Use orogastric tube.
- Release the fat around angle of His to expose the left crus.
- Commence dissection on lesser curvature of stomach at about 6–7cm from GOJ. Create a window to gain access to lesser sac.
- Use a stapler to divide the stomach transversely and then continue upwards towards angle of His taking care to avoid injury to the oesophagus. Release any posterior adhesions to the stomach pouch for mobility.

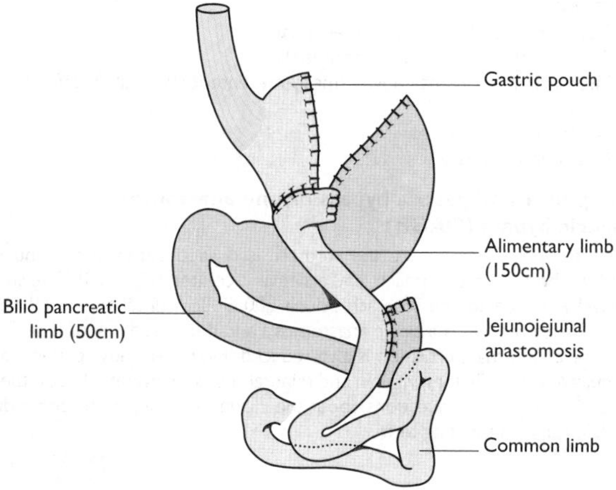
Gastric pouch
Alimentary limb (150cm)
Bilio pancreatic limb (50cm)
Jejunojejunal anastomosis
Common limb

Fig. 2.19 Roux-en-Y gastric bypass.

- Divide greater omentum in its full length to prevent traction on the anastomosis when performing antecolic anastomosis.
- Lift colon to show the DJ flexure. To create a gastro-jejunostomy, measure 50cm of jejunum (biliopancreatic limb) from DJ flexure and anastomose to gastric pouch using a stapler. Close the enterotomy with 2-0 Vicryl®.
- The length of the bypass is variable (100–150cm). Measure this distally from the GJ anastomosis (alimentary limb). Rejoin the jejunum here to the biliary limb with a stapler producing an omega configuration. Complete the Roux limb by dividing the biliary limb close to the stomach pouch.
- Close both the mesenterico-mesenteric and Petersen's defect (defect between transverse mesocolon and the alimentary limb) with either non-absorbable suture or stapling clips.
- Inject diluted methylene blue through the orogastric tube to check luminal patency and anastomotic leak of GJ anastomosis.
- Close all the port sites with subcuticular sutures.

Postoperative care

- Clear fluids are allowed from the following day and patients are encouraged to mobilize as soon as possible to prevent DVT.
- Soft diet is allowed on the 2nd day.
- May be discharged if making satisfactory progress on 2nd day.
- Soft diet continued for 4–6 weeks.
- For diabetic patients a specific postoperative plan should be in place by the diabetology team.

RYGB patients require lifelong vitamin B12, folic acid, and trace elements (magnesium, calcium, zinc, selenium).

Complications

- Staple line bleeding (primary/secondary).
- Anastomotic leak (GJ/JJ anastomosis).
- Internal hernia of small bowel (meso-mesenteric/Petersen's defect).
- Marginal ulcers.
- Nutritional deficiencies.
- Gastrogastric fistula.

Loop or 'mini' gastric bypass or one anastomosis gastric bypass (OAGB)

This is a procedure where the stomach is divided between the antrum and the body of the stomach, and a sleeve is created (Fig. 2.20). The small bowel is joined to the stomach pouch 200–300cm distal to the DJ flexure. The advantage is a single anastomosis and decreased risk of leak. The chance of internal herniation is also reduced. However, these patients are required to take lifelong vitamin and mineral supplements. In addition there are still unanswered questions about the incidence of stomach cancer due to bile reflux in the long term.

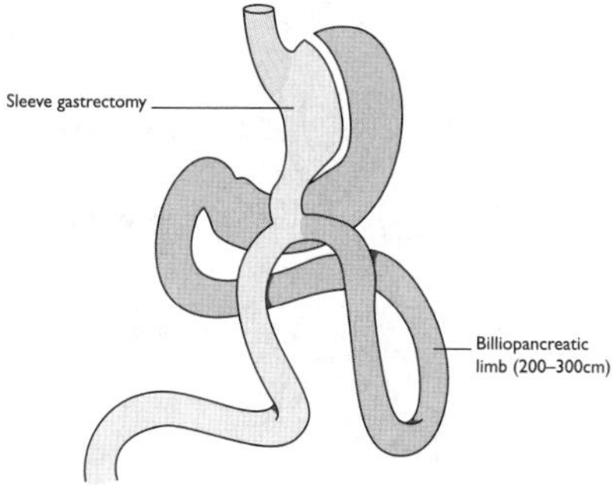
Sleeve gastrectomy
Billiopancreatic
limb (200–300cm)

Fig. 2.20 Loop or 'mini' gastric bypass or one anastomosis gastric bypass (OAGB).

Bilio-pancreatic diversion (BPD)

This is 'purely' a malabsorption procedure. It involves division of the ileum about 250cm proximal to ileo-caecal junction. The distal ileum is anastomosed to a stomach pouch, which is created by subtotal gastrectomy. The volume of stomach is tailored as per patient's BMI (average 200–300ml capacity). The bilio-pancreatic limb is then connected to the distal ileum about 50cm proximal to the ileo-caecal junction. Since the common channel is very small, it wouldn't absorb many calories and fats; hence there is significant malabsorption of food. This procedure is preferred in patients with significantly high BMI or when other surgical procedures have failed to lower the BMI.

These patients require dedicated close follow-up as they can develop significant fat, protein, vitamin, and mineral deficiencies. All fat-soluble vitamins should be replaced to avoid night blindness (vitamin A deficiency) and bleeding disorders (vitamin K deficiency).

BPD+ duodenal switch (BPD+DS)

This is a modified version of BPD, where instead of subtotal gastrectomy a long gastric sleeve is performed like a loop bypass (preserve antrum and pylorus). The duodenum is divided about 5cm distal from the pylorus. Similar to BPD, the ileum is divided about 250cm from ileo-caecal (IC) junction and is joined to the proximal duodenum. The BP limb is then joined to the ileum leaving a long (100cm) common channel (Fig. 2.21). Unlike BPD, addition of sleeve gastrectomy acts as a restrictive procedure and hence malabsorption is less significant compared to BPD.

Laparoscopic BPD+DS is a highly technically demanding operation and carries significant morbidity and mortality. Selection of suitable cases and surgeon's acquaintance with the procedure are crucial.

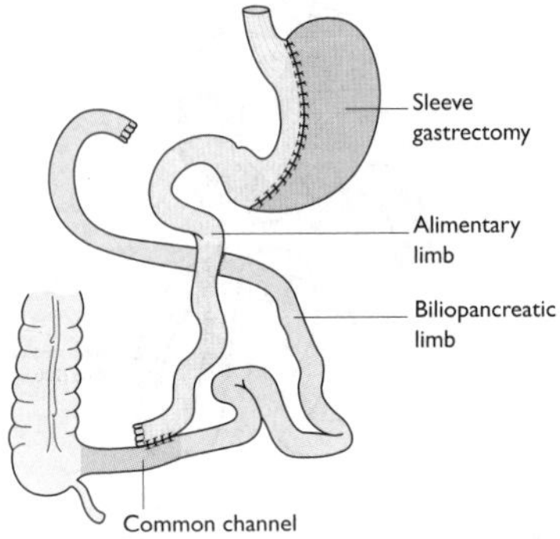
Sleeve
gastrectomy
Alimentary
limb
Biliopancreatic
limb
Common channel

Fig. 2.21 Bilio-pancreatic diversion with duodenal switch.

Tips and tricks

- Patient selection is important for all outcomes.
- Rule out endocrine causes for obesity before surgical intervention.
- Patient and port positioning are important for successful operation.
- Take care to close hernia spaces created.
- Perform leak test.
- Use staplers according to guidelines from manufacturer.
- Check the staple line bleeding by elevating the systolic blood pressure to 130mmHg.
- Surgery is a small part of the overall care. All bariatric patients should be followed up and have monitoring of nutritional parameters.

Oesophageal rupture and perforation

Perforation of the oesophagus is a rare, life-threatening condition associated with significant morbidity and mortality. Causes of perforation include:
- Boerhaave's syndrome (post-vomiting/barogenic spontaneous rupture).
- Iatrogenic perforation (endoscopic or operative).
- Traumatic injury (penetrating gun/stab wounds or blunt compression injury).
- Ingestion of corrosive agent or foreign body.

Anatomical considerations

'Spontaneous' perforation of the oesophagus is usually due to severe barotrauma when a person vomits against a closed glottis. Due to increased intraluminal pressure, the oesophagus perforates at its weakest point, which is in its lower third and invariably on the left side. However, the commonest cause of oesophageal perforation is iatrogenic, especially from dilatation of strictures.

Preoperative evaluation

- Clinical history is important; suspect a perforation if pain follows vomiting or endoscopic therapy.
- CXR may show surgical emphysema/pneumo-mediastinum/hydropneumothorax, or pleural effusion.
- Video endoscopy by a highly skilled endoscopist can be useful to assess site/size of injury and associated pathology.
- A NJ tube can be placed at endoscopy for feeding purposes.
- Water-soluble contrast swallow to assess the site, extent of any leak.
- CT is an alternative to contrast X-rays

General considerations and non-operative management

- The aim of treatment is to minimize the mediastinal contamination and to control the existing infection. Most of the endoscopic perforations have minimal contamination and therefore are ideal for non-operative management.
- Perforations that are contained within the mediastinum and without any signs of mediastinitis or small perforations with minimal contamination (no solid contamination of pleural cavity or mediastinum) can usually be treated conservatively as long as there is no distal obstruction. These usually occur after instrumental perforation in a starved patient.
- Conservative management is also considered in patients with delayed diagnosis who have demonstrated good tolerance, especially with a range of antibiotics available, advanced radiological drainage procedures, and enteral tube feeding.
- Malignant perforation in the presence of advanced disease is treated with a covered endo-prosthesis.

Surgical management

Carry out surgery on injuries with heavy contamination, free uncontained leakage, or distal luminal obstruction.

Primary repair

This is suitable only for injuries recognized early prior to infection and necrosis of local tissues. Ideally this treatment should be reserved for patients who were diagnosed and operated within 24h of injury, beyond which the tissue become oedematous and friable, and less suitable for primary repair.

- Boerhaave's syndrome usually affects the lower left oesophagus and septic load is expected to be high due to food debris. Explore chest via a left low (8th or 9th interspace) postero-lateral thoracotomy. Extensive lavage and debridement of devitalized tissue is required. Open the mediastinal pleura widely and perform a long myotomy to expose the whole length of the mucosal tear, which is longer than the muscular breach.
- Carry out repair in two layers. To strengthen the repair, patch it using an intercostal flap, diaphragm, or gastric fundus for further reinforcement to prevent on-going leakage.
- Insert large-bore intercostal drains and close the chest.
- Insert a feeding jejunostomy for prolonged enteral nutrition via a mini laparotomy.

T-tube repair

This is the standard approach for those perforations or ruptures that are associated with worse contamination (Boerhaave's), tissue necrosis, and local sepsis.

- After initial debridement, wash, and myotomy, insert a large-bore T-tube (8–10mm) into the oesophageal defect, with each limb lying beyond the defect. Secure the T tube in place by longitudinal approximation sutures using 3-0 PDS. This creates a controlled oesophago-cutaneous fistula. Place a large-bore intercostal drain next to the repair and another apically before closing the chest.
- Insert a feeding jejunostomy via mini-laparotomy for prolonged enteral nutrition.
- Perform contrast radiographs and CT scan to monitor the progress of healing. In majority of cases, remove the T-tube between 3 and 6 weeks.

Postoperative care

- These high-risk patients should be managed in HDU/ITU.
- Watch out for signs of chest infections and mediastinitis. Assess by serial CXR or CT scans.
- Continue enteral/parenteral nutrition, as required.
- Remove the chest drains when appropriate.
- If further collections develop, consider radiological drainage with antibiotic coverage.

Complications

- Mediastinitis.
- Pleural effusion/empyema.
- Severe sepsis and multi-organ failure
- Chronic non-healing fistula.

- Oesophageal stricture/stenosis.
- Severe nutritional deficiencies.
- High mortality ≈20% (10% if early diagnosis and treatment, 60–70% if late presentation).

Tips and tricks

- Early diagnosis and resuscitation is important.
- HDU/ITU care with multidisciplinary approach is paramount.
- Give antibiotics cover and nutritional support.
- If facilities or expertise is not available, consider referring to specialist upper GI unit.
- Carry out prompt radiological drainage of new collections.

Chapter 3

Hepato-pancreato-biliary (HPB) surgery

Introduction

- Major liver and pancreatic resections are now the preserve of specialist units with not only the surgical experience, but also endoscopic and interventional radiology support.
- The fact that there are increasing numbers of elderly patients with multiple co-morbidities undergoing major HPB surgery has highlighted the importance of anaesthetic evaluation.
- For the junior surgeon, the challenge of managing these patients in the perioperative period is considerable.

Endoscopic retrograde cholangio-pancreatography (ERCP)

Endoscopic retrograde cholangio-pancreatography (ERCP)

Surgical anatomy

(See Fig. 3.1)

- Second part of the duodenum.
- Ampulla of Vater.
- Pancreatic and biliary ductal system.

Indications

- No longer diagnostic—magnetic resonance cholangiography (MRCP) or endoscopic ultrasound are more appropriate.
- Extraction of biliary stones.
- Relieve jaundice due to benign and malignant strictures with placement of stents (metal, covered metal, plastic).
- Ampullary biopsy, biliary brushings for cytology.

Pre-op preparation

- Ensure hydration.
- Check bilirubin, prothrombin time (PT), and platelet count.
- Administer vitamin K parenterally, if jaundiced or coagulopathic.
- Group and save.
- Radiology request.

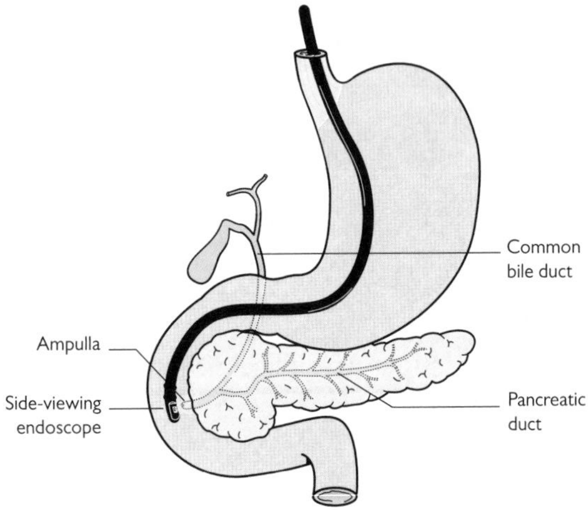
Common bile duct
Ampulla
Side-viewing endoscope
Pancreatic duct

Fig. 3.1 Upper gastrointestinal anatomy (with reference to ERCP and pancreatic/biliary ductal system).

- Pregnancy test, if appropriate.
- Place cannula in right hand for administration of antibiotics and sedation.
- Consent:
  - Risks of pancreatitis, cholangitis, bleeding, perforation.
  - 1 in 50 risk of major complications.

Positioning and theatre setup

- Patient left lateral with right hand up.
- Radiological image intensifier and endoscopic monitor in view.

Steps of surgery

- Advance side-viewing endoscope into 2nd part of duodenum.
- Locate and cannulate ampulla.
- Do sphincterotomy (knife/balloon), as required.
- Do definitive procedure.

Post-op care and instructions

- If the patient has abdominal pain, check amylase.

Complications

- Pancreatitis: ↑ amylase/lipase.
  - The most common complication; early hydration is critical with HDU care for patients with predicted severe disease on scoring (Ranson's, APACHE, etc.).
- Bleeding: melaena, hypotensive shock.
  - Normally from the sphincterotomy site in a jaundiced patient.
  - Definitive management requires either endoscopic adrenaline injection or radiological angio-embolization.
- Duodenal perforation: abdominal/flank pain, shock.
  - Linear tear of D1 and D2 on anti-mesenteric border from scope trauma—the most common pathology.
  - Diagnose with contrast CT.
  - Treat either nil by mouth (NBM), total parental nutrition (TPN), and antibiotics or if shocked/peritonitic ► laparotomy, washout, drains then NBM/TPN.
- Cholangitis: abdominal pain and shock.
  - Intravenous fluids, antibiotics—if the biliary system is still obstructed, percutaneous trans-hepatic cholangiographic (PTC) drain may be required.

Tips and tricks

Recent evidence suggests there may be a role for prophylactic rectal indomethacin to reduce the risks of ERCP pancreatitis (1).

Liver resection

Resection of the liver was considered highly dangerous, with most patients succumbing to the complications of massive blood transfusion. With modern resection techniques, mortality, for even major resections, is now only 1–3%.

Surgical anatomy

- Knowledge of the segmental liver anatomy essential (Fig. 3.2).
- Major liver resection involves removal of three or more segments (left/right/central).
- Extended resection leaves only two or three segments (extended right or left).
- The caudate lobe (segment 1) can be removed in isolation and should always be removed in resections for hilar cholangiocarcinoma.

Indications

- 1° and 2° malignant liver tumours.
    - hepatocellular carcinoma (HCC), cholangiocarcinoma, angiosarcoma.
    - Metastases (colorectal most common).
- Benign tumours.
    - Hepatic adenoma (risk of malignant transformation), massive haemangioma (mass effect).
- Intrahepatic biliary stones, congenital choledochal cysts, or infectious hydatid cysts.

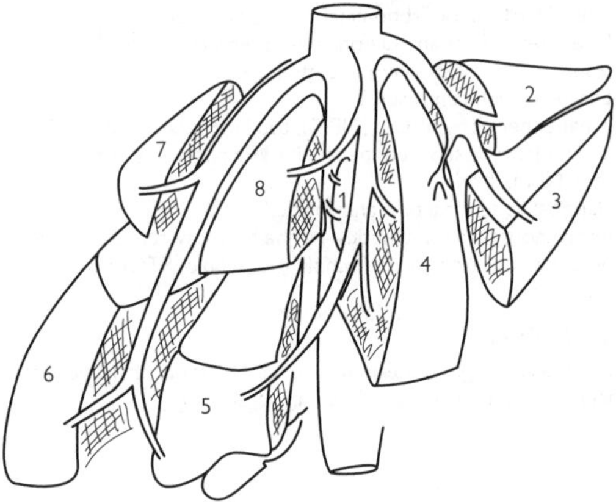
2
7
8
3
1
4
6
5

Fig. 3.2 Segmental anatomy of the liver.

Pre-op preparation

- Ensure no extrahepatic disease with metastatic tumours.
- Consider staging laparoscopy and cardiopulmonary fitness testing.
- Check bilirubin, PT, and platelet count.
- Administer vitamin K parenterally, if jaundiced or coagulopathic.
- If bilirubin >100μmol/l consider PTC or ERCP and stent.
- Crossmatch 2–4 units of packed cells and fresh frozen plasma (FFP).
- Tumour markers: carbohydrate antigen 19.9 (Ca19.9), carcinoembryonic antigen (CEA), alphafetoprotein (AFP).

Positioning and theatre setup

- Operator stands on the patient's right, assistant and scrub nurse on the left.
- Urinary catheterization.
- Give induction antibiotics.
- Patient supine with arms out.
- Expose abdomen from xiphisternum to pubis.

Steps of surgery

- Make reverse 'L' incision or rooftop according to resection/surgical preference.
- Mobilize liver fully by dividing coronary/triangular ligaments and posterior peritoneal attachments to adrenal gland.
- For major right-sided resections, ligate the caudate veins on the right of the IVC and pass a sling around the right hepatic vein.
- Extrahepatic ligation of the right hepatic artery and portal vein aid in identifying Cantlie's line (middle hepatic vein) and reduce blood loss during transection.
- The left portal triad has a longer extrahepatic course and can also be secured prior to transection, although the left hepatic vein is intrahepatic.
- Mark resection line with intraoperative ultrasound having confirmed lesion location, margins of resection, and vascular anatomy
- Sling portal structures in preparation for clamp (Pringle manoeuvre), if required.
- Transect parenchyma with ultrasonic or hydro dissector; the Kelly crush/clamp is an older technique.
- Tie, clip, or staple biliary radicles and larger vascular structures.
- Remove specimen.
- Confirm haemostasis after raising CVP to +5 or +10mmHg. Inspect resection margin to confirm no biliary leaks or bleeding.

Closure

- Monofilament (PDS or nylon) running suture, single layer fascia.
- Continuous absorbable subcuticular or surgical clips.

Post-op care and instructions

- Check Hb, bilirubin, PT, and platelet count.
- Administer FFP only if PT >30s with evidence of bleeding.
- Consider further doses of antibiotics, if evidence of biliary obstruction.
- Proton pump inhibitor for peptic ulcer prophylaxis.
- Heparin for DVT prophylaxis, if not coagulopathic.

Complications

- Bleeding ❗.
  - Urgent re-exploration is required, most often from the resection margin.
- Bile leak (collection or fistula).
  - ↑ Bile in the drain or if no drain, pyrexia/abdominal pain (▶ radiological drainage).
  - Most settle spontaneously; however, if the bile duct has been damaged or there is distal obstruction (i.e. stone, stricuture), then ERCP may be required.
- Liver failure (day 3 onwards).
  - 'Small for size'. ↑ Bilirubin, ↑ PT, ↓ albumin leading to ascites, coagulopathy and encephalopathy.
  - ▶ Doppler ultrasound scan (USS) to confirm patency of hepatic artery, and hepatic and portal veins in the remnant. If thrombosed, consider radiological thrombectomy.
  - Often precipitated by sepsis, bile leak.
- ✍ Multiorgan support in ICU.

Tips and tricks

- Prior to transection, ask anaesthetist to ↓ CVP to 0 by administering vasodilators. However, negative venous pressures incur a risk of air embolism.
- Liver remnant volume estimation is critical in larger resections or patients with compromised liver function (chemotherapy, steatosis, frank cirrhosis) to prevent development of liver failure.
- Laparoscopic or robotic approach to the anterior segments (6, 5, 4, left lateral; Fig 3.2) is practical and associated with reduced morbidity.

Pancreatico-duodenectomy

Pancreatico-duodenectomy (classical Whipple's procedure) remains the gold standard of treatment for tumours of the proximal pancreas, duodenum, and distal bile duct. However, most centres now aim to preserve the gastric pylorus in most patients (pylorus preserving pancreatico-duodenectomy, PPPD). This gives a better long-term result with reduced incidence of 'dumping' syndrome, biliary reflux, and stomal ulceration. Morbidity is dependent on recipient fitness and forms a critical part of the multidisciplinary team meeting (MDT) assessment.

Surgical anatomy

- The resection includes all parts of the duodenum, head of the pancreas proximal to the portal vein, common bile duct, and gall bladder (Fig. 3.1).
- Extended lymph node resections have not shown any improvement to long-term survival.

Indications

- Pancreatic ductal adenocarcinoma.
- Distal bile duct cholangiocarcinoma.
- Duodenal adenocarcinoma (high-grade dysplasia).
- Intra-pancreatic mucinous neoplasia (IPMN).
- Functioning and non-functioning neuroendocrine tumours.
    - Arterial (common hepatic artery/superior mesenteric artery) involvement is a contraindication in most centres.

Pre-op preparation

- Ensure no extra-pancreatic disease with endoscopic ultrasound (EUS), triple-phase CT.
- Consider staging laparoscopy, cardiopulmonary fitness testing.
- Check bilirubin, PT, and platelet count.
- Administer vitamin K parenterally, if jaundiced or coagulopathic.
- Consider ERCP and stent if bilirubin >300μmol/l.
- Crossmatch 2–4 units of packed cells and FFP.
- Tumour markers (Ca19.9, CEA).

Positioning and theatre setup

- Operator stands on the patient's right, assistant and scrub nurse on the left.
- Urinary catheterization.
- Give induction antibiotics (include aminoglycoside if biliary stent *in situ*).
- Patient supine with arms out.
- Expose abdomen for thorough laparotomy.

Steps of surgery

(See Fig. 3.3)

- Bilateral subcostal incision (rooftop).
- Check for extra-pancreatic disease (liver, peritoneum).
- Do Kocherization of the duodenum (Fig. 3.3).
- Open lesser sac and expose pancreas.

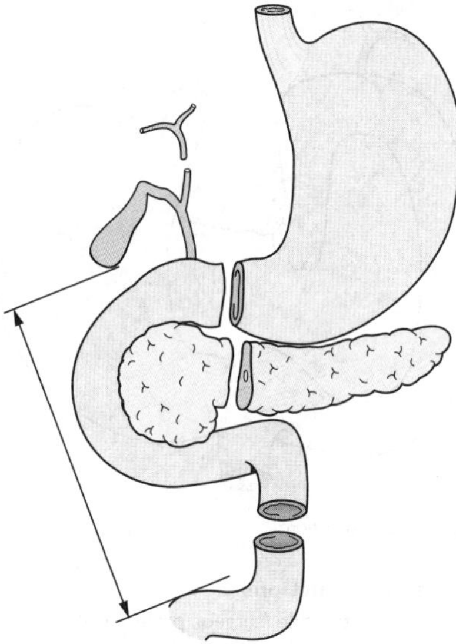

Fig. 3.3 Resection specimen in a Whipple's pancreatico-duodenectomy.

Resection

- Cholecystectomy but keep cystic duct in continuity with common bile duct (CBD).
- Divide common hepatic duct.
- Beware of the right hepatic artery behind the duct.
- Portal lymphadenectomy.
- Decide if the tumour can be cleared from the vessels.
- Divide gastroduodenal artery.
- Divide stomach (classical) or D1 (PPPD) and proximal jejunum with stapler.
- Transect pancreas in front of portal vein and remove specimen (Fig. 3.3).

Reconstruction

- Pancreatico-jejunostomy (PJ) or pancreatico-gastrostomy (Fig. 3.4).
- Hepatico-jejunostomy (HJ).
- Gastro-jejunostomy.
- Check position of nasojejunal tube (NJ)/NG tube or place percutaneous jejunostomy.
- Place drains around PJ and HJ.

Closure

- Monofilament (PDS or nylon) running suture, single layer fascia.
- Continuous absorbable subcuticular or surgical clips.

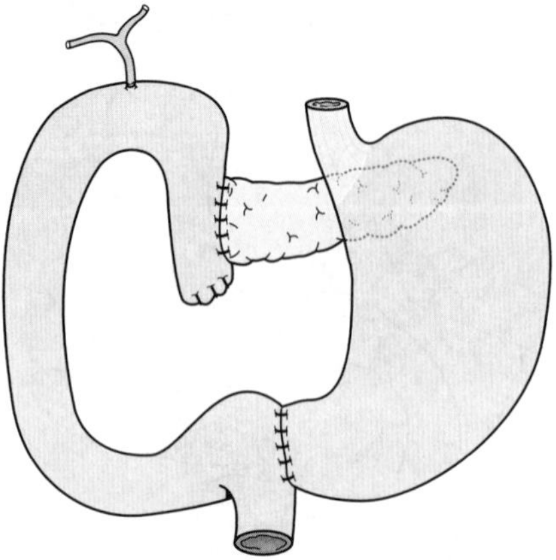

Fig. 3.4 Completed reconstruction.

Post-op care and instructions

- Start subcutaneous octreotide (surgeon preference).
- Consider further doses of antibiotics if biliary stent or recent cholangitis.
- Check drain amylase at 48 h.
- Start pancreatic enzyme replacement.
- Start feed via NJ tube.

Complications

- Pancreatic leak/fistula/collection.
- Presentation varies from high amylase in drains (>500 Unit/l) with no clinical signs or symptoms through to the patient being in hypotensive shock.
    - Treatment depends on the condition of the patient. For a patient with biochemical evidence of a leak only, then stopping oral intake and placing them on a parental feed may be sufficient. Intravenous octreotide may also be helpful. If the patient is clinically shocked then a return to the operating theatre may be required for laparotomy, washout, completion pancreatectomy and placement of multiple peritoneal drains.
- Bile leak.
    - Less common, normally resolves with NBM, TPN.
- Delayed gastric emptying.
    - More common with PPPD, check for collection (CT).
    - ► Give prokinetics, normally self-limiting.
- Bleeding ❗.
    - Day 7 onwards commonly from ruptured arterial (gastroduodenal artery) pseudoaneurysm as a result of pancreatic leak.
    - Radiological angio-embolization is treatment of choice.

Late complications

- Steatorrhea, diabetes (up to 30%), 'dumping' syndrome, tumour recurrence.

Tips and tricks

- Multiple techniques for reconstruction have been described and surgeon preference is based on experience.
- Stents can be placed across the PJ to reduce pancreatic leaks in high-risk patients (small duct, soft pancreas).

Necrosectomy

Classical open pancreatic necrosectomy is being challenged with minimal access procedures using radiological, endoscopic, or laparoscopic techniques. Utilizing a combination of these techniques, all areas of the gland can normally be accessed and debrided.

Surgical anatomy

- The body of the gland is best accessed either via an endoscopic or an open approach.
- Tail: left-sided percutaneous drainage, followed by retroperitoneal minimal access approach may be the best option (Fig. 3.5).
- Head/uncinate/periduodenal pancreatic and right-sided retroperitoneal fat tissue is the most difficult to access and debride (minimal access either endoscopic or right-sided radiological drain).
- ❗ Splenic or portal vein thrombosis 2° to pancreatitis—be aware of the potential for variceal haemorrhage. Relative contraindication for open surgery.

Indications

- Infected pancreatic and/or retroperitoneal fat necrosis.
- Pancreatic abscess.

Pre-op preparation

- Treat systemic sepsis with antibiotics/antifungals.
- Ensure nutrition and hydration.
- Consider placement of feeding tube under anaesthetic.
- Check bilirubin, platelets, PT.
- Administer vitamin K parenterally, if jaundiced or coagulopathic.

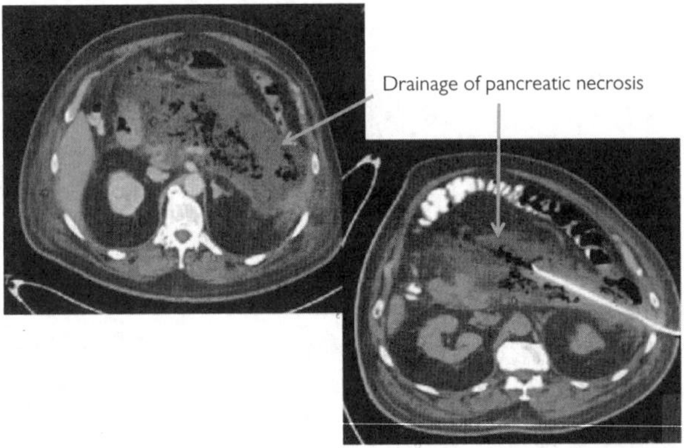
Drainage of pancreatic necrosis

Fig. 3.5 Surgical drain in a CT scan of a patient with complicated necrotizing pancreatitis.

- Consider ERCP and stent if bilirubin >300μmol/l.
- Crossmatch or group and save serum.

Positioning and theatre setup

Open necrosectomy

- Operator stands on the patient's right, assistant and scrub nurse on the left.
- Urinary catheterization.
- Give induction antibiotics (include aminoglycoside if biliary stent *in situ*).
- Patient supine with arms out.
- Expose abdomen from xiphisternum to pubis.

Steps of surgery

- Bilateral subcostal incision (rooftop).
- Kocherization of the duodenum (Fig.3.6).
- Open lesser sac and expose pancreas
- Blunt (finger fracture) dissection of necrotic pancreatic material.
- Copious lavage.
- If heavy bleeding, pack the cavity with gauze.
- Place irrigation catheters and large-bore drains.
- Check position of NJ/NG tube.

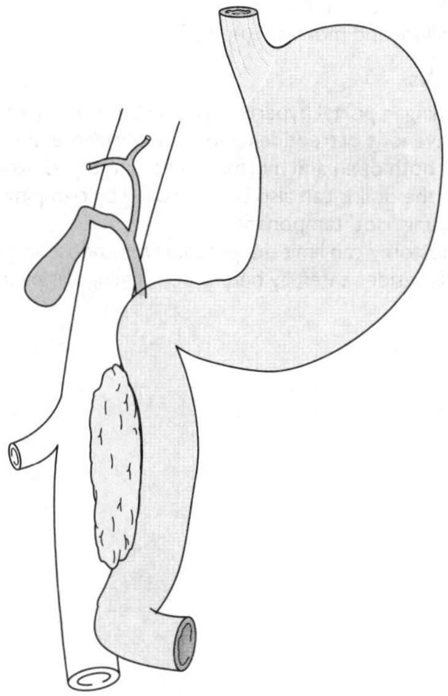

Fig. 3.6 Kocher's manoeuvre with duodenum elevated and IVC exposed posteriorly.

Consider

- Gastro-jejunostomy if gastric outlet obstruction and poor nutrition.
- Hepatico-jejunostomy if jaundiced and no portal hypertension.
- Cholecystectomy and common bile duct (CBD) clearance in gallstone disease.

Closure

- Consider temporary closure with Bogota bag if cavity packed.
- Monofilament (PDS or nylon) running suture, single layer fascia.
- Continuous absorbable subcuticular or surgical clips.

Post-op care and instructions

- Continue antibiotics.
- Transfuse red cells and FFP, as required.
- Start elemental fluid feed to maintain nutrition.

Complications

- Ongoing bleeding (!).
  - Consider urgent re-exploration.
- Biliary obstruction.
- Gastric outlet obstruction.
- Multiple procedures.
- Fistulae.
  - Biliary, enteric, or colonic.
- Multiorgan failure and mortality (up to 30%).

Tips and tricks

- Venous bleeding in portal hypertension can be torrential and difficult to control. Intravenous octreotide lowers the portal pressure and reduces blood loss in both open and minimal access surgery. Ongoing rapid blood loss in the drains can also be controlled by clamping the drains and precipitating 'clot' tamponade.
- Gastro-jejunostomy can limit the potential for endoscopic access to the duodenum. Consider carefully before performing this procedure.

Surgery for chronic pancreatitis

Multiple procedures have been described to help alleviate the signs and symptoms of this debilitating condition. The choice of procedure depends on the predominant symptoms and the results are often compromised by opiate dependency and chronic malnutrition.

Surgical anatomy

- Pain can be due to calculi, collections, pseudocyst, or ductal obstruction.
- In cases of pancreatic atrophy, alternative pain-relieving procedures include thoracosopic splanchnectomy, celiac axis plexus block, and spinal stimulators.
- Total pancreatectomy and islet auto transplantation is an option in patients with hereditary pancreatitis and preserved endocrine function.
- ! Portal hypertension can be severe and often contraindicates open surgery. Endoscopic procedures (drainage of collections, coeliac plexus ablation, pancreatic duct stent) may still be possible.

Indications

- Pain associated with pancreatic parenchymal or ductal calculi, ductal obstruction, or small duct disease (Izbicki).
- Jaundice or gastric outlet obstruction 2° to pancreatitis.

Pre-op preparation

- Treat systemic sepsis with antibiotics/antifungals.
- Ensure nutrition and hydration.
- Consider placement of feeding tube under anaesthetic.
- Epidural anaesthesia to facilitate opiate weaning post-op.
- Check platelets, PT.
- Crossmatch or group and save serum.

Pre-op preparation

- Ensure nutrition and hydration.
- Consider placement of feeding tube under anaesthetic.
- Check bilirubin, platelets, PT.
- Administer vitamin K parenterally, if jaundiced or coagulopathic
- Consider ERCP and stent if bilirubin >300.

Positioning and theatre setup

- Operator stands on the patient's right, assistant and scrub nurse on the left.
- Urinary catheterization.
- Give induction antibiotics (include aminoglycoside if biliary stent *in situ*).
- Patient supine with arms out.
- Expose abdomen from xiphisternum to pubis.

Steps of surgery

- Bilateral subcostal incision (rooftop).
- Kocherization of the duodenum (Fig. 3.6).
- Cholecystectomy.
- Open lesser sac and expose pancreas.

Table 3.1 Procedures

Procedure name	*Description*
Beger	Pancreatic head resection with distal PJ
Berne	Pancreatic head jejunostomy
Cyst-jejunostomy	Chronic pseudocyst drainage/Roux-en-Y
Frey's	Pancreatic head resection with lateral PJ
Izbicki	V-shaped resection and lateral PJ
Partington–Rochelle	Lateral PJ
Puestow	Distal pancreatectomy and lateral PJ
Whipple's	Pancreatico-duodenectomy

- Perform appropriate resectional/drainage procedure, dependent on anatomy/pathology.
- Consider simultaneous hepatico-jejunostomy/gastro-jejunostomy.
- See Table 3.1 for procedure names and descriptions.

Closure

- Monofilament (PDS or nylon) running suture, single layer fascia.
- Continuous absorbable subcuticular or surgical clips.

Post-op care and instructions

- Continue antibiotics.
- Wean off opiates.
- Start elemental fluid feed to maintain nutrition.

Complications

As for Whipple's:

- Pancreatic leak/fistula/collection.
- Varies from just high amylase in drains (>500) to hypotensive shock.
  - Treat NBM, TPN, and antibiotics or if shocked/peritionitic, ► laparotomy, washout, completion pancreatectomy/drains, then NBM/TPN.
- Bile leak.
  - Less common, normally resolves with NBM, TPN.
- Delayed gastric emptying.
- Bleeding ❗
  - Radiological angio-embolization is the treatment of choice.

Late complications

- Steatorrhea, diabetes (up to 70%), 'dumping' syndrome, tumour recurrence.

Tips and tricks

- Pancreatic head resection can be combined with choledocotomy to relieve jaundice.
- A probe placed down the CBD via the cystic duct at the time of cholecystectomy facilitates identification of the duct within the pancreatic head.

References

1 Elmunzer, B.J., James, M.D., Scheiman, M. et al., for the U.S. Cooperative for Outcomes Research in Endoscopy (USCORE). A Randomized Trial of Rectal Indomethacin to Prevent Post-ERCP Pancreatitis 2012. N Engl J Med 2012; 366:1414–22 April 12, 2012DOI: 10.1056/NEJMoa1111103.

Further reading

International Hepato-pancreato-biliary Society (IHPBA). Liver resection guidelines. http://www.ihpba.org/90_Guidelines-.html2012 [cited 2016 21st September].

Bassi C, Dervenis C, Butturini G, Fingerhut A, Yeo C, Izbicki J, et al. Postoperative pancreatic fistula: an international study group (ISGPF) definition. Surgery. 2005;138(1):8–13. Epub 2005/07/09.

Elmunzer BJ, Scheiman JM, Lehman GA, Chak A, Mosler P, Higgins PD, et al. A randomized trial of rectal indomethacin to prevent post-ERCP pancreatitis. The New England journal of medicine. 2012;366(15):1414–22. Epub 2012/04/13.

Rahbari NN, Garden OJ, Padbury R, Brooke-Smith M, Crawford M, Adam R, et al. Posthepatectomy liver failure: a definition and grading by the International Study Group of Liver Surgery (ISGLS). Surgery. 2011;149(5):713–24. Epub 2011/01/18.

Rahbari NN, Garden OJ, Padbury R, Maddern G, Koch M, Hugh TJ, et al. Post-hepatectomy haemorrhage: a definition and grading by the International Study Group of Liver Surgery (ISGLS). HPB: the official journal of the International Hepato Pancreato Biliary Association. 2011;13(8):528–35. Epub 2011/07/19.

Tol JA, Gouma DJ, Bassi C, Dervenis C, Montorsi M, Adham M, et al. Definition of a standard lymphadenectomy in surgery for pancreatic ductal adenocarcinoma: a consensus statement by the International Study Group on Pancreatic Surgery (ISGPS). Surgery. 2014;156(3):591–600. Epub 2014/07/26.

Wente MN, Bassi C, Dervenis C, Fingerhut A, Gouma DJ, Izbicki JR, et al. Delayed gastric emptying (DGE) after pancreatic surgery: a suggested definition by the International Study Group of Pancreatic Surgery (ISGPS). Surgery. 2007;142(5):761–8. Epub 2007/11/06.

Wente MN, Veit JA, Bassi C, Dervenis C, Fingerhut A, Gouma DJ, et al. Postpancreatectomy hemorrhage (PPH): an International Study Group of Pancreatic Surgery (ISGPS) definition. Surgery. 2007;142(1):20–5. Epub 2007/07/17.

Chapter 4

Colorectal surgery

Rigid sigmoidoscopy

Overview

A rigid sigmoidoscope is a 25cm-long and 2cm-wide tube with an attached light source and insufflating bellows (Fig. 4.1). In the past a rigid stainless steel instrument was used, now replaced by disposable equipment. Using a disposable instrument not only reduces transmittable infections, but also reduces the burden of cleansing and sterilization. The examination allows the assessment of the anal canal and rectum (15cm from anal verge):

- Quick outpatient assessment tool for rectal bleeding.
- To obtain biopsy from visible lesions and to remove small polyps.
- Preoperative assessment of rectal tumour.
- Assessment of fistula-ano.

Preoperative preparation

- Enquire if patient is on anticoagulants.
- Prescribe phosphate enemas to empty rectum for clear views.
- Ensure that chaperon is present.
- Check the equipment before use.
- Explain the procedure and obtain verbal consent.

Procedure

- WHO checklist.
- Position the patient in left lateral position or in lithotomy if under general anaesthesia.

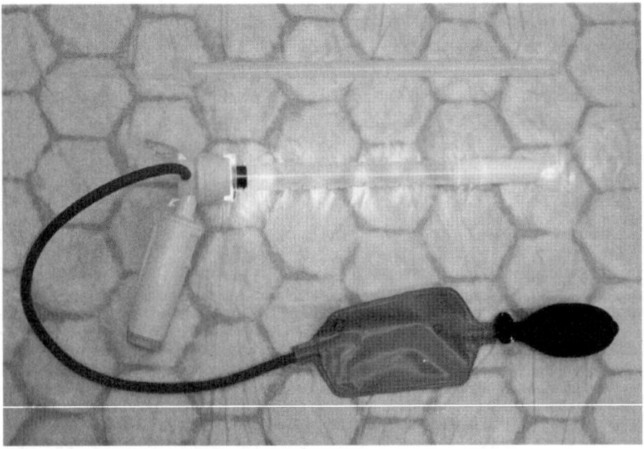

Fig. 4.1 Rigid sigmoidoscopy.

- Bear in mind the slight anterior direction of the anal canal and then sharp posterior angulation of the rectum, followed by the curve of the sacrum.
- Perform a digital rectal examination. Exclude anal fissure, palpable tumour, and/or any tenderness.
- When pain is encountered, consider abandoning the procedure.
- Lubricate the instrument tip, insert into anal canal, remove obturator, and close the cap.
- Insufflate just enough to visualize the lumen, as you advance the scope.
- Assess the mucosa in clockwise or anti-clockwise pattern.
- The scope allows assessment up to 15cm only. Do not attempt to assess further, as it can cause significant discomfort to the patient.

Complications

- Vasovagal syncope if procedure is painful.
- Bleeding from biopsy site.
- Perforation of rectal wall if full thickness biopsy taken (especially anterior).

Tips and tricks

- Check the equipment before starting procedure.
- Always perform a digital rectal examination before the sigmoidoscopy.
- Don't push the scope further if uncomfortable to the patient.
- Beware—the biopsy forceps is longer than the scope. Be cautious not to cause full-thickness damage to the rectal wall, especially anteriorly.
- Ensure patient is not on anticoagulation before taking biopsy.

Flexible sigmoidoscopy

Overview

A flexible sigmoidoscope is a 60cm-long instrument with fibre-optic digital imaging technology. It is used to examine the rectum, sigmoid, and descending colon. Commonly a colonoscope is used instead of a flexible sigmoidoscope. It requires training and skill to perform this diagnostic/therapeutic procedure. Either air or carbon dioxide is used to stretch the bowel wall, so that lesions within the mucosal folds can be visualized. The tip of the scope is turned up, down, and sideways by manipulating two wheels that are attached to pulleys in the head of the scope.

Indications

- Diagnosis of distal anorectal type per rectal bleeding.
- Investigation of lower colorectal symptoms.
- Screening for colorectal cancer (bowel scope screening).
- Preoperative evaluation and marking of rectal and sigmoid/descending colon cancers.
- Removal of foreign bodies.
- Excision of polyps or biopsy of a lesion.
- Decompression of sigmoid volvulus.

Contraindications

- Bowel perforation.
- Acute diverticulitis.
- Peritonitis.
- Significant anorectal bleeding.
- Inadequate bowel preparation.
- Severe cardiopulmonary disease.

Pre-procedure preparation

- Phosphate enema (30min before procedure) to empty the rectum and sigmoid colon for clear visualization of mucosal lesions.
- This is an invasive procedure, informed consent is mandatory.
- Obtain brief relevant history, including drug history (anticoagulants).
- Usually this procedure is done without sedation. Cannulation is required if patient choses to have sedation. Usually Midazolam or Pethidine/Fentanyl is used. Ensure that antagonists to both opiates (Naloxone) and Benzodiazepam (Flumazenil) are available.

Steps of procedure

- Ensure patient's checklist is completed (WHO).
- Ask patient to lie in left lateral position.
- Using insufflation and torque, negotiate the scope tip under vision.
- If a lesion or abnormality is detected, note the distance from anal verge. Take photographs. Take biopsies. Tattoo by injecting India ink close to the area of interest.
- If a large diverticulum is found, slow down the procedure. Pull back the instrument and renegotiate under vision. Do not push against resistance.

- If excising a lesion, ensure that bleeding has stopped. If necessary use one of the haemostatic methods (clips/adrenaline injection).
- This procedure can be difficult or uncomfortable to patients who have had previous pelvic surgery (colonic adhesions). Consider radiological alternative investigations (CT colonography or barium enema).
- Suction all the air at the end of procedure to reduce post -procedural discomfort.
- Patients are kept under observation if they had sedation (2–3h). Otherwise they are discharged. Discuss the findings.

Complications

- Complications related to sedation (hypoxia, bradycardia, anaphylaxis, hypotension).
- Perforation (1/10,000).
- Bleeding.
- Missed lesions.
- Vasovagal symptoms.

Colonoscopy

Overview

This test allows examination of the entire large bowel and terminal ileum using a long (120–180cm) flexible fibre-optic scope (Fig. 4.2). The technology is similar to 'Flexible sigmoidoscopy' (p. 142). Compared to other imaging modalities, colonoscopy can detect very small mucosal abnormalities. In addition, biopsies can be taken and therapeutic interventions can be done at the same time (polypectomy).

Indications

- Symptoms suggestive of colorectal cancer (red flag symptoms). Refer to British Society of Gastroenterology guidelines.
- Patients with maelena when UGI cause is excluded.
- Patients with chronic diarrhoea (microscopic colitis).
- Positive faecal occult blood on screening test.
- Abnormal or suspicious lesions found on radiological tests (CT scan/CT colonography).
- Persistent abdominal pain with raised C reactive protein or raised faecal calprotectin.
- History suggestive of inflammatory bowel disease (IBD).
- For IBD surveillance.
- Surveillance after colorectal cancer resection or in familial adenomatous polyposis (FAP).
- Insertion of stents.

Contraindications

- These are similar to 'Flexible sigmoidoscopy' (p. 142).

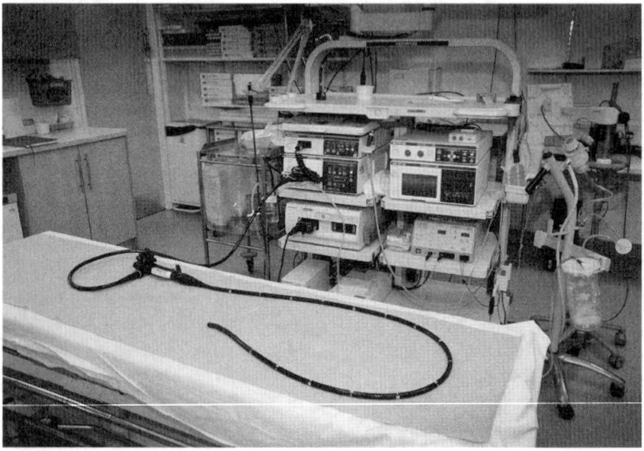

Fig. 4.2 Colonoscope.

Preoperative preparation

- This procedure requires thorough planned bowel preparation. The endoscopy department will send a detailed dietetic advice with bowel preparation agents (Picolax/Moviprep/Kleanprep/Fleet).
- Oral iron supplements, constipating agents, and anticoagulants are stopped before the procedure.
- Bowel preparation commenced on the previous day with different timings for different preparation agents.
- As the procedure can be uncomfortable, sedation is advised.

Procedure

- WHO checklist.
- Patient in left lateral position. Using torque and gentle hand–eye co-ordination skills, manoeuvre the colonoscope.
- In sigmoid colon, the colonoscope may form a loop (N or alpha loop), withdraw the scope with a clockwise torque to reduce the loop. Advance with clockwise/anticlockwise torque (either technique should work).
- Transverse colon is another potential area to form a loop. Overcome this by further withdrawing scope and turning the patient on either side before advancing under vision.
- Try not to over insufflate the colon, regular withdrawal and suction will 'concertina' the colon over the colonoscope.
- Recognize the caecum by identifying appendicular orifice or ileo-caecal valve.
- Take biopsies where necessary.
- Tattoo the polyp excision site by injecting permanent India ink solution.
- Suction the insufflated air as the scope is withdrawn. Examine the mucosa carefully during withdrawal. Perform retro-flexion in the rectum to assess the anorectal lining.
- Severe pain and discomfort despite adequate sedation is a warning sign to abandon the procedure (high risk of perforation). Alternative assessment methods should be used (CT colonography/barium enema).
- Patients who have had sedation should be observed for next 2–3h and are discharged as per progress. Patients who complain of severe uncontrolled abdominal pain should be re-assessed and investigated further or admitted if necessary.

Complications

- Similar to 'Flexible sigmoidoscopy' (p. 142).

Tips and tricks

- Keep the scope short and straight by withdrawing with low suction.
- Risk of perforation—do not push the scope against resistance.
- If no progress—change patient position/technique quickly.

Surgery for fissure-in-ano

Overview

This is a linear ulcer occurring below the dentate line. May be due to an increase in anal resting pressure from overactivity of the internal anal sphincter causing hypoperfusion and fissuring at sites of 'watershed' vascular supply. They occur in the anterior and posterior midline and are more common in the posterior midline (90%). Consider possible underlying pathology such as Crohn's disease, infection, trauma, or malignancy.

Conservative measures like using bulk laxatives, stool softeners, and topical application of local anaesthetic assist in the spontaneous healing of most acute fissures. Topical glyceryl trinitrate 0.2%, 0.4%, or Diltiazem 2% applied locally, reduces anal pressure and achieves healing in 50–70% of all fissures. Intra-sphincteric injection of botulinum toxin (Botox) to paralyse sphincter gives sufficient time to heal the fissure and is successful in >70% of cases.

Lateral internal sphincterotomy

Indication

Surgery is indicated when medical therapy fails. Anal dilatation has been abandoned in favour of lateral internal sphincterotomy (Figs 4.3 and 4.4) because the latter procedure is more controlled and incontinence is less common.

Position

Lithotomy.

Procedure

This is done as a day procedure under general anaesthesia.

- WHO checklist.
- Perform a digital rectal examination and sigmoidoscopy.
- Introduce a bivalve anal speculum. Open it gradually to put the fibres of the internal sphincter on the stretch.
- Ask the assistant to apply traction to peri-anal skin.
- Palpate the inter-sphincteric groove in 3 o'clock position.
- Infiltrate local anaesthetic with 1:200,000 adrenaline in the groove and make a 1cm incision along the groove.
- The lower border of the internal sphincter is identified as a white band. Using blunt-ended scissors develop the inter-sphincteric and submucosal planes. Divide the internal sphincter to the level of the dentate line.
- Excise any skin tag or hypertrophied internal papilla.
- Apply pressure to achieve haemostasis.
- Leave the wound open.

In the closed technique, insert a scalpel in the same position with the blade parallel to the internal sphincter. Advance it along the inter-sphincteric groove. Rotate the scalpel towards the internal sphincter and divide it.

Local advancement flap of peri-anal skin may be used for recurrent fissure after sphincterotomy and where risk to continence is high.

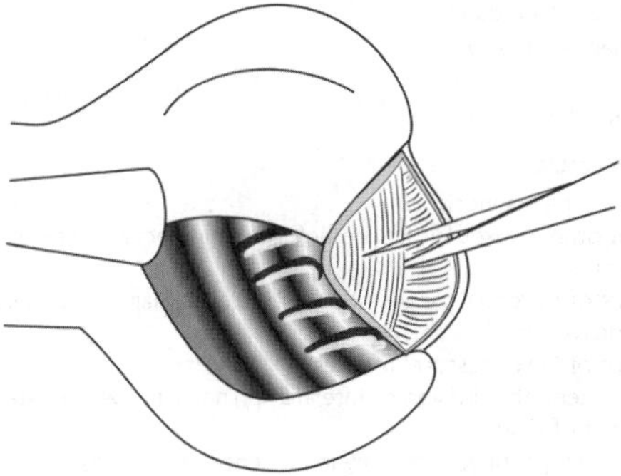

Fig. 4.3 Lateral internal sphincterotomy. Reproduced with permission from McLatchie, G, and Leaper, D. Operative Surgery 2nd edition, Oxford University Press: 2006.

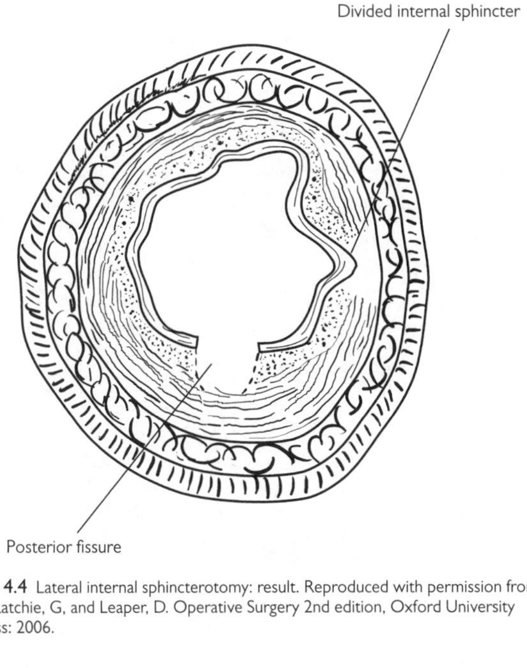
Divided internal sphincter
Posterior fissure

Fig. 4.4 Lateral internal sphincterotomy: result. Reproduced with permission from McLatchie, G, and Leaper, D. Operative Surgery 2nd edition, Oxford University Press: 2006.

Postoperative complications

- Incontinence—passive.
- Recurrence/persistence.
- Bleeding/haematoma.

Tips and tricks

- Be sure of the diagnosis.
- Rule out other causes for fissure before commencing conservative treatment.
- Be aware of potential for previous sphincter damage—anal surgery, vaginal deliveries.
- Be aware of 'low pressure' fissures.
- Do not extend the division of internal sphincter above dentate line or upper limit of fissure.
- Do not attempt sphincterotomy in presence of proctitis.

Procedures for haemorrhoids

Overview

Degeneration of the supporting structures of the three anal cushions causes them to prolapse, leading to development of haemorrhoids. The majority of patients present with intermittent, small rectal bleeds and require no treatment other than reassurance and dietary advice, but thorough evaluation is necessary to exclude other pathologies such as inflammatory bowel disease and malignancies. Examination should include inspection of the perineum, digital rectal examination, proctoscopy, and sigmoidoscopy. A full colonic examination may be required by colonoscopy or CT colonography.

Injection sclerotherapy

Indications

Persistent haemorrhoidal bleeding or small anterior mucosal prolapse. The aim of the procedure is to cause submucosal fibrosis.

Position

Left lateral.

Procedure

- Done as an outpatient procedure.
- Discuss procedure and obtain consent.
- Draw up 10–15ml of 5% phenol in almond oil into a Luer lock syringe with a shouldered Gabriel needle.
- Pass a proctoscope and identify the left lateral, right anterior, and right posterior internal haemorrhoids.
- Inject 3–5ml of the solution under vision into the submucosa above each haemorrhoid (Fig. 4.5) The correct plane of injection is indicated by elevation of the mucosa.
- Review the patient at 6 weeks and repeat the procedure if necessary.

Rubber band ligation

Indication

Persistent bleeding and prolapsing haemorrhoids The aim of the procedure is to fix the mucosa thereby preventing prolapse. This treatment is reserved for grade II haemorrhoids.

Contraindications

Anticoagulation, immunocompromised patient.

Position

Left lateral.

Procedure

- Outpatient procedure. Discuss procedure and obtain consent.
- Pass a proctoscope and identify the internal haemorrhoids.
- Use suction banding apparatus (Fig. 4.6) to put a rubber band over the mucosa of lower rectum above the haemorrhoidal tissue at 3, 7, and 11 o' clock positions (Fig. 4.5).

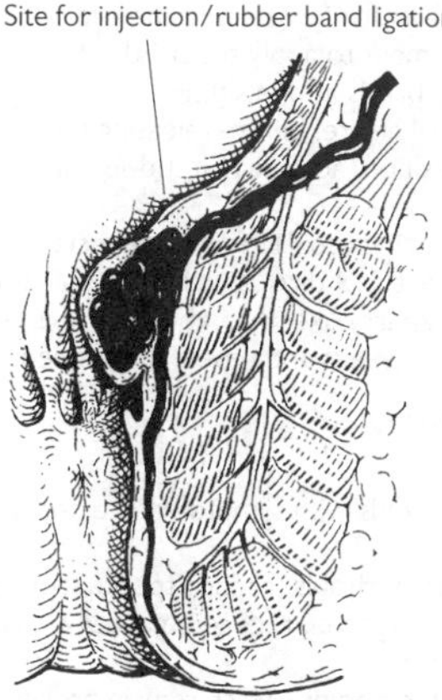
Site for injection/rubber band ligation

Fig. 4.5 Site for injection/rubber band ligation. Reproduced with permission from McLatchie, G, and Leaper, D. Operative Surgery 2nd edition, Oxford University Press: 2006.

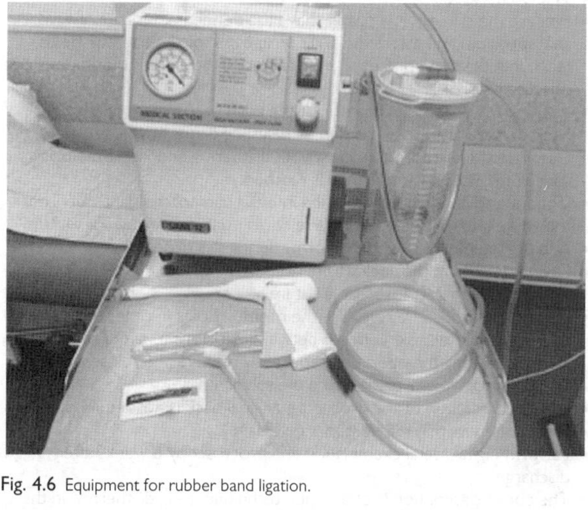

Fig. 4.6 Equipment for rubber band ligation.

- Apply suction and wait for few seconds before completely pulling the handle of the instrument to apply the band.
- Apply two or three bands at one sitting.
- It is important to make sure, before releasing the band, that the suction on the mucosa does not cause pain. If it does, apply the band to a more proximal position.

Warn the patient that it is usual to feel some rectal discomfort and a desire to defecate for the next 2–3 days and that a small amount of bleeding or the passage of a 'blackberry-like' thrombosed pile is common (4–10 days). Review the patient at 6 weeks and repeat the procedure if necessary.

Haemorrhoidectomy

Indications

- Prolapsing haemorrhoids with symptomatic external haemorrhoids (pain, swelling).
- Second-degree haemorrhoids (reduce spontaneously) and third-degree haemorrhoids (needing to be reduced manually) that do not respond to outpatient procedures.
- Fourth-degree haemorrhoids (which remain prolapsed permanently).

Position

Lithotomy or prone jack-knife with general/spinal anaesthetic.

Procedure (Milligan–Morgan technique)

Usually done as a day-case procedure

- WHO checklist.
- Prepare the skin, towel up, and shave the perineum. Insert a bivalve anal speculum and assess the position and size of the haemorrhoids. Start with the most posterior lying haemorrhoid so that blood does not obscure vision.
- Apply artery forceps to the skin at the edge of the external haemorrhoid and incise the skin with cutting diathermy.
- Continue the dissection medially with diathermy and insert the bivalve speculum once the anal margin is reached.
- Continue to carefully separate the internal haemorrhoidal tissue from the white internal sphincter muscle fibres using diathermy (Fig. 4.7).
- Achieve haemostasis with diathermy during this dissection.
- Divide mucosa at the apex of the haemorrhoid with diathermy or by transfixing with 2/0 absorbable suture.
- Repeat the procedure to excise the haemorrhoids in other positions, taking care to keep skin bridges between excisions to avoid anal stenosis. During the operation repeatedly remove and reinsert the speculum to avoid overstretching the sphincter.
- At the completion of the procedure an anal pack is not required.
- Stool softeners may aid postoperative pain.
- Perform digital rectal examination and proctoscopy 6 weeks after discharge.
- The above description is of an open technique using diathermy. In the closed technique, the skin edges and the mucosa are sutured together.

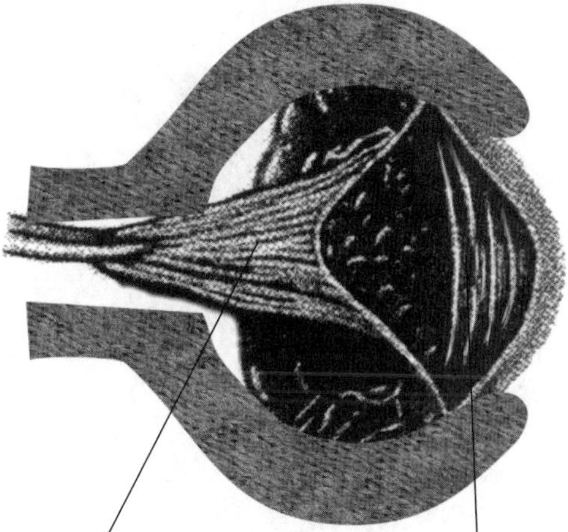
Haemorrhoid dissected
off the internal sphincter
Internal sphincter
muscle fibres

Fig. 4.7 Haemorrhoidectomy. Reproduced with permission from McLatchie, G, and Leaper, D. Operative Surgery 2nd edition, Oxford University Press: 2006.

Postoperative complications

- Bleeding/haematoma.
- Acute urinary retention.
- Sepsis is uncommon, but can be serious.
- Recurrence/persistence.
- Incontinence.
- Stenosis.

Circular stapled haemorrhoidectomy

Another technique, where a circular stapling device is introduced per-anally, is used to excise a rim of rectal mucosa above the haemorrhoids (Fig. 4.8). The result is that the prolapsed haemorrhoidal tissue is drawn back into a more physiological position and its blood supply is interrupted (Fig. 4.9). The procedure is claimed to be less painful and allows rapid postoperative recovery.

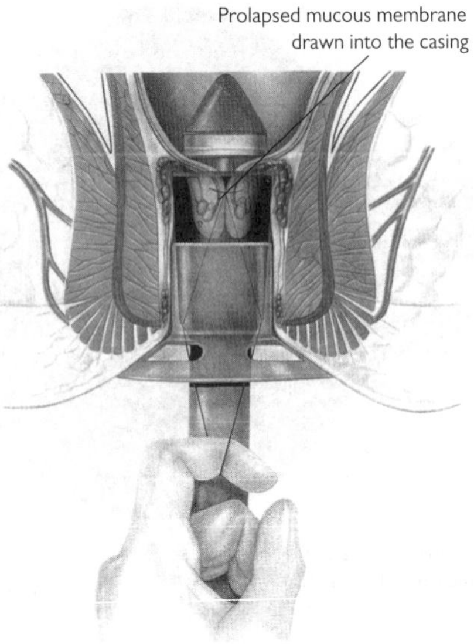
Prolapsed mucous membrane
drawn into the casing

Fig. 4.8 Circular stapled haemorrhoidectomy—insertion of stapling device. Reproduced with permission from McLatchie, G, and Leaper, D. Operative Surgery 2nd edition, Oxford University Press: 2006.

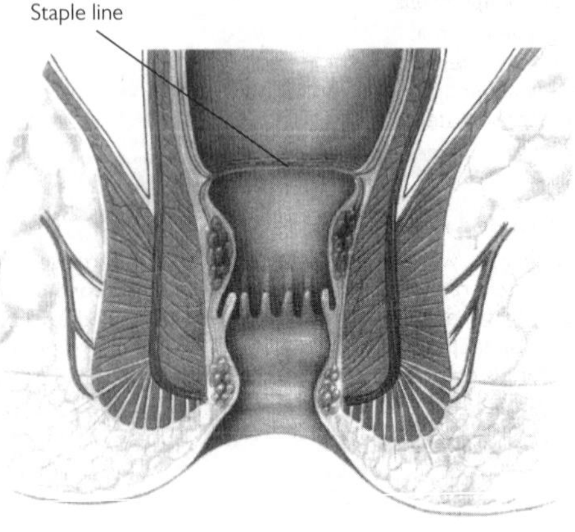
Staple line

Fig. 4.9 Circular stapled haemorrhoidectomy—final result. Reproduced with permission from McLatchie, G, and Leaper, D. Operative Surgery 2nd edition, Oxford University Press: 2006.

Haemorrhoidal artery ligation operation (HALO), trans-anal haemorrhoidal dearterialization (THD)

This is a novel, less invasive, and non-excisional technique. This technique consists of ligation of terminal haemorrhoidal branches of the superior rectal artery using a specifically designed proctoscope with a Doppler probe to locate the vessels. The vessels are ligated by figure-of-8 sutures at 1, 3, 5, 7, 9, and 11 o'clock positions. This results in a thrombosis of the vessel and shrinkage/fibrosis of haemorrhoidal tissue with reduced or no wound complications. An additional procedure of mucopexy can be added to deal with large or prolapsing haemorrhoids after ligation of vessels. Success rate is reported to be >90%.

Peri-anal haematoma

Haematoma due to rupture of an anal venule. Surgery is indicated if the patient presents early with a painful lump. Incise the skin over the swelling and evacuate the clot. This can be done under local or general anaesthesia.

Thrombosed or strangulated haemorrhoids

Conservative treatment is usually successful. Immediate surgery, if undertaken, should be under antibiotic cover and carried out by an experienced surgeon.

Tips and tricks

- Haemorrhoids may coexist with other conditions like inflammatory bowel disease or malignancy.
- Non-excisional procedures should be considered first, if appropriate.
- Choice of technique should be tailor-made to patient's symptoms and severity of prolapse.
- Keep skin bridges between haemorrhoids being excised and always safeguard sphincter complex.

Surgery for fistula-in-ano

Overview

The majority of fistulae-in-ano arise from a diseased anal gland in the inter-sphincteric space. They are classified as crypto-glandular. Crohn's disease, infections, hydradenitis suppurativa, and malignancy may be associated with fistulas.

Preparation

Examination under anaesthesia is very important before planning for operation. Endoanal ultrasound/MRI scan is recommended for complex fistulae. Warn the patient of the possibility of further procedures if a complex or high fistula is encountered. A phosphate enema is administered 1h prior to the procedure.

Position

Lithotomy.

Procedure

- WHO checklist.
- Carried out under general anaesthetic, usually as a day-case procedure.
- Perform rigid procto-sigmoidoscopy.
- Identify the position of the external opening (or openings). Goodsall's rule (Fig. 4.10) is helpful in predicting the direction of tract. It states that a fistula where the external opening is situated behind the transverse anal line has a curved tract and opens in the posterior midline, whereas anteriorly placed openings have straight tracts with an internal opening in the corresponding quadrant of the anal canal.
- Palpate the peri-anal skin carefully for induration. This helps to indicate the course of the fistulous tract.
- Perform a digital examination of the anorectum to feel for the internal opening and any supra-levator induration.
- Insert an Eisenhammer proctoscope and look for the internal opening.
- Gently insert a Lockhart–Mummery fistula probe in the external opening and ascertain the direction and depth of the tract (Fig. 4.11). Look for secondary tracts. Allow the tip to exit through the internal opening. Bend the probe to bring the tip outside the anal orifice.
- Using diathermy cut onto the probe to lay open superficial, inter-sphincteric and low trans-sphincteric tracts (Fig. 4.12).
- Use self-retaining retractors to expose the tract. Curette the granulation tissue away. Consider sending tissue from the tract for histological examination.
- Cut away any overhanging skin edges. Lay open any secondary extensions.
- When the exact position and level of the tract in relation to the external sphincter is not clear, insert a loose Seton such as a vascular sling or non-absorbable suture.

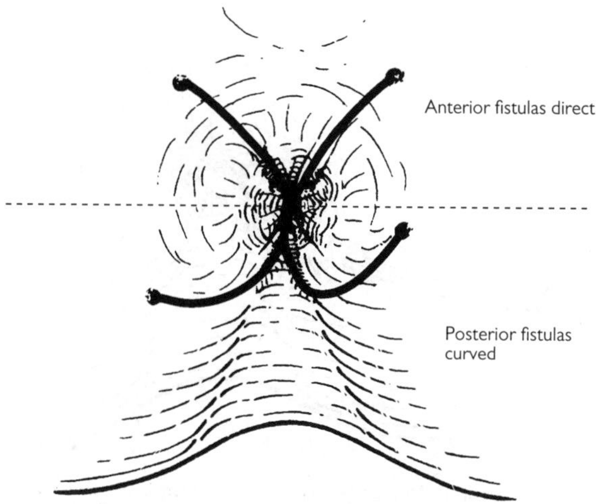
Anterior fistulas direct
Posterior fistulas curved

Fig. 4.10 Goodsall's law. Reproduced with permission from McLatchie, G, and Leaper, D. Operative Surgery 2nd edition, Oxford University Press: 2006.

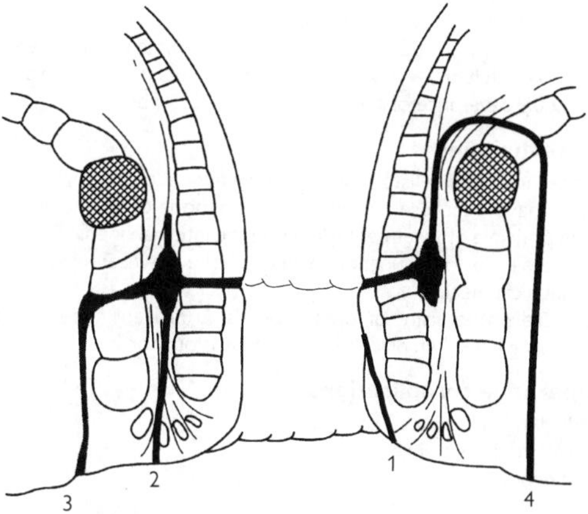
1
2
3
4

Fig. 4.11 Types of fistula-in-ano: (1) superficial; (2) inter-sphincteric; (3) trans-sphincteric; (4) supra-sphincteric. Reproduced with permission from McLatchie, G, and Leaper, D. Operative Surgery 2nd edition, Oxford University Press: 2006.

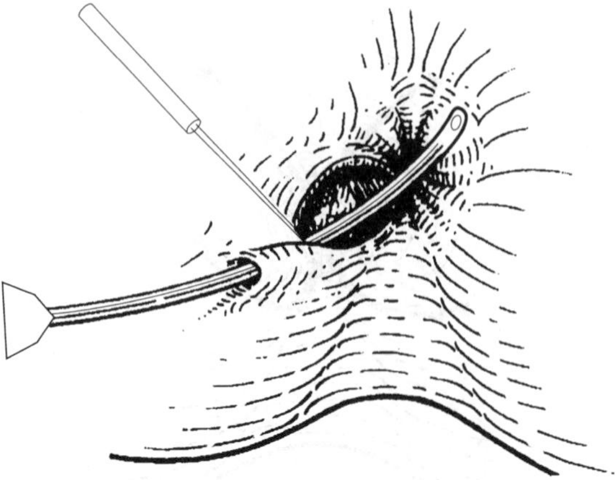

Fig. 4.12 Laying open of fistula tract. Reproduced with permission from McLatchie, G, and Leaper, D. Operative Surgery 2nd edition, Oxford University Press: 2006.

- Seton can similarly be used to drain acute infection secondary to a fistula-in-ano with definitive surgery being deferred until the acute inflammation settles.
- Lay open the tract outside the sphincters when you encounter a high trans-sphincteric or supra-sphincteric tract. Encircle the muscle with a Seton. Tighten it at 2-weekly intervals until it cuts through. This allows the gradual severance of the muscle followed by fibrosis.

Other techniques

Various techniques like fistula plug, advancement flap, and regenerative cell infiltration have been used as alternative methods of sphincter preservation. The principle of treatment is to close the internal opening of the fistula so that there is no contamination from inside the bowel and external tracts, and wounds can heal.

Emphasize proper care of open wounds to prevent superficial healing before healing has taken place from the depths outwards.

Postoperative complications

- Bleeding/haematoma.
- Recurrence/persistence.
- Incontinence.

Tips and tricks

- Don't force the probe—you may create a false passage.
- Look for multiple extensions and deal with them individually.
- It is possible to feel the fistula tract by palpating the peri-anal skin with a lubricated finger.

Pilonidal sinus

Overview

Pilonidal sinus occurs most commonly in the natal cleft. Enlargement of hair follicles, with ingress of exogenous hairs, results in the sinus, which may be asymptomatic. Treatment is only indicated when there is symptomatic disease. It may present acutely with cellulitis or as an abscess. The former may resolve with the use of antibiotics but an abscess requires drainage of pus, which can be done under local anaesthetic using a stab incision. The sinus is treated electively once the acute infection has settled.

Surgical options

Pilonidal sinus may also present with discharge as a result of chronic infection. The options are laying open of the tracts, wide excision with or without primary midline closure, asymmetric closure using Karydakis or Bascome's technique, and Rhomboid flaps and Z-plasty. Low recurrence and high primary healing rates have been achieved by techniques that result in the main wound being placed away from the midline and which obliterate the natal cleft.

Bascome's cleft closure technique can be done under local anaesthetic as a day-case procedure (Fig. 4.13).

Mark the line of contact between buttocks with patient standing in a relaxed position.

Position

Prone with table jack-knifed; the buttocks may be separated using tapes to expose the natal cleft, if necessary.

Procedure

- WHO checklist.
- Mark an island of skin, asymmetrically placed off the midline according to whichever side is most affected by skin sinuses/previous sepsis—the excision will need to be asymmetrical and with a 'tear drop' extension on the anal end to allow for equal skin-edge lengths.
- Excise the island of skin.
- All sinuses and associated scar tissue should be identified and cleared or excised/ablated. It is not necessary to excise tissue in the midline down to the pre-sacral fascia.
- Elevate a flap of skin off to one side of the cleft.
- Remove the tapes if present.
- Close the natal cleft by suturing together the exposed fat from deep to superficial in multiple levels, if necessary.
- A drain may be left for 2–3 days.
- Advance the flap across the middle of the cleft and suture in place.
- Use subcuticular monofilament sutures to oppose skin margins.

Postoperative complications

- Bleeding/haematoma.
- Wound infection and dehiscence.
- Recurrence.

Tips and tricks

- Look for and excise secondary tracts.
- Mobilize flaps adequately to prevent tension on suture line.

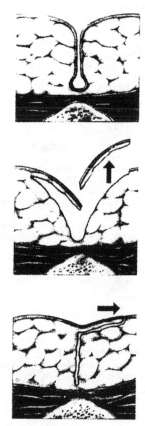

Fig. 4.13 Bascome's cleft closure technique. Reproduced with permission from McLatchie, G, and Leaper, D. Operative Surgery 2nd edition, Oxford University Press: 2006.

Surgery for rectal prolapse

Full-thickness rectal prolapse can be treated by perineal and abdominal procedures.

Delorme's procedure

This procedure involves resection of redundant rectal mucosa and plication of rectal muscle wall without resection (Fig. 4.14). The functional results are good if the prolapse is small or incomplete. This procedure is particularly tolerated by elderly people who are unfit for intra-abdominal surgery. Though the recurrence rate is reported to be 5–25%, the morbidity and mortality is low.

Position

Prone jack-knife/left lateral/lithotomy.

Procedure

- WHO checklist.
- This procedure is done under either general or regional anaesthesia.
- Prescribe enema to empty rectum.
- Allow the rectum to prolapse to its full extent.
- Infiltrate saline containing 1 in 200,000 adrenalin in the sub-mucosal plane to facilitate dissection and haemostasis.
- Make a circumferential incision in the mucosa, 1cm proximal to the dentate line.
- Using diathermy, carefully separate the mucosa circumferentially from muscle. Continue until the apex of the prolapse is reached (Fig. 4.14).
- Plicate the muscle tube using four to eight individual absorbable sutures.
- Divide the mucosal cylinder in stages and approximate the mucosal ends with interrupted absorbable sutures (Fig. 4.15).
- Prescribe laxatives postoperatively.

Postoperative complications

- Bleeding.
- Infection.
- Recurrence.

Laparoscopic posterior rectopexy

In this procedure, the rectum is mobilized and is fixed to the sacrum either using non-absorbable sutures or using a mesh.

Preoperative preparation

- Phosphate enema.
- Intravenous antibiotics at induction of anaesthesia.

Position

Lloyd–Davis.

Procedure

- Perform WHO checklist.
- Catheterize the patient.
- Make a vertical skin incision below the umbilicus. Expose the linea alba. Place two anchoring fascial sutures and incise linea alba between them.

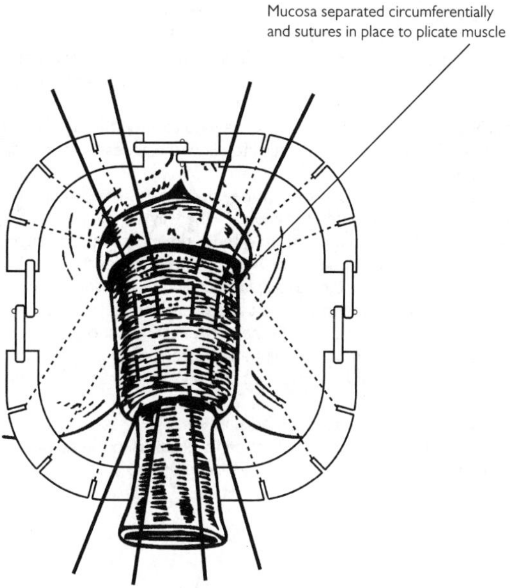
Mucosa separated circumferentially
and sutures in place to plicate muscle

Fig. 4.14 Delorme's procedure. Reproduced with permission from McLatchie, G, and Leaper, D. Operative Surgery 2nd edition, Oxford University Press: 2006.

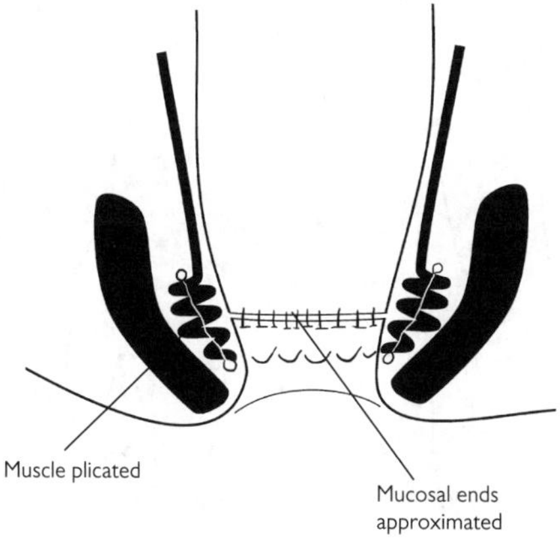
Muscle plicated
Mucosal ends
approximated

Fig. 4.15 Delorme's procedure. Reproduced with permission from McLatchie, G, and Leaper, D. Operative Surgery 2nd edition, Oxford University Press: 2006.

- Open peritoneum and insert a 10 mm blunt port.
- Create pneumoperitoneum.
- Under laparoscopic vision, insert a 5mm cannula in both iliac fossae. If necessary insert an additional 5mm suprapubic port to keep the sigmoid colon in left upper quadrant (Fig. 4.16).
- Usually 30–40° of head-down tilt is needed to keep the small bowel out of the pelvis. Achieve this in stages to allow the anaesthetist to adjust ventilation.
- Insert two transcutaneous straight-needled sutures to encircle the Fallopian tubes to elevate uterus out of the way.
- Grasp the recto-sigmoid junction to tense the root of the mesocolon.
- Dissect with harmonic scalpel or hook diathermy over the sacral promontory. Enter the bloodless plane behind the mesorectum.
- Divide the peritoneum on the right and dissect down to the pelvic floor. There is no need to divide the peritoneal reflection anteriorly, but complete mobilization on the right and posteriorly.
- Swing the sigmoid colon to the right and divide the peritoneum on the left.
- Identify the ureter and dissect medial to it.
- Choose the points in the mesorectum for fixation to the sacral promontory after pulling on the mobilized rectum.

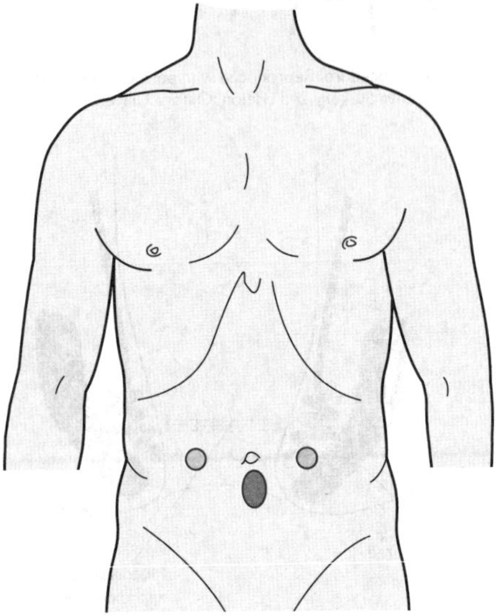

Fig. 4.16 Port placement for laparoscopic abdominal rectopexy (two 5mm and one infra-umbilical 10mm port).

- Place a suture through the mesorectum and sacral promontory on each side. Alternatively, anchor the top end of a mesh to the sacral promontory with tackers and suture the mesorectum to the lateral edge of the mesh.
- Remove uterine sutures.
- Close the fascia of the 10mm port site and approximate the skin with steristrips/subcuticular suture.
- Infiltrate wounds with local anaesthetic.

Open abdominal rectopexy can similarly be carried out using sutures or mesh.

Postoperative complications

- Bleeding.
- Infection.
- Inadvertent bowel injury.
- Recurrence.

Tips and tricks

- Perineal approach may be preferred in elderly and high-risk patients.
- Patient selection is important when deciding the type of operation offered.
- Put the patient in steep head-down position, if small bowel is in the operating field.

Ventral mesh rectopexy

Preoperative preparation

- Phosphate enema.
- Intravenous antibiotics at induction of anaesthesia.

Position

Lloyd–Davies.

Procedure

- WHO checklist.
- General anaesthesia.
- Achieve pneumoperitoneum by open Hasson technique in umbilical region. Under vision place a 10mm port in right iliac fossa. Place a 5mm port in left iliac fossa. An additional 5mm port is occasionally needed for retraction of bowel (left flank).
- Use Trendelenberg position to displace the small bowel loops out of pelvis.
- Give gentle traction at recto-sigmoid junction to straighten the rectum.
- Make hockey stick-shaped incision on the peritoneum along anterior and right lateral side of the rectum up to the sacral promontory.
- Commence the dissection in the anterior part of the incision and continue it deeper to enter the rectovaginal space till the pelvic floor.
- Suture a strip of suitable mesh (biological or synthetic) to the distal rectovaginal septum/perineal body and to the anterior rectal wall.
- Keeping the traction on the rectum, anchor the top end of the mesh to the fascia over the sacral promontory by tackers or sutures.
- Close the peritoneal incision to cover the mesh.
- Close laparoscopic port sites.

Postoperative care

Laxatives for 2 weeks.

Complications

- Bleeding.
- Injury to rectum.
- Infection of mesh.
- Rectovaginal fistula.
- Recurrent symptoms.
- Erosion of mesh into rectum/vagina.

Tips and tricks

- Do not deepen the lateral peritoneal incision to avoid injury to lateral pelvic ligaments.
- Continue anterior dissection to the perineal body.
- Prevent undue tension while fixing the mesh to the sacral promontory.

Surgery for acute anorectal infection (abscess)

Overview

Anorectal infection is usually linked to anal gland infection and is commonly associated with a fistula. Anorectal infection may also be seen in association with Crohn's disease, hydradenitis suppurative, and malignancy. Patients with peri-anal abscesses present with pain and a palpable tender lump at the anal margin. Those with an ischiorectal abscess have tenderness, induration, and fullness in the ischiorectal fossa. An inter-sphincteric or submucous abscess should be suspected in a patient with persistent anal pain and no obvious peri-anal abnormality (Fig. 4.17).

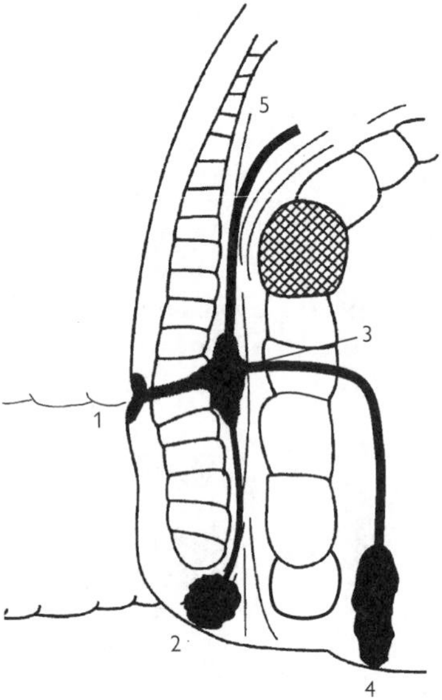
5
3
1
2
4

Fig. 4.17 Spread of infection from anal gland infection: (1) submucous; (2) peri-anal; (3) inter-sphincteric; (4) ischiorectal; (5) pelvirectal. Reproduced with permission from McLatchie, G, and Leaper, D. Operative Surgery 2nd edition, Oxford University Press: 2006.

Position

Lithotomy.

Procedure

The procedure is performed under general anaesthetic.

- WHO checklist.
- Make a cruciate incision over the swelling and deepen it to the abscess cavity.
- Take a swab for bacteriology.
- Gently break down the fibrous septa in the ischiorectal fossa.
- Remove the corners of the incisions so that free drainage is provided and the final opening represents the entire floor of the abscess cavity (Fig. 4.18).
- Loosely pack the cavity with an alginate dressing.
- Do not attempt to probe for a fistula tract or to lay it open.

Aftercare with loose packing and dressing ensures that healing occurs from deep to superficial, and lessens risk of a further abscess.

Postoperative complications

- Bleeding/haematoma.
- Development of fistula-in-ano.

Tips and tricks

- Adequate/generous drainage is very important
- Do not probe the abscess cavity with force, this will result in a false tract.

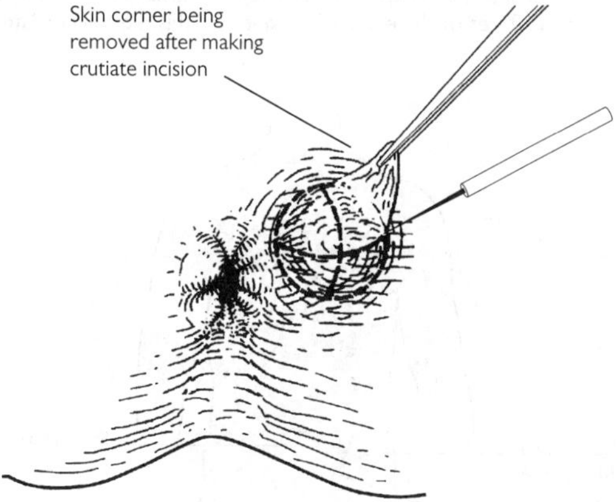
Skin corner being
removed after making
crutiate incision

Fig. 4.18 Incision and drainage of peri-anal abscess. Reproduced with permission from McLatchie, G, and Leaper, D. Operative Surgery 2nd edition, Oxford University Press: 2006.

Appendicectomy

Appendicitis is the most common major abdominal condition necessitating an emergency operation. The exception to this is when an appendix mass is found without evidence of general peritonitis.

Preoperative preparation

- Give intravenous antibiotics to cover anaerobes and Gram-negative bacilli (usually cefuroxime and metronidazole) at induction of anaesthesia.
- If a generalized peritonitis is suspected due to perforation, commence IV fluids, regular IV antibiotics, and NG aspiration.

Open appendicectomy

Position

Supine.

Incision

Lanz (Fig. 4.19).

Procedure

Palpate the abdomen again with the patient anaesthetized, as it may help to locate the position of the appendix. If a circumscribed lump or a diffuse thickening is felt, plan the incision accordingly.

- Perform WHO checklist.
- Divide the aponeurosis of the external oblique in line with its fibres and split the internal oblique and transversus muscles. Retract the muscles to expose the peritoneum.
- Open the peritoneum between artery forceps. If wider access is required, the internal oblique and transversus muscles can be divided in line with the fibres of the external oblique. Do this medially or laterally, as required.

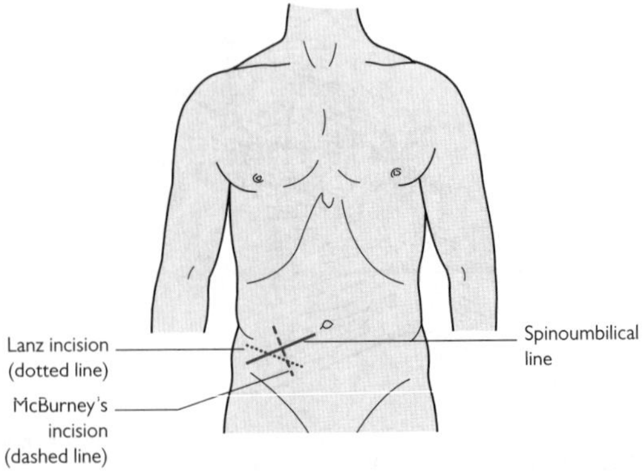
Lanz incision (dotted line)
McBurney's incision (dashed line)
Spinoumbilical line

Fig. 4.19 Incisions for appendicectomy.

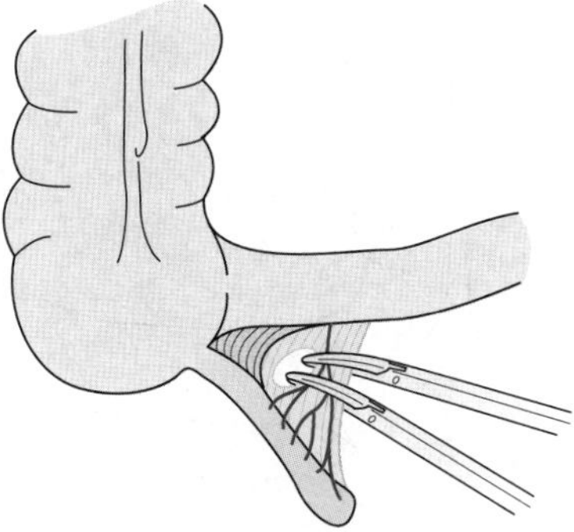

Fig. 4.20 Ligation of meso-appendix.

- Aspirate serous exudate or frank pus and send a sample for culture and sensitivity.
- Identify the caecum. Pick it up with fingers or Babcock's forceps applied to the tinea coli, and slowly and carefully draw the caecum to the surface. If the appendix does not come into view, pass an index finger along one of the tinea to their junction at the appendix base and then lift it out.
- Hold up the appendix with tissue forceps applied around it. Divide the meso-appendix with the appendicular artery between forceps and ligate it (Fig. 4.20). Identify the base of the appendix, apply artery forceps to the base to crush it then apply again more distally. Ligate the crushed appendix area (Fig. 4.21).
- Pass a purse-string seromuscular suture in the caecum about 1cm from the base of the appendix using a 3/0 absorbable suture. Divide the appendix flush with the under-surface of the artery forceps. Place the appendix and the instruments in a dirty dish taking care during and after division not to soil the wound or the peritoneum.
- Invaginate the stump and tie the purse-string suture. If the caecal wall is oedematous and friable, this is not necessary.

Complicated appendicitis

- If the inflamed appendix is retro-caecal and cannot be delivered into the wound, carry out a retrograde appendicectomy.
- Dividing the appendix first at its base, invaginating the stump, and then dividing the meso-appendix in small segments.
- If the omentum is adherent to the inflamed appendix, remove it with the appendix.

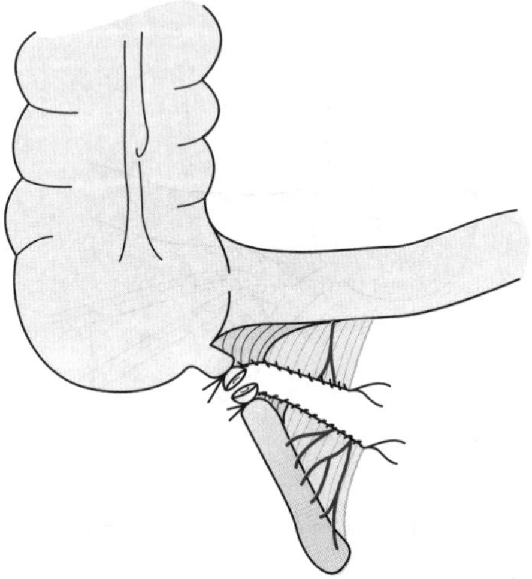

Fig. 4.21 Ligation and division of the stump of appendix.

- If a mass is encountered after opening the peritoneum, surround it with moist packs and gently explore the mass with a finger.
- Aspirate any pus, isolate the appendix, and remove it in the usual way.
- If the appendix is disintegrated at the site of the perforation, take care to remove the entire appendix to the base.
- If the diagnosis of acute appendicitis was incorrect, most local abnormalities can be dealt with by extending the incision.
- Make an appropriate vertical laparotomy incision if exposure is still inadequate or the abnormality lies outside the reach of the Lanz incision.
- If normal appendix is found, search for an inflamed Meckel's diverticulum.

Closure

- Close the peritoneum with absorbable suture.
- Allow the split muscles to fall together. Suture the external oblique aponeurosis.
- Close the skin incision with interrupted or subcuticular sutures.
- Drainage is not generally used after appendicectomy, unless there is an abscess with pus.

Postoperative complications

- Haemorrhage.
- Wound infection.
- Pelvic or abdominal abscess.
- Paralytic ileus.
- Incisional hernia.

Laparoscopic appendicectomy

Especially useful in women of child-bearing age when the diagnosis of acute appendicitis is in doubt.

Position

Lithotomy.

Procedure

- WHO checklist.
- Empty bladder before commencing the operation.
- Make a vertical skin incision within the umbilicus. Expose the linea alba. Place two anchoring fascial sutures and incise the linea alba between them.
- Open peritoneum and insert blunt trocar.
- Create pneumoperitoneum.
- Under laparoscopic vision, place a 10mm and 5mm port in the left iliac fossa and suprapubic area, respectively, avoiding the inferior epigastric vessels (Fig. 4.22).
- Have the table tilted head-down and right-side up.
- Expose the appendix by displacing the ileum and caecum using atraumatic grasping forceps.

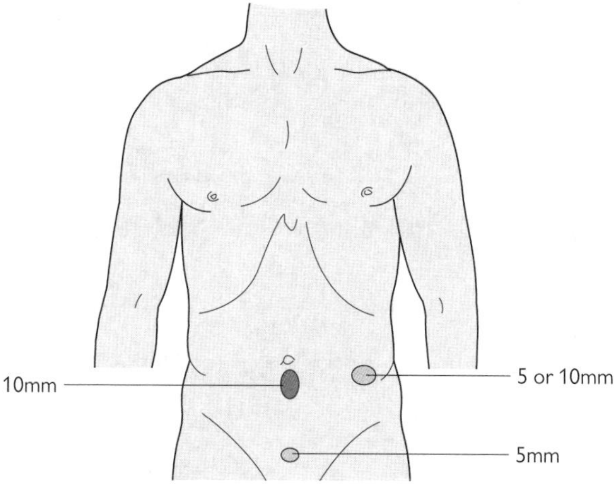
10mm
5 or 10mm
5mm

Fig. 4.22 Port sites for laparoscopic appendicectomy.

- Ligate or clip the meso-appendix and its artery.
- Apply two ligatures at the base of the appendix and transect the appendix between them. There is no need to bury the stump of the appendix.
- Visualization of the Fallopian tubes and ovaries is aided by manipulating the uterus with fingers placed in vaginal fornices.
- The appendix is removed through the 10mm cannula or by placing it in an endo bag, if bulky/friable.
- Lavage with normal saline.
- Remove carbon dioxide and take out the ports.
- Close fascia of 10mm port sites.
- Use steristrips to approximate skin.
- Infiltrate wounds with local anaesthetic.

Postoperative complications
- Wound infection.
- Pelvic or intra-abdominal abscess.

Tips and tricks
- Re-examine the abdomen under anaesthesia, plan your operation and incision accordingly.
- Do not hesitate to extend the incision or convert from laparoscopic to open procedure, if the anatomy is not clear or no progress in operation.
- If appendix is normal, always look for other pathology.

Excision of Meckel's diverticulum

Meckel's diverticulum is the persistence of a segment of vitello-intestinal duct on the anti-mesenteric border of the ileum. It is found in 2% of the population within 60cm of the caecum and is ~5cm long.

Indications

- Acute inflammation.
- Bleeding from ectopic gastric mucosa.
- Intestinal obstruction—volvulus around a persistent band or adhesion, intussusception.
- An incidental finding at laparotomy. Consider excision because of the risk of associated pathology. A wide-mouthed, thin-walled unattached diverticulum in an adult patient may be left alone.

Position

Supine.

Procedure

The choice is between either diverticulectomy or excision of the segment of ileum carrying the diverticulum.

- WHO checklist.
- Isolate the segment of ileum containing the diverticulum. Ligate any supplying vessels.
- Apply light occlusion clamps to the ileum and divide the diverticulum at its base and close the bowel wall transversely (Fig. 4.23). The diverticulum can also be removed by a single firing of a transverse stapler.
- Resect the segment of ileum in patients with peptic ulceration or diverticulitis affecting the base.
- Restore intestinal continuity by a single- or two-layer anastomosis (Fig. 4.24).

Postoperative complications

- Wound infection.
- Pelvic or intra-abdominal abscess.
- Ileus.
- Incisional hernia.
- Anastomotic leak.

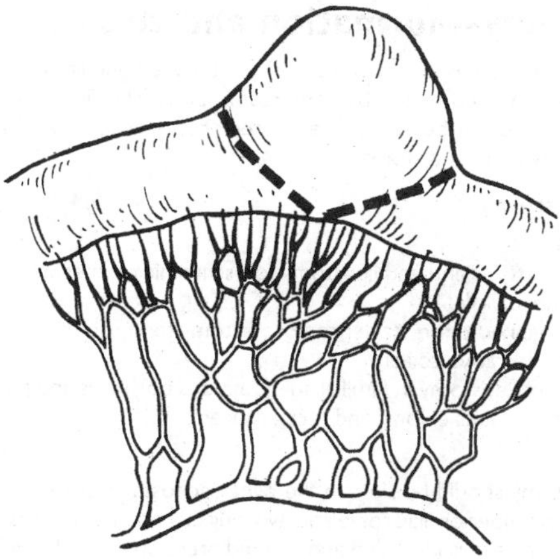

Fig. 4.23 Excision of Meckel's diverticulum—extent of excision. Reproduced with permission from McLatchie, G, and Leaper, D. Operative Surgery 2nd edition, Oxford University Press: 2006.

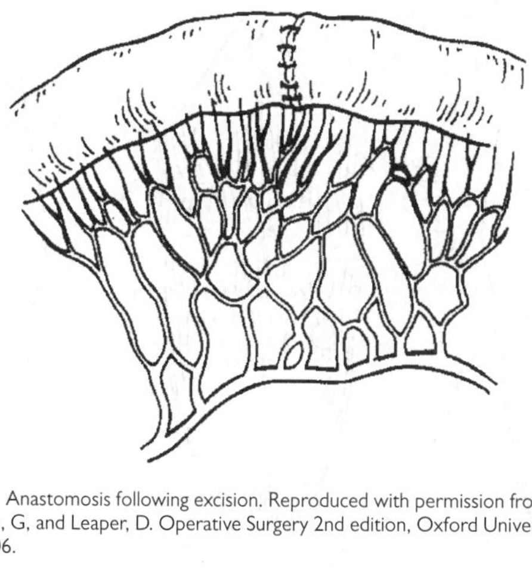

Fig. 4.24 Anastomosis following excision. Reproduced with permission from McLatchie, G, and Leaper, D. Operative Surgery 2nd edition, Oxford University Press: 2006.

Ileostomy—formation and closure

The terminal ileum is exteriorized as a spout in the right iliac fossa. Effluent is collected in a collecting bag (ileostomy bag). The ileostomy may be formed as a loop of bowel to divert enteric contents temporarily or more permanently as an end stoma.

End ileostomy

Indications

- Total colectomy and end ileostomy for ischaemic or infective colitis like *Clostridium difficile*.
- Part of planned three-stage proctocolectomy for inflammatory bowel disease (ulcerative colitis).
- Permanent ileostomy in familial adenomatous polyposis and patients with synchronous colonic and rectal cancers.

Preparation

The ileostomy should be sited in the right iliac fossa clear of the umbilicus and anterior superior iliac spine and avoiding any scars or depressions. The optimal stoma site is identified and marked preoperatively (Fig. 4.25).

Position

Supine or Lloyd–Davies position to allow a combined abdomino-perineal procedure to be carried out.

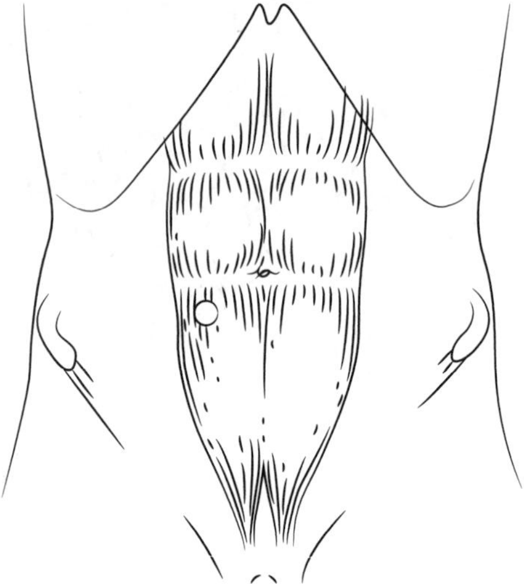

Fig. 4.25 Site of ileostomy. Reproduced with permission from McLatchie, G, and Leaper, D. Operative Surgery 2nd edition, Oxford University Press: 2006.

Procedure

- WHO checklist.
- In addition to laparotomy for the major procedure, make a trephine by excising a circular area of skin over the marked stoma site. Pick up the skin with a Littlewood's forceps and excise a disc ~2cm in diameter. Alternatively, make a cruciate incision and trim the edges using a cutting diathermy point.
- Excise a disc of subcutaneous fat to expose the anterior rectal sheath. Make a cruciate incision on the sheath.
- Use artery forceps to split the rectus abdominis muscle. Do this carefully to avoid injury to the inferior epigastric vessels.
- Expose the peritoneum by retracting the split muscle. Open the peritoneum between artery forceps. The trephine must admit the tips of two fingers to ensure there will be no obstruction to the blood supply of the bowel.
- Divide the ileum close to the ileo-caecal junction using a linear stapler.
- Divide the adjacent mesentery and partially remove the mesentery of about 5cm of terminal ileum.
- Deliver this length of ileum through the trephine onto the skin surface.
- The ileal mesentery should lie in a cephalad direction. Stitch the cut edge of the mesentery to the parietal peritoneum; it is not necessary to close the lateral gutter.
- Close and cover the abdominal incision.
- Excise the staple line on the small-bowel end.
- Insert 3/0 Monocryl® sutures through the skin edge, the adjacent seromuscular wall of the ileum (6cm proximal to distal end) and full thickness of the open bowel end at three or four levels, avoiding the vessels of the mesentery (Fig. 4.26).
- Clip the sutures long and tie them once all have been inserted. This everts the bowel end and results in a 3cm spout (eversion manoeuvre) (Fig. 4.27). This permits close application of the ileostomy bag with discharge of effluent away from the skin.

Postoperative complications

- Bleeding.
- Necrosis.
- Retraction.
- Stenosis.
- Prolapse.
- Parastomal herniation.

Loop ileostomy

Indication

To divert faecal stream or protect large bowel anastomosis or ileal pouch anal anastomosis.

Preparation

As for 'End ileostomy' (p. 178).

Position

Lloyd–Davies position to allow stapling or suturing to be carried out peri-anally.

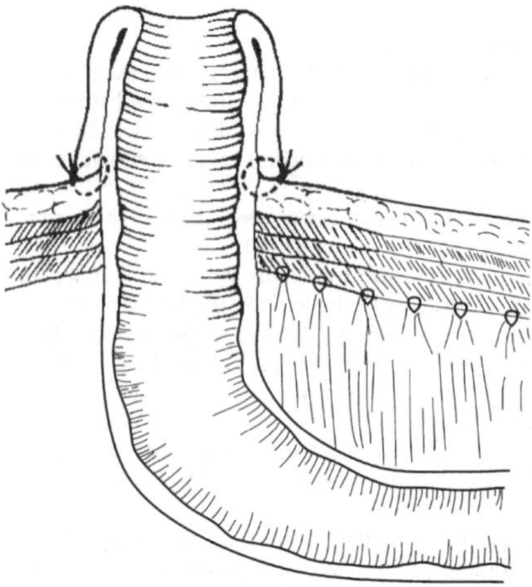

Fig. 4.26 End ileostomy. Reproduced with permission from McLatchie, G, and Leaper, D. Operative Surgery 2nd edition, Oxford University Press: 2006.

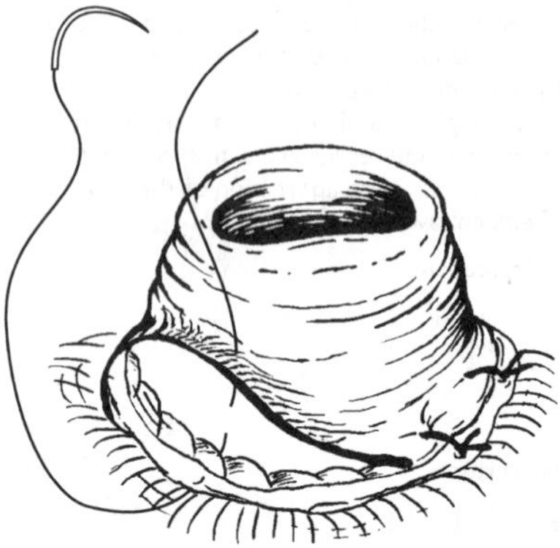

Fig. 4.27 End ileostomy. Reproduced with permission from McLatchie, G, and Leaper, D. Operative Surgery 2nd edition, Oxford University Press: 2006.

Procedure

- WHO checklist.
- Select a loop of terminal ileum close to the ileo-caecal junction. This should be of sufficient length to be brought out without tension.
- Mark the distal limb with a suture.
- Deliver the loop through a trephine incision, as described in 'Ileostomy—formation and closure' (p. 178).
- Close and cover the abdominal incision.
- Make a transverse enterotomy in the distal limb at the junction with the skin using a diathermy point.
- Insert three 3/0 Monocryl® sutures through the superior skin edge, adjacent to seromuscular wall of the ileum and full thickness of the open proximal bowel end.
- On the distal limb open end, insert a further four interrupted 4/0 Vicryl® sutures through full thickness of bowel and subcuticular skin so that the distal lumen is flush with the skin (Fig. 4.28).
- Tie the sutures after all of them are in place. This forms a spout and avoids forceful grasping of the mucosa with forceps to evert the bowel.
- Put extra sutures from open end of ileum to skin edge, as required. A gentle push with a Langenbeck retractor on the serosal side helps to form a spout.

Postoperative complications

- Bleeding.
- Necrosis.
- Retraction.
- Prolapse.
- Parastomal herniation.

Laparoscopic loop ileostomy

Indications and preparation

As for 'Ileostomy—formation and closure' (p. 178).

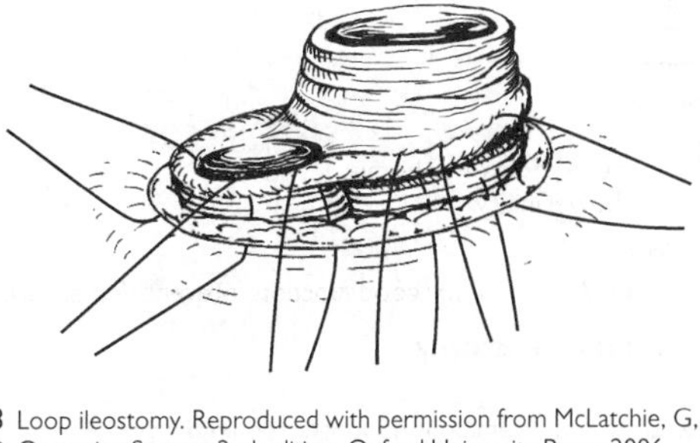

Fig. 4.28 Loop ileostomy. Reproduced with permission from McLatchie, G, and Leaper, D. Operative Surgery 2nd edition, Oxford University Press: 2006.

Position

Supine.

Procedure

- WHO checklist.
- Create pneumoperitoneum using Hasson technique at umbilicus.
- A 5mm suprapubic working port is placed under vision.
- The table can be tilted head-down and left lateral position to facilitate visualizing the caecum.
- Identify the ileo-caecal junction and work proximally up the small bowel using atraumatic grasping forceps to identify a convenient loop of terminal ileum that can be brought out easily and without tension. Orientate this loop carefully under vision so that the proximal bowel lies superiorly with the ileal mesentery lying in a cephalad direction.
- Make an open trephine by excising a circular area of skin over the marked stoma site. Ensure that the trephine admits two fingers to ensure there will be no obstruction to the blood supply of the bowel.
- Excise subcutaneous fat to expose the anterior rectal sheath. Make a cruciate incision on the sheath and use artery forceps to split the rectus abdominis muscle. Do this carefully to avoid injury to the inferior epigastric vessels.
- Expose the peritoneum by retracting the split muscle.
- Before opening the peritoneum, grasp the loop of ileum laparoscopically and hold up to the surface just away from the trephine.
- Open the peritoneum between artery forceps and immediately grasp and deliver the ileal loop through the trephine incision with Babcock forceps.
- Remove carbon dioxide and withdraw the ports.
- Close fascia of 10mm port sites.
- Subcuticular sutures or steristrips to approximate skin.
- Infiltrate wounds with local anaesthetic and dress the wounds.
- Continue with fashioning the loop ileostomy as for an open procedure.

Postoperative complications

- Bleeding.
- Necrosis.
- Retraction.
- Stenosis.
- Prolapse.
- Development of parastomal hernia.
- Inadvertent bowel injury.

Tips and tricks

- Aim to create 3cm spout for good function (prevent skin excoriation).

Closure of loop ileostomy

Indication

When faecal stream diversion is no longer required.

Preoperative preparation

Check for anastomotic integrity and patency using contrast radiology and endoscopic examination prior to reversal.

Position

Supine.

Procedure

- WHO checklist.
- Insert four muco-cutaneous stay sutures to help in mobilization. Hold the long ends on an artery forceps.
- Using cutting diathermy, incise the skin circumferentially close to the muco-cutaneous junction.
- Use sharp dissection to free the ileal loops from the parieties.
- Insert a finger in the peritoneal cavity and sweep it carefully around to separate adhesions and to allow withdrawal of sufficient length of small bowel for anastomosis.
- Separate the loops and divide the mesentery adjacent to the site chosen for anastomosis.
- Divide the ileum and carry out a single- or two-layered anastomosis or a stapled functional end–end anastomosis.
- Return the segment of bowel into the peritoneal cavity.
- Close with a single layer of interrupted PDS or non-absorbable sutures.
- Oppose the skin margins with interrupted non-absorbable sutures or apply a purse string suture and tighten it leaving a gap in the centre.

Postoperative complications

- Acute obstruction.
- Anastomotic leakage.

Tips and tricks

- Check that the loops are not twisted/rotated.
- Create space for the joined bowel loop to easily return into peritoneal cavity.

Colostomy—formation and closure

The colon may be exteriorized temporarily or permanently as an end or loop colostomy. Faeces are collected in a colostomy bag.

End colostomy

Usually formed from the sigmoid or lower descending colon, which is brought to the surface through a trephine in the left side of the abdominal wall.

Indications

- After abdomino-perineal excision for distal rectal cancers and some anal cancers.
- After a Hartmann's procedure (potentially reversible).
- Irremediable faecal incontinence.

Preparation

The patient is counselled both in elective and emergency situations. The optimal site is identified and marked preoperatively (Fig. 4.30). It is sited in the left iliac fossa clear of the umbilicus and anterior-superior iliac spine and avoiding any scars or depressions.

Position

Lithotomy.

Procedure

- WHO checklist.
- In addition to laparotomy for the major procedure, make a trephine by excising a circular area of skin over the marked stoma site. Pick up the skin with a Littlewood's forceps and excise a disc of skin ~2cm in diameter. Alternatively make a cruciate incision and trim the edges using a cutting diathermy point.
- Excise a disc of subcutaneous fat exposing the anterior rectal sheath.
- Make a cruciate incision on the anterior rectal sheath to expose the rectus abdominis muscle.

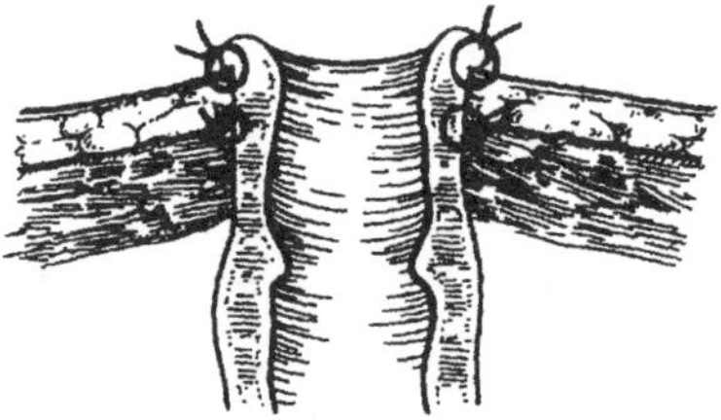

Fig. 4.29 End colostomy. Reproduced with permission from McLatchie, G, and Leaper, D. Operative Surgery 2nd edition, Oxford University Press: 2006.

- Split the rectus muscle using artery forceps gently to avoid injury to the inferior epigastric vessels.
- Retract the muscle and open the peritoneum between artery forceps. The aperture should allow the tips of two fingers through it.
- The divided, proximal end of the mobilized colon is brought through the abdominal wall aperture using Babcock forceps (Fig. 4.29).
- Close and cover the main wound.
- Excise the staple line and suture the skin edge to full thickness of bowel end using interrupted 3/0 Monocryl® sutures.

Postoperative complications

- Bleeding.
- Necrosis.
- Retraction.
- Stenosis.
- Prolapse.
- Parastomal hernia.

Loop colostomy

This is used to divert the faecal stream. The most commonly selected sites are the transverse and sigmoid colon (Fig. 4.30). Transverse colostomy should be avoided if an alternative is possible as it is prone to many complications.

Indications

- In patients with distal colonic obstruction as first part of a staged resection.
- As palliation for unresectable lesions.
- To defunction distal anastomosis.
- To protect anal operations, e.g. anal fistula or sphincter repair.

Preparation

The patient is counselled regarding the stoma. The optimal site is identified and marked preoperatively.

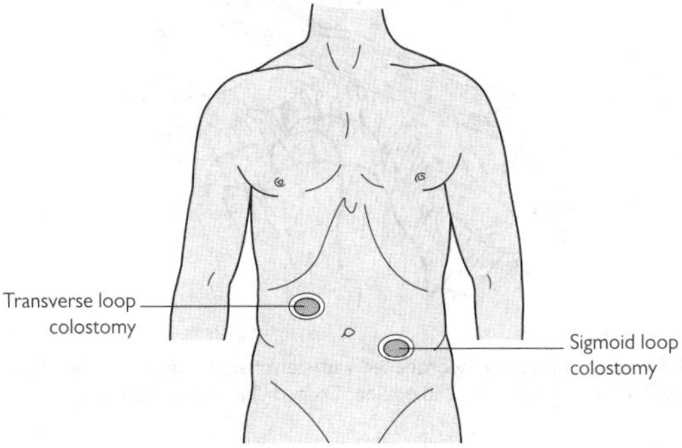
Transverse loop colostomy
Sigmoid loop colostomy

Fig. 4.30 Common sites of colostomy.

Procedure

A formal laparotomy may not be needed.

- WHO checklist.
- For a transverse colostomy, make a horizontal incision midway between the umbilicus and the costal margin in the right upper quadrant.
- Incise all the layers of the abdominal wall. Divide the muscle fibres of the rectus abdominis.
- Mobilize the transverse colon from omental adhesions. Preserve the marginal vasculature.
- Make a window close to the bowel in the transverse mesocolon. Pass a nylon tape through the window. Use this to bring the loop to the surface.
- Replace the tape with a rod. The latter supports the loop.
- Attach the bowel to the anterior rectus sheath with interrupted absorbable sutures.
- If a midline incision has been made close and cover it.
- Open the colon longitudinally. Suture the margin of the open colon to the adjacent skin edge with interrupted absorbable sutures (Fig. 4.31).
- An appropriate sized hole is cut in the stoma bag to accommodate the rod and the looped colon.

For a sigmoid loop colostomy make a left grid-iron incision. Carefully identify the sigmoid colon to make sure it is not small bowel. It has no omentum but has appendices epiploicae and taenia. Orient the loop to avoid rotation. The loop may be tethered with congenital adhesions that may need to be divided. The rest of the procedure is as described for a transverse loop colostomy (p. 185).

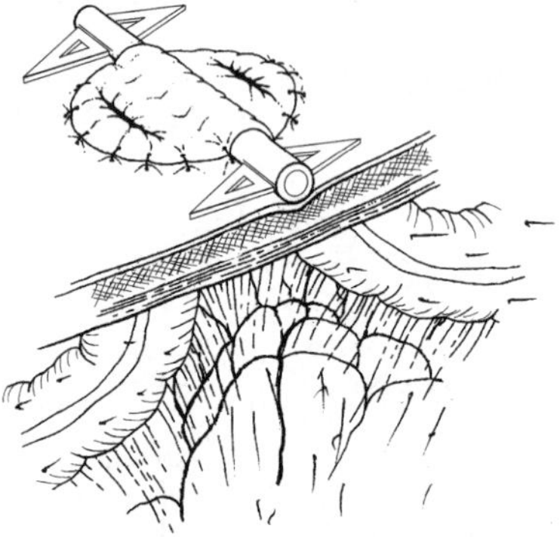

Fig. 4.31 Loop colostomy. Reproduced with permission from McLatchie, G, and Leaper, D. Operative Surgery 2nd edition, Oxford University Press: 2006.

Postoperative complications
- Bleeding.
- Necrosis.
- Retraction.
- Prolapse.
- Parastomal hernia.

Closure of loop colostomy

Indications
- When faecal stream diversion is no longer required. Check for anastomotic integrity and patency using contrast radiology and endoscopic examination prior to reversal.
- Prepare proximal colon as for any colonic anastomosis.

Procedure
- Preoperative investigations (contrast study/colonoscopy) to rule out distal obstruction are necessary.
- WHO checklist.
- Insert four muco-cutaneous stay sutures to help in mobilization. Hold the long ends on an artery forceps.
- Using cutting diathermy, incise the skin close to the muco-cutaneous junction.
- Use sharp dissection and retraction to free the colon loops from the parieties.
- Close the colostomy transversely using one-layer interrupted seromuscular extra-mucosal sutures.
- Replace the colon into the peritoneal cavity.
- Close the abdominal wall in one layer using interrupted PDS sutures. Close the skin with interrupted sutures or skin staples.

Postoperative complications
- Bleeding.
- Wound infection.
- Anastomotic leakage.

Tips and tricks
- Preoperative marking is important to select appropriate site.
- Check the orientation of colon, ensure not twisted or rotated (insufflation of air in rectum).
- Rule out distal obstruction before reversal of colostomy.

Intestinal anastomosis

The essentials for any bowel anastomosis are:
- Tension free.
- Adequate blood supply (pulsating mesenteric vessels).
- Accurate apposition using good surgical techniques.
- Minimal local spillage.

Single-layer interrupted seromuscular (extra-mucosal) technique

Mobile anastomosis (ileo-ileal, ileo-colic anastomosis)
- Line up the ends of the bowel.
- Ensure that the ends to be anastomosed are roughly equal in circumference. To achieve this make an incision on the anti-mesenteric aspect of the bowel or do an end–side anastomosis.
- Use non-crushing bowel clamps to prevent spillage.
- Isolate the operative field using moist packs.
- Use 3/0 absorbable suture material with an atraumatic round-bodied needle.
- Insert stay sutures at the mesenteric and anti-mesenteric borders; do not ligate them but place them in haemostats.
- Starting from the mesenteric aspect, place interrupted sutures along the anterior wall of the bowel 4mm apart and tie as they are placed. Each suture should perforate the bowel from the serosal surface, penetrating the muscle layer and sub-mucosa, and emerging between the mucosa and sub-mucosa (Fig. 4.32).
- Include the sub-mucosa, as this is the strongest layer of the bowel wall.
- On completion, tie both stay sutures; do not cut but replace in haemostats.

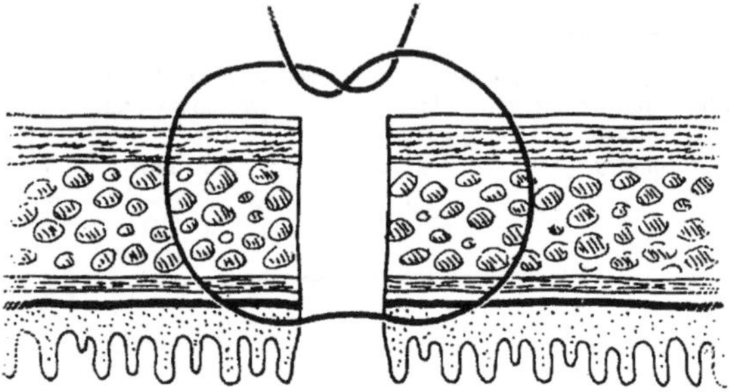

Fig. 4.32 Seromuscular suture. Reproduced with permission from McLatchie, G, and Leaper, D. Operative Surgery 2nd edition, Oxford University Press: 2006.

- Use the stay sutures to reverse the bowel. The posterior wall will now lie anteriorly.
- Suture the new front wall in a similar manner. Ensure the angles are adequately sutured.
- On completion return the stay sutures to their original position and cut them.
- Close the mesenteric defect with absorbable sutures taking care not to damage the mesenteric vessels.

Immobile anastomosis (colorectal or ileo-rectal)

- Insert stay sutures at the lateral ends of the cut end of the bowel walls. Do not ligate them but place them in haemostats.
- Insert the posterior row of seromuscular sutures, hold suture ends in individual artery forceps. Thread the artery forceps to a forceps' holder to avoid tangling. After insertion of the whole row 'parachute' the proximal bowel down to the rectum. Tie the knots; they will lie on the luminal side of the anastomosis (Fig. 4.33). Cut the knot tails.
- Perform the anterior anastomosis in a similar fashion; the knots will lie on the serosal side of the anastomosis.

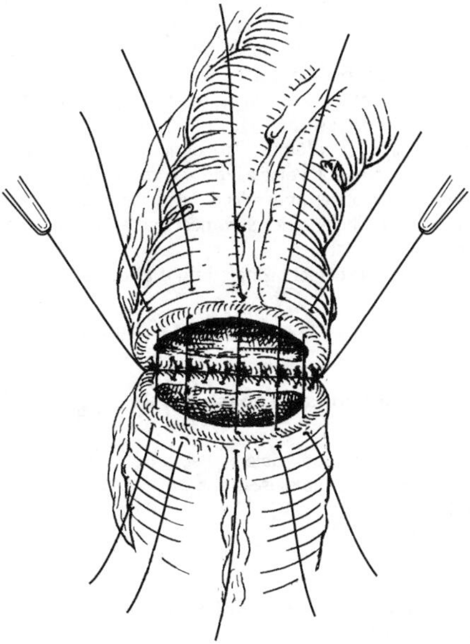

Fig. 4.33 Interrupted seromuscular single-layer anastomosis. Reproduced with permission from McLatchie, G, and Leaper, D. Operative Surgery 2nd edition, Oxford University Press: 2006.

Two-layer anastomosis

- Line up the ends of the bowel.
- Ensure that the ends to be anastomosed are roughly equal in circumference. To achieve this, make an incision on the anti-mesenteric aspect of the bowel or do an end–side anastomosis.
- Use non-crushing bowel clamps to prevent spillage.
- Isolate the operative field using moist packs.
- Use 3/0 absorbable suture material with an atraumatic round-bodied needle.
- Insert stay sutures at the mesenteric and anti-mesenteric borders; do not ligate them but place them in haemostats.
- Place a stitch between the adjacent cut edges of the bowel in the middle of the posterior wall. Continue towards one corner with full thickness over-and-over stitches. The stitches should be less than 4mm apart and pick up about 4mm of bowel wall. To turn the corner, pass the needle from the mucosa outwards on one corner to the serosa inwards on the other, followed by the mucosa outwards on the same side to the serosa inwards on the other, thus forming a series of loops on the mucosal surface (Connell suture).
- Once around the corner, leave this stitch and return to the middle of the posterior wall. Using a new length of suture insert and tie a stitch close to the site of the previous ligature. Proceed towards the opposite side turn around the corner using the technique described in the above paragraph (Connell suture). Oppose the anterior walls using over-and-over stitches and tie off the ends of the suture in the middle (Figs 4.34 and 4.35). Remove the bowel clamps.
- Place a second layer of seromuscular continuous or interrupted sutures, starting at one corner and going all the way round by rotating the bowel. The posterior layer of seromuscular sutures can be placed before the full-thickness layer. The anterior seromuscular layer being completed subsequently.
- Close the mesenteric defect taking care not to damage the mesenteric vessels.

Anastomosis using staplers is described in the topics Right hemicolectomy and Anterior resection.

Small-bowel resection and anastomosis

Indications

- Obstruction leading to non-viable bowel.
- Irreducible small-bowel intussusception.
- Mesenteric ischaemia.
- Meckel's diverticulum.
- Crohn's stricture.
- Traumatic damage.
- Tumours—primary or adherent small-bowel loop to large-bowel tumour.

Preparation

In cases of small-bowel obstruction: NG aspiration, re-hydration with intravenous fluids, correction of electrolyte abnormality.

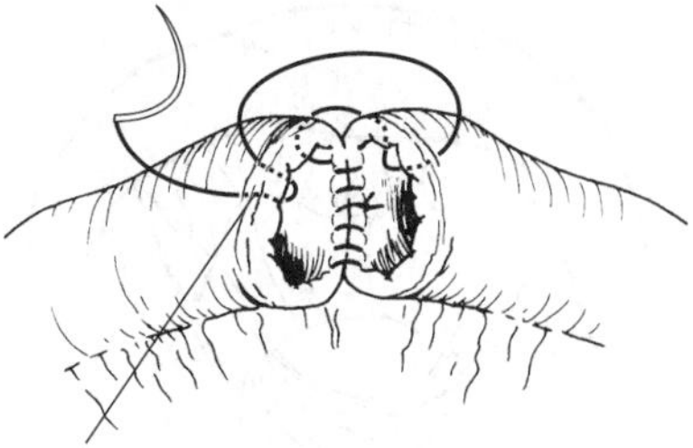
Connell inverting suture

Fig. 4.34 Two-layer anastomosis. Reproduced with permission from McLatchie, G, and Leaper, D. Operative Surgery 2nd edition, Oxford University Press: 2006.

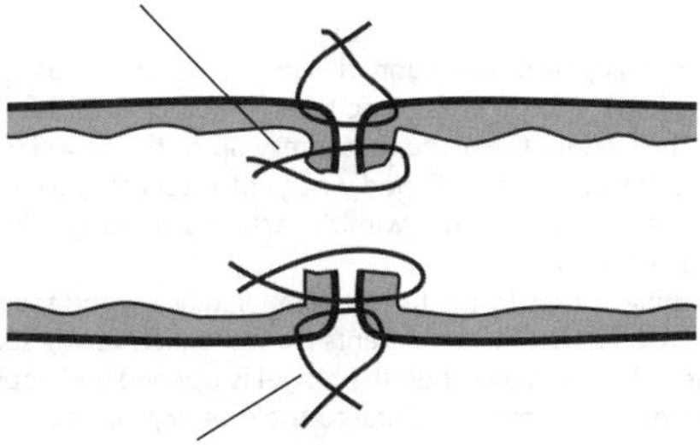
Full thickness suture
Inverting seromuscular
Lembert suture

Fig. 4.35 Two-layer anastomosis. Reproduced with permission from McLatchie, G, and Leaper, D. Operative Surgery 2nd edition, Oxford University Press: 2006.

Position

Supine.

Incision

Midline; in case of strangulated external hernia make the appropriate incision.

Procedure

- Inspect the bowel requiring resection and also the remaining bowel. Choose the resection margins (Fig. 4.36).
- Trans-illuminate the mesentery by shining a light from behind. This may not be helpful in Crohn's disease because of thickened mesentery.

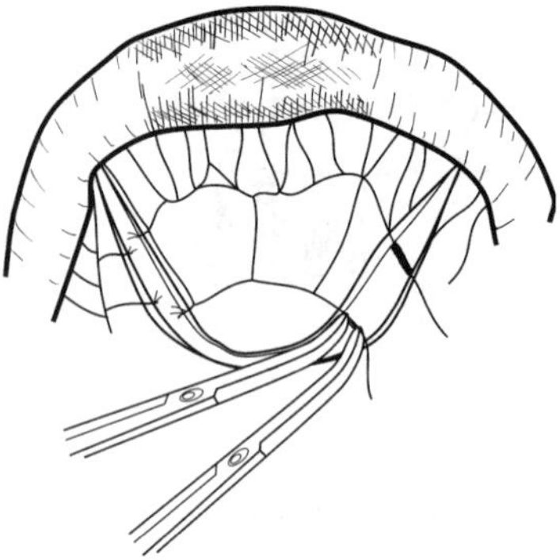

Fig. 4.36 Resection of small bowel. Reproduced with permission from McLatchie, G, and Leaper, D. Operative Surgery 2nd edition, Oxford University Press: 2006.

- Between the margins of resection, divide the mesentery using diathermy or scissors, leaving the vessels to be taken between artery forceps. Cut and ligate the vessels. Clear the mesentery up to the bowel wall. In malignant disease, take a V-shaped wedge of mesentery to remove the local lymphatic tissue that runs with the arteries. In benign disease keep close to the bowel wall.
- Apply crushing clamps to the bowel immediately beyond the point of resection. Milk the bowel contents from the intervening section to reduce the risk of spillage when the bowel is opened and apply non-crushing clamps proximal and distal to the crushing clamps.
- Divide bowel flush with the crushing clamp using a knife.
- Anastomose the two ends in one or two layers.
- Close the defect in the mesentery taking care not to damage the mesenteric vessels (Fig. 4.37).

Closure

Single-layer 1/0 PDS/Prolene® and subcuticular Monocryl®.

Postoperative complications

- Bleeding.
- Ileus.
- Small-bowel obstruction/stricture.
- Anastomotic leak.

Tips and tricks

- Ensure good vascularity of both the bowel ends.
- If there is disparity of lumens consider carrying out a side–side anastomosis

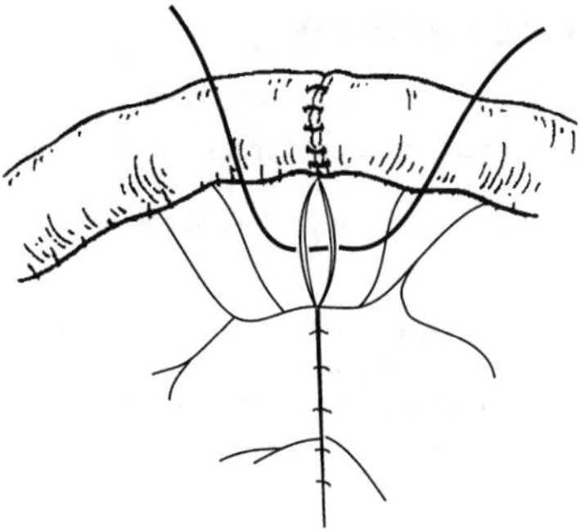

Fig. 4.37 Closure of mesentery after small-bowel resection. Reproduced with permission from McLatchie, G, and Leaper, D. Operative Surgery 2nd edition, Oxford University Press: 2006.

Right hemicolectomy

Indications

- Malignant disease affecting the caecum, ascending colon, and hepatic flexure.
- Inflammatory conditions such as Crohn's disease.

Preparation

- Bowel preparation is not necessary.
- Thromboembolism prophylaxis.
- Antibiotics administered after induction of anaesthesia.
- Urethral catheter inserted after patient has been anaesthetized.

Position

Supine.

Incision

Midline with two-thirds of the incision above the umbilicus to ease mobilization of hepatic flexure or transverse incision in right upper quadrant just above the level of umbilicus.

Procedure

- WHO checklist.
- Carry out a full laparotomy to assess resectability and metastatic spread to the liver and peritoneum. Synchronous tumours should have been excluded by preoperative colonoscopy and CT scan. If not, palpate the colon carefully (Fig. 4.38).
- Cover the small bowel with wet packs and keep it away from the operative field by tilting the table to the patient's left.
- Stand on the left side of the table and retract the right colon.
- Using diathermy, divide the peritoneum on the right para-colic gutter from the caecum to the hepatic flexure and continue this dissection to develop the plane between the mesocolon and the posterior abdominal wall. In doing so the ureter and gonadal vessels will safely fall away.
- Carefully divide the vascular omental attachments of the hepatic flexure close to the colon.
- Identify the duodenum behind the right colon and gently dissect this away. Do not dissect medial to the duodenal loop to avoid injury to the small vessels around the pancreas.
- Enter the lesser sac distal to the hepatic flexure.
- Divide the greater omentum below the gastro-epiploic arcade to the junction between proximal third and distal two-thirds of the transverse colon.
- Now move to the right side of the table.
- Lift the terminal ileum and right colon.
- Trans-illuminate the mesentery and clamp, divide and ligate the ileo-colic and right colic vessels at their origin from the superior mesenteric. Clamp, divide, and ligate the right branch of the middle colic artery.
- Clear the bowel wall at the sites of transection and apply crushing clamps.

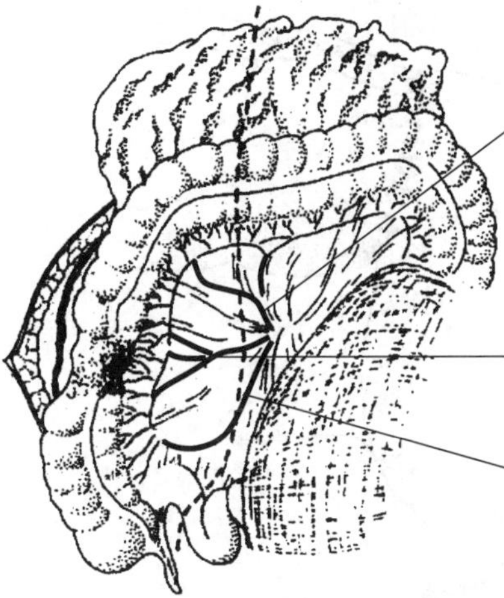
Middle colic
artery
Right colic
artery
Ileocolic
artery

Fig. 4.38 Right hemicolectomy. Reproduced with permission from McLatchie, G, and Leaper, D. Operative Surgery 2nd edition, Oxford University Press: 2006.

- Apply occlusion clamps on the proximal small bowel and distal large bowel.
- Divide the bowel on the crushing clamps leaving them on the specimen.
- An end–end anastomosis is commonly performed but end–side with closure of the end of the colon is another option (Fig. 4.39). Carry out the anastomosis either using a single layer of interrupted seromuscular 3/0 Vicryl® or PDS sutures or alternatively as a two-layer suturing technique.
- Alternatively, a stapled one-stage functional end–end anastomosis and resection can be performed.
- Loop the portion of bowel to be resected and approximate the antimesenteric borders with stay sutures.
- Make a 1cm stab wound into the lumen of both the proximal and distal limbs and insert one fork of a GIA instrument (linear cutter stapling devise) into each lumen. Routinely, a GIA80 stapler is used (Fig. 4.40).
- Apply downward traction on the stay sutures to keep the mesentery out of the stapler.
- Close the instrument and fire the staples. Two double staggered rows of staples join the bowel; simultaneously, the knife blade cuts between the two staple lines creating a stoma.
- Inspect the anastomotic staple lines for completeness and haemostasis.
- Use a Babcock forceps to oppose the ends of the staple lines.

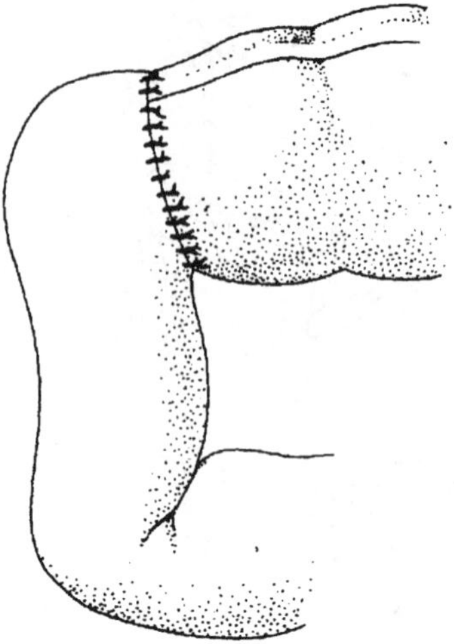

Fig. 4.39 End–end anastomosis. Reproduced with permission from McLatchie, G, and Leaper, D. Operative Surgery 2nd edition, Oxford University Press: 2006.

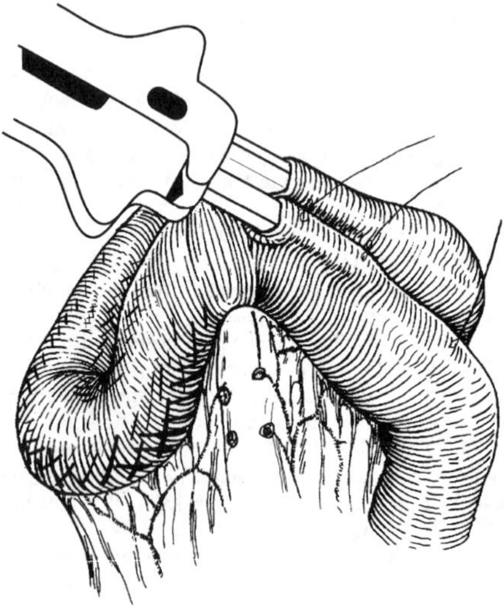

Fig. 4.40 Stapled anastomosis. Reproduced with permission from McLatchie, G, and Leaper, D. Operative Surgery 2nd edition, Oxford University Press: 2006.

- Apply another stapling devise like TA90 or GIA80 instrument across both limbs of the bowel, distal to the Babcock forceps, and fire the stapler to transect the bowel.
- Close the mesenteric window; avoid taking the vessels in the bites.
- Ensure that haemostasis is achieved and wash the peritoneal cavity with warm saline, if there was peritoneal contamination.

Closure
- Single-layer mass closure using 2/0 loop PDS.
- Skin with subcuticular Monocryl® to approximate the edges.

Postoperative complications
- Bleeding.
- Wound infection.
- Anastomotic dehiscence.
- Postoperative paralytic ileus.
- Incisional hernia.

Lesions of the transverse colon, splenic flexure, and descending colon can be treated by *extended right hemicolectomy*.

Laparoscopic right hemicolectomy
Position of patient
- In laparoscopic colorectal procedures, extreme positional changes may be required during the operation.
- A gel mattress should be present between patient and the operating table to prevent sliding.
- Straps are placed over the chest and on the thighs to prevent the patient sliding during extreme position tilt.
- Supine position with both arms wrapped at the side of the patient.
- Surgeon and assistant stand on patient's left-hand side.

Steps of operation
- WHO checklist.
- This procedure usually requires three to four ports. Achieve pneumoperitoneum after inserting a 12mm umbilical port using an open technique. Insert a 12mm port in left upper quadrant, another 5mm port in left iliac fossa. An additional 5mm port may be required in right iliac fossa (Fig. 4.41).
- This procedure is done either lateral to medial dissection (like open right hemicolectomy) or medial to lateral approach. The difference being, the ileo-colic vessels are divided first in a medial to lateral approach, which has gained in popularity.
- Tilt the table head-down and patient's right side up.
- Give gentle traction on the mesentery next to the caecum. This creates a small groove below the ileo-caecal vessels. Using a harmonic scalpel, make an incision just below the vessels and create a window.
- Continue dissection till you see the duodenum. Safeguard the duodenum. Do not dissect medial to the duodenum.
- Divide the ileo-colic vessels by a vascular stapler gun or in between vascular clips near its origin from the superior mesenteric vessels.

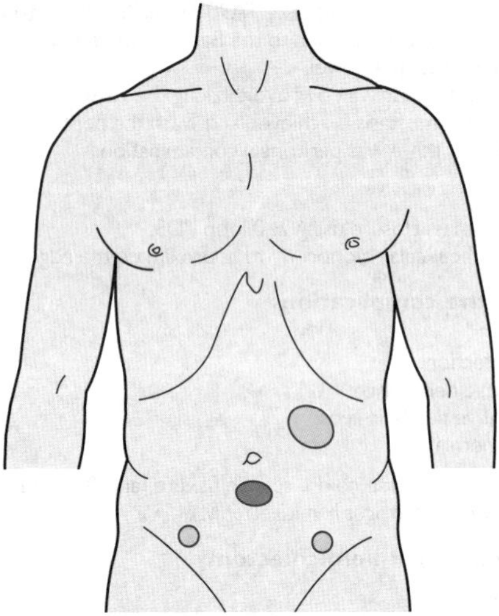

Fig. 4.41 Port sites for Laparoscopic right hemicolectomy.

- Continue the dissection laterally in the avascular plane above Gerota's fascia, safeguarding the ureter and gonadal vessels.
- Mobilize the caecum and ascending colon by incising the lateral peritoneal reflection and pulling it towards the midline.
- Continue to mobilize hepatic flexure, safeguarding the duodenum. A head-up tilt facilitates this step. Separate the greater omentum from the proximal transverse colon and hepatic flexure.
- Divide right colic vessels and the right branch of middle colic vessel.
- For an *intracorporeal ileo-colic anastomosis* divide the terminal ileum and transverse colon with an endoscopic linear cutter stapling devise. Move the completely freed specimen up towards the liver. Place the divided terminal ileum and transverse colon side by side. Make a stab incision in the transverse colon about 8cm from its cut end and in the terminal ileum about 2cm from its cut end.
- Insert the ends of a linear cutter stapling devise into the colon and ileum and create a stoma between the two. Close the enterotomy with continuous 3/0 Vicryl® extramucosal seromuscular sutures.
- Remove the specimen after extending the port site at the umbilicus or left iliac fossa and placing an Alexis wound protector.
- For *extra corporeal ileo-colic anastomosis* extend the umbilical port incision to about 4–5cm and open the peritoneum. Place an Alexis wound protector in the wound to avoid any tumour seedlings during extraction of the specimen.

- Extract the specimen outside and perform a functional end–end stapled or end–end/side–side hand-sewn anastomosis.
- Usually it is not necessary to close the mesenteric defects and drains are not necessary.
- Close the wounds in layers.
- Follow enhanced recovery protocol.

Postoperative complications

Similar to open surgery, as discussed in 'Right hemicolectomy' (p. 197).

Tips and tricks

- Small transverse incision in right upper quadrant gives good access and better recovery compared to midline incision.
- Maintain traction of tissues while dissecting to find appropriate planes.
- Small and thready vessels in retro-peritoneum are the best guide to finding the correct plane.

Sigmoid colectomy/left hemicolectomy

Indications

- Neoplastic lesions involving descending colon or sigmoid colon.
- Complex, symptomatic diverticular disease.

Preparation

- Thromboembolism prophylaxis.
- Prophylactic antibiotics administered after induction of anaesthesia.
- Urethral catheter inserted after patient has been anaesthetized.

Position

Lloyd–Davies.

Incision

Lower midline with some extension above umbilicus.

Procedure

- WHO checklist.
- Ascertain resectability of tumour, presence of liver metastases, peritoneal deposits, and synchronous tumours (Fig. 4.42).

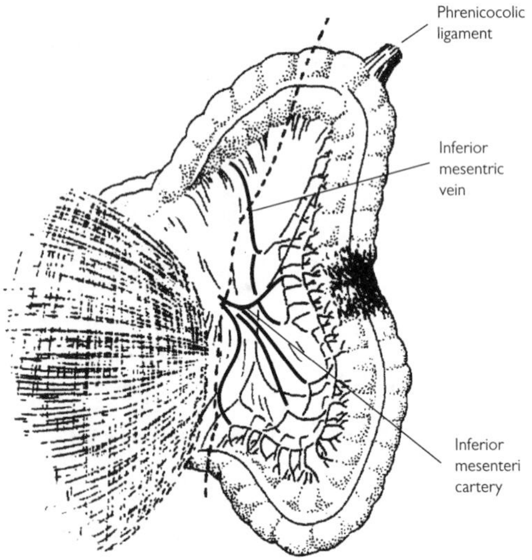
Phrenicocolic ligament
Inferior mesentric vein
Inferior mesenteri cartery

Fig. 4.42 Left hemicolectomy. Reproduced with permission from McLatchie, G, and Leaper, D. Operative Surgery 2nd edition, Oxford University Press: 2006.

- Cover the small bowel with wet packs and keep it away from the operative field by tilting the table to the patient's right.
- Stand on the right side of the table and retract the sigmoid colon medially.
- Ask the assistant to retract the lower left abdominal wall.
- Divide the peritoneum lateral to the sigmoid and descending colon along the 'white line' of fusion using diathermy.
- Develop the plane between the mesentery and the retro-peritoneum. In the process, sigmoid mesocolon is swept away from retro-peritoneal structures behind it like gonadal vessels and ureter (Fig. 4.43). Identify and safeguard the hypo-gastric nerves.
- Lift the descending colon and its mesentery off Gerota's fascia.
- Separate the greater omentum from the distal transverse colon.
- Continue the incision along the left para-colic gutter upwards towards the splenic flexure.
- For splenic flexure tumours the gastro-colic omentum is divided and the omentum removed with the specimen.
- Now grasp both limbs of the colon and under vision divide the peritoneum at the flexure. Bring the colon out of its splenic bed. Take care during the mobilization of the splenic flexure that the tip of the retractor held by the assistant does not damage the spleen and avoid undue traction on the omentum during this manoeuvre as the splenic capsule can be torn.

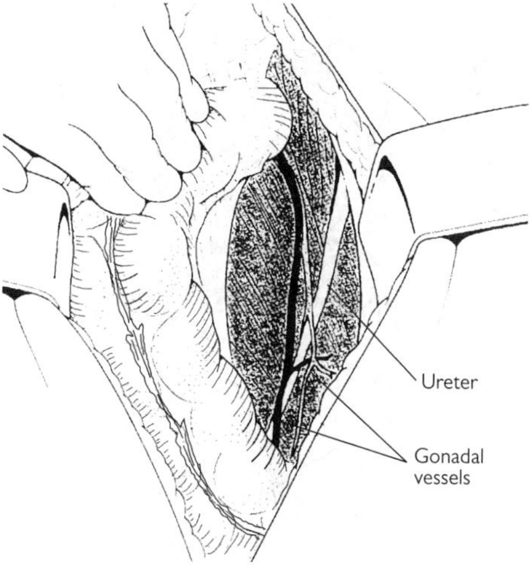
Ureter
Gonadal vessels

Fig. 4.43 Mobilization of left colon. Reproduced with permission from McLatchie, G, and Leaper, D. Operative Surgery 2nd edition, Oxford University Press: 2006.

- Lift up the sigmoid colon and divide the peritoneum on the right side from the origin of the inferior mesenteric artery down to the level of the sacral promontory.
- Pass a finger under the sigmoid colon and define the origin of the inferior mesenteric artery.
- Double clamp, divide, and doubly ligate the inferior mesenteric artery.
- Then clamp, divide, and ligate the inferior mesenteric vein below the inferior border of the pancreas, taking care not to tear this vessel.
- Divide the transverse mesocolon at a convenient point. Isolate and ligate the marginal artery.
- Divide the transverse colon between occlusion and crushing clamps.
- Similarly divide the colon at the recto-sigmoid junction between Hayes' clamps.
- Move to the left side of the table.
- Make sure there is no tension at the bowel ends and that it is adequately vascularized.
- Restore bowel continuity by using a single layer of 3/0 PDS interrupted seromuscular sutures (Fig. 4.44).

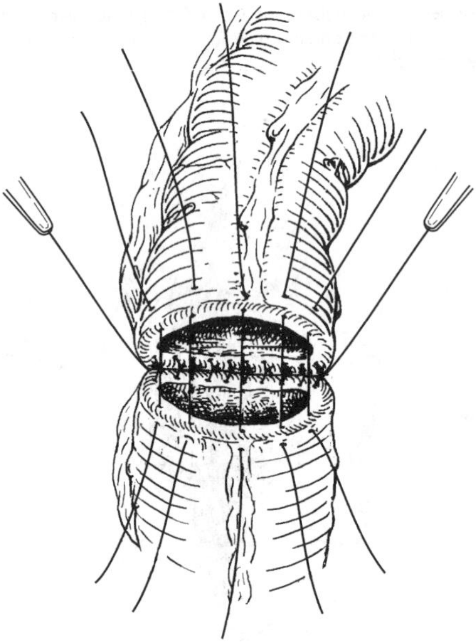

Fig. 4.44 Interrupted seromuscular single-layer anastomosis. Reproduced with permission from McLatchie, G, and Leaper, D. Operative Surgery 2nd edition, Oxford University Press: 2006.

- For a *stapled anastomosis* divide the rectosigmoid junction of the colon with stapler device. Insert 2/0 Prolene® purse-string suture to the proximal cut end of the colon and tie it around the anvil of the circular stapler.
- Insert circular stapling gun through the anus to create a colorectal anastomosis (Fig. 4.45).
- Check the donuts for completeness.
- Perform a leak test by insufflating air through a sigmoidoscope introduced per-anally and filling the peritoneal cavity with normal saline.
- Do a washout of the peritoneal cavity. Water is preferred for cytotoxic properties in cases of malignancy.
- Usually there is no need for a drain.

Closure

In a single layer, using number 1 Prolene® and the skin with subcuticular Monocryl®.

Laparoscopic sigmoid colectomy

Position of the patient

Lloyd–Davies.

Procedure

- WHO checklist should be performed.
- The surgeon and assistant stand on right side of the patient.
- Achieve pneumoperitoneum after inserting a 10 mm umbilical port using an open technique. Place a 12mm port in right iliac fossa. Insert a 5mm port in the right upper quadrant or epigastric region. Put a 5mm port in left iliac fossa.

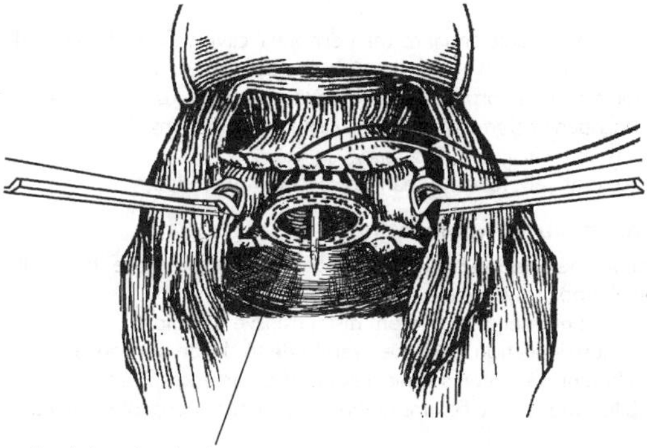
Anvil placed in distal segment

Fig. 4.45 Stapled anastomosis. Reproduced with permission from McLatchie, G, and Leaper, D. Operative Surgery 2nd edition, Oxford University Press: 2006.

- Tilt patient head-down and right-side down to keep small bowel away from dissection site.
- In order to avoid injury to the bowel, it is helpful to stack the small bowel loops in the right upper quadrant by flip technique, rather than pushing with instruments.
- Retract sigmoid colon upwards and laterally.
- Identify sacral promontory and sigmoid mesocolon clearly.
- Incise the peritoneum at the base of the mesocolon near the sacral promotary and extend towards the origin of the inferior mesenteric vessels.
- Dissect through the loose areolar tissue just behind the inferior mesenteric vessels.
- Isolate inferior mesenteric vessels. Divide with Endo GIA vascular stapler or between vascular clips about 2cm distal to its origin.
- Using retraction, identify tissue plane and continue dissection upwards and laterally between the mesocolon and Toldt's fascia.
- Divide inferior mesenteric vein between vascular clips lateral to duodeno-jejunal flexure.
- Divide lateral attachments of sigmoid and descending colon and meet the dissection plane created from medial side.
- Dissect the sigmoid colon below the pelvic reflection and divide with Endo GIA at a suitable site, after dividing the mesocolon/mesorectum with a harmonic scalpel.
- For sigmoid colectomy, usually there is no need to mobilize the splenic flexure, but it is necessary for left hemicolectomy.
- Extend the incision at one of the port sites, umbilical or left iliac fossa.
- Use an Alexis™ wound protector. Extract the specimen.
- Divide the colon and apply a purse string. Insert the anvil of the circular stapler.
- Return the colonic end into the peritoneal cavity. Twist the wound protector to obtain a seal. Regain pneumoperitoneum.
- Perform an intra-corporeal end-to-end anastomosis using a circular stapler, as described in 'Sigmoid colectomy/left hemicolectomy' (p. 200).
- Drains are usually not necessary.
- Postoperatively, follow enhanced recovery protocol.

Splenic flexure mobilization

- Change the position of the patient to head up and move the small-bowel loops towards the right iliac fossa.
- Dissect the omentum off from distal transverse colon.
- Continue dissection from the lateral side to divide peritoneal attachments between splenic flexure of colon and spleen.
- Mobilize the splenic flexure down, keeping the mesocolon intact.

Postoperative complications

- Bleeding.
- Anastomotic dehiscence.
- Postoperative paralytic ileus.
- Wound infection.
- Incisional hernia.

Tips and tricks

- Stacking up the small bowel and keeping it away from the field of operation is key to progress the operation.
- Avascular plane between mesocolon and retroperitoneal structures is found in front of the thready vessels.
- Traction in right direction and counter-traction is key to finding the correct tissue planes.

Transverse colectomy

Transverse colectomy in isolation is performed rarely. It is done usually as a part of extended right hemicolectomy for tumours in transverse colon or splenic flexure.

Indications

Malignant tumour of the mid-transverse colon.

Preparation

As described in 'Sigmoid colectomy/left hemicolectomy' (p. 200).

Position

Supine.

Incision

Upper midline or transverse.

Procedure

- WHO checklist.
- Ascertain resectability of tumour, presence of liver metastases, peritoneal deposits, and synchronous tumours (Fig. 4.46).
- Separate the omentum from the stomach below the gastro-epiploic vessels.
- Mobilize the hepatic and splenic flexures of the colon. The latter step may not be needed if there is a long transverse colon.
- A wedge resection based on the middle colic vessels is then undertaken with at least 5cm clearance from a malignant tumour.
- Clamp, divide, and ligate the middle colic artery at its origin.

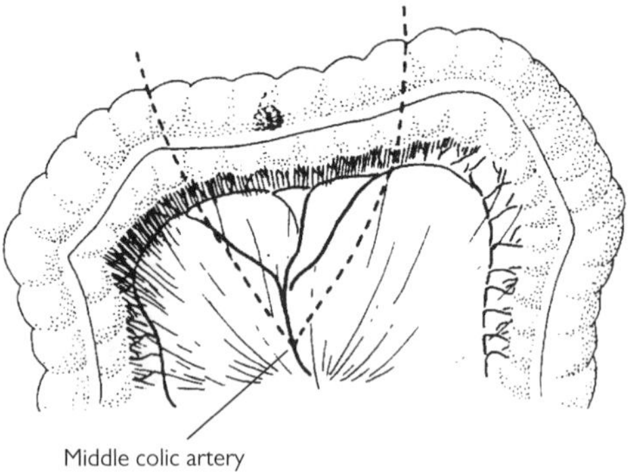
Middle colic artery

Fig. 4.46 Transverse colectomy. Reproduced with permission from McLatchie, G, and Leaper, D. Operative Surgery 2nd edition, Oxford University Press: 2006.

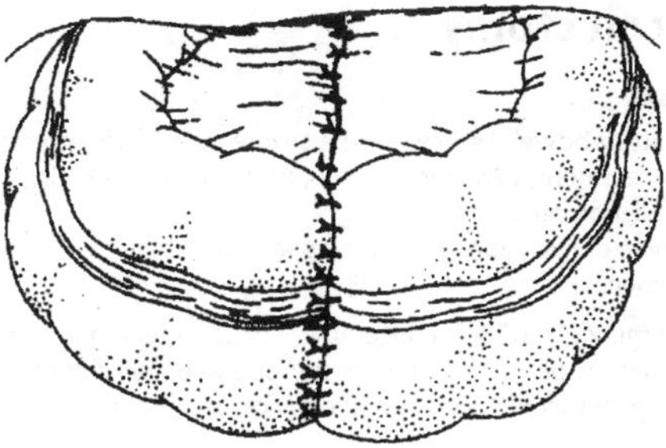

Fig. 4.47 Single layer interrupted anastomosis. Reproduced with permission from McLatchie, G, and Leaper, D. Operative Surgery 2nd edition, Oxford University Press: 2006.

- Clamp, divide, and ligate the mesocolon and marginal vessels up to the sites of bowel resection.
- Restore bowel continuity by using a single layer of 3/0 PDS interrupted seromuscular sutures (Fig. 4.47).
- Drain is usually not necessary.

Closure

Close the abdominal wall using single layer number 1 loop PDS, skin with subcuticular Monocryl®.

Postoperative complications

- Bleeding.
- Anastomotic dehiscence.
- Postoperative paralytic ileus.
- Wound infection.
- Incisional hernia.

Total colectomy

Indications

- Inflammatory bowel disease—acute severe colitis failing to respond to medical treatment, toxic mega-colon, perforation, bleeding.
- Familial adenomatous polyposis.
- Left colonic obstruction with caecal perforation.
- Colonic inertia.

In the emergency setting for ulcerative colitis, colectomy with ileostomy and preservation of rectal stump is the operation of choice. Subsequent restorative proctocolectomy and avoidance of permanent ileostomy is a possibility.

Preparation

- Carry out adequate resuscitation when procedure done as an emergency.
- Administer prophylactic antibiotics.
- Thromboembolism prophylaxis.
- Catheterize.
- Counsel patient and have ileostomy site marked by stoma nurse.
- Bowel preparation is not required for total colectomy.

Position

Lloyd–Davies.

Incision

Midline.

Procedure

- WHO checklist.
- When carrying out emergency colectomy for inflammatory bowel disease, insert proctoscope to deflate bowel.
- Make the trephine for the ileostomy before opening the abdomen.
- Handle bowel with care to avoid perforation.
- Start with mobilizing the right colon.
- Divide bowel at the ileo-caecal junction with a linear stapler.
- Continue mobilizing the colon, ligating or transfixing relevant vessels (Fig. 4.48).
- Divide bowel at recto-sigmoid junction or at pelvic brim. Leaving part of sigmoid colon (usually the most diseased part of the bowel) increases the morbidity and risk of stump blow out.
- Wash the rectal stump with betadine and saline solution and leave a Foley's catheter for drainage.

Colectomy with ileo-rectal anastomosis can be carried out in selected cases of chronic inflammatory bowel disease, slow transit constipation, and for familial adenomatous polyposis. Follow the steps for colectomy. Carry out a hand-sutured or stapled ileo-rectal anastomosis.

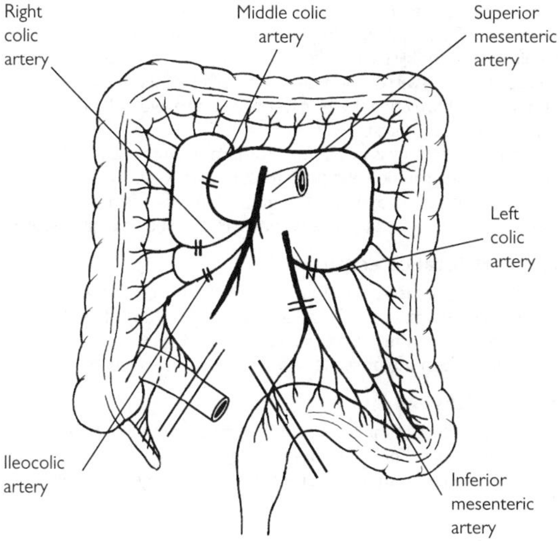
Right
colic
artery
Middle colic
artery
Superior
mesenteric
artery
Left
colic
artery
Ileocolic
artery
Inferior
mesenteric
artery

Fig. 4.48 Total colectomy. Reproduced with permission from McLatchie, G, and Leaper, D. Operative Surgery 2nd edition, Oxford University Press: 2006.

Postoperative complications

- Bleeding.
- Wound infection.
- Anastomotic dehiscence.
- Stoma complications.
- Rectal stump suture line breakdown.

Laparoscopic total colectomy

Preparation and position

As described in 'Total colectomy' (p. 208).

Procedure

- This procedure requires a minimum of five ports. Using an open technique, insert 11mm port at the umbilicus. Create pneumoperitoneum. Place another 11mm port in the right iliac fossa under vison. Place a further three 5mm ports in the right upper quadrant, left upper quadrant, and left iliac fossa.
- The procedure can be started with mobilizing the right colon, as described in 'Right hemicolectomy' (p. 194) or mobilizing sigmoid colon, as described in 'Sigmoid colectomy/left hemicolectomy' (p. 200).

- Many surgeons prefer to mobilize the sigmoid colon first and divide the rectum. Then mobilize the descending colon upwards to complete splenic flexure mobilization.
- Mobilize the transverse colon taking the middle colic vessels. Maintain caution while mobilizing the transverse colon to avoid damage to the duodenum and stomach.
- If the total colectomy is performed for inflammatory bowel disease, the dissection plane can be kept close to the bowel wall.
- The specimen can be extracted from the right iliac fossa port by extending the 11mm port. This wound can be used to create ileostomy.

Single port total colectomy

A multichannel port is inserted at the site of the ileostomy. Procedure is performed as described in 'Total colectomy' (p. 208). The dissection is started by mobilizing the left colon and continued proximally. The specimen is taken out through the port site. An end ileostomy is created.

Tips and tricks

- Divide the rectum at the level of the sacral promontory to preserve the pelvic tissue planes for future pouch surgery.
- Wash out the rectal stump to prevent mucus spillage in case of stump blowout.

Anterior resection

When part of rectum (high anterior resection) or complete rectum (low anterior resection) is removed along with sigmoid colon, it is called anterior resection.

Indication

Carcinoma of the rectum, where sphincter preservation is possible. High anterior resection is done for tumours of rectosigmoid junction and upper rectum. Low anterior resection entails the removal of complete rectum and mesorectum. For low anterior resections, defunctioning stoma is made.

Preparation

As described in 'Sigmoid colectomy/left hemicolectomy' (p. 200). The stoma nurse marks the ileostomy site (for defunctioning).

Position

Lloyd–Davies.

Incision

Long midline.

High anterior resection

Procedure

(See Fig. 4.49)

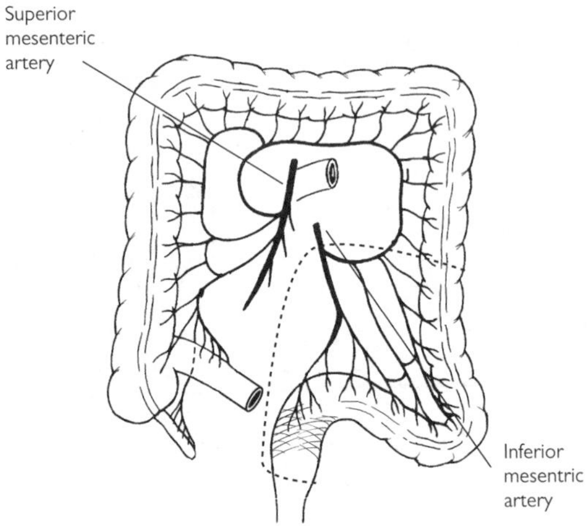
Superior mesenteric artery
Inferior mesentric artery

Fig. 4.49 Anterior resection. Reproduced with permission from McLatchie, G, and Leaper, D. Operative Surgery 2nd edition, Oxford University Press: 2006.

- WHO checklist.
- Stand on the right side of the table.
- Assess the position and resectability of the tumour. Assess liver and peritoneum for metastatic deposits and colon for synchronous tumours.
- Keep the small bowel away from operating field by tilting the patient to the right and covering the small bowel with moist packs.
- Retract the sigmoid colon to the midline and have the assistant retract the lower left abdominal wall.
- Using diathermy, divide the peritoneum along the 'white line'.
- Develop a plane between the mesentery and retro-peritoneum. In the process, the mesocolon is swept away from the ureter and the gonadal vessels. Identify and preserve these along with the hypo-gastric nerves.
- Lift the descending colon and its mesentery off Gerota's fascia.
- Separate the greater omentum from the distal transverse colon and continue the dissection laterally towards the flexure.
- Extend the dissection along the left para-colic gutter towards the splenic flexure.
- Grasp both limbs of the colon and, under vision, divide the peritoneum at the flexure. The colon can now be brought out of its splenic bed. Take care during the mobilization of the splenic flexure that the the retractor tip held by the assistant does not damage the spleen. Avoid undue traction on the omentum during this manoeuvre as the splenic capsule can be torn.
- Hold the sigmoid colon and descending colon up; divide the peritoneum on the right side from the origin of the inferior mesenteric artery to the level of the sacral promontory.
- Identify and preserve the right ureter.
- Pass a finger under the sigmoid colon and define the origin of the inferior mesenteric artery. Apply three artery forceps and divide the vessel between the two proximal forceps. This allows double ligation of the artery remnant.
- Clamp, divide, and ligate the inferior mesenteric vein below the inferior border of the pancreas.
- Divide the mesocolon at the descending sigmoid colon junction ligating and dividing the marginal vessels.
- Transect the colon at this level using a side–side stapler.
- Now pack the small bowel and mobilized colon into the upper abdomen using two large moist packs. Place a Goligher's retractor to retract the wound edges, using the central blade to hold the bowel in place.
- Remove the side tilt to the table and apply a head-down tilt.
- Move to the patient's left side to carry out the pelvic dissection.
- When present, the uterus can be hitched up by two sutures inserted through each broad ligament.
- Hold the sigmoid colon up and, using diathermy, develop the plane behind the superior rectal vessels.
- Identify and preserve the pre-sacral nerves as they cross the pelvic brim medial to the ureters.

- Carry on the dissection in the avascular plane between the mesorectum and the pre-sacral fascia posteriorly. Keeping in this plane dissect the lateral aspects of the mesorectum.
- Having reached the level of the peritoneal reflection, assess whether further mobilization is needed.
- Aim for a 2cm clearance below the distal margin of the tumour and a 5cm clearance of the mesorectum.
- Then dissect anterior to Denonvillier's fascia, between the rectum and the bladder, seminal vesicles and prostate in men and the bladder and vagina in women.
- Divide the mesorectum at the selected level. Pinch the mesorectum between the index finger and the thumb off the rectum. Insert two right-angled clamps through this window and cut between them. Transfix the mesorectum held in the clamps.
- Then apply a right-angled clamp across the rectum.
- Irrigate the rectum with Betadine or another tumouricidal aqueous antiseptic agent using a Foley's catheter introduced per-anally.
- Apply another right-angled clamp below the previous one.
- Transect the rectum between the clamps.
- Remove the clamp on the rectal stump and apply Babcock's forceps to the cut edge. Suck any Betadine from the lumen.
- Place a purse-string suture using 2/0 Prolene®, no more than 2.5mm from the cut edge to avoid tissue bunching.
- Remove the staple line on the colonic end and, similarly, place a purse-string suture. Insert the detached anvil of an end–end type circular stapler into the lumen and securely tie the purse-string suture around the shaft.
- Insert the stapler per-anally and unwind the stapler so the rod exits completely through the open rectal end. Secure the purse-string suture around the rod.
- Mate the central shaft of the anvil with the instrument shaft by pushing firmly until the shaft clicks into its fully seated position. Turn the wing nut clockwise to approximate the tissue and to close the space between the cartridge and anvil (Fig. 4.50).
- Fire the stapler when close approximation is obtained (green colour appears on the window—adhere to manufacturer's instructions) (Fig. 4.51). Unwind and remove the stapler.
- Check to see the doughnuts are complete.
- Fill the pelvis with normal saline. Check for any leaks by insufflating air through a sigmoidoscope inserted into the rectum.
- Irrigate the peritoneal cavity.
- Leave a drain in close proximity to the anastomosis.
- The rectum can be divided with a right-angled stapling device below the clamp after rectal wash. Anastomosis is completed using a circular stapling devices as described in 'Low anterior resection' (p. 215).
- Alternatively, a hand-sewn anastomosis can be performed using interrupted seromuscular extra-mucosal 3/0 PDS sutures.

Closure

Close the abdomen in a single 'mass' layer using number 1 loop PDS, with subcuticular Monocryl® for the skin.

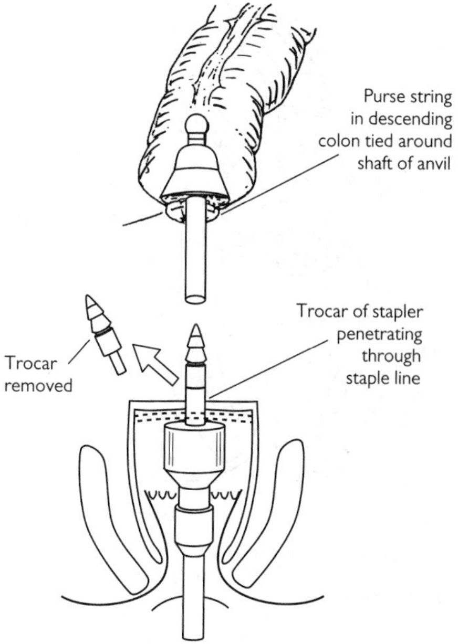
Purse string
in descending
colon tied around
shaft of anvil
Trocar of stapler
penetrating
through
staple line
Trocar
removed

Fig. 4.50 Stapled anastomosis: after anterior resection. Reproduced with permission from McLatchie, G, and Leaper, D. Operative Surgery 2nd edition, Oxford University Press: 2006.

Low anterior resection

Procedure

- Continue the rectal mobilization to the pelvic floor performing a total mesorectal excision.
- Cross-staple the rectum using a TA30 or 45.
- Carry out a Betadine washout of the rectum.
- Cross-staple the rectum below the previous staple line.
- Transact the rectum flush on the stapler.
- Open and remove the stapler.
- Insert the anvil of the circular stapler in to the cut end of the colon and tie purse string suture around the anvil.
- Insert the end–end stapler with the sharpened point retracted into the rectal stump and bring it up to the staple line.
- Advance the spike so that it appears posterior to the staple line.
- Mate the central shaft of the anvil with the instrument shaft and approximate the two ends.

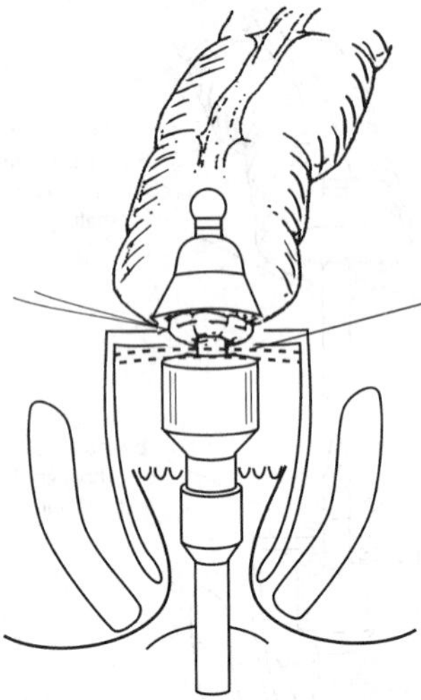
Stapler
approximated
and ready for
firing

Fig. 4.51 Stapled anastomosis: after approximation of end–end stapler. Reproduced with permission from McLatchie, G, and Leaper, D. Operative Surgery 2nd edition, Oxford University Press: 2006.

- Fire the stapler after the green spot appears in the window (check manufacturer's instructions).
- Check for completeness of the doughnuts.
- Perform a leak test, as described in 'High anterior resection' (p. 212). A 5cm colonic pouch can be fashioned by linear cutter stapler and a colo-pouch anal anastomosis made instead of the straight colo-anal anastomosis described. Colopouch-anal anastomosis provide better function.
- Leave a suction drain in the hollow of the pelvis.
- Washout the peritoneal cavity.
- Make a trephine in the marked site in the right iliac fossa and pull out a loop of terminal ileum to create a defunctioning stoma after closing the abdomen.

Closure

Close the abdomen in a single mass layer using number 1 Prolene®, with subcuticular Monocryl® for the skin. Make the *loop ileostomy* as described in 'Ileostomy—formation and closure' (p. 178).

Laparoscopic anterior resection

Position

Lloyd–Davies.

Port position

An 11mm port is placed parallel to the umbilicus in the mid-clavicular line on the right side. One more 11mm port is placed in the right iliac fossa to introduce the stapling device for dividing the rectum. Three 5mm ports are introduced under vision in the right upper quadrant, parallel to the first 11mm port on the opposite side and one in the left iliac fossa.

Procedure

- Initial steps of the operation are same as for 'Sigmoid colectomy/left hemicolectomy' (p. 200) to mobilize left colon and divide the inferior mesenteric artery and vein.
- Completely mobilize the splenic flexure by continuing the dissection on the lateral side of the descending colon. Free the omentum from the distal transverse colon.
- Retract the rectosigmoid area upwards and anteriorly to see loose areolar tissue plane outside mesorectal fascia. Dissect this plane with hook diathermy and gentle retraction.
- Divide the peritoneum on the right lateral side of the rectum and extend the posterior dissection to the lateral side.
- Divide the peritoneum anteriorly 1cm above the peritoneal reflexion and dissect in front of Denonvillier's fascia.
- Divide the peritoneum on the left lateral side and complete the dissection all around.
- Depending on the level of resection planned, the mesorectum is divided using an harmonic scalpel.
- Divide the rectum with endo stapler at required level after rectal washout.
- For low anterior resection, continue dissection around mesorectum down to the pelvic floor. Divide rectum with a laparoscopic stapler.
- Extend the incision at the port site. Protect the wound. Extract the specimen. Divide the mesocolon and colon at required level.
- Apply a purse string to the cut end of the colon. Tie the purse string around the anvil of the circular stapler.
- The colo-rectal/colo-anal (low anterior resection) anastomosis is completed, as described in 'Anterior resection' (p. 212).

Postoperative complications

- Bleeding.
- Wound infection.
- Postoperative paralytic ileus.
- Anastomotic dehiscence.
- Anastomotic stricture.
- Urinary and sexual dysfunction.
- Incisional hernia.

Tips and tricks

- Mobilize the splenic flexure completely for tension-free anastomosis.
- Stay close to the inferior mesenteric artery when entering the total mesorectal excision (TME) plane to prevent injury to pelvic nerves.
- Give rectal washout before division.

Panproctocolectomy

Removal of the colon, rectum, and anus.

Indications

- Ulcerative colitis where medical treatment fails or there is malignant transformation, performed in patients where a sphincter-saving procedure is not desirable or suitable.
- Colonic Crohn's disease.
- Synchronous colonic and rectal cancers.
- Familial adenomatous polyposis (for those with low rectal cancers).

Preparation

As described in 'Sigmoid colectomy/left hemicolectomy' (p. 200). Ileostomy site marked by stoma nurse.

Position

Lloyd–Davies with perineum protruding 5cm from lower edge of table.

Incision

Midline.

Procedure

(See Fig. 4.52)

- Make the trephine for the ileostomy before opening the abdomen.
- Start with mobilizing the right colon.
- Divide the bowel at the ileo-caecal junction with a linear stapler.
- Follow the steps as described in the topics Right hemicolectomy, Sigmoid colectomy/left hemicolectomy, Transverse colectomy, and Anterior resection, when mobilizing the colon and rectum. Preservation of the greater omentum is not necessary.
- When carcinoma or dysplasia is present, perform wide clearance with high ligation of the lympho-vascular pedicle.
- Mobilize the rectum performing a total mesorectal excision, preserving the pre-sacral nerves. In benign cases the rectum can be removed by close (peri-muscular) dissection.
- Do the perineal dissection by entering the inter-sphincteric plane.
- Follow the steps as described in 'Ileostomy—formation and closure' (p. 178).

Postoperative complications

- Bleeding.
- Wound Infection.
- Paralytic ileus.
- Delayed healing of perineal wound.
- Urinary or sexual dysfunction.
- Ileostomy related complications.

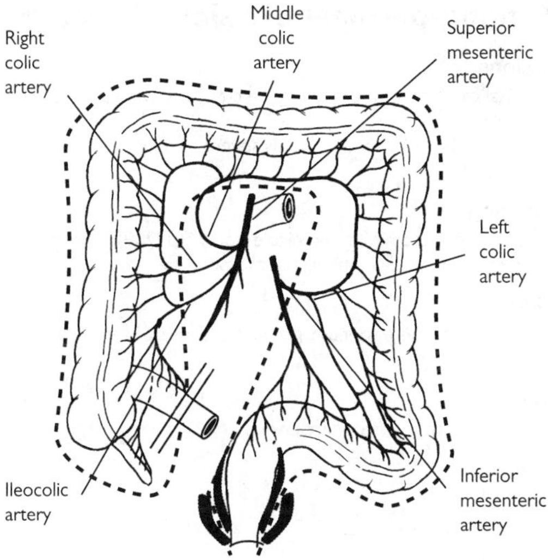
Middle colic artery
Right colic artery
Superior mesenteric artery
Left colic artery
Ileocolic artery
Inferior mesenteric artery

Fig. 4.52 Proctocolectomy and Ileostomy. Reproduced with permission from McLatchie, G, and Leaper, D. Operative Surgery 2nd edition, Oxford University Press: 2006.

Abdomino-perineal excision of rectum

Indications

- Low rectal carcinoma where adequate clearance will not be obtained by anterior resection.
- Inflammatory bowel disease, such as severe Crohn's disease with multiple fistulae.

Preparation

As in 'Sigmoid colectomy/left hemicolectomy' (p. 200). The stoma nurse marks the colostomy site in the left iliac fossa.

Position

Lloyd–Davies with the perineum projecting 5cm from the lower edge of the table.

Incision

Midline or lower transverse (Pfannenstiel).

Procedure

(See Fig. 4.53)

- Stand on the right side of the table.

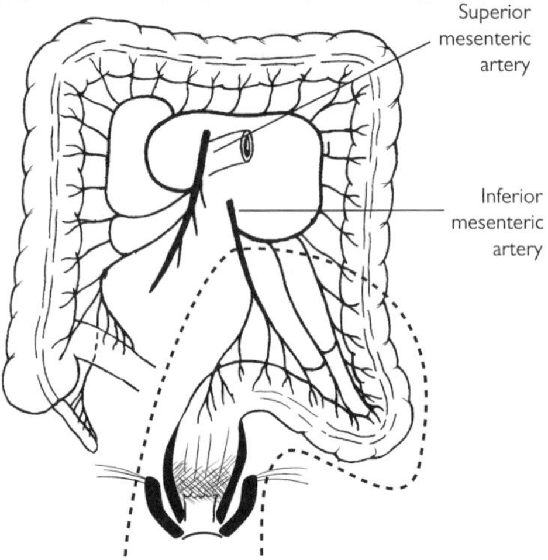
Superior
mesenteric
artery
Inferior
mesenteric
artery

Fig. 4.53 Abdomino-perineal excision of rectum. Reproduced with permission from McLatchie, G, and Leaper, D. Operative Surgery 2nd edition, Oxford University Press: 2006.

- Assess the liver and peritoneum for metastatic deposits and the colon for synchronous tumours.
- Keep the small bowel away from the operating field by tilting the patient to the right and covering the small bowel with moist packs.
- Retract the sigmoid colon to the midline and have the assistant retract the lower left abdominal wall.
- Using diathermy, divide the peritoneum along the 'white line'. Develop a plane between the mesocolon and the retro-peritoneum. In the process the mesocolon is swept away from the retroperitoneum. Identify the gonadal vessels and ureter. Safeguard these along with the hypo-gastric nerves.
- Lift the descending colon and its mesentery off Gerota's fascia.
- The splenic flexure mobilization is not routinely required.
- Hold the sigmoid colon and descending colon up. Divide the peritoneum on the right side from the origin of the inferior mesenteric artery to the level of the sacral promontory.
- Identify and preserve the right ureter.
- Pass a finger under the sigmoid colon and define the origin of the inferior mesenteric artery. Apply three artery forceps and divide the vessel between the two proximal forceps. This allows double ligation of the artery remnant.
- Clamp, divide, and ligate the inferior mesenteric vein.
- Divide the mesocolon at the descending sigmoid junction, ligating and dividing the marginal vessels.
- Transect the colon at this level using a GIA stapler.
- Now pack the small bowel and mobilized colon into the upper abdomen using two large moist packs.
- Place a Goligher's retractor to retract the wound edges, use the central blade to hold the bowel in place.
- Remove the side tilt to the table and apply a head-down tilt.
- Move to the patient's left side to carry out pelvic dissection.
- When present the uterus can be hitched up by two stitches inserted through each broad ligament.
- Hold the sigmoid colon up and, using diathermy, develop the plane behind the superior rectal vessels.
- Identify and preserve the pre-sacral nerves as they cross the pelvic brim medial to the ureters.
- Carry on the dissection in the avascular plane between the mesorectum and pre-sacral fascia posteriorly. Keeping in this plane, dissect the lateral aspects of the mesorectum.
- Incise the peritoneal reflection anteriorly.
- Dissect anterior to Denonvillier's fascia, between the rectum and the bladder, seminal vesicles and prostate in men, and the bladder and vagina in women.
- Continue the rectal mobilization to the pelvic floor, performing a total mesorectal excision.

While doing pelvic dissection from above, the second team can do the perineal dissection simultaneously as a combined synchronous approach.

- Close the anal orifice with a 0 or 1 silk purse-string suture. Apply an artery forceps to the ends of the suture, which is left long.
- Make an elliptical incision from the midpoint of the perineal body, in the male or the posterior aspect of the vaginal introitus, in the female, to a point over the coccyx.
- Deepen the incision laterally into the ischio-rectal fossa. Control bleeding from the pudendal vessels.
- Use retractors to help dissect to the level of the levator ani.
- Carry the incision posteriorly to expose the anococcygeal ligament. Incise the ligament in front of the coccyx.
- Dissect behind the external sphincter to reach the levator muscles.
- Use the tip of the scissors to traverse the muscle—ask the abdominal operator to help to direct the scissors tip correctly. Avoid lifting the pre-sacral fascia from the sacrum and entering the pre-sacral venous plexus.
- Insert a finger into the pelvis and divide the levator muscles over it on either side.
- Continue the dissection anteriorly making a transverse incision in the anterior decussating fibres of the external sphincter, exposing the posterior fibres of the superficial and deep transverse perineal muscles. Deep to the latter, identify the median raphe in the rectourethralis and puborectalis muscles. Follow the median raphe with blunt scissor dissection into the pelvis with the abdominal operator guiding with his finger. Divide the remaining tissues to free the rectum and then remove it.
- Close the perineal wound in layers—approximating levator muscles and fibro-fatty tissue in the midline. Close the skin.
- Extra levator abdomino perineal excision (ELAPE) can be performed by continuing the dissection outside the muscle with removal of levator muscles. Closure of the pelvic defect wound requires a mesh or a flap.
- Irrigate the pelvis and leave a suction drain. It is not essential to reperitonize the pelvis.
- Make a trephine at the marked site and deliver the colon end.
- Follow the steps as described for construction of colostomy.

Closure

In single mass layer using 1/0 PDS. Subcuticular Monocryl® for skin.

Postoperative complications

- Bleeding.
- Wound infection.
- Paralytic ileus.
- Urinary or sexual dysfunction.
- Colostomy related complications.

Laparoscopic abdomino-perineal excision of rectum (APER)

The steps are the same as described in 'Sigmoid colectomy/left hemicolectomy' (p. 200) and 'Anterior resection' (p. 212). The perineal dissection is same as described in open procedure.

Tips and tricks

- Stay behind superficial transverse perineal muscles to avoid injury to the urethra.
- Stay close to sphincter complex and do not excise surrounding fibro-fatty tissue, which can devascularize the perineal skin flap.

Restorative proctocolectomy (ileal pouch surgery)

Proctocolectomy with ileal pouch–anal anastomosis.

Indications

- Chronic ulcerative colitis where medical therapy fails and patient wants to avoid permanent ileostomy.
- As a second procedure after colectomy in patients with acute severe ulcerative colitis.
- Familial adenomatous polyposis.

Patient should be highly motivated and have an adequate anal sphincter.

Preparation

As for 'Sigmoid colectomy/left hemicolectomy' (p. 200). Ileostomy site marked by stoma nurse.

Position

Lloyd–Davies.

Incision

Midline.

Procedure

(See Fig. 4.54)

- Follow the steps as described in the 'Panproctocolectomy' section (p. 218).
- Mobilize the rectum to anorectal junction.
- For stapled anastomosis, apply a transverse stapler at this level. For hand-sutured anastomosis, divide the bowel to leave an open anal stump.
- Select the point on the ileum for ileo-anal anastomosis and attempt a trial descent to the anal canal level.
- Make a J or W ileal reservoir.
- Perform a stapled pouch–anal anastomosis or a hand-sutured anastomosis after mucosectomy.
- Fashion a defunctioning ileostomy.

Postoperative complications

- Pelvic sepsis.
- Stricture of the anastomosis.
- Intestinal obstruction.
- Pouchitis.
- Excessive frequency of defecation.
- Pouch–vaginal, pouch–perineal fistula.
- Failure—need to remove the pouch and establish a permanent ileostomy.

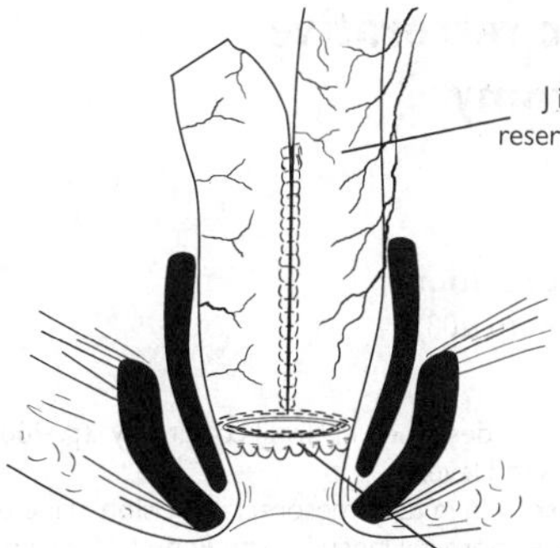
J ileal
reservoir
Stapled pouchanal
anastomosis

Fig. 4.54 Restorative proctocolectomy. Reproduced with permission from McLatchie, G, and Leaper, D. Operative Surgery 2nd edition, Oxford University Press: 2006.

Laparoscopic restorative proctocolectomy

Position

Lloyd–Davies.

Laparoscopic port position

As for 'Total colectomy' (p. 208).

Procedure

- Mobilize entire colon as described in 'Total colectomy' (p. 208). Ligate named vessels at desired levels.
- Carry out rectal dissection in total mesorectal excision plane down till pelvic floor. Divide anorectal junction with Endo GIA or equivalent stapler.
- Take out specimen. Construct a 20cm 'J' pouch from terminal ileum using a stapling device.
- The pouch-anal anastomosis is carried out as described in open technique.
- Single port laparoscopic restorative proctocolectomy is possible and can be done through potential ileostomy site. There would be no scar on abdomen, apart from ileostomy at the end of the procedure.

Tips and tricks

- Ensure that the pouch reaches the pelvic floor to form a tension-free anastomosis.
- Do not leave excess blind loop at the top of the pouch.
- Make sure that the pouch is not twisted before doing the anastomosis.

Hartmann's procedure (sigmoid colectomy and end colostomy)

Indications

A safe option when dealing with left-sided colonic emergencies (obstruction, perforation). The diseased colon is resected, divided colon is brought out as an end colostomy in the left lower quadrant, and the rectal stump is closed. The procedure is performed when conditions are unfavourable for immediate anastomosis (faecal peritonitis, obstruction, unprepared bowel, unstable patient, inexperience of surgeon).

Preparation

- Ensure adequate resuscitation.
- Prophylactic antibiotics.
- Thromboembolism prophylaxis.
- Catheterize.
- Forewarn the patient about colostomy and mark the site.

Position

Lloyd–Davies.

Incision

Midline.

Procedure

(See Fig. 4.55)

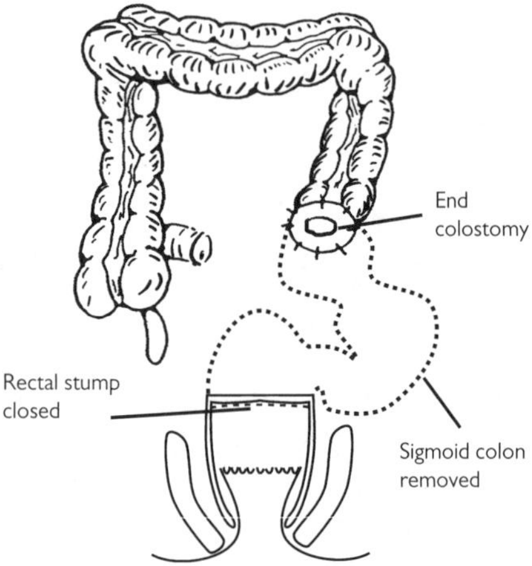
End
colostomy
Rectal stump
closed
Sigmoid colon
removed

Fig. 4.55 Hartmann's procedure. Reproduced with permission from McLatchie, G, and Leaper, D. Operative Surgery 2nd edition, Oxford University Press: 2006.

- As for the topics 'Sigmoid colectomy/left hemicolectomy' (p. 200) and 'Colostomy—formation and closure' (p. 184).
- Close the rectal stump by cross stapling or suturing.

Postoperative complications

- Bleeding.
- Wound infection.
- Breakdown of rectal stump.
- Colostomy complications.

Reversal of Hartmann's procedure

Usually considered 3 months after the initial surgery.

Position

Lloyd–Davies.

Preparation

As for 'Sigmoid colectomy/left hemicolectomy' (p. 200).

Procedure

- Mobilize colostomy and re-open laparotomy incision.
- Mobilize adherent small-bowel loops and identify the rectal stump. Introduce a rigid sigmoidoscope/sizers to aid identification if locating the stump is difficult.
- Mobilize proximal colon to bring it close to the rectum without tension. The splenic flexure may need to be brought down.
- Perform a stapled or a hand-sewn anastomosis, as described in 'Anterior resection' (p. 212).
- The operation also can be performed laparoscopic-assisted.

Single port laparoscopic reversal of Hartmann's

- Mobilize colostomy by dissecting from skin and abdominal wall.
- Excise the end and insert the anvil of a circular stapling device chosen for anastomosis (end—end or side—end anastomosis).
- Reduce the colonic end back into the peritoneal cavity and place the single port device.
- Using laparoscopic instruments, divide the adhesions with both blunt and sharp dissection. Take out small-bowel loops from pelvis.
- Continue dissection in the pelvis till the rectal stump is free of adhesions.
- Consider mobilizing the descending colon and splenic flexure for a tension-free anastomosis.
- The anastomosis is completed using a circular stapler, as described in 'Anterior resection' (p. 212).
- Closure of colostomy site with 1 Prolene®, continuous, or interrupted sutures.
- Skin clips or sutures.

Tips and tricks

- Preoperative endoscopic assessment of both rectal stump and colon is necessary.
- Mobilize the colon adequately to perform tension free anastomosis.

Procedures for large-bowel obstruction

Preparation

- Resuscitate the patient adequately.
- Perform CT scan to exclude pseudo-obstruction, to determine cause of obstruction, to stage if malignant.
- Cross-match two units of blood.
- Thromboembolism prophylaxis.
- Prophylactic antibiotics at induction.
- Catheterize patient.

Position

Lloyd–Davies.

Incision

Midline.

Procedures

- Consider decompression of gaseous large-bowel distension. Insert a 14 or 16G needle through a tinea into the lumen of the bowel and attach to suction.
- If obstruction is due to a right-sided lesion, consider a right hemicolectomy, or for a fixed tumour, an ileo-transverse anastomosis (hand-sutured single or two-layered anastomosis or a stapled anastomosis).
- If obstruction is due to left-sided lesion, options are: three-stage approach (defunctioning loop colostomy, resection and anastomosis, closure of stoma); two-stage approach (Hartmann's procedure and reversal of Hartmann's); one-stage approach (sub-total colectomy with ileo-colic or ileo-rectal anastomosis or left hemicolectomy after an on-table colonic irrigation). Choice of operation depends on patient fitness, stage of disease if malignancy, and local conditions for primary anastomosis.

On-table colonic irrigation

- Make a colotomy proximal to the lesion causing the obstruction.
- Insert anaesthetic scavenging tubing and secure with heavy suture around the bowel. Connect tubing into a plastic bag and place this into a bucket.
- Insert a large Foley catheter into the caecum via appendix stump or an enterotomy in the terminal ileum.
- Infuse 2–3l or more of warm saline into the caecum and manipulate colonic contents into anaesthetic tubing. Mobilize colonic flexures, if necessary, to achieve this. Continue this until effluent is clear (Fig. 4.56).
- Carry out a left hemicolectomy, as described in 'Sigmoid colectomy/left hemicolectomy' (p. 200).

There are kits available on the market for carrying out on-table colonic irrigation.

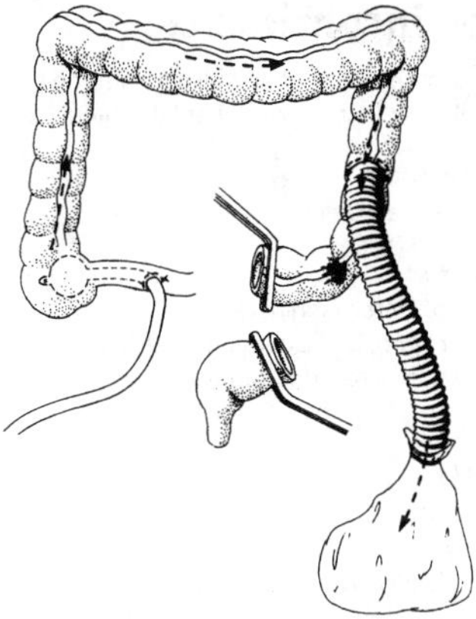

Fig. 4.56 On-table colonic lavage. Reproduced with permission from McLatchie, G, and Leaper, D. Operative Surgery 2nd edition, Oxford University Press: 2006.

Tips and tricks

- Decompress the colon with a needle or via the appendix stump before commencing mobilization.
- Self-expanding metal stents are now being used in large-bowel obstruction secondary to malignancy, either for palliation or as a temporary bridge to surgery (stent decompression followed by elective resection).

Surgery for incontinence

Faecal incontinence is potentially a disabling condition (physical and psychological) with variable involuntary loss of solid or liquid stool.

Indication for surgery

- Failed conservative treatment.

Types of surgery

- Direct repair of sphincter (sphincteroplasty).
- Anal neosphincter (graciloplasty, artificial sphincter).
- Augmentation of sphincter function (sacral nerve stimulation/ bulking agents).

Sphincteroplasty

Preoperative preparation

- Phosphate enema.
- IV antibiotic at induction of anaesthesia.

Position

Lloyd–Davies.

Procedure

- WHO checklist.
- Make a curvilineal incision from 10 to 2 o'clock position on the outer border of the external sphincter and raise an anodermal flap.
- Dissect the sphincter complex cephaled till anorectal ring. Dissect the scar tissue and the external anal sphincter muscle ends from surrounding structures.
- Excise scar tissue at the dehiscence area. Overlap both muscle ends with 2/0 PDS sutures.
- Close the wound with interrupted absorbable sutures, preferably in longitudinal orientation to increase the distance between vaginal introitus and anus. Leave the central area open to allow drainage. Alternatively leave a suction drain.

Post-operative care

- Remove drain after 24–48h.
- Wound care.
- Laxatives.
- Metronidazole for 1 week.

Complications

- Injury to pudendal nerve.
- Wound infection.
- Anal canal stenosis.
- Fistulae.

Tips and tricks

- Patient selection is paramount for good results.
- Care must be taken while dissecting the sphincter complex to avoid damage to pudendal nerve.

Graciloplasty

This highly technical procedure should be done in high-volume institutes for better outcomes. Usually indicated in patients with extensive sphincter disruption, severe neurological damage, or in patients with congenital disorders.

The gracilis muscle from the leg is mobilized (with or without electrical stimulation) and is translocated into a circum-anal position. Success rates of 45–85% have been reported from high-volume centres. The implantation of electrically stimulated gracilis muscle functions better and hence is called '*dynamic graciloplasty*'.

Artificial bowel sphincter (ABS)

A silicon implantable device is used to restore continence. An inflatable cuff is placed around the lower rectum and upper anal canal. Patients with Crohn's disease, morbid obesity, diabetes, and previous pelvic sepsis/radiation injury are not suitable for this procedure.

A fluid-filled reservoir is implanted in the scrotum or labia. It is connected to a cuff that encircles the anal canal. A pressure-regulated balloon is implanted in the retropubic space. To initiate defaecation, the pump is manually squeezed to empty the cuff by transferring the fluid from the cuff to the balloon, allowing the passage of faeces. After a few minutes, the cuff re-inflates spontaneously. It is paramount that patients are motivated and have sufficient skills to operate the device independently.

Sacral nerve stimulation (SNS)

This is an emerging procedure and is becoming widely popular. An electrode is placed using fluoroscopy in the sacral foramina (usually S3). It is connected to a portable external stimulator. Patients who have a success rate of at least 50% clinical improvement in faecal incontinence during the 'testing phase' are selected for permanent implant. A permanent stimulator is placed in the subcutaneous plane in the gluteal area. The electrode delivers an intermittent electrical stimulus to the anal sphincter complex and pelvic floor muscles. In addition, it also affects colonic motility and increases blood flow in the perineal structures including rectum.

This expensive procedure is contraindicated in patients with poor access to the sacral area (skin disease, pathological conditions of sacrum), severe sphincter complex damage, bleeding diathesis, non-compliance, and cardiac pacemaker or defibrillator.

Surgery for defecatory disorders

Obstructive defecation syndrome (ODS) is characterized by an impaired ability to expel the faecal bolus. The symptom complex includes unsuccessful faecal evacuation attempts leading to a sense of incomplete emptying, pain due to excessive straining attempts, and sometimes bleeding. ODS is usually associated with intrarectal intussusception, rectocele, and rectal mucosal prolapse.

Indications

- Failed conservative treatment (diet, biofeedback, pelvic floor exercise).
- Demonstrable underlying structural abnormality on contrast studies.

Preoperative investigations

- Flexible sigmoidoscopy.
- Defecation proctogram/MR procto-defecography.
- Anorectal manometry.

Surgical procedures

Stapled trans-anal rectal resection (STARR) and laparoscopic ventral mesh rectopexy (LVMR).

STARR

Preoperative preparation

- Phosphate enema.

Position

Lithotomy.

Procedure

- General/regional anaesthesia.
- Introduce a circular anal dilator and secure with skin sutures.
- Place three to four sutures in the anterior wall at intervals above the anorectal junction in a semi-circular fashion.
- Place a spatulated retractor to protect the posterior wall.
- Introduce a circular stapler into the rectum and position the anvil above the level of the sutures.
- Apply traction on the sutures to retract as much redundant rectal wall as possible into the holding of the stapler.
- After ensuring that the vaginal wall is free, fire the stapler. The anterior wall of rectum is resected.
- In a similar fashion, resect the posterior rectal wall.
- Check the circumferential staple line for bleeding. Interrupted haemostatic sutures are occasionally needed.

Postoperative care

- Watch for primary and secondary haemorrhage.
- Laxatives.

Complications
- Retroperitoneal sepsis secondary to infected haematoma.
- Persistant peri-anal pain.
- Faecal incontinence.
- Rectovaginal fistula.

Tips and tricks
- Select patients carefully—pelvic floor dyssynergia is a predictor of poor outcome.
- Avoid technical errors like stapling too close to the dentate line and inclusion of vaginal wall in the staple line.

LVMR

This procedure is described as ventral rectopexy in 'Surgery for rectal prolapse' (p. 162).

Trans-anal endoscopic microsurgery/ trans-anal endoscopic operation (TEMS/TEO)

Trans-anal endoscopic microsurgery (TEMS) is a minimally invasive surgical procedure that uses a specialized magnifying resectoscope (40mm diameter, 12 and 20cm length) with a light source and camera viewing system (Fig. 4.57). Rectal insufflation is achieved with carbon dioxide. There is a sealing system, three operative ports, and a channel for suction/irrigation.

Indications

- Large sessile benign polyps.
- Early rectal cancers.
- Small carcinoid tumours.
- Palliative resection for advanced rectal cancers.
- Patients with rectal cancer who are unfit for major pelvic surgery.

Preoperative preparation

- Detailed assessment of lesion is mandatory—size, location, extent of spread (if cancer).
- Phosphate enema.
- Broad-spectrum antibiotic at induction of anaesthesia.

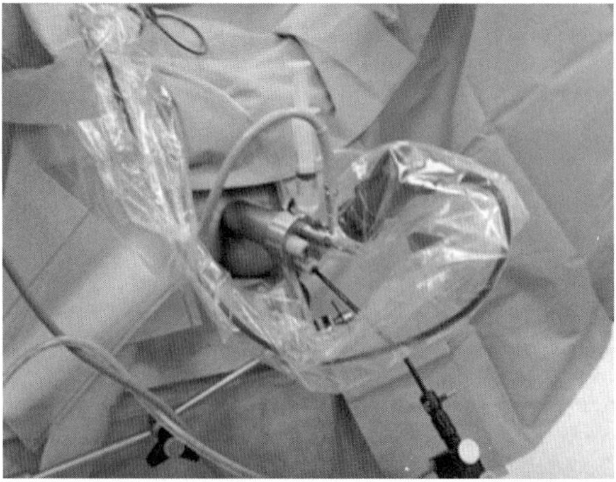

Fig. 4.57 Trans-anal endoscopic operation.

Position

Lithotomy/lateral/prone.

Steps of operation

- WHO checklist.
- General anaesthesia.
- Hold the resectoscope in position by fixing it to the operating table.
- Using specially designed microsurgical instruments, excise the tumour along with a cuff of normal tissue all around (Figs 4.58 and 4.59).
- Dissect either in a submucosal plane or a plane outside the rectal wall (full thickness). Retrieve the specimen.
- Achieve haemostasis with diathermy or harmonic instrument.
- Wash the excised area with a weak solution of Betadine.
- Close the defect with absorbable sutures.

Postoperative care

- Fluids and diet is commenced on the same day.
- Laxatives.
- Patients are usually discharged the following day.

Complications

- Bleeding.
- Infection.
- Severe retroperitoneal sepsis.
- Recurrence.

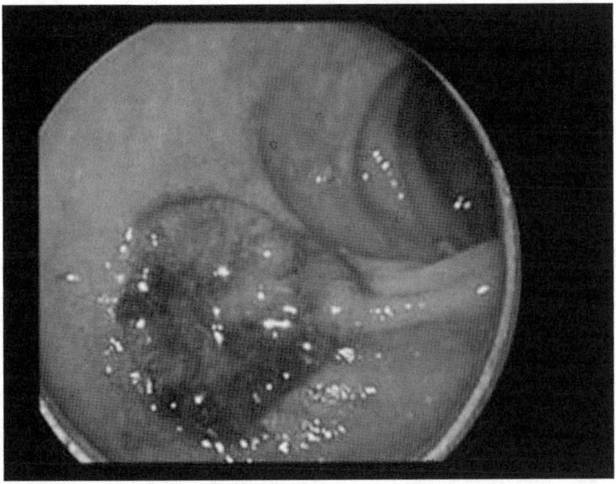

Fig. 4.58 Tumour at 6 o'clock position.

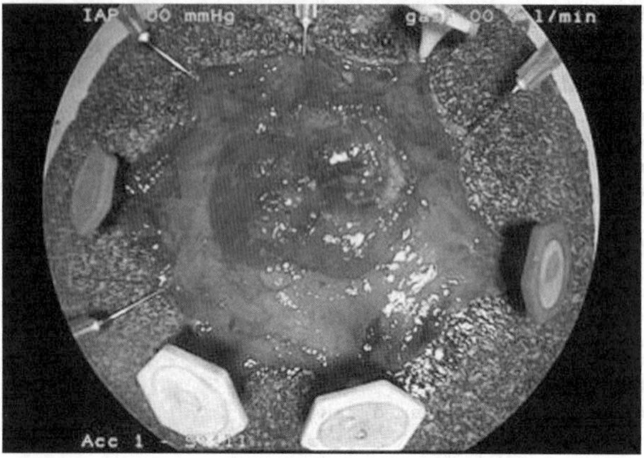
1/min
Acc 1

Fig. 4.59 Cuff of normal tissue is excised along with the tumour for clearance.

Tips and tricks

- Position the patient in such a way that the tumour is at the 6 o'clock position.
- Haemostasis in mesorectal plane is crucial.

Chapter 5

Breast surgery

Fine-needle aspiration cytology (FNAC)

FNAC is a quick, technically simple, accurate, and atraumatic method for diagnosing breast masses and axillary lymph nodes. Results can be reported at a 'one-stop clinic' as part of triple assessment. Impalpable lesions or axillary nodes can be sampled under stereotactic mammography or ultrasound guidance.

Fine-needle aspirates are graded as follows:

- AC1—insufficient sample.
- AC2—benign.
- AC3—indeterminate.
- AC4—suspicious of malignancy.
- AC5—malignant.

Reliability depends upon the experience of the cytopathologist. It cannot discriminate between in situ or invasive malignancy. False-negative rates of up to 5% are reported. Failure to reach a diagnosis in the presence of suspicious clinical and radiological findings requires further investigation (repeat FNAC or core biopsy).

Indications

- Triple assessment of breast mass.
- Screen-detected breast lesions.
- Assessment of axillary lymph nodes.

Consent

Take verbal consent, explaining the risks (e.g. bruising, haematoma, pneumothorax).

Position

Supine, arm behind the head.

Procedure

Use 21G (green) to 23G (blue) needle, 10 or 20ml syringe, syringe holder, glass slides, and slide holder. Local anaesthesia is not generally required. Injection may be more uncomfortable than FNAC.

- Use one hand to fix the mass, the other to direct the needle. Needle should be held parallel to the chest wall in as much as possible (Fig. 5.1).
- Clean overlying skin with alcohol wipe.
- Insert needle into lump, apply suction, and pass through lesion four to five times. Only a small amount of cells are harvested, so you will not always see aspirate into needle hub or syringe.
- Release suction before withdrawing the needle from the lesion.
- Ask patient to apply pressure over the area.
- Disconnect needle and fill syringe with air. Expel contents onto a slide. Repeat procedure if necessary.
- Spread the aspirate using another clean slide.
- Prepare one dry and wet slide. Dry-fixed slides must be spread thinly and air dried. Wet-fixed slides must be fixed immediately with alcohol-based fixative supplied by the laboratory. Label the slides (AD for 'air-dried' and WF for 'wet-fixed') and place in slide container.

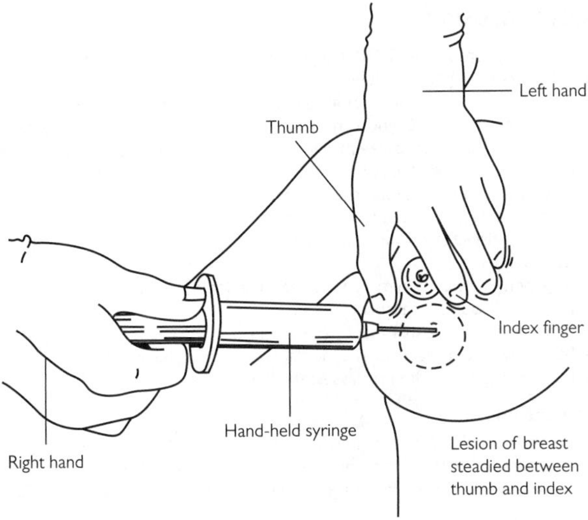
Left hand
Thumb
Index finger
Hand-held syringe
Right hand
Lesion of breast
steadied between
thumb and index

Fig. 5.1 Fine-needle aspiration of the breast. A handheld syringe holder can also be used (not illustrated). Reproduced with permission from McLatchie, G, and Leaper, D. Operative Surgery 2nd edition, Oxford University Press: 2006.

Complications

Bruising, haematoma, pneumothorax (rare).

Tips and tricks

- Before inserting the needle into the lesion withdraw the plunger 2–3ml and then perform the biopsy as described. You can then expel the contents onto a slide.
- You can wash out the needle and syringe with a preservative solution (i.e. CytoLyt) and send the washout specimen to the lab.

Core biopsy

Core biopsy removes a 12–18-gauge cylindrical 'core' of the sampled tissue. This allows for histopathological analysis (ability to differentiate between in situ and invasive carcinoma) and immunohistochemical staining for hormone receptors, Her2, and other markers. False-positives are very rare. Confirmation of diagnosis—malignant or benign—avoids the need for excision biopsy. Core biopsy can be done freehand for palpable or image-guided (stereotactic mammography or ultrasound) for impalpable lesions.

Core biopsies are graded as follows:

- B1—unsatisfactory or normal tissue only.
- B2—benign.
- B3—benign, uncertain malignant potential. Indeterminate.
- B4—suspicious of malignancy.
- B5a—non-invasive malignancy (i.e. DCIS).
- B5b—invasive malignancy (i.e. ductal carcinoma, lobular carcinoma, etc.).
- B5c—malignancy with non-assessable invasiveness.

Indications

- Breast lesions (palpable or impalpable).
- Indeterminate (AC3) or suspicious (AC4) lesions on FNAC.
- Alternative to FNAC. Preferred investigation method in many centres.

Consent

Verbal consent is sufficient. Explain the risk of bruising, haematoma, and infection.

Position

Supine, head slightly raised, arm above head (if comfortable). Raise couch to avoid back strain.

Procedure

- Materials: disposable dressing/wound pack, spring-loaded core biopsy gun, local anaesthetic infiltration, scalpel, alcohol swabs, formalin specimen pot, adhesive strips, and adhesive dressing.
- Palpate lump. Choose needle entry point so that needle track is parallel to the chest wall (to minimize the risk of pneumothorax). Ideally, entry point should be placed in a location that will be easy to excise if the mass proves malignant.
- Clean area with alcohol swab and infiltrate local anaesthetic into skin and subcutaneous tissue.
- Stabilize lump with non-dominant hand. Make a stab incision with the scalpel over the planned entry point.
- Introduce the needle into the mass and fire the biopsy gun. Remember to keep the needle parallel to chest wall.
- Withdraw needle and place specimen into formalin specimen pot. You can use scalpel to gently scrape specimen off the needle. Adipose tissue tends to float, whereas lesional tissue tends to sink.

- Repeat biopsy two to five times.
- Apply adhesive strips and adhesive dressing followed by pressure for a few minutes. Alternatively, a pressure dressing can be used.
- Label the specimen.

Complications

- Bruising (very common), haematoma, infection, mastitis.
- Pneumothorax (rare).

Incision and drainage of breast abscess

Incision and drainage of a breast abscess is no longer the mainstay of treatment of a pus collection within the breast. Antibiotic therapy with repeat ultrasound-guided aspiration is often preferred. However, failure of such treatment will require formal incision and drainage.

Skin lesions, such as epidermal/sebaceous cysts and the tubercles of Montgomery (a modified sweat gland) on the areola, can become infected and lead to a superficial abscess. These do not originate from within the breast parenchyma.

Parenchymal breast abscesses can occur during pregnancy, the early postnatal period, or lactation. As a rule of thumb these tend to be peripheral. When not associated with pregnancy, abscesses are most often related to periductal mastitis and tend to have a central location (periductal mastitis affects main/central lactiferous ducts). In such cases, incision and drainage may result in a mammary duct fistula. Recurrence is also higher since the infection is related to a chronic inflammatory condition.

Indications

Breast abscess that has failed antibiotic and/or ultrasound-guided aspiration.

Consent

Written consent. Explain the risk of bleeding, recurrence, mammary duct fistula requiring further surgery, scarring, unpredictable healing, and poor cosmesis.

Preoperative preparation

Mark incision over area of maximal fluctuance. Aim for a curvilinear incision circumferential to nipple–areolar complex.

Position

Supine. General anaesthetic often used.

Procedure

- Incise over the area of maximal fluctuance.
- Take a pus swab for culture and sensitivity.
- Break down loculations with your finger. Part of the cavity wall can be sent for histology if there is a suspicion of inflammatory breast cancer.
- Wash out abscess cavity with saline.
- Loosely pack the cavity with a calcium alginate dressing (Kaltostat, Aquacel, Sorbisan, etc.).
- A soft corrugated drain (e.g. Yeates) can also be used if the abscess is not in a dependent part of the breast.

Closure

- Leave wound open and apply a gauze and adhesive dressing.
- Regular dressing changes until cavity heals by secondary intent.
- Delayed primary wound closure can be considered once cellulitis resolves.

Complications

Recurrence, delayed healing, deformity, mammary duct fistula.

Benign or diagnostic breast lump excision

This refers to the surgical removal of the entire breast mass either for diagnostic purposes or because the patient wants the mass removed even if it is benign.

Indications

- Indeterminate FNAC and/or core biopsy results.
- Patient choice.

Consent

Written consent. Explain risks of bleeding, infection, scarring, unpredictable healing, and potential for further breast surgery depending on results.

Preoperative preparation

- Confirm side with patient, palpate lump, and mark site and laterality.
- When marking incision, ensure patient is in the same position as on the operating table (Fig 5.2).
- Aim for incision along skin tension lines (Kraissl's lines).
- There are some exceptions: closer to the areola, circumareolar curvilinear incisions are preferred. Peri-areolar incisions can be used if it allows good access to the lesion. In the lower meridian of the breast, consider radial incisions as these tend to cause less nipple–areolar distortion. Inframammary or axillary incisions can also be used if they allow good access to the lesion. Ideally, the incision should be placed so that it can be included in a subsequent mastectomy, if necessary.

Position

Supine with arm abducted on an arm board (no more than 90° to avoid plexus neuropathy).

Procedure

- Incise skin, subcutaneous fat, and deepen into breast tissue. No need to excise skin.
- Stay close to lesion. Resection of normal tissue should be limited. (i.e. this is not a wide local excision).
- Orientate the specimen according to local preference, e.g. short stitch for superior, long stitch for lateral, and double stitch for posterior.
- Ensure haemostasis.

Closure

- Close the wound in two layers: interrupted inverted dermal sutures (e.g. 3.0 absorbable undyed monofilament) followed by a subcuticular stitch (e.g. 3.0 or 4.0 absorbable undyed monofilament).
- Apply adhesive strips (e.g. Steristrips) and an adhesive absorbent dressing.

Complications

Haematoma, infection, seroma formation, altered appearance, further surgery.

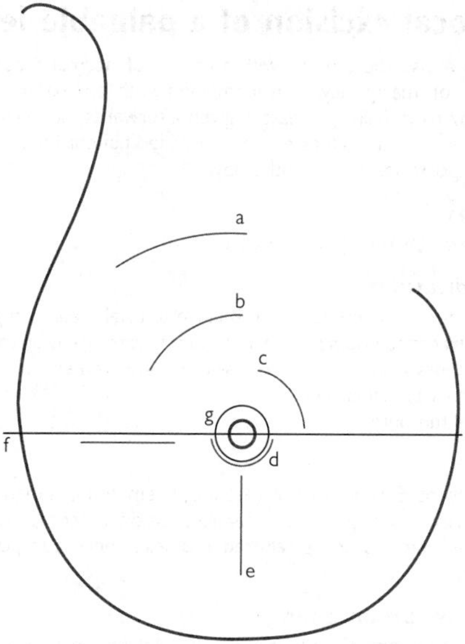
a
b
c
g
f
d
e

Fig. 5.2 Preferred incisions for a breast lump/wide, local excision: (a) skin tension line incision; (b) curvilinear incision; (c) circumareolar incision; (d) peri-areolar incision; (e) radial incision; (f) imaginary line separating upper and lower breast meridian; (g) areolar edge.

Wide local excision of a palpable lesion

Intended to excise the tumour with a margin of normal tissue (Fig. 5.3). In the case of malignancy, it is combined with an axillary procedure. Radiotherapy to remaining breast is given afterwards. Survival and recurrence rates are similar to mastectomy, provided patient receives adequate surgery and postoperative radiotherapy.

Indications

Invasive or non-invasive (DCIS) breast cancer.

Contraindications

- Tumours >4cm (in practice this is relative to total breast size).
- Centrally placed tumours (in selected cases a central excision can be done).
- Large tumours with obvious/extensive skin involvement.
- Inflammatory breast cancer.
- Multi-focal tumours.

Consent

Written consent. Explain risks of bleeding, haematoma, infection, seroma, positive margins leading to need for re-excision or completion mastectomy, unpredictable scarring, altered cosmesis, need for postoperative radiotherapy.

Preoperative preparation

- Mark circumference of tumour and additional 1cm margin. This helps to define the extent of skin flap dissection.
- When marking incision, ensure patient is in the same position as on the operating table.
- Aim for incision along skin tension lines.

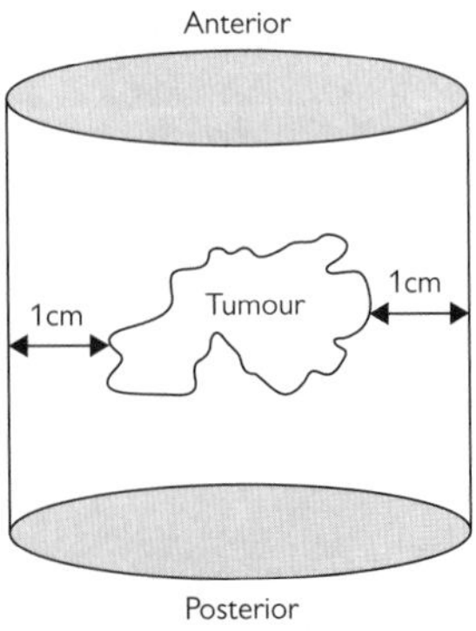
Anterior
1cm
Tumour
1cm
Posterior

Fig. 5.3 Diagram of a wide, local excision specimen. Reproduced with permission from McLatchie, G, and Leaper, D. Operative Surgery 2nd edition, Oxford University Press: 2006.

- There are some exceptions: closer to the areola circumareolar curvilinear incisions are preferred. Peri-areolar incisions can be used if it allows good access to the lesion. In the lower meridian of the breast, consider radial incisions as these tend to cause less nipple–areolar distortion. Inframammary or axillary incisions can also be used if they allow good access to the lesion. Ideally, the incision should be placed so that it can be included in a subsequent mastectomy, if necessary (Fig. 5.2). Combining all these factors is not always possible.
- If the tumour involves the skin, mark a skin ellipse over tumour.

Position

Supine with arm abducted on arm board (no more than 90° to avoid plexus neuropathy).

Procedure

- Ask assistant to support breast.
- Incise skin with scalpel. Aim for a single, clean incision perpendicular to the skin surface.
- Raise the 'skin flaps' over the lesion. The ideal plane is demarcated by the layer of investing fascia (called Scarpa's fascia in the groin) separating subcutaneous fat from breast tissue.
- Adopt a methodical approach to tumour dissection. Place fingers over superior aspect of lesion, apply downward traction, and cut breast tissue down to the pectoral fascia with scalpel or diathermy. Once on the pectoral fascia, extend the incision so as to undermine/lift lesion off the pectoral fascia. Repeat the same to the inferior border of the tumour. Repeat the same steps to the lateral edges of the tumour. Remove the lesion and place a swab in the cavity.
- Orientate the specimen according to local preference, e.g. short stitch for superior, long stitch for lateral, and double stitch for posterior.
- Ensure haemostasis.
- Apply clips to edges of the cavity. This demarcates excision area and helps radiation oncologist in planning subsequent delivery of radiotherapy.

Closure

- Larger cavities may benefit from mobilization of remaining breast tissue and oncoplastic procedures to reshape the breast.
- Close the wound in two layers: interrupted inverted dermal sutures (e.g. 3.0 absorbable undyed monofilament) followed by a subcuticular stitch (e.g. 3.0 or 4.0 absorbable undyed monofilament).
- Apply adhesive strips (e.g. Steristrips) and an adhesive absorbent dressing.

Complications

Haematoma, infection, seroma formation, altered appearance, further surgery.

Tips and tricks

When cutting through breast parenchyma it is often easy to 'cone in' as the dissection is deepened. This can take you too close to the tumour. Aim to cut by angling the diathermy or knife away from the fingers holding the lesion.

Mastectomy

Simple mastectomy is the removal of the entire breast tissue with overlying skin ellipse and the nipple–areolar complex. 'Skin sparing' techniques (with or without nipple/areola preservation) are modifications of the simple mastectomy. This involves performing a mastectomy through a smaller incision so as to preserve the skin and subcutaneous envelope (with or without nipple/areolar preservation) of the breast. These can be performed through peri-areolar, transverse lateral, axillary, or inframammary incisions. The operation is technically more challenging as the field of dissection and tissue retraction are more limited. However, preserving the natural skin envelope allows for more anatomically accurate reconstructions (Fig. 5.4).

Indications

- Tumours >4cm (in practice this is relative to whole breast size).
- Patient preference.
- Central tumours (relative indication).
- Multicentric tumours.
- Inflammatory breast cancer.

Consent

Written consent. Explain risks of bleeding, haematoma, infection, seroma, need for further treatment, unpredictable scarring, altered cosmesis, further surgery or reconstruction.

Preoperative preparation

- Mark skin ellipse, inframammary fold, and midline.
- Aim to include previous scars if possible (e.g. previous wide local excision scar). Ellipse can be orientated transversely or obliquely based on breast size, body habitus, size, and location of tumour.
- A skin ellipse encompassing the inframammary fold, and only a small amount of skin superior to the nipple, will create a larger superior flap and result in an aesthetically favourable scar.
- Skin ellipse should be wide enough to avoid redundant skin but allow for closure without excessive tension.

Position

Supine with arm abducted on arm board (no more than 90° to avoid plexus neuropathy).

Procedure

- Ask assistant to support breast.
- Incise skin with scalpel. Aim for a single, clean incision perpendicular to the skin surface.
- Incise subcutaneous fat down to investing layer of fascia until breast tissue is evident. Several superficial veins will require haemostasis.
- Place tissue forceps (Allis, Littlewood, skin hooks) onto dermis of flap to be raised and ask assistant to retract vertically. The key to raising the flaps is adequate traction. Place gauze onto breast tissue to avoid slipping and apply counter-traction.

(a)

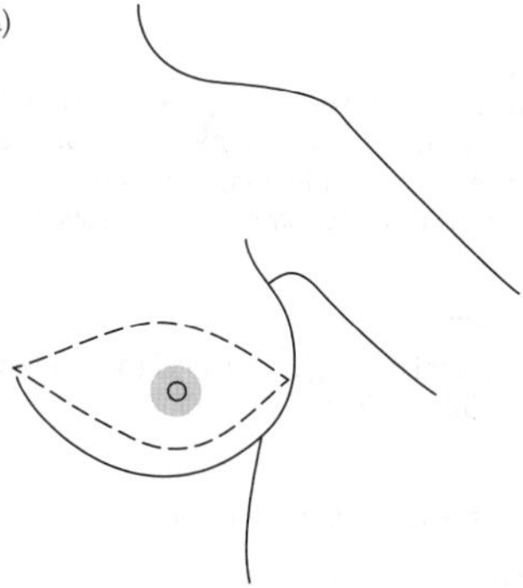

(b)

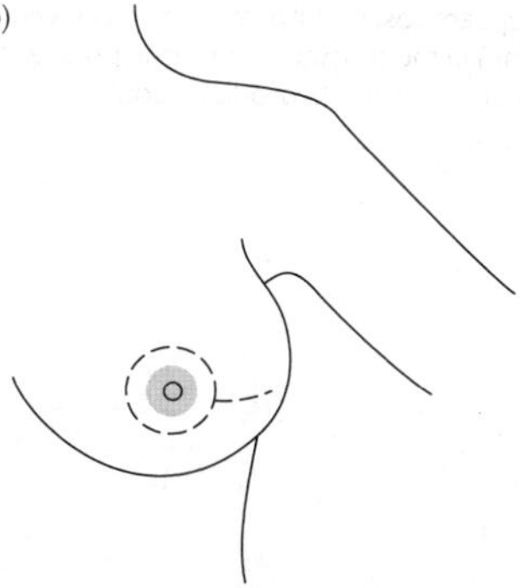

Fig. 5.4 Mastectomy markings. Example of: (a) simple mastectomy; (b) skin sparing mastectomy. Reproduced with permission from McLatchie, G, and Leaper, D. Operative Surgery 2nd edition, Oxford University Press: 2006.

- Create flaps with diathermy (or scissors, scalpel) by separating breast parenchyma from skin and subcutaneous tissue. It is relatively easy to stray, check flap thickness regularly and re-adjust traction.
- When flaps are dissected, cut down to the pectoral fascia. Take care not to undermine inframammary fold.
- Excise breast from underlying pectoralis muscles. Start medially, lift breast up, retract laterally, and dissect breast off pectoralis fascia. With adequate traction you will see a loose areolar plane, which will facilitate dissection. Medial perforating branches will require meticulous haemostasis as you go along. Continue dissection to lateral border of pectoralis major muscle to include axillary tail.

Closure

- Place a suction drain.
- Close the wound in two layers: interrupted inverted dermal sutures (e.g. 3.0 absorbable undyed monofilament) followed by a subcuticular stitch (e.g. 3.0 or 4.0 absorbable undyed monofilament).
- Apply adhesive strips (e.g. Steristrips) and an adhesive absorbent dressing.

Postoperative care

Drains are left in situ until drainage is minimal (depends on local preference, usually less than 30–50ml in 24h).

Complications

Haematoma, seroma, infection, scarring/delayed healing.

Tips and tricks

The fascial plane, although anatomically constant, is not always easy to see and sometimes appears absent. Infiltration of saline with 1:400,000 adrenaline (2.5mcg per mL) in the subcutaneous plane prior to dissection can facilitate identification of the plane (hydrodissection).

Sentinel node biopsy (dual technique)

Minimally invasive procedure designed to identify and remove the first axillary nodes draining lymph from the breast cancer (the sentinel nodes). It predicts the nodal status of the axilla. If the sentinel lymph nodes are negative, the patient does not require further axillary clearance. Identification of the nodes is performed with the help of blue dye and radioactive tracer injected into the breast preoperatively. Blue and/or 'hot' nodes should be removed.

Indications

Axilla that has been proven 'node negative' by clinical and ultrasound assessment +/– fine-needle aspiration of suspicious nodes.

Consent

Written consent. Explain risks of failure to localize nodes, haematoma, seroma, painful scar, allergy to blue dye, blue discoloration of skin and urine (temporary), risk of lymphoedema (very low), need for further axillary clearance, chemotherapy, and/or radiotherapy.

Preoperative preparation

Patient will have had the radioactive tracer injected preoperatively by the nuclear medicine department. Check lymphoscintigram (if performed by your department) to assess the number of potential sentinel nodes.

Position

Supine with arm abducted on arm board (no more than 90° to avoid plexus neuropathy).

Procedure

- Inject 2ml of patent blue dye under the areolar dermis. As there is a risk of allergic reaction/anaphylaxis this is best done once the patient is anaesthetized. Massage for 1–2min with a gauze swab to help diffusion.
- Use gamma detector probe to localize 'hot' spots in the axilla.
- Make 2–3cm incision over 'hot' spot.
- Aim to place incision in a natural crease, often below the axillary hairline. The incision should be able to be incorporated into a subsequent axillary clearance procedure if necessary.
- Cut down through subcutaneous fat, identify lateral border of pectoralis major, and incise axillary fascia (either longitudinally or transversely).
- Use combination of auditory clues from the gamma probe and visual clues (i.e. blue discoloration) to guide you towards the node. Dissect tissues onto node with a combination of blunt and sharp techniques.
- Use a non-traumatic tissue forceps to grab node(s) and dissect with diathermy. Ensure haemostasis.

Closure

- Close the wound in two layers: interrupted inverted dermal sutures (e.g. 3.0 absorbable undyed monofilament) followed by a subcuticular stitch (e.g. 3.0 or 4.0 absorbable undyed monofilament).
- Apply adhesive strips (e.g. Steristrips) and an adhesive absorbent dressing.

Complications

Failure to localize sentinel nodes, haematoma, seroma, infection, painful scar/axillary skin owing to injury to intercostobrachial nerves.

Tips and tricks

The intercostobrachial nerves will often be seen running from the chest wall into the skin of the axilla. Care must be taken to preserve these nerves and/or to avoid undue stretching as it can lead to chronic axillary pain.

Axillary clearance

Involves 'en bloc' resection of level I, II, and sometimes III axillary lymph nodes. It is a procedure that offers local control (by virtue of removing diseased nodes) and staging information. It does not affect overall survival.

Surgical anatomy

The axillary space has a somewhat pyramidal shape, its base being the axillary skin and its apex abutting the first rib (thoracic outlet). It is bound anteriorly by the pectoralis muscles, medially by the serratus anterior muscle (chest wall), and posteriorly by the latissimus dorsi muscle. Within the axillary tissue, level I nodes are lateral, level II nodes are behind, and level III nodes medial to the pectoralis minor muscle. This tissue has to be dissected off some important structures: the axillary vein, the thoracodorsal artery, vein, and nerve, which run together and form the thoracodorsal neurovascular bundle and the long thoracic nerve of Bell (Fig. 5.5). Sensory intercostobrachial nerves run from the chest wall to the skin of the axilla. These are often cut, although they should be preserved if they are not in the direct path of the specimen.

Indications

- Breast malignancy with axillary node involvement.
- Positive sentinel lymph node biopsy (this is currently a relative indication only).

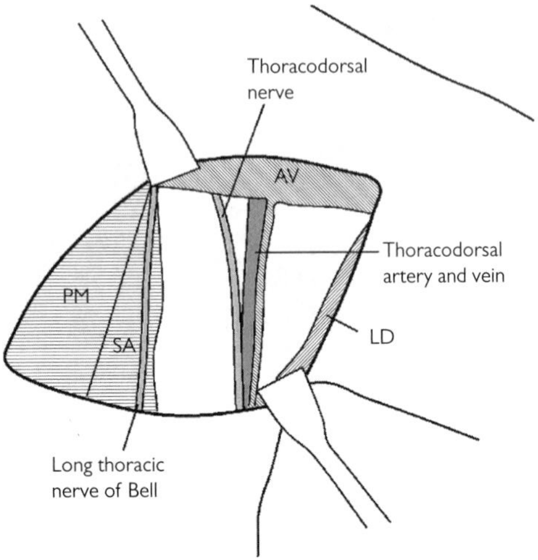
Thoracodorsal nerve
AV
Thoracodorsal artery and vein
PM
SA
LD
Long thoracic nerve of Bell

Fig. 5.5 Important structures of the axilla: AV, axillary vein; LD, latissimus dorsi; PM, pectoralis major; SA, serratus anterior. Reproduced with permission from McLatchie, G, and Leaper, D. Operative Surgery 2nd edition, Oxford University Press: 2006.

Consent

Written consent. Explain risks of bleeding, infection, seroma, lymphoedema, numbness/pain over axillary skin due to intercostobrachial nerve damage, painful scar, 'frozen shoulder', risk of injury to axillary vein and brachial plexus, need for further medical treatment (chemo/radiotherapy).

Preoperative preparation

- Mark site. Place incision in a natural crease below axillary hair bearing area from lateral border of pectoralis major to anterior border of latissimus dorsi.
- If a mastectomy is performed at the same time, no separate incision is necessary.

Position

Supine with arm abducted on arm board (no more than 90° to avoid plexus neuropathy).

Procedure

- Incise skin as previously marked. Continue dissection onto axillary fascia.
- Expose lateral border of pectoralis major muscle by cutting laterally along its length. Retract pectoralis major and continue in similar fashion to expose lateral border of pectoralis minor, taking care not to damage the medial pectoral neurovascular bundle.
- Continue dissection until axillary vein is exposed. This marks upper limit of dissection.
- Sweep axillary tissue off antero-inferior portion of axillary vein downwards using dissecting scissors. Small arteries and veins are given off by the axillary artery/vein and thoracodorsal bundle. Apply clips or ligate and cut them as you progress with the dissection.
- In addition to the axillary artery, identify and protect thoracodorsal neurovascular bundle laterally, long thoracic nerve of Bell medially (runs close to chest wall), and intercostobrachial nerves, which run from the chest wall to the axillary skin (Fig. 5.5).
- Remove axillary content 'en bloc' with mastectomy specimen if applicable.
- Ensure haemostasis.

Closure

- Place suction drain in axilla.
- Close the wound in two layers: interrupted inverted dermal sutures (e.g. 3.0 absorbable undyed monofilament) followed by a subcuticular stitch (e.g. 3.0 or 4.0 absorbable undyed monofilament).
- Apply adhesive strips (e.g. Steristrips) and an adhesive absorbent dressing.

Postoperative care

- Drains are left in situ until drainage is minimal (depends of local preference, usually less than 30–50ml in 24h).
- Patient should be encouraged to perform regular shoulder exercises to prevent 'frozen shoulder'.

Complications

- Haematoma, seroma, lymphedema, painful axillary skin, restriction of shoulder movement.
- Nerve damage—brachial plexus injury is rare but can occur if tissue is dissected superior to axillary vein.
- Intercostobrachial nerves are often removed with the specimen. This leads to numb axillary skin and the risk of neuropathic pain.
- Long thoracic nerve of Bell—loss of serratus anterior muscle function: winging of scapula.
- Thoracodorsal nerve—loss of latissimus dorsi muscle function: weakness of shoulder extension and adduction. In practice it may not be clinically apparent unless patient is active: golf, rock climbing, swimming.

Image-guided surgery—fine-wire localization

Screening mammography has led to the detection of impalpable lesions. In such cases a wire-localized wide local excision will be necessary. Using stereotactic mammography or USS, a thin, flexible wire is inserted through a rigid introducer into the breast lesion.

Indications

Impalpable breast lesions.

Consent

Written consent. Explain risks of bleeding, haematoma, infection, seroma, positive margins leading to need for re-excision or completion mastectomy, unpredictable scarring, altered cosmesis, need for postoperative radiotherapy.

Preoperative preparation

- Patient will come to theatre with wire in situ.
- Wire does not usually follow a straight path from skin to lesion.
- Check craniocaudal and mediolateral mammograms to orientate yourself and ascertain where wire is in relation to the lesion. Read the wire insertion report.

Position

- Supine with arm abducted on arm board (no more than 90° to avoid plexus neuropathy).

Procedure

- Because the wire rarely follows a straight path from skin to lesion, the incision does not need to be placed over the wire entry point.
- Ask assistant to support breast.
- Incise skin with scalpel. Aim for a single, clean incision perpendicular to the skin surface.
- Raise the 'skin flaps' over the lesion. The ideal plane is demarcated by the layer of investing fascia (called Scarpa's fascia in the groin) separating subcutaneous fat from breast tissue.
- Once flaps are dissected, identify shaft of wire and bring it out through the wound. You can cut excess wire so it does not get in the way. Take care not to dislodge the wire.
- Once you have established direction of dissection, place a tissue forceps (Babcock/Allis) onto the wire/lesion and resect the tissue around the wire.
- Adopt a methodical approach to tumour dissection. Place fingers over superior aspect of lesion, apply downward traction, and cut breast tissue down to pectoral fascia with scalpel or diathermy. Once on pectoral fascia, extend incision so as to undermine/lift lesion off pectoral fascia. Repeat the same to the inferior border of the tumour. Repeat the same steps to the lateral edges of the tumour. Remove the lesion and place a swab in the cavity.

- Orientate the specimen according to local preference, e.g. short stitch for superior, long stitch for lateral, and double stitch for posterior.
- Ensure haemostasis.
- Apply clips to edges of the cavity. This demarcates excision area and helps radiation oncologist in planning subsequent delivery of radiotherapy.

Closure

- Larger cavities may benefit from mobilization of remaining breast tissue and oncoplastic procedures to reshape the breast.
- Close the wound in two layers: interrupted inverted dermal sutures (e.g. 3.0 absorbable undyed monofilament) followed by a subcuticular stitch (e.g. 3.0 or 4.0 absorbable undyed monofilament).
- Apply adhesive strips (e.g. Steristrips) and an adhesive absorbent dressing.

Complications

Haematoma, infection, seroma formation, altered appearance, further surgery.

Microdochectomy

Procedure aims to excise a single terminal lactiferous duct.

Indications

Single duct nipple discharge either suspicious (bloody) or persistent.

Consent

Written consent. Explain risk of bruising, haematoma, infection, loss of nipple/areola sensation, nipple/areola necrosis (rare), scarring, inability to locate duct, further surgery, inability to breast feed.

Preoperative preparation

- Mark site. Do not express discharge at this point.
- Mark a peri-areolar incision to encompass one-third and no more than half of the circumference. Another option is to make a radial incision over the suspected duct (smaller incision limits operating field).

Position

Supine.

Procedure

- Identify duct by gently squeezing the nipple to identify discharge.
- Cannulate duct using a lacrimal probe.
- Sub-areolar infiltration of a local anaesthetic (without adrenaline) will often help dissection in the right plane.
- Ask assistant to stretch the skin and make the incision with a 15 blade.
- Place skin hooks and ask assistant to apply upward traction.
- Dissect areolar flap down to main ducts with blunt tenotomy scissors or diathermy, taking extra care not to buttonhole the skin.
- Identify and dissect the duct using fine artery forceps and scissors. Dissect about 2–3cm of the duct with a small margin of breast tissue around it.
- Ensure meticulous haemostasis.

Closure

- Close the wound in two layers: interrupted inverted dermal sutures (e.g. 3.0 absorbable undyed monofilament) followed by a subcuticular stitch (e.g. 3.0 or 4.0 absorbable undyed monofilament).
- Apply adhesive strips (e.g. Steristrips) and an adhesive absorbent dressing.

Complications

Haematoma, scarring, distortion of nipple, loss of nipple sensation, nipple necrosis, failure to excise the lesion.

Tips and tricks

In addition to the lacrimal probe, a small amount of patent V blue dye can be injected into the offending duct by cannulating the duct with a 23G (blue) cannula. Remove the needle and simply use the plastic catheter.

Total duct excision (Hadfield–Adair procedure)

Total excision of the terminal lactiferous ducts.

Indication

- Suspicious or persistent multiple duct discharge (patient choice) or similar single duct discharge that cannot be localized.
- Suspicious intraductal lesion.
- Recurrent peri-ductal mastitis.

Consent

Written consent. Explain risk of bruising, haematoma, infection, loss of nipple/areola sensation, nipple inversion, nipple/areola necrosis (rare), scarring, further surgery, inability to breast feed.

Preoperative preparation

- Mark site.
- Mark a peri-areolar incision to encompass one-third and no more than half of the circumference.

Procedure

- Sub-areolar infiltration of a local anaesthetic (preferably without adrenaline) will often help dissection in the right plane.
- Ask assistant to stretch the skin and make the incision with a 15 blade.
- Place skin hooks on skin edge, ask assistant to apply vertical traction, dissect areola down to terminal lactiferous ducts using blunt tenotomy scissors or diathermy, taking extra care not to buttonhole the skin.
- Use artery forceps to 'hook' around the terminal ducts. Gently probe from either side until you tunnel through. Take care not to create false passages (i.e. only including part of the ducts).
- Hook artery forceps around the ducts and disconnect them from the nipple with a scalpel or diathermy. Pay attention not to injure/buttonhole the nipple.
- Place a tissue forceps onto the ducts and pull upwards. Using diathermy, excise 3–4cm of ductal and breast tissue. The excision should cone outwards so you end up with a pyramidal-shaped tissue sample.
- Ensure haemostasis.
- Place a suture or clip on the terminal ducts to orientate the specimen.

Closure

- Often the nipple becomes inverted. Place two interrupted absorbable sutures (3.0 or 4.0) onto nipple dermis to maintain it everted.
- Close the wound in two layers: interrupted inverted dermal sutures (e.g. 3.0 absorbable undyed monofilament) followed by a subcuticular stitch (e.g. 3.0 or 4.0 absorbable undyed monofilament).
- Apply adhesive strips (e.g. Steristrips) and an adhesive absorbent dressing.

Complications

Haematoma, scarring, distortion of nipple, loss of nipple sensation, nipple necrosis, nipple inversion, failure to excise the lesion.

Breast reconstruction

The goals of surgical therapy for breast cancer are not only local tumour control but also restoration of an acceptable cosmetic outcome. The choice and timing of reconstruction must be balanced with the need for systemic adjuvant therapy and radiation. The cosmetic concerns should not compromise the surgical/medical oncological therapy.

Breast reconstruction can be broadly divided into two types: implant-based and autologous (patient's own tissue). Because of inherent complexity we only aim to provide an overview. It is not possible to detail the panoply of oncological/reconstructive procedures or combinations thereof in this book.

Implant-based reconstruction

- In broad terms, technically it is 'easier' and the initial recovery is swift. Generally, the cosmetic result is not as good or anatomical when compared to myocutaneous flaps. Revision surgery is common (implants do not last for life). Contralateral balancing surgery (lift, reduction) may also be necessary. Some of the more complex implant-based techniques (skin sparing or skin reducing, dermal and prosthetic slings) are not covered in this chapter.
- At times placement of a tissue expander (Fig. 5.6) under the pectoralis major muscle precludes that of the implant. It allows for gradual expansion of tissues and the creation of an adequate-sized 'pocket'. It can be placed at the time of initial surgery (immediate) or at a later date (delayed). Over 2 months it is gradually inflated about 25% more than the desired implant volume and maintained for 4–6 months.

Indications

Immediate or delayed implant-based reconstruction.

Contraindications

- Infection.
- Radiotherapy is a relative contraindication. It is acceptable to place a tissue expander, to allow the patient to have their adjuvant radiation therapy, and to perform final implant-based reconstruction later. This is an area of on-going discussion.

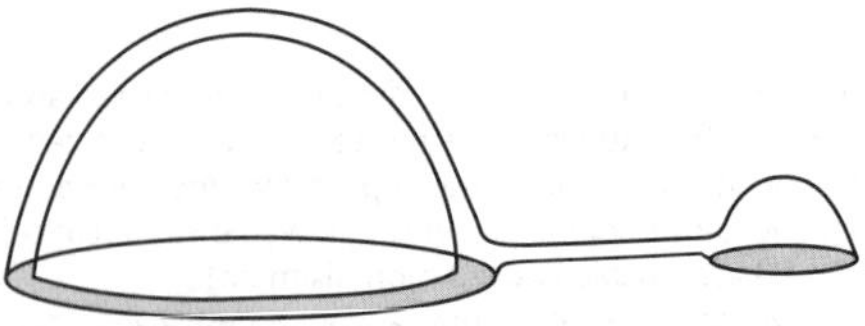

Fig. 5.6 Temporary tissue expander, connecting tube and reservoir dome. Reproduced with permission from McLatchie, G, and Leaper, D. Operative Surgery 2nd edition, Oxford University Press: 2006.

Consent

Written consent. Explain risks or bleeding, infection, implant failure, skin flap necrosis, scarring, delayed healing, poor cosmesis, asymmetry, capsular contracture, implant leak, further surgery.

Preoperative preparation

- Mark midline, inframammary fold, breast outline. This marks the limits of your flap dissection.
- If the patient has had a mastectomy, then copy the markings from the 'normal' side.
- Mark old mastectomy scar for subsequent excision.

Position

- Supine, with both arms out on arm boards (no more than 90° to avoid plexus neuropathy).
- Prepare and drape upper chest, exposing contralateral breast.

Procedure

- If patient has had a mastectomy, excise old mastectomy scar.
- Cut down onto the pectoralis major muscle.
- Separate the pectoralis major from the underlying serratus anterior, apply upward traction to the muscle, and create the sub-pectoral pocket with a combination of blunt and diathermy dissection, taking care to stop bleeding from perforating branches. Continue dissection to previously marked landmarks.
- Laterally dissect the serratus anterior fascia. It is thin; however, if intact, it provides good lateral support and helps to prevent lateral implant migration.
- Fully deflate the expander, part fill with saline, and insert into the pocket.
- Tunnel the inflation port (usually laterally a few cm below inframammary fold).

Closure

- A suction drain can be inserted behind the implant.
- Make sure there is no undue tension on the skin flaps. If so, deflate the expander as required.
- Close the wound in three layers: interrupted sutures to subcutaneous layer (2.0 or 3.0 absorbable suture), interrupted inverted dermal sutures (e.g. 3.0 absorbable undyed monofilament), and a subcuticular stitch (e.g. 3.0 or 4.0 absorbable undyed monofilament).
- Apply adhesive strips (e.g. Steristrips) and an adhesive absorbent dressing.

Once the expansion period is finished, the expander is replaced with a definitive implant following broadly the same steps.

Complications

Haematoma, infection, skin flap necrosis, implant migration, implant extrusion, implant failure (leak), capsular contracture, deformity.

Autologous flaps

The patient's own tissues are used to re-create the breast mound. The reconstruction is softer, more anatomical; it enables recreation of a ptotic mound, which will age at the same rate as the contralateral side. Autologous reconstruction can be performed immediately or delayed. These are long and complex surgical procedures; however, revisions tend to be shorter and less frequent. Because the vascular supply is paramount to flap health, co-morbidities, such as diabetes, heart disease, obesity, severe lung disease, and smoking, pose risks to a successful outcome.

Latissimus dorsi myocutaneous flap

Uses the latissimus dorsi muscle with or without skin/subcutaneous fat island (Fig. 5.7). It can be augmented with an implant to bolster the reconstructive volume. The thoracodorsal vascular pedicle needs to be intact.

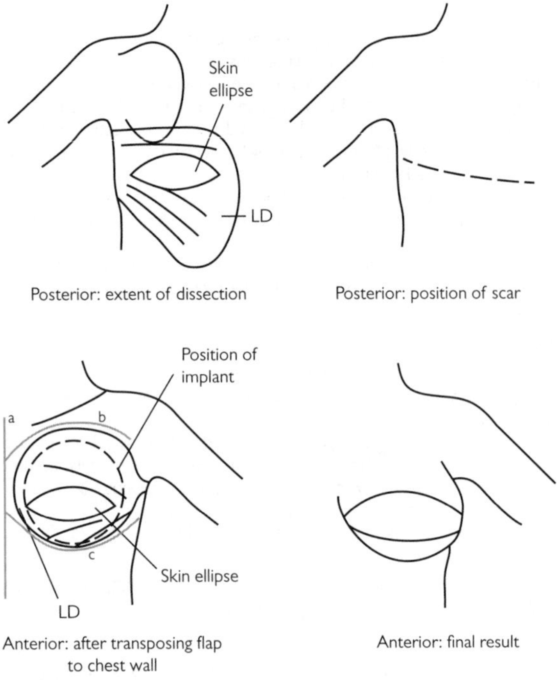
Skin
ellipse
LD
Posterior: extent of dissection
Posterior: position of scar
Position of
implant
a
b
c
Skin ellipse
LD
Anterior: after transposing flap
to chest wall
Anterior: final result

Fig. 5.7 Outline of latissimus dorsi flap. Landmarks: (a) midline; (b) breast contour; (c) inframammary fold. Reproduced with permission from McLatchie, G, and Leaper, D. Operative Surgery 2nd edition, Oxford University Press: 2006.

Indications

- Immediate or delayed breast reconstruction.
- Volume replacement following a high-volume, wide local resection (immediate or delayed).
- Salvage procedure for previously failed flaps or local recurrence.

Contraindications

- Relative contraindications: obesity, diabetes, lung disease, smoking, poor performance status, postoperative radiotherapy.
- Previous posterior thoracotomy (severed thoracodorsal pedicle).

Consent

Written consent. Explain risk of bleeding, infection, seroma, scarring, partial or complete flap failure, donor site scarring and pain, poor cosmesis, asymmetry, further surgery, as well as implant-based complications if you are using an implant.

Preoperative preparation

- Patient in upright position.
- Breast: mark midline, breast contour, inframammary fold.
- Back: mark midline, iliac crest, lateral border of latissimus dorsi, and feel tip of the scapula. Mark elliptical skin island (approximately four fingers below tip of scapula) along tension lines and ensure tension-free closure by pinching the skin island.

Position

A lateral position is necessary to harvest the flap. Excision of the mastectomy scar can also be done in this position. To insert the flap, move the patient to a supine position with both arms out on arm boards and expose the chest. If performing a mastectomy and immediate reconstruction, start with the patient in the supine position unless two operating teams are working together (simultaneous mastectomy and flap harvest).

Procedure

- Either perform a mastectomy/skin sparing mastectomy or excise old mastectomy scar and raise skin flaps to preoperative markings.
- Dissect into the axilla to identify the thoracodorsal pedicle and anterior border of the latissimus dorsi muscle.
- Incise skin ellipse markings, cut through superficial fascial layer and fat onto the latissimus dorsi muscle. Continue dissecting the superficial tissue plane off the muscle down to the iliac crest, medially, laterally, and up to scapula tip.
- Dissection of the muscle is classically done caudal to cranial. Inferio-laterally, develop a plane between the external oblique and latissimus dorsi muscle. Medially the muscle will have to be dissected off the thoracolumbar fascia. Supero-laterally the muscle has to be separated from the underlying serratus posterior. Supero-medially the muscle has to be separated as it dips below the trapezius. Further up you will also see the teres major muscle running horizontally at the inferior border of the scapula. This marks the upper limit of the LD (latissimus dorsi) dissection.

- Some ligate the serratus branch of the thoracodorsal pedicle, as it can sometimes hinder full mobilization of the muscle.
- Identify thoracodorsal pedicle.
- Tunnel flap through the axilla to the mastectomy defect, cover with a swab and adhesive film dressing.
- Return patient to supine position.
- Suture the edge of the myocutaneous flap to the chest wall. An implant can be placed under the flap at this time.
- Adjust flap position and shape.

Closure

- Place two suction drains—one in the LD donor site and the other posterior to the breast reconstruction.
- The back wound can be closed in three layers: interrupted sutures to subcutaneous fascial layer (2.0 absorbable suture), interrupted inverted dermal sutures (3.0 absorbable undyed monofilament), and a subcuticular stitch (3.0 absorbable undyed monofilament).
- The reconstruction can be closed in two layers: interrupted inverted dermal sutures (e.g. 3.0 absorbable undyed monofilament) and a subcuticular stitch (e.g. 3.0 or 4.0 absorbable undyed monofilament).
- Apply adhesive strips and an adhesive absorbent dressing.

Complications

Wound infection, haematoma, donor site seroma, partial or total flap loss, implant-based complications if using an implant, donor site scarring and pain.

Transverse rectus abdominis myocutaneous pedicled flap (pedicled TRAM)

The procedure harvests a flap of skin and abdominal fat supported by perforators that course through the underlying rectus abdominis muscle. It can either be tunnelled through to the chest in a 'pedicled' TRAM (Fig. 5.8) or the blood supply disconnected and anastomosed to the internal mammary artery in the case of a 'free' TRAM. A pedicled TRAM uses the superior epigastric artery pedicle, a 'free' TRAM the inferior epigastric artery pedicle.

Indications

Immediate or delayed breast reconstruction in patients with moderate/large breast size and sufficient abdominal tissue.

Contraindications

- Very obese patients (owing to increased risk of fat necrosis).
- Bilateral reconstruction (high abdominal wound related morbidity).
- Previous abdominal surgery (liposuction, abdominoplasty, transverse abdominal incisions).
- Smoking.
- Radiotherapy following reconstruction (relative).

Consent

Explain risk of bleeding, infection, seroma, scarring, partial or complete flap failure, fat necrosis, umbilical necrosis, incisional hernia over donor site, poor cosmesis, asymmetry, and further surgery.

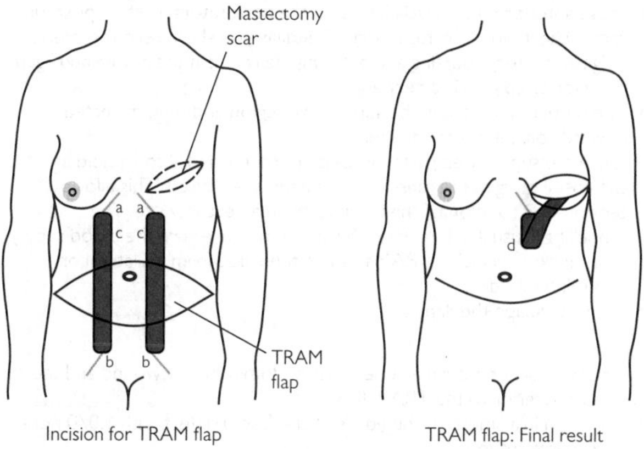
Mastectomy
scar
a
a
c
c
b
b
TRAM
flap
Incision for TRAM flap
d
TRAM flap: Final result

Fig. 5.8 Pedicled TRAM flap: (a) superior epigastric vessels; (b) inferior epigastric vessels; (c) rectus muscles; (d) rectus muscle with skin island tunnelled on superior epigastric artery pedicle. Adapted with permission from McLatchie, G, and Leaper, D. Operative Surgery 2nd edition, Oxford University Press: 2006.

Preoperative preparation

- Patient in the standing position.
- Breast: mark midline, breast contour, inframammary fold.
- Abdomen: mark midline from xyphysternum to pubic symphysis. Mark the ellipse of tissue to be harvested. Upper line includes umbilicus. Ideally the height of the flap should correspond to the distance from the inframammary fold to the upper breast line, but being able to close the abdominoplasty wound takes precedence.
- Doppler can be used to mark perforators.

Position

Supine, arms out on arm boards, chest and abdomen exposed.

Procedure

- Either perform a mastectomy or excise old mastectomy scar and raise skin flaps to preoperative markings.
- Incise abdominal markings (Fig. 5.8) and cut down to the abdominal wall fascia.
- Dissect flap off abdominal wall proceeding lateral to medial. The lateral and medial rows of perforators emerge through the anterior rectus sheath; these will support the flap so they need to be preserved. On the contralateral side they can be sacrificed, ensuring haemostasis.
- The umbilicus is circumcised.

- Incise anterior rectus fascia lateral to the perforators. Dissect posterior rectus sheath from rectus muscle. Caudally you should see the inferior epigastric artery coursing and entering the rectus muscle. Clip and ligate the inferior epigastric artery and vein.
- The muscle is divided in the suprapubic region and then dissected upwards off the posterior sheath.
- Once the superior epigastric vessels are seen (medial to xiphoid at the costal margin) the muscle attachments are incised. This allows tension-free rotation of the flap into the mastectomy site. The tunnelling is usually done over the sternum. Make sure the blood supply is not kinked. Pedicled TRAMs can be tunnelled from ipsilateral or contralateral side.
- Trim and shape the flap.

Closure

- Place two suction drains—one in the abdominoplasty wound and the other posterior to the TRAM flap.
- Suture an inlay mesh to the edges of the fascial defect with 1.0/0 non-absorbable sutures.
- Create an opening in the superior flap, which will accommodate the umbilicus. Suture the umbilicus with interrupted 4.0 absorbable sutures.
- Perform closure of the abdominoplasty wound in three layers: interrupted sutures to subcutaneous fascial layer (2.0 absorbable suture), interrupted inverted dermal sutures (3.0 absorbable undyed monofilament), and a subcuticular stitch (3.0 absorbable undyed monofilament).
- Suture flap in two layers: interrupted inverted dermal sutures (e.g. 3.0 absorbable undyed monofilament) and a subcuticular stitch (e.g. 3.0 or 4.0 absorbable undyed monofilament).
- Apply adhesive strips and dressings.

Complications

Partial or total flap loss/necrosis, fat necrosis of the flap (usually lesser perfused areas), delayed healing, scarring, seroma (abdominoplasty), infection, incisional hernia.

Free TRAM and deep inferior epigastric perforator (DIEP) free flap

Free flaps are harvested with their respective blood supply and re-anastomosed to the desired site employing microvascular techniques (microvascular instruments and magnification).

DIEP free flap is an evolution of the free TRAM flap and aims at reducing the morbidity associated with the resection of the rectus abdominis muscle and overlying anterior sheath: loss of abdominal wall strength and formation of incisional hernia. As a consequence a bilateral reconstruction using free DIEP flap can be done.

Indications

Immediate or delayed breast reconstruction.

Absolute contraindications

- Systemic disease: cardiovascular, autoimmune, COPD (chronic obstructive pulmonary disease), diabetes.
- Smoking.

Contraindications

- Transverse abdominal incisions.
- Previous liposuction.
- Postoperative radiotherapy.
- Obese patients.

Consent

Written consent. Explain risk of bleeding, infection, seroma, scarring, partial or complete flap failure/loss, fat necrosis, umbilical necrosis, poor cosmesis, asymmetry, further surgery.

Preoperative preparation

- As per pedicled TRAM.
- DIEP: the perforators are marked with Doppler on both sides. Some surgeons perform a preoperative CT angiogram.

Position

Supine, arms out on arm boards (no more than 90° to avoid plexus neuropathy), chest and abdomen exposed.

Procedure

- Free TRAM: harvested in the usual way, however, both superior/inferior epigastric vessels are mobilized and ligated.
- A DIEP flap: flap harvested in usual way to pre-marked perforators bilaterally.
- The largest perforator is chosen by clinical examination and intraoperative Doppler; the others can be clamped temporarily to assess perfusion through chosen perforator.
- The anterior rectus sheath is incised around the perforator and the rectus muscle split along the line of its fibres. The perforator is dissected through the muscle down to the inferior epigastric artery and vein. The inferior epigastric vessels are ligated and cut at their origin onto the external iliac vessels.
- The flap is flushed with a heparin/saline solution. A single systemic heparin dose is often also given.
- Microvascular anastomoses are fashioned between superior epigastric and internal mammary vessels. The internal mammary vessels course over the parietal pleura, lateral to the sternum. Access is by splitting the pectoralis muscle and excising a small section of the 3rd or 4th parasternal rib.
- In the case of a free TRAM, the inferior epigastric vessels can also be anastomosed to the thoracodorsal vessels to 'supercharge' the flap.
- Flaps are trimmed and shaped.

Closure

- Place two suction drains in the abdominoplasty wound.
- DIEP: a mesh is sutured to the fascial edges of the rectus muscle with interrupted 1.0 non-absorbable sutures; the anterior rectus sheath is closed over the mesh with continuous 2.0 non-absorbable sutures.
- Rest of closure as per pedicled TRAM.

Complications

Venous congestion of flap, arterial or venous flap thrombosis, partial or complete flap loss, fat necrosis, delayed healing, scarring, seroma.

Reduction mammoplasty

This describes a variety of surgical techniques that aim at reducing breast volume and skin envelope, whilst retaining or improving breast shape and preserving the nipple–areolar complex.

From an oncoplastic point of view, reduction mammoplasty allows for larger tumour resection volumes and/or resection of tumours in cosmetically unfavourable locations (e.g. superior, central, inferior). This can avoid the need for mastectomy in selected patients (depending on breast size and shape, and tumour location).

The concept of breast reduction involves creation of a dermo-glandular (parenchymal) 'pedicle' to support the nipple–areolar complex, excision of the redundant tissue, and reduction of the skin envelope if necessary. Inferior, superior, medial, and lateral pedicles have been described. We outline two common techniques: inferior pedicle and medial pedicle breast reductions.

Inferior pedicle mammoplasty

Indications

- Breast reduction (cf. NICE guidelines for criteria).
- Oncoplastic resection in patients with medium, large, or ptotic breasts.

Contraindications

Consider impact of cardiorespiratory co-morbidities, diabetes, and smoking.

Consent

Written consent. Explain risks of bleeding, infection, seroma, loss of nipple–areolar sensation, full or partial nipple–areolar necrosis, scarring, delayed healing, asymmetry, need for further surgery.

Preoperative preparation

- Patient in upright/standing position.
- Mark midline, inframammary fold, breast contour, and breast meridian (draw line from mid-clavicular point through nipple and inframammary fold).
- Mark new nipple position at the intersection of the inframammary fold with the breast meridian.
- Draw an inverted V with its peak at the previously marked new nipple position. The limbs of the V are ~8–9cm long. The angle of the V limbs determines the amount of parenchyma to be resected. A wide V angle will make skin closure difficult and also result in a flatter breast (i.e. less projection). Pinch the skin to ensure closure.
- Some measure angles between 70 and 120°, depending on breast size and tissue to be removed.
- Draw horizontal lines from the V limbs to the inframammary fold.
- Draw inferior pedicle with a base of 8–10cm.
- See Figs 5.9 and 5.10.

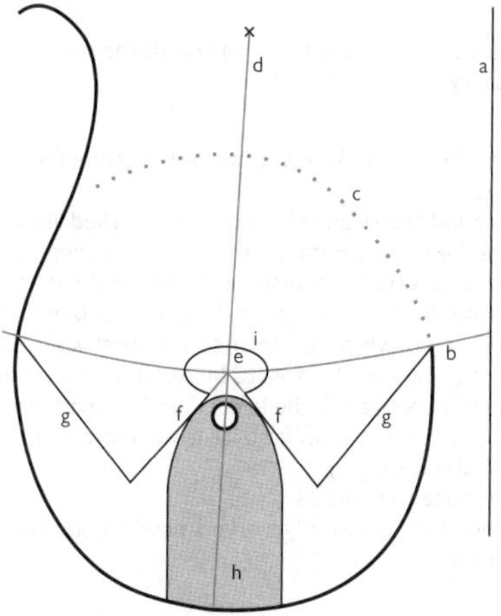
x
d
a
c
i
e
b
g
f
f
g
h

Fig. 5.9 Inferior pedicle breast reduction markings: (a) midline; (b) inframammary fold; (c) breast contour; (d) breast meridian; (e) new nipple position; (f) V limbs (measured from the new nipple position); (g) line from V limb to inframammary fold; (h) inferior pedicle base; (i) new areolar opening (elipse circumference measures ~16cm).

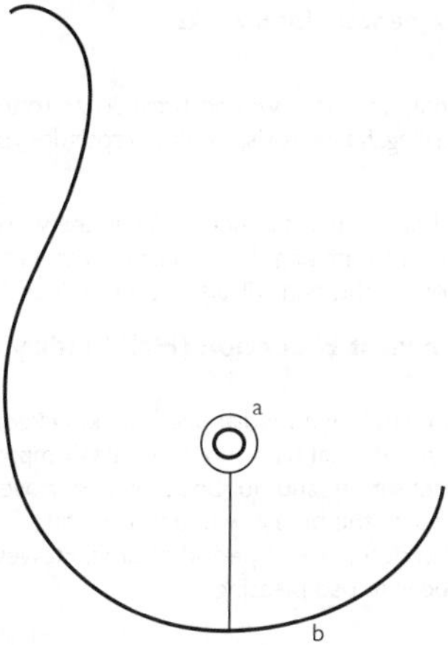
a
b

Fig. 5.10 Closure of the skin results in a peri-areolar and an 'inverted-T' scar: (a) peri-areolar scar; (b) inverted-T scar. The inferior portion of the scar is in the inframammary fold.

Position

Supine, chest exposed, arms out on arm boards (no more than 90° to avoid plexus neuropathy).

Procedure

- Use nipple marker to mark new nipple–areola complex over previously marked point.
- Incise skin around areola and skin along pre-marked lines.
- De-epithelize the skin over the pedicle as per marking.
- Raise skin flaps superiorly, medially, and laterally down to the pectoralis fascia but do not incise it (minimizes disruption of blood supply).
- Cut into parenchyma vertically down to the chest wall and excise redundant breast tissue. The area to be excised is essentially the area between the V markings and the inferior pedicle markings. Leave a small amount of breast tissue/fat over the pectoralis fascia (minimizes disruption of blood supply).
- Do not undermine the pedicle.
- Excise the skin of the previously marked 'new' areolar opening (Fig. 5.9e).
- Ensure haemostasis.

Closure

- Place a suction drain.
- Re-shape breast, bring out nipple–areolar complex through into new position, use skin clips to provisionally bring skin flaps together.
- Close in two layers: interrupted inverted dermal sutures (e.g. 2.0 or 3.0 absorbable) and a subcuticular stitch (e.g. 3.0 or 4.0 absorbable undyed monofilament).
- Adhesive strips and adhesive dressing.
- Supportive bra to be worn for 6 weeks.

Complications

Haematoma, seroma, infection, wound breakdown (often the T-junction), scarring, delayed healing, fat necrosis, nipple necrosis, loss of nipple sensation.

Tips and tricks

- When de-epithelizing skin it is easier to divide the work area into narrow strips by gently incising the epidermis with a knife.
- Generous traction on the skin will also help the dissection.

Medial pedicle breast reduction (Hall Findlay or snowman technique)

Nipple–areola supported by a medial pedicle. Skin excision pattern is also different, resulting in a vertical scar only. It results in improved breast shape, projection, nipple sensation, and no 'bottoming' out over time. Bottoming out describes a drop of the breast with ensuing lifting up of the inframammary fold, which can occur over a period of time. However, the immediate postoperative shape is not so pleasing.

Indications

- Breast reduction: small or medium-sized breasts. Not suited for large volume resections (>800g).
- Oncoplastic resections.

Contraindications

Consider impact of cardiorespiratory co-morbidities, diabetes, and smoking.

Consent

Written consent. Explain risks of bleeding, infection, seroma, loss of nipple areolar sensation, full or partial nipple–areolar necrosis, scarring, delayed healing, asymmetry, need for further surgery.

Preoperative preparation

- Mark midline, inframammary fold, breast contour, and breast meridian. Mark new nipple position at the intersection of the inframammary fold with the breast median.
- Mark the new areolar opening 2cm above the new nipple position. The drawing will look like an inverted fishbowl. The circumference of this drawing should be ~16–18cm.
- The skin resection pattern is then marked: draw a wide 'U-shape' or 'upright fishbowl' connecting it to the limbs of the nipple–areola marking. Pinch it to make sure the skin will come together without tension. The resulting drawing (areolar opening and U-shape marking) will look like a snowman, hence the name. The bottom of the snowman should be 2–4cm above inframammary fold. This will prevent the ensuing scar from crossing the fold.
- Draw the medial pedicle; its base (width) should be about 8cm.
- See Figs 5.11 and 5.12.

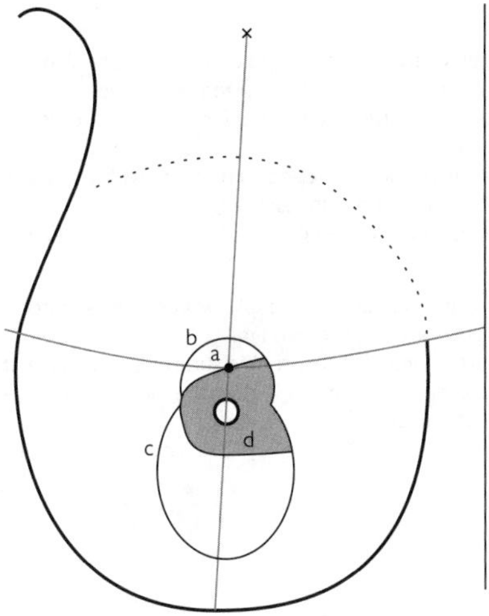
x
b
a
c
d

Fig. 5.11 Medial pedicle breast-reduction markings: (a) new nipple position; (b) new areolar opening ('inverted fishbowl'); (c) skin resection pattern ('U-shape'); (d) medial pedicle base.

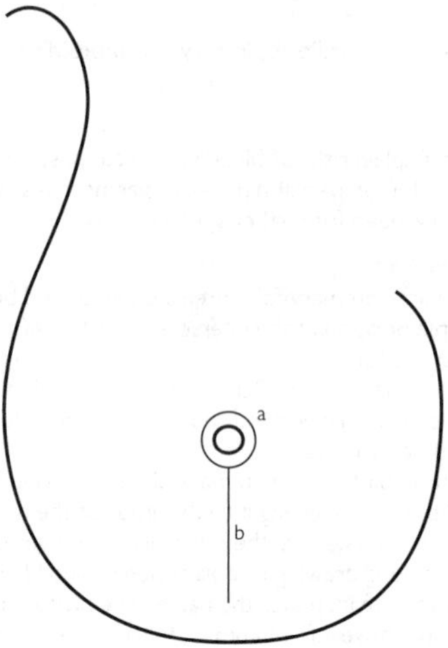
a
b

Fig. 5.12 Closure of the skin results in a peri-areolar and a vertical scar: (a) peri-areolar scar; (b) vertical scar. The vertical scar should be 2–4cm above the inframammary fold.

Procedure

- Mark the nipple–areola with a nipple marker. Incise skin around areola and incise skin markings. De-epithelize the pedicle.
- Create pedicle by cutting down to the chest wall. Do not incise pectoral fascia.
- Skin and parenchyma are excised as marked, with more tissue being excised by bevelling under the skin edges.
- More parenchyma is removed under the inferior skin flaps.

Closure

- Join the areolar opening with a staple or interrupted stitch and bring out the nipple–areolar complex through.
- Place few interrupted 3.0 absorbable sutures to approximate the lateral and medical breast parenchyma below the nipple. These are called the medial and lateral 'pillars'.

- Close in two layers: interrupted inverted dermal sutures (e.g. 2.0 or 3.0 absorbable) and a subcuticular stitch (e.g. 3.0 or 4.0 absorbable undyed monofilament). The inferior portion of the vertical scar is 'gathered up'. To help you visualize: the head of the snowman becomes the nipple–areola and the body of the snowman a vertical scar (Fig 5.12).
- Adhesive strips and adhesive dressing.
- Supportive bra to be work for 6 weeks.

Complications

Haematoma, seroma, infection, wound breakdown (often the T-junction), scarring, delayed healing, fat necrosis, nipple necrosis, loss of nipple sensation.

Chapter 6

Endocrine surgery

Ultrasound-guided fine-needle aspiration cytology of a thyroid nodule

Various techniques are described for thyroid fine-needle aspiration cytology (FNAC) using different types and gauges of needle, aspiration versus no aspiration, even core biopsy. The author prefers not to use aspiration (unless aspirating cysts), relying on the forward cutting motion of the needle and capillary action to obtain sufficient cells for cytological analysis. Whichever technique is employed, the clinician should aim to achieve >90% adequacy rate with minimum complications.

Thyroid FNAC should be done under ultrasound guidance to limit the rate of insufficient biopsies, reduce false-negative biopsies, and target the solid component of solid/cystic nodules.

Indications

- Cytological diagnosis of a:
  - symptomatic thyroid nodule
  - incidentally found thyroid nodule if solid >1–1.5cm, suspicious ultrasound features, or risk factors for thyroid cancer
  - suspicious/dominant nodule in multinodular goitre.
- In cystic nodules aspirate cystic component and perform FNAC of any solid component.

Consent

- Explain possibility of yielding insufficient number of cells for cytological diagnosis, cyst recurrence, and risk of bleeding (almost always managed conservatively).
- Ensure the patient is aware of the potential need for surgery, depending on biopsy results.

Procedure

- Position the patient supine in slight neck extension.
- A high resolution (7.5–15MHz) linear array transducer with a sterile cover is used.
- Clean the skin and place a small amount of sterile gel on the ultrasound probe.
- Infiltrate 2ml of local anaesthetic subcutaneously.
- Place the ultrasound probe over the nodule, usually in a transverse plane, and plan the trajectory of the needle from the point of insertion in the skin to the thyroid nodule, avoiding any major vessels.
- The author prefers a 21-gauge needle (though narrower diameter 23–27-gauge needles are often used) and does not attach a syringe to the needle unless cystic components of the nodule need to be aspirated.
- Monitor the trajectory of the needle to the target lesion with ultrasound (US) and aim to perform a series of quick (3/s) advance–withdraw oscillations for 2–5s in the nodule.

- Withdraw the needle, fill syringe with air, attach to the needle, and expel the aspirate onto glass slides. Smear aspirate onto slides and fix with 95% ethyl alcohol (for Papanicolaou stains) or air dry (Giemsa or Diff-Quik stains).
- Ask the patient to apply pressure to the biopsy site with a cotton-wool bud and place a small adherent dressing if necessary.

Complications

- Insufficient sample for cytological diagnosis.
  - This should occur in <10% of aspirates.
- Recurrence of cystic nodules if aspirated.
- Bleeding.
  - Rare but important as can cause airway compromise.
  - Consider stopping anticoagulation prior to FNAC.

Tips and tricks

FNAC is well tolerated by most patients and not associated with significant pain or distress. However, patients may be reassured by the use of local anaesthetic. Having a cytopathologist examine the aspirate immediately to assess whether there are sufficient cells for diagnosis is very useful.

Thyroidectomy

Anatomy

(See Figs 6.1 and 6.2)
Embryologically derived from the primitive pharynx and ultimobranchial body, the thyroid gland is a dark red bi-lobed encapsulated endocrine gland connected by a central isthmus. The distal remnants of embryological descent of the thyroid gland from the floor of the mouth may also result in a pyramidal lobe extension from the isthmus. Posterolaterally a protuberance of thyroid called the tubercle of Zuckerkandl lies next to a thickening of pre-tracheal fascia, known as the ligament of Berry, through which the recurrent laryngeal nerve (RLN) passes to reach the larynx. The thyroid gland lies anterior to, and is attached to, the trachea by the pre-tracheal fascia. It weighs about 20g.

Arterial supply is via the superior thyroid artery (a branch of the external carotid artery) and inferior thyroid artery (a branch of the thyrocervical trunk). Occasionally a thyroid ima artery may be present as a direct branch of the aorta or brachiocephalic trunk.

Venous drainage is via superior thyroid and inferior thyroid veins to the internal jugular and brachiocephalic veins, respectively. A middle thyroid vein is also commonly present that drains to the internal jugular vein. Lymphatic drainage mainly occurs to the peri-thyroid, pre-/para-tracheal, and pre-laryngeal lymph nodes before passing laterally to the internal jugular and posterior triangle nodes.

Anatomical position and relations

- Anterior—strap muscles of the neck, deep cervical fascia.
- Posterior—parathyroid glands, recurrent laryngeal nerves, trachea, pre-tracheal fascia.
- Lateral—carotid sheath and contents.
- Superior—larynx, external branch of the superior laryngeal nerve.
- Inferior—thymus/thyrothymic ligament, brachiocephalic vessels.

External branch of the superior laryngeal nerve (EBSLN)

This branch of the vagus nerve innervates the cricothyroid muscle. It runs from the vagus nerve to the cricothyroid muscle in close proximity to the branches of the superior thyroid artery and superior pole of the thyroid gland. Care must be taken to identify the EBSLN when mobilizing the superior pole of the thyroid gland to avoid injuring this nerve during thyroidectomy.

Recurrent laryngeal nerve (RLN)

The RLN is a branch of the vagus nerve that innervates all the muscles of the larynx except the cricothyroid. On the right it passes behind the subclavian artery before running obliquely to lie in the tracheo-oesophageal groove in close proximity to Berry's ligament (at which site it is most prone to injury during thyroidectomy) before entering the larynx. On the left side, the RLN passes behind the arch of the aorta before following a more vertical course to the tracheo-oesophageal groove. On the right side, a non-RLN very rarely occurs passing across to the larynx from the cervical vagus.

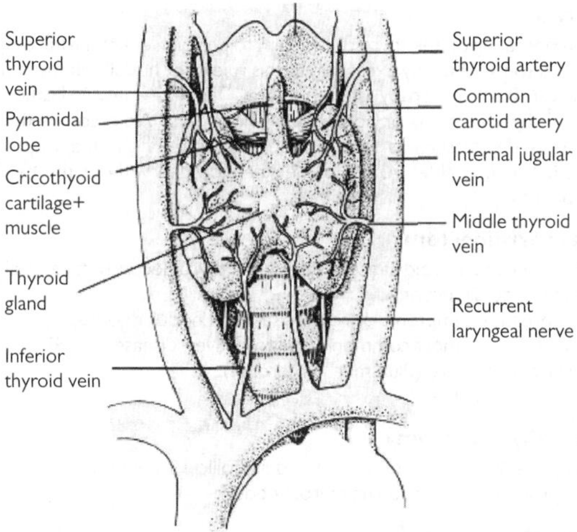
Superior
thyroid
vein
Pyramidal
lobe
Cricothyoid
cartilage+
muscle
Thyroid
gland
Inferior
thyroid vein
Superior
thyroid artery
Common
carotid artery
Internal jugular
vein
Middle thyroid
vein
Recurrent
laryngeal nerve

Fig. 6.1 Thyroid anatomy. Reproduced with permission from McLatchie, G, and Leaper, D. Operative Surgery 2nd edition, Oxford University Press: 2006.

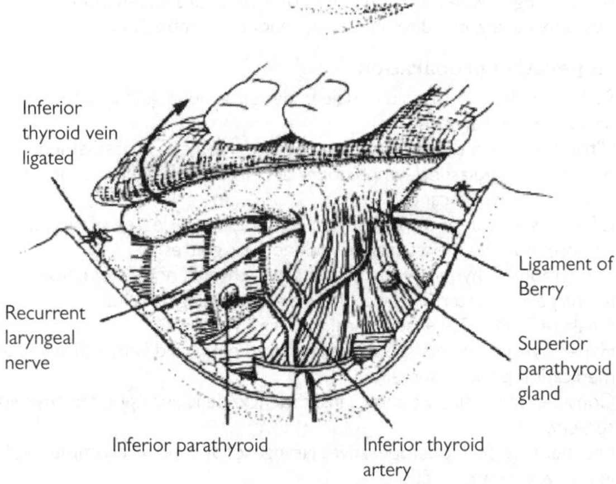
Inferior
thyroid vein
ligated
Recurrent
laryngeal
nerve
Ligament of
Berry
Superior
parathyroid
gland
Inferior parathyroid
Inferior thyroid
artery

Fig. 6.2 Anterior dislocation of the left thyroid lobe showing the RLN and parathyroids. Reproduced with permission from McLatchie, G, and Leaper, D. Operative Surgery 2nd edition, Oxford University Press: 2006.

Indications

When operating on the thyroid gland aim to perform either a total or hemi-thyroidectomy. The only exception to this rule is for nodules in the isthmus, which can be removed by isthmusectomy. There are few indications for subtotal thyroidectomy or nodulectomy nowadays. We recommend using an energy device such as the Harmonic® scalpel for the majority of the dissection as it enables vessels to be safely divided without the need for multiple ties.

Total thyroidectomy

- Differentiated thyroid cancer usually total thyroidectomy ± cervical lymph node dissection.
- Compression symptoms or cosmesis in multinodular goitre.
- Thyrotoxicosis most commonly due to Graves' disease or toxic multinodular goitre (Plummer's syndrome).
- Retrosternal goitre.

Hemi-thyroidectomy

- Diagnose indeterminate thyroid nodule/follicular neoplasm.
- Symptomatic or functioning thyroid nodule.

Consent

- The patient must understand the need for lifelong thyroxine supplementation following total thyroidectomy and occasionally hemi-thyroidectomy.
- Discuss complications, in particular emphasizing potential for voice change, need for calcium and/or vitamin D supplementation postoperatively, bleeding, infection, venous thromboembolism.

Preoperative preparation

- Perform FNAC of thyroid nodule under ultrasound guidance for preoperative diagnosis.
- Ultrasound/non-contrast computed tomography (CT) assessment of cervical/mediastinal lymph nodes ± FNAC and evidence of local invasion in thyroid cancer.
- CT to assess extent of retrosternal extension and degree of airway compression/deviation in large multinodular goitres.
- Scintigraphy in hyperthyroid patients with thyroid nodule(s) considered for surgery to determine site of hyper-functioning nodules.
- Measure TSH, T3, T4, serum calcium, and vitamin D.
- Hyperthyroid patients should be rendered euthyroid with anti-thyroid medication prior to surgery.
- Consider correcting vitamin D insufficiency/deficiency prior to thyroid surgery.
- Preoperative (and postoperative) laryngoscopy is now recommended to assess vocal cord function.

Position

- Supine with arms at side, padded bolster beneath shoulders, neck extended, and head resting on padded head-ring (see Fig. 6.3).
- Head of operating table elevated to empty neck veins.

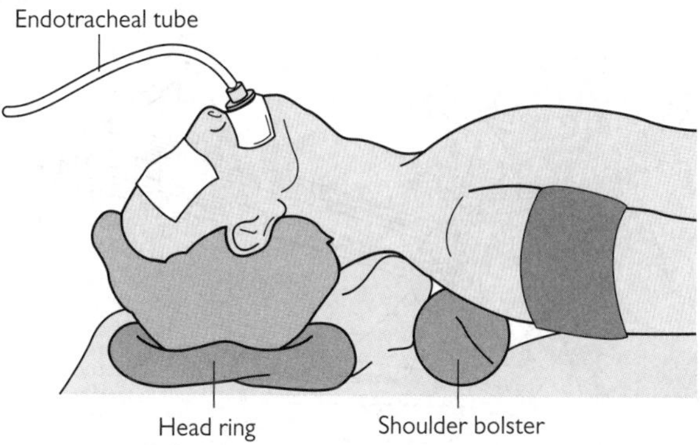
Endotracheal tube
Head ring
Shoulder bolster

Fig. 6.3 Position of patient for thyroidectomy or parathyroidectomy.

Incision

- Mark a symmetrical collar incision midway between the sternal notch and the cricoid cartilage, ideally in a skin crease extending to the medial border of the sternomastoid muscle.
- Consider infiltration of local anaesthetic with adrenaline or cervical plexus block.

Procedure

- Deepen the incision with diathermy through platysma.
- Dissect subplatysmal plane from thyroid cartilage to sternal notch.
- Use Joll's retractor to separate wound edges.
- Either separate strap muscles in the midline (Fig. 6.4) or divide them. If dividing the strap muscles do so as far cranially as possible due to an inferiorly based nerve supply from the ansacervicalis.
- Open the plane between the strap muscles and thyroid gland by blunt/diathermy dissection (Fig. 6.4).
- Ligate and divide the middle thyroid vein, if present, using an energy device (harmonic scalpel or ligasure) or Ligaclips®/ties and retract the strap muscles laterally.
- Divide the loose areolar tissue in the lateral thyroid recess down to the prevertebral fascia.
- Develop the avascular plane (of Reeve) between the larynx medially and superior thyroid vessels laterally with Lahey forceps. Pass blunt forceps laterally behind the superior pole vessels and gently pull caudally.
- The superior thyroid vessels can then be divided with an energy device such as the Harmonic® scalpel or Ligasure (Fig. 6.5) or tied/divided close to the upper thyroid pole to avoid damaging the external branch of the superior

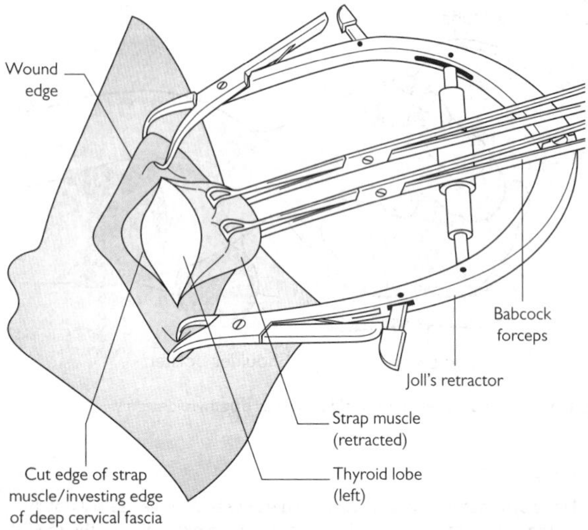
Wound
edge
Babcock
forceps
Joll's retractor
Strap muscle
(retracted)
Thyroid lobe
(left)
Cut edge of strap
muscle/investing edge
of deep cervical fascia

Fig. 6.4 Dissection plane beneath retracted strap muscles to expose left thyroid lobe.

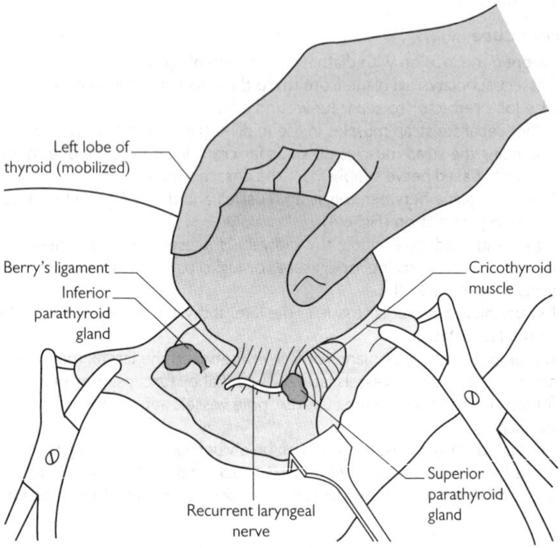
Left lobe of
thyroid (mobilized)
Berry's ligament
Inferior
parathyroid
gland
Cricothyroid
muscle
Superior
parathyroid
gland
Recurrent laryngeal
nerve

Fig. 6.5 Left hemi-thyroidectomy—view of RLN.

laryngeal nerve, which lies on/supplies the cricothyroid muscle—this nerve can interdigitate with branches of the superior thyroid artery and should ideally be identified before ligating these vessels.
- Reflect the thyroid lobe upwards and perform a capsular dissection dividing the branches of the inferior thyroid artery (ITA) close to the thyroid to avoid damaging the blood supply to the parathyroid glands.
- The parathyroid glands should be identified, dissected free, and gently swept away from the thyroid gland with a pledget. If the blood supply to the parathyroid gland is divided during this manoeuvre, and the gland becomes ischaemic, place the gland in saline, cut into small pieces, and transplant into a small pocket in the sternomastoid muscle at the end of the procedure (close the pocket with a non-absorbable suture).
- The RLN should be identified lying deep to the tubercle of Zuckerkandl passing from the tracheo-oesophageal groove to the larynx. It is usually situated behind the ITA but may pass in front or between the branches of the ITA. Rarely the RLN is non-recurrent on the right side and the surgeon should be aware of this possibility. If it is difficult to identify the RLN at this site, the superior pole of the thyroid can be reflected downwards until the RLN is encountered entering the larynx.
- Intraoperative nerve monitoring maybe used as an adjunct to map the course of the RLN, confirm its presence, or warn of impending traction/compression injury to the nerve.
- Use the energy device to divide the small vessels in the thickening of pre-tracheal fascia (Berry's ligament), being careful to avoid thermal injury to the RLN, which passes just below this fascia (Fig. 6.2).
- Reflecting the thyroid upwards, divide its attachments to the trachea. Divide the isthmus with the energy device or over-sew with absorbable sutures in hemi-thyroidectomy. Repeat above steps on contralateral side for a total thyroidectomy.
- Dissect out a pyramidal lobe extension if present in total thyroidectomy, which may extend to the hyoid bone.
- Ensure haemostasis and place a drain if a large dead-space is left.

Closure

Close strap muscles, platysma, and skin separately with a continuous suture (the author uses a 3.0 braided absorbable suture for the deep layers and a 4.0 absorbable monofilament subcuticular suture for skin).

Postoperative care

- Monitor for neck haematoma.
- Remove drain on first postoperative day.
- Check serum calcium daily following total thyroidectomy until stable (48h is sufficient if normal and no significant downwards trend).
- A protocol should be agreed to guide calcium replacement if hypocalcaemia occurs.
- Start thyroxine replacement on first postoperative day after total thyroidectomy.
- Discharge usually on first postoperative day following hemi-thyroidectomy and second postoperative day after total thyroidectomy.

Complications

- Hypocalcaemia.
  - Temporary need for calcium and vitamin D supplementation occurs in up to 30% of patients after total thyroidectomy.
  - Chronic hypoparathyroidism requiring long-term calcium/vitamin D supplements occurs in <10% following total thyroidectomy.
- Voice change due to recurrent RLN or EBSLN injury.
  - Unilateral RLN injury occurs in 1–2% of patients after thyroid surgery and may cause hoarse voice and swallowing difficulties.
  - Bilateral RLN is thankfully extremely rare but can cause aphonia and stridor necessitating tracheostomy.
  - EBSLN injury may result in difficulty singing high notes and voice projection.
- Haematoma.
  - Occurs in <1% of thyroidectomies in experienced hands but can be life-threatening due to airway compromise necessitating emergency evacuation.

Tips and tricks

- Careful positioning of the patient is essential.
- Meticulous dissection is needed to avoid bleeding that may obscure the view of the RLN and parathyroid glands.
- Capsular dissection is necessary to avoid RLN/EBSLN injury.
- The RLN is most commonly damaged superior to its intersection with the ITA at Berry's ligament. Ensure you have identified it fully before dividing the ligament.

Parathyroidectomy—bilateral neck exploration (BNE)

Anatomy

(See Figs 6.6–6.8)

The parathyroid glands are paired yellow-brownish glands lying in the space around the thyroid gland. Normal weight for an individual gland is 30–70mg. In the majority, there are four glands: a superior and an inferior on each side, usually located in symmetrical positions within a 1cm radius of the intersection of the RLN, and an ITA. The number and position of the parathyroid glands is variable. The parathyroid glands usually receive their blood supply from branches of the inferior thyroid artery, though blood supply may be from the superior thyroid artery in 10–15% of glands.

Superior parathyroid glands

- Embryologically from the ultimobranchial body located in the 4th branchial (pharyngeal) arch.
- Most commonly found above and lateral to the intersection of the RLN and the ITA; the superior glands are more constant in position than the inferior glands.
- Large superior parathyroid adenomas may migrate posteriorly to a para-oesophageal position and inferiorly to lie from the level of the lower pole of the thyroid gland to the posterior mediastinum.
- Retropharyngeal or retro-oesophageal spaces are more unusual locations of the superior parathyroid glands.

Inferior parathyroid glands

- From the 3rd branchial arch, therefore closely related embryologically to the thymus.
- Position less constant than the superior glands but usually found around the lower pole of the thyroid gland below and medial to the intersection of the RLN and ITA.
- Embryological descent of the thymus may result in the inferior parathyroid gland being present in the thyrothymic tract/thymus or anterior mediastinum.
- Rarely inferior parathyroid glands are located behind/above the superior thyroid lobe or within the thyroid gland.

Indications

- Secondary/tertiary hyperparathyroidism in renal failure.
- Primary hyperparathyroidism (PHPT) with:
  - negative or discordant localization on preoperative imaging
  - familial parathyroid disease as in multiple endocrine neoplasia (MEN) syndrome.

Consent

- Warn about potential failure of the operation to control hyperparathyroidism, i.e. persistent disease. This should occur in <2–3% of patients in experienced hands, and is more common following negative preoperative localization.

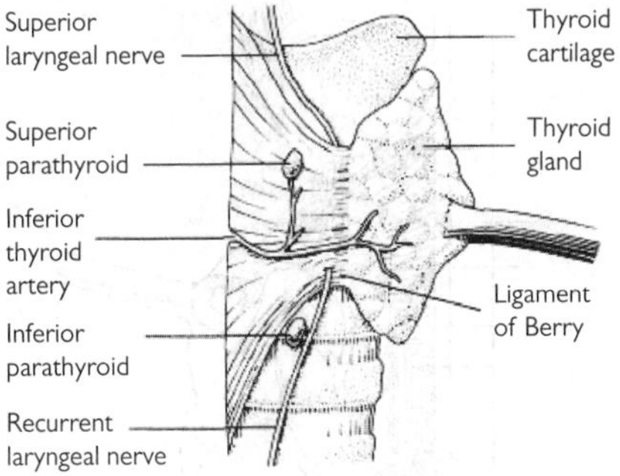
Superior laryngeal nerve
Thyroid cartilage
Superior parathyroid
Thyroid gland
Inferior thyroid artery
Ligament of Berry
Inferior parathyroid
Recurrent laryngeal nerve

Fig. 6.6 Anterior dislocation of the right thyroid lobe to show the RLN and parathyroids. Reproduced with permission from McLatchie, G, and Leaper, D. Operative Surgery 2nd edition, Oxford University Press: 2006.

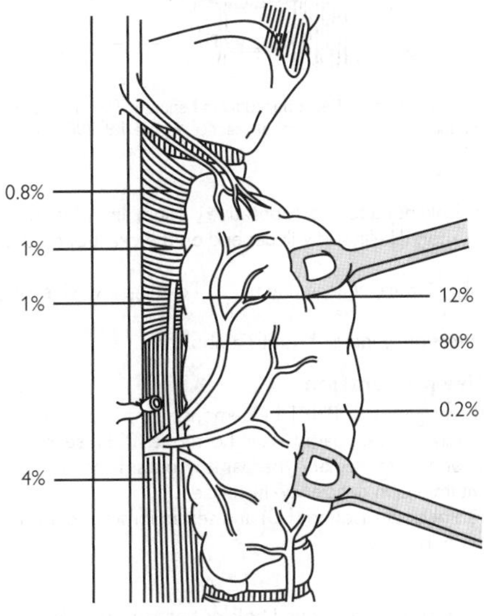
0.8%
1%
1%
4%
12%
80%
0.2%

Fig. 6.7 Superior parathyroids. Reproduced from Lennard, Tom, Endocrine Surgery: a companion to specialist surgical practice, Figure 1.9, 2009, with permission from Elsevier.

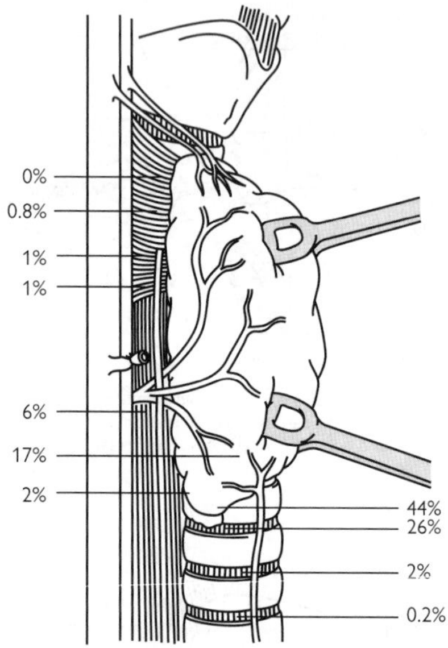
0%
0.8%
1%
1%
6%
17%
2%
44%
26%
2%
0.2%

Fig. 6.8 Inferior parathyroids. Reproduced from Lennard, Tom, Endocrine Surgery: a companion to specialist surgical practice, Figure 1.9, 2009, with permission from Elsevier.

- Discuss possible need for postoperative calcium and vitamin D supplementation (likelihood will depend on the exact operation and indication).
- Warn of risk of voice change due to RLN damage, which should be <1%.
- Bleeding, infection, venous thromboembolism.

Preoperative preparation

- Confirm the diagnosis of PHPT by demonstrating hypercalcaemia with inappropriately elevated parathyroid hormone (PTH) secretion.
- Exclude secondary causes of hyperparathyroidism and consider replacing vitamin D in deficiency/insufficiency.
- Imaging with neck ultrasound (US) and sestamibi scan to localize the disease preoperatively.

Position

- Supine with arms at side, padded bolster beneath shoulders, neck extended, and head resting on padded head-ring (see Fig. 6.3).
- Head of operating table slightly elevated to empty neck veins.

Incision and access

- Mark a symmetrical collar incision midway between the sternal notch and the cricoid cartilage, ideally in a skin crease extending to the medial border of the sternomastoid muscle.
- Consider infiltration of local anaesthetic with adrenaline or cervical plexus block.

Procedure

- Divide the middle thyroid vein between Ligaclips® and retract the strap muscles laterally off the thyroid gland.
- Use blunt/sharp dissection to divide the loose areolar tissue in the lateral thyroid recess down to the prevertebral fascia.
- The parathyroid glands are generally located within a 1cm radius of the intersection of the RLN and the ITA, and are identified as yellow-brown structures with a distinct vascular pedicle. They are quite mobile and bruise easily, both of which can be useful in identification.
- Delicate dissection is essential to avoid bleeding from small vessels, which can otherwise obscure the view. Divide small vessels between Ligaclips® or with diathermy.
- Begin to look for the inferior parathyroid glands around the lower pole of the thyroid gland. If not here, they can often be found in the thyrothymic tract or the thymus.
- Cervical thymectomy is performed by applying artery clips to the thyrothymic tract and gently pulling the thymus cranially out of the anterior mediastinum. It may be done to retrieve a parathyroid adenoma in the thymus.
- The superior parathyroid glands should be sought above and posterior to the RLN/ITA intersection. If not here, they may be found behind/above the upper thyroid pole, which may need to be mobilized by ligating and dividing the superior thyroid vessels to identify the superior parathyroid gland in this location. Large superior parathyroid glands may prolapse posteriorly to the prevertebral fascia where they then can descend to lie in an inferior position anywhere from behind the thyroid lobe to the superior mediastinum.
- More unusual locations to find parathyroid glands include the carotid sheath and retro-pharyngeal/oesophageal space. Intra-thyroidal parathyroid glands are very rare. Avoid performing a blind hemi-thyroidectomy in the hope of removing an adenoma in this location.
- In BNE aim to identify all four parathyroid glands. Parathyroid tumours are dissected free from the surrounding structures and excised after applying a Ligaclip® to the vascular pedicle. Take care not to breach the capsule, which can cause seeding of parathyroid tissue throughout the neck (parathormotosis).
- In multi-gland disease, the number of glands removed is a matter of judgement/experience but must balance the risk of recurrent disease with the need for long-term calcium supplements. Normal parathyroid glands should not be excised.

- Subtotal parathyroidectomy is generally performed for secondary/tertiary hyperparathyroidism in renal failure, particularly if the patient is going to have a renal transplant. In this operation, either a normal-sized remnant of a single gland is left behind with a Ligaclip® applied across its body or a total parathyroidectomy is undertaken with re-implantation of a normal-sized remnant of parathyroid (cut into small pieces) into muscle—either the sternomastoid muscle in the neck or the brachioradialis in the forearm.
- Frozen section or intraoperative PTH measurement may be used as an adjunct to parathyroid surgery.
- Intraoperative monitoring of PTH levels takes advantage of the short half-life (3–5min) of PTH. Monitoring venous PTH levels and comparison to preoperative levels can allow a more focused, quicker operation, and is predictive of postoperative success. Commonly a reduction of over 50% is accepted as an indication of adequate excision of hyperfunctioning parathyroid tissue.

Closure

Close strap muscles, platysma, and skin separately with a continuous suture (the author uses a braided 3.0 absorbable suture for the deep layers and a 4.0 absorbable monofilament subcuticular suture for skin).

Postoperative care

- Monitor for haematoma.
- Measure serum calcium postoperatively (daily or more frequently if low or symptomatic) and treat with oral/intravenous calcium ± vitamin D supplements. Each unit should have an agreed protocol for managing hypocalcaemia following parathyroid surgery.
- Patients can be discharged once serum calcium is stable and they are asymptomatic.

Complications

- Hypocalcaemia.
- Voice change.
- Bleeding.
- Infection.
- Persistent disease.

Tips and tricks

- If you are experiencing difficulty locating a gland, stay calm and logical. Make sure the gland is not in its usual location, as a missed parathyroid gland is more often found in its normal site than in an abnormal one.
- Superior and inferior parathyroid glands are usually found in symmetrical positions in the neck, therefore finding the contralateral gland may be helpful.
- Avoid blind hemi-thyroidectomy if you cannot locate a parathyroid gland.

Parathyroidectomy—minimally invasive parathyroidectomy (MIP)

Minimally invasive parathyroidectomy (MIP) is undertaken through a small central or lateral neck incision. Various approaches have been described, including MIP, minimally invasive video-assisted parathyroidectomy (MIVAP), and endoscopic parathyroidectomy. MIP via a lateral incision over the site of the parathyroid adenoma is the most popular approach and is described under 'Incision' (p. 296).

Indications

- Primary hyperparathyroidism with concordant preoperative localization of the adenoma on at least two imaging modalities (ultrasound/ sestamibi scan/computed tomography/magnetic resonance imaging).
- If minimally invasive surgery is undertaken with only a single preoperative scan identifying an adenoma, then intraoperative PTH measurement should be done to exclude multi-gland disease.

Consent

- Warn about the small possibility of persistent hyperparathyroidism due to failure to identify the causative gland or unrecognized multi-gland disease.
- Explain possible need to convert to BNE if unable to find the causative parathyroid gland at MIP or if findings suggest multi-glandular disease.
- Discuss possible need for postoperative calcium and vitamin D supplementation (likelihood will depend on the exact operation and indication).
- Warn of risk of voice change due to RLN damage, which should be <1%.
- Bleeding, infection, venous thromboembolism.

Position

- Supine with arms at side, padded bolster beneath shoulders, neck extended, and head resting on padded head-ring (see Fig. 6.3).
- Head of operating table elevated to empty neck veins.

Incision

2cm transverse incision, ideally centred over the site of the adenoma (located perioperatively with ultrasound) or on the side of the adenoma extending from the midline laterally.

Procedure

- Deepen incision with diathermy through platysma.
- Dissect subplatysmal plane using diathermy inferiorly and superiorly.
- Medial and lateral approaches to access the adenoma can be used, depending on surgeon-preference.
    - *Medial approach*: the midline between the strap muscles is identified after incising the investing layer of deep cervical fascia. The sternohyoid and sternothyroid muscles are retracted laterally off the thyroid gland.

  - *Lateral approach*: dissect along the medial border of the sternomastoid and retract laterally, identify the lateral border of the sternohyoid and the sternothyroid, and retract medially off the thyroid gland (the omohyoid is usually superior to the operative area).
- Ligate the middle thyroid vein, if present, between Ligaclips®.
- Retract the thyroid gland medially with a pledget, while the assistant retracts the sternomastoid laterally with a Langenbeck retractor.
- Perioperative ultrasound is particularly useful to identify the precise location of the parathyroid adenoma with relation to the surrounding neck structures. Dissection can then proceed directly to the target, while being aware of the path of the recurrent laryngeal nerve in relation to the adenoma/operative field.
- Staying close to the capsule, dissect out the parathyroid adenoma from the surrounding tissue and apply a Ligaclip® across its pedicle.

Closure

- Close strap muscles (in medial approach) with a continuous 3.0 absorbable suture.
- Close platysma and skin (the author uses a 3.0 braided absorbable suture for the deep layer and a 4.0 absorbable monofilament subcuticular suture for the skin).

Postoperative care

- Measure serum calcium on first postoperative day and give supplements if hypocalcaemia occurs (see ➔ 'Parathyroidectomy—bilateral neck exploration (BNE)', p. 290).
- Hypocalcaemia is less common than after BNE and so patients who are eucalcaemic and asymptomatic may be discharged on the first postoperative day.

Complications

- Hypocalcaemia.
- Voice change.
- Bleeding.
- Infection.
- Persistent disease.

Tips and tricks

- Tailor the incision to your approach and the location of the parathyroid adenoma (perioperative US is useful here).
- Removing a parathyroid adenoma through a small incision requires a meticulous technique and attention to haemostasis.
- Enlarge the incision, if necessary, for large/deeply situated parathyroid adenomas or in large necks.
- Stay close to the capsule when dissecting out a parathyroid adenoma to minimize damage to nearby structures such as the RLN.
- By spacing out your subcuticular skin suture bites the wound will 'concertina' leaving a smaller scar.

Adrenalectomy

Introduction

Minimally invasive surgery is now the standard surgical approach to the adrenal gland. Open surgery is usually reserved for malignant adrenal tumours to enable safe, compartmental tumour resection along oncological principles, and for large tumours (>8–12cm, depending on expertise) and multiple tumours, particularly synchronous adrenal and extra-adrenal tumours. Open approaches to the adrenal gland include anterior, lateral, and posterior.

The open posterior approach to the adrenal gland, although historically important, has been largely superseded by minimally invasive techniques, as it provides only limited access for larger tumours. The open anterior approach provides excellent access for major vessel control and en bloc resection of adjacent organs in malignant adrenal tumours, and access to both adrenal glands in bilateral and synchronous adrenal/extra-adrenal phaeochromocytoma. The open lateral approach, although providing more limited access than the open anterior approach remains an option for large, benign, unilateral adrenal tumours.

Anatomy

(See Fig. 6.9)

The adrenal glands are paired retroperitoneal glands of the neuroendocrine system, weighing 5–7g. They have a characteristic golden colour due to their cholesterol content. The left is semilunar in shape and lies superomedial to the left kidney. The right is pyramidal in shape and lies superior to the right kidney.

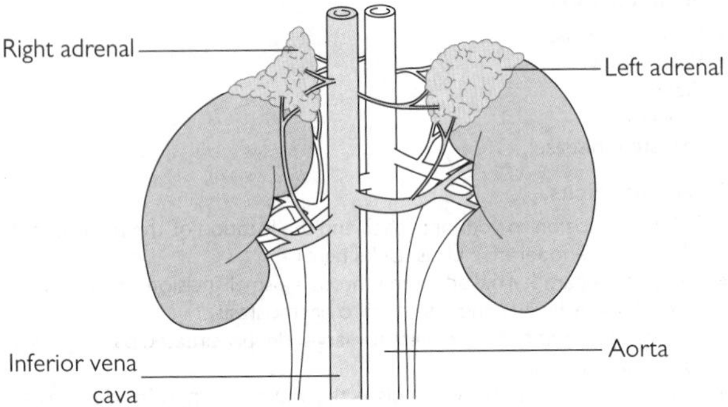
Right adrenal
Left adrenal
Aorta
Inferior vena
cava

Fig. 6.9 The adrenal glands.

The adrenal glands have two distinct parts:

- The outer cortex, derived from mesoderm, is divided into three zones called the zona glomerulosa, zona fasciculate, and zona reticularis, which secrete aldosterone, cortisol, and sex steroids, respectively.
- The inner medulla, derived from neural crest tissue, synthesizes catecholamines, including noradrenaline and adrenaline.

Vascular supply

The arterial supply is from small branches of the inferior phrenic artery, aorta, and renal artery, and the venous drainage via a single adrenal vein—the right adrenal vein drains directly to the inferior vena cava (IVC) and the left adrenal vein drains to the left renal vein.

Nerve supply

Secretion of hormones from the adrenal medulla occurs via activation of the sympathetic nervous system and the adrenal medulla can be considered a specialized ganglionic synapse directly receiving sympathetic preganglionic fibres from T5-9 spinal roots. In normal circumstances synthesis of cortisol and sex steroids from the adrenal cortex is regulated by trophic hormones from the hypothalamic–pituitary–adrenal axis and aldosterone via renin/ angiotensin II.

Anatomical position and relations

- Left adrenal gland: anterior—splenic artery, pancreas, peritoneum of the lesser sac; posterior, superior—diaphragm; medial—aorta; lateral, inferior—left kidney, renal vessels.
- Right adrenal gland: anterior, superior—bare area of the liver; posterior, lateral—diaphragm; medial—inferior vena cava; inferior—right kidney, renal vessels.

Anterior open adrenalectomy

Indications

- Malignant tumours of the adrenal cortex or medulla.
- Large adrenal tumours >8–12cm.
- Bilateral adrenal tumours or synchronous adrenal/extra-adrenal phaeochromocytoma.

Preoperative preparation

- Careful preoperative clinical, biochemical, and radiological work-up are essential prior to adrenal surgery to avoid perioperative complications.
- Appropriate biochemical investigation should be undertaken to confirm (or exclude) tumour functionality, including (but not limited to) serum electrolytes and sex hormones, plasma renin/aldosterone (Conn's syndrome), plasma and urine overnight metanephrines (phaeochromocytoma), 24h urine cortisol, and overnight dexamethasone suppression test (Cushing's syndrome).
- Adrenal venous sampling may be needed to confirm laterality of the tumour in Conn's adenoma.
- Radiological investigation should include computed tomography (CT) with adrenal protocol to characterize and stratify the risk of malignancy.
- Meta-iodobenzylguanidine (MIBG) scan is done in phaeochromocytoma to confirm functionality of the causative lesion seen on cross-sectional imaging and to exclude extra-adrenal lesions/metastases.
- Hypertension and electrolyte abnormalities due to mineralocorticoid excess in Conn's adenoma needs to be corrected prior to surgery.
- Catecholamine excess in phaeochromocytoma needs to be pharmacologically blocked prior to surgery and any complications of this, such as cardiac arrhythmia/failure, addressed.
- Medical complications of glucocorticoid secretion in Cushing's syndrome, such as diabetes mellitus, hypertension, and osteoporosis, need to be managed prior to surgery.

Consent

- In malignant tumours with radiological evidence/suspicion of invasion of surrounding structures (e.g. kidney), consent for the possibility of en bloc resection of these structures.
- Discuss complications, including bleeding, damage to nearby structures (bowel, spleen, pancreas, inferior vena cava), infection, wound problems, venous thromboembolism, and cardiovascular events.
- In surgery for Cushing's syndrome explain the need for perioperative steroid replacement, and that symptoms and signs of cortisol excess will take months to fully resolve.
- Following surgery for phaeochromocytoma or aldosterone producing tumour, antihypertensive medication can be reduced and often discontinued.

Position

Supine with arms at side or at 90°.

Incision

Rooftop, subcostal, or vertical midline ± transverse extension on side of the tumour.

Procedure

Right

- Mobilize the hepatic flexure of the colon inferiorly and the liver superiorly, dividing the right triangular ligament of the liver if necessary. Consider using a table-mounted retractor such as the Omni-tract®.
- Divide the posterior parietal peritoneum in the hepatorenal pouch to expose the retroperitoneal fat, kidney, adrenal gland, and IVC.
- Dissect along the lateral border of the IVC from the liver to the renal pedicle, identifying the short, right adrenal vein passing transversely from the lateral border of the IVC to the medial border of the adrenal gland.
- Ligate the right adrenal vein between ties, Ligaclips®, or using an energy device such as the Harmonic scalpel®.
- Complete the dissection of the adrenal tumour before lifting the tumour forward to divide its posterior attachments.
- Often a small extension of the adrenal gland passes behind the IVC at the superior–medial extent of the dissection. This needs to be excised if a total adrenalectomy is performed.
- The adrenal gland is supplied with blood from small branches of the inferior phrenic, aorta, and renal arteries, which are easily ligated during this dissection.
- In malignant lesions the whole retroperitoneal compartment is resected, along with any adjacent organs invaded by the tumour (such as the kidney) to achieve an R0 resection. In this operation the retroperitoneal compartment containing the adrenal tumour from the lateral border of the IVC (medially), kidney (inferiorly), diaphragm (postero-laterally), and liver (superiorly) is excised en bloc.

Left

- Pack small bowel inferiorly and mobilize the splenic flexure of the colon inferiorly.
- Divide the parietal peritoneum lateral to the spleen, the lienorenal and splenophrenic ligaments to allow mobilization of the spleen and tail of the pancreas medially.
- Consider the use of a table-mounted retractor such as Omni-Tract®.
- Usually open adrenalectomy is done for large adrenal tumours that are easily identified in the retroperitoneum.
- Dissect the adrenal tumour from the surrounding tissue and ligate the left adrenal vein, which passes upwards from the renal vein to the inferior border of the adrenal gland, with ties, Ligaclips®, or an energy device.
- Complete the dissection of the inferior border of the gland and, lifting the tumour, divide its posterior attachments. As on the right, the small arterial branches supplying blood to the adrenal gland are easily ligated during this dissection.

- In malignant lesions en bloc excision of the retroperitoneal compartment containing the tumour and retroperitoneal fat is recommended from the lateral border of the aorta (medially), diaphragm (superolaterally), and kidney (inferiorly). Adjacent organs invaded by the tumour, including the kidney, spleen, and tail of the pancreas, may need to be excised en bloc with the tumour to achieve an R0 resection.

Closure
- Ensure haemostasis and consider using a drain if any concern regarding pancreatic injury.
- Close abdominal wall fascia in layers for transverse or as a single layer in vertical incisions.
- Close skin with an absorbable subcuticular suture.

Postoperative care
- Ensure venous thromboembolism prophylaxis is prescribed.
- Invasive blood pressure monitoring is required intraoperatively in patients with phaeochromocytoma and anaesthetic expertise to control variations in blood pressure that accompany tumour manipulation and excision. These patients, as well as any with significant co-morbidity (e.g. Cushing's syndrome), should be admitted to the HDU postoperatively.
- Give prophylactic antibiotics in surgery for Cushing's syndrome.
- Blood glucose needs to be monitored closely following surgery for phaeochromocytoma and Cushing's syndrome.
- In surgery for Cushing's syndrome, perioperative parenteral steroids are needed to prevent an Addisonian crisis in the immediate postoperative period. These can then be substituted with oral steroids, which are weaned over months as an outpatient.
- Alpha-blockers can be stopped following surgery for phaeochromocytoma.
- Antihypertensives may be reduced or discontinued following surgery for Conn's adenoma.

Complications
- Bleeding.
  - This can be severe and life-threatening if from the IVC.
- Damage to surrounding structures.
  - Such as the kidney, spleen, bowel, liver, or pancreas.
- Infection.
- Wound complications.
  - Dehiscence, hernia, scar.

Tips and tricks

- Adequate access for vascular control and en bloc resection of surrounding organs in large malignant tumours is essential—plan your incision to allow for this.
- A table-based mechanical retraction system can be very useful in gaining adequate exposure.
- Although a single adrenal vein is described, it is not unusual to see multiple veins.
- Inform the anaesthetist before dividing the adrenal vein in surgery for phaeochromocytoma, as hypotension and cardiovascular instability can result.

Laparoscopic adrenalectomy—transperitoneal

Indications

- Non-functioning adrenal tumours with indeterminate clinical or radiological features.
- Benign functioning adrenal tumours (Conn's adenoma, Cushing's syndrome, and phaeochromocytoma).
- Bilateral adrenalectomy in Cushing's disease or ectopic adrenocorticotropic hormone (ACTH) production.

Consent

- Explain possible need for conversion to open surgery.
- Discuss complications, including bleeding, damage to nearby structures (bowel, spleen, pancreas, IVC), infection, wound problems, venous thromboembolism, and cardiovascular events.
- In surgery for Cushing's syndrome explain the need for perioperative steroid replacement and that symptoms and signs of cortisol excess will take months to fully resolve.
- Following surgery for phaeochromocytoma or aldosterone-producing tumour, antihypertensive medication can be reduced and often discontinued.

Preoperative preparation

- Careful preoperative clinical, biochemical, and radiological work-up are essential prior to adrenal surgery to avoid perioperative complications.
- Appropriate biochemical investigation should be undertaken to confirm (or exclude) tumour functionality, including (but not limited to) serum electrolytes and sex hormones, plasma renin/aldosterone (Conn's syndrome), plasma and urine overnight metanephrines (phaeochromocytoma), 24h urine cortisol, and overnight dexamethasone suppression test (Cushing's syndrome).
- Adrenal venous sampling may be needed to confirm laterality of the tumour in Conn's adenoma.
- Radiological investigation should include CT with adrenal protocol to characterize and stratify the risk of malignancy.
- MIBG scan is done in phaeochromocytoma to confirm functionality of the causative lesion seen on cross-sectional imaging and to exclude extra-adrenal lesions/metastases.
- Hypertension and electrolyte abnormalities due to mineralocorticoid excess in Conn's adenoma needs to be treated prior to surgery.
- Catecholamine excess in phaeochromocytoma needs to be pharmacologically blocked prior to surgery and any complications of this, such as cardiac arrhythmia/failure, addressed.
- Medical complications of glucocorticoid secretion in Cushing's syndrome, such as diabetes mellitus, hypertension, and osteoporosis, need to be managed prior to surgery.

Position

- Lateral position with side of the adrenal to be removed facing upwards (see Fig. 6.10).
- Both knees flexed to 45°.
- Table broken to 30° to open the space between the iliac crest and costal margin.
- Upper arm flexed at 90° and supported on an arm board.
- Lower arm resting in slight elbow flexion.
- Padded support/roll behind gluteal fold and mid-thoracic spine.
- Secure patient to the operating table with Sleek®/Gamgee and/or straps at the level of the knees, iliac crest, and mid-thoracic spine.
- Tilt table 5–10° backwards so the patient rests against the padded support—this manoeuvre with aid mobilization of the intra-abdominal organs.

Incision

- Insert 12mm laparoscopic port in the upper quadrant of the abdomen below the costal margin at approximately the mid-clavicular line, using either a cut-down technique/blunt trocar or optical port such as Visiport™.
- Insufflate pneumoperitoneum to 12–15mmHg.
- Insert two further 12mm laparoscopic ports under direct vision in the upper quadrant for the laparoscope and to enable triangulation of instruments to the adrenal tumour.
- In right laparoscopic adrenalectomy a fourth port may be required further laterally for a liver retractor.
- Use a 10mm 30° laparoscope.

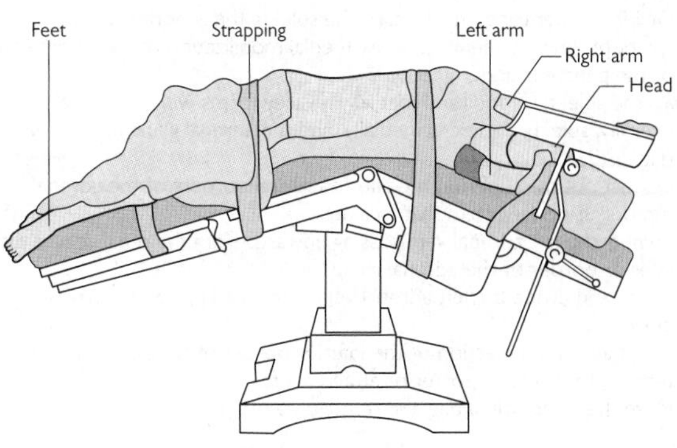
Feet
Strapping
Left arm
Right arm
Head

Fig. 6.10 Positioning for laparoscopic transperitoneal adrenalectomy.

Procedure

Right

- Using an energy device such as the Harmonic® scalpel divide the right triangular ligament to mobilize the liver and if necessary mobilize the hepatic flexure of the colon.
- Incise the parietal peritoneum transversely in the hepatorenal pouch to expose the retroperitoneal fat and adrenal tumour.
- Lifting the upper divided flap of the peritoneum cranially start dissecting the superior border of the adrenal tumour.
- Identify the lateral border of the IVC and continue the dissection inferiorly along the lateral border from the liver to the renal vessels.
- Identify the short, right adrenal vein passing transversely from the lateral border of the IVC to the medial border of the adrenal tumour (Fig. 6.11).
- Ligate and divide the right adrenal vein with care using Ligaclips® or an energy device.
- Complete the dissection of the adrenal tumour along its medial, inferior, lateral, and superior borders (not necessarily in this order) before lifting the tumour and dividing its posterior attachments.
- A small tongue of normal adrenal gland may pass behind the IVC at the superomedial aspect of this dissection that needs to be excised in a total adrenalectomy (particularly in Cushing's disease/ectopic ACTH production).
- Place the tumour in a bag and remove via the port site (this may need enlarging, depending on the size of the mass).

Left

- Mobilize the splenic flexure of the colon, allowing the colon to fall safely out of the operative field.
- Divide the peritoneum lateral to the spleen, the lienorena and splenophrenic ligaments to allow medial mobilization of the spleen/tail of the pancreas under gravity.
- As the spleen is mobilized medially a valley forms with the kidney laterally, spleen/pancreas medially, and the adrenal gland at the bottom (Fig. 6.12).
- Dissect out the superior, medial, and lateral borders of the adrenal tumour using the Harmonic® scalpel.
- Identify the left adrenal vein passing upwards from the renal vein at the inferior border of the adrenal gland.
- Ligate and divide the left adrenal vein with Ligaclips® or an energy device.
- Complete the dissection of the inferior border of the gland then lift the tumour to divide its posterior attachments.
- Place the tumour in a bag and remove via the port site.

Closure

- Ensure haemostasis and close abdominal wall fascia under direct vision.
- Close skin with an absorbable suture.

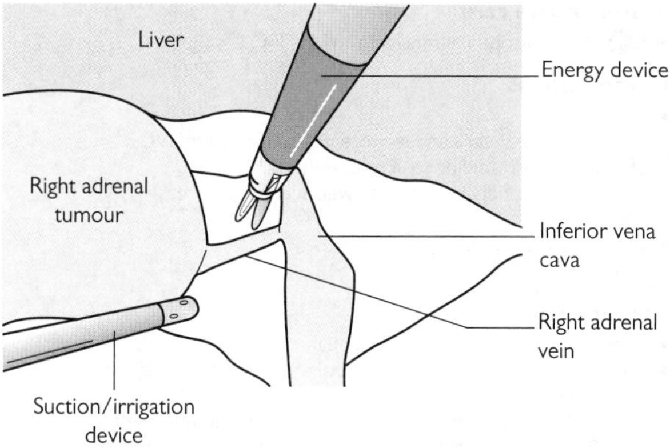
Liver
Energy device
Right adrenal tumour
Inferior vena cava
Right adrenal vein
Suction/irrigation device

Fig. 6.11 Laparoscopic right adrenalectomy.

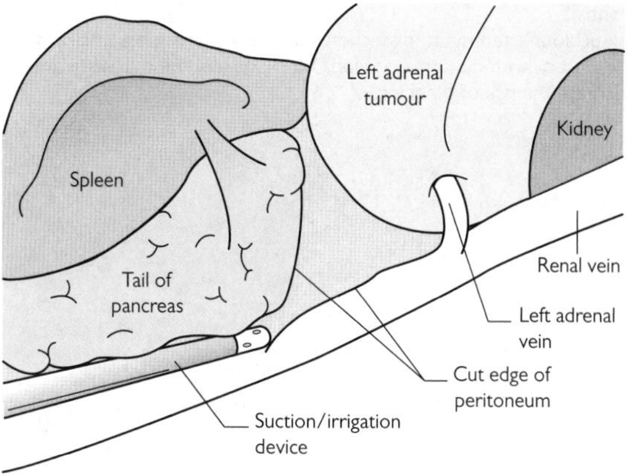
Left adrenal tumour
Kidney
Spleen
Renal vein
Tail of pancreas
Left adrenal vein
Cut edge of peritoneum
Suction/irrigation device

Fig. 6.12 Laparoscopic left adrenalectomy.

Postoperative care

See ➲ 'Anterior open adrenalectomy', p. 300.

Complications

- Bleeding.
  - This can be severe and life-threatening if from theIVC.
- Damage to surrounding structures.
  - Such as the kidney, spleen, bowel, liver, or pancreas.
- Infection.
- Wound complications.
  - Dehiscence, hernia, scar.

Tips and tricks

- Careful patient positioning is essential.
- Take care when inserting the first port to avoid damaging intra-abdominal viscera.
- Fully mobilize the spleen along the lienorenal ligament in left laparoscopic adrenalectomy to allow this to fall inferiorly.
- Inform the anaesthetist when dividing the adrenal vein in surgery for phaeochromocytoma, as this can lead to haemodynamic instability.
- Take care when dissecting out and ligate the adrenal vein, particularly a short, right adrenal vein, as bleeding from this vessel can be difficult to control.
- Meticulous attention to dissection and haemostasis is essential in surgery for phaeochromocytoma, as alpha blockade and tumour vascularity increase the risk of bleeding.

Endoscopic retroperitoneal adrenalectomy

This approach has similar indications to laparoscopic transabdominal adrenalectomy, though it is particularly suitable for patients with intra-peritoneal adhesions, bilateral tumours (as the patient does not need to be repositioned), and smaller tumours (due to the more limited working space). The experience and preference of the surgeon has a major influence on which approach is undertaken.

Indications

- Non-functioning adrenal tumours with indeterminate clinical or radiological features.
- Benign functioning adrenal tumours (Conn's adenoma, Cushing's syndrome, and phaeochromocytoma).
- Bilateral adrenalectomy in Cushing's disease or ectopic ACTH production.

Contraindications

- Limited operative working space makes this approach less suitable for larger tumours (>8cm).
- Obesity may preclude adequate ventilation in the prone position.
- Previous nephrectomy/renal surgery makes this approach difficult.

Consent

- Explain the possible need for conversion to open surgery—turning the patient to a supine position and using an anterior approach may be needed.
- Warn the patient of possible postoperative surgical emphysema.
- Discuss complications, including pneumothorax, bleeding, damage to other structures, infection, wound problems, pneumonia, venous thromboembolism, cardiovascular events.
- In surgery for Cushing's syndrome, explain the need for steroid replacement postoperatively, and that symptoms and signs of cortisol excess will take months to fully resolve.
- Following surgery for phaeochromocytoma or aldosterone producing-tumour, antihypertensive medication can be reduced and often discontinued.

Position

- Prone (see Fig. 6.13), knees and hips flexed to 90°.
- Knees resting on step, abdomen resting on padded support, and head on padded head-ring.

Incision

- Mark the position of the 11th and 12th ribs with a skin marker.
- Make an incision below the tip of the 12th rib just long enough to insert a 12mm laparoscopic port.

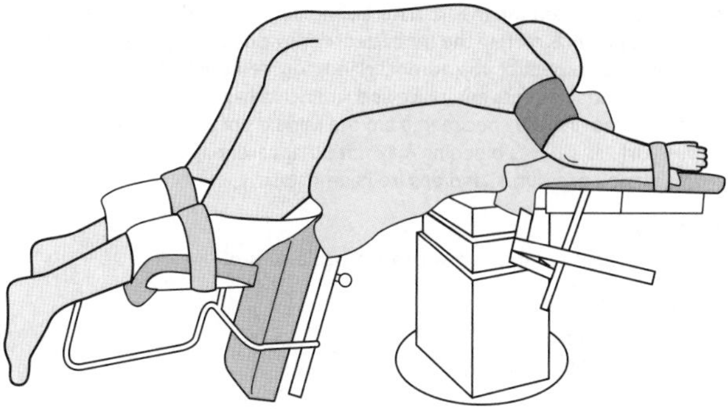

Fig. 6.13 Positioning for endoscopic retroperitoneal adrenalectomy.

- Dissect through muscle of posterior abdominal, enter the retroperitoneum, and sweep an index finger around under the muscle to create a working space.
- Insert a 5mm port below the tip of the 11th rib, guiding the port into the working space with an index finger. Similarly guide a 12mm port into the retroperitoneum three fingerbreadths medial to 1st port (lateral to erector spinae).
- Insert a cuffed 12mm laparoscopic port into the middle port site, inflate the cuff beneath the muscle, and insufflate to 20–25mmHg.

Procedure

- Using blunt dissectors and a 30° 10mm laparoscope in the medial port, open Gerota's fascia to enter the perinephric space.
- Define landmarks that are the spine medially, peritoneum covering spleen (left side), or liver (right side), and kidney inferiorly. The adrenal tumour will be in the retroperitoneal fat above the kidney, but will not usually be visible at this stage.
- Begin by dissecting along the superior and lateral borders of the kidney using an energy device such as the Harmonic® scalpel. Mobilizing the kidney enables it to be retracted to get access to the inferior aspect of the adrenal gland.
- Dissect the retroperitoneal fat containing the adrenal tumour off the superior pole of the kidney and continue the dissection along the medial and lateral borders of the adrenal gland. Be sure not to divide the superior attachments of the gland at this stage as these keep the adrenal tumour suspended during the dissection.
- Divide the right adrenal vein (medially) and left adrenal vein (inferiorly) with an Harmonic® scalpel (or similar device) or between Ligaclips®. The blood supply to the adrenal gland via small branches of the aorta, inferior phrenic, and renal artery will be divided with an energy device during the dissection.

- Having mobilized the medial, lateral, and inferior borders of the tumour (if necessary retracting the mobilized kidney posteriorly to get access to the inferior aspect of the adrenal gland), divide its anterior then finally superior attachments and place specimen in a bag.
- After removing the specimen from the middle port, reduce insufflation pressure, as venous bleeding may not be apparent at these high insufflation pressures, and ensure haemostasis.

Closure

Close muscle layer and skin with absorbable suture.

Complications

- Pneumothorax.
- Surgical emphysema.
- Bleeding.
  - This can be life-threatening if from the IVC.
- Infection.
- Wound complications.

Tips and tricks

- Careful patient positioning is important to allow good access.
- Correct port placement is essential as the working space is small.
- Adequate mobilization of the kidney is needed to allow access to the inferior aspect of the adrenal gland.
- Do not divide the superior attachments of the adrenal gland until the rest of the gland has been dissected out.
- Insufflation pressures exceed venous pressure, so to prevent postoperative venous bleeding, reduce the insufflation pressure first and inspect the operative field prior to wound closure.

Chapter 7

Paediatric surgery

Abscess drainage

Surgical anatomy

Neck

Abscesses arise in the neck following bacterial lymphadenitis or, more rarely, in the context of atypical mycobacterial infection. They can also occur at the site of a branchial remnant (2nd branchial cleft, anterior to sternomastoid) or pre-existing thyroglossal cyst (midline).

Peri-anal

The anal canal is lined with crypto-glandular epithelium. The internal sphincter can be breached by these crypts, allowing bacteria from the gut lumen to migrate into perirectal tissues, thereby generating an abscess. There are two peaks: <1yr and teenagers. In older children, Crohn's disease should be considered.

Indications

Red, fluctuant, tender swelling.

Preoperative preparation

- If unusual location or consistency, consider US imaging.
- Consent.
- Usually GA, but in neonates, can consider aspiration under topical local anaesthetic.
- Check blood glucose.
- If recurrent check immunological function.

Position and theatre set-up

- For neck abscesses, supine on table with neck extended, head tilted to opposite side.
- For peri-anal abscesses in most children, lateral position with knees drawn up to chest.
- Larger children may need to be placed in lithotomy.

Procedure

- Stab incision and irrigation/gentle curettage to express all pus.
- Pus sent for microbiology.
- Cavity gently packed with absorbable dressing (e.g. Aquacel™).

Postoperative care

- Remove dressing and irrigate at 24h, can then be followed up in community if tolerating dressing changes.
- If first abscess, no routine follow-up.
- For recurrent abscess, consider checking immune function.

Complications

- Recurrent abscess.
- Fistula-in-ano—will require EUA, probe, fistulotomy.

Tips and tricks

- Peri-anal: send skin biopsy if any suspicion of Crohn's disease.
- Incision and drainage only, do not probe for fistula initially.

Appendicectomy

Surgical anatomy

Appendix may be retrocaecal, pelvic, sub-ileal.

Indications

Suspected acute appendicitis, can be diagnostic, e.g. Meckel's, ovarian pathology.

Preoperative preparation

IV antibiotic prophylaxis as per local hospital policy.

Position and theatre set-up

- Supine, GA. Urinary catheter is usually placed, may be removed at end of procedure if not required postoperatively.
- Once ports are in place, patient positioned head-down and right side up. Lap stack placed on patient's right side, facing surgeon and assistant (both on patients left).

Procedure

- Open insertion of umbilical port (11 or 12mm), either supra- or infra-umbilical. Use 5mm laparoscope and instruments.
- After visual inspection, place 1st additional 5mm port in LIF. Use atraumatic grasper to manipulate caecum and inspect appendix to confirm pathology. If appendix is normal, plan to walk the small bowel to exclude Meckel's and inspect ovaries in female patients. For simple appendicitis with mobile appendix a two-port procedure can be performed. The laparoscope can be placed in the LIF port and the appendix grasped via the umbilical port and withdrawn (with the port) into the umbilical wound. The meso-appendix can be diathermied or ligated with Vicryl® sutures and the appendix excised as for an open appendicectomy.
- 3rd laparoscopic port:
  - Suprapubic (older child). Laparoscope is moved to the LIF. Right and left hands operate via umbilical and supra-pubic ports, respectively.
  - RUQ (right upper quadrant)—(small child).
- Any free pus or fluid is aspirated with laparoscopic suction/irrigation, and sent for microbiological analysis.
- The tip of the appendix is grasped and elevated to display the meso-appendix. Hook monopolar diathermy (starting at the tip) is used to diathermy the meso-appendix to its base. If it is difficult to identify or mobilize the appendix, the caecum is mobilized from lateral to medial. Usually hook diathermy alone is sufficient to divide the meso-appendix.
- The appendix is released. A 0 loop PDS (Ethicon) is introduced via 5mm port. An atraumatic grasper is passed through the loop and grasps and elevates the tip of the appendix. The loop is manoeuvred to the base of the appendix, pulled tight, and cut. This step is repeated twice to leave three sutures over the appendix. The last suture is left uncut to aid in

retrieval of the appendix. The appendix is amputated between the 2nd and 3rd sutures to leave two on the appendix base, the 3rd suture uncut and passing through the port it was inserted through. The laparoscope is moved into a port other than the umbilical port. The appendix (or its final suture) can be grasped with an atraumatic grasper and retrieved directly through the larger umbilical port, thus avoiding contact with any of the wounds.
- Final inspection of the appendix base is performed. Any pus (or spilled faecolith) is aspirated.
- Ports are removed and sites closed under lap vision.

Postoperative care

- Antibiotics as per local guidelines.
- Will vary as to whether simple or perforated appendicitis.

Complications

Intra-abdominal abscess. Stump blow-out, paralytic ileus, small bowel obstruction (including adhesions).

Tips and tricks

Mobilize caecum lateral to medial of appendix difficult to identify or mobilized directly. Two-port procedure (lap-assisted appendicectomy) is advantageous for simple appendicitis with a mobile appendix. Shorten the loop PDS before inserting through port makes it easier to pass the grasper through it and then place around the appendix.

Diagnostic laparoscopy

Umbilical port insertion as on p. 316.

To 'walk' the small bowel to look for a Meckel's diverticulum or a duplication cyst; two atraumatic graspers are used. Starting at the caecum, the ileum is held by the graspers spaced apart by a few cm. The bowel is then followed proximally and inspected on both sides, in a stepwise fashion, ensuring that both graspers do not release the bowel simultaneously. If a Meckel's or duplication cyst is found, the bowel can be exteriorized via the umbilicus and an extra-corporeal resection and anastomosis performed.

If ovarian pathology is encountered, a gynaecology opinion can be sought. Options include cyst aspiration, cystecytomy, de-torsion or oophorectomy.

Congenital diaphragmatic hernia

Surgical anatomy

(See Fig. 7.1)

Subtypes:

- 95% are left-sided.
- 95% are postero-lateral diaphragmatic defect.
- 5% are central Morgagni defect.

Indications

- Majority are antenatally-diagnosed—repair deferred until >24h age minimum and haemodynamic/cardiorespiratory physiology normalized.
- Postnatal presentation—respiratory distress.
- Incidental finding.

Preoperative preparation

- Elective paralysis and intubation at delivery.
- Cross-match blood.
- Pass NG tube.
- Echocardiography—structural anomalies, pulmonary hypertension.
- Pre- and post-ductal saturation levels.
- CXR.
- Ventilatory strategies aimed at minimizing barotrauma, permissive hypercapnia.
- Nitric oxide, inotropic support may be required. Extra-corporeal membrane oxygenation (ECMO) maybe required in a small proportion.

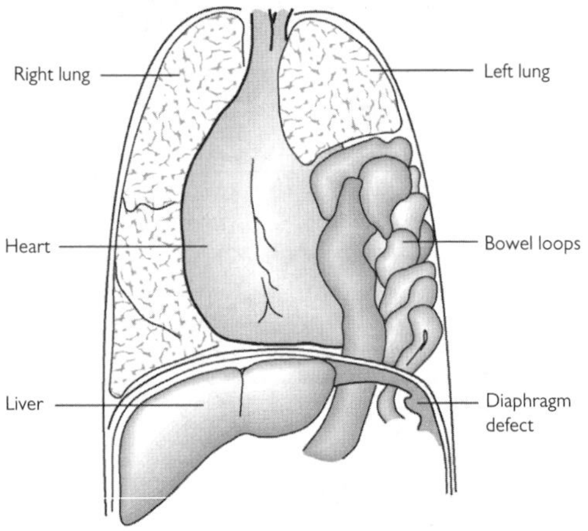
Right lung
Left lung
Heart
Bowel loops
Liver
Diaphragm defect

Fig. 7.1 Diaphragmatic hernia. Reproduced with permission from McLatchie, G, and Leaper, D. Operative Surgery 2nd edition, Oxford University Press: 2006.

Position

- Supine.

Procedure

- Left (or right) subcostal muscle-cutting incision (open repair).
- Thoracoscopic approach favoured by some, but higher recurrence rates reported.
- Herniated contents are carefully withdrawn back into the abdomen (may include stomach, small bowel, colon, spleen, left lobe liver).
- Anterior and posterior rims of diaphragm delineated. Maybe deficient postero-laterally.
- Assess for rotational anomaly—Ladd's procedure may be performed if small-bowel mesentery narrow.
- Primary repair of diaphragm with interrupted non-absorbable sutures (3/0).
- Patch repair (e.g. Porcine collagen) required of primary closure not possible.

Closure

- 4/0 Vicryl® figure of eight interrupted all layers.
- Subcut fat layer 5/0 Vicryl®.
- Skin 5/0 Monocryl® subcuticular.

Postoperative care

- NG tube left on free drainage for 24–48h or while patient is still intubated.
- Enteral feed introduced when bowel function returns.
- Neonatal management of pulmonary hypoplasia and pulmonary hypertension.

Complications

- Recurrence.
- Adhesive small-bowel obstruction.
- Survival dependent on pulmonary hypoplasia and pulmonary hypertension.

Tips and tricks

- Place diaphragmatic sutures and leave untied until all placed.
- Use paper template to estimate size of patch (if used).

Gastrostomy insertion—open/lap-assisted

Surgical anatomy

Usually there is no underlying anatomical abnormality. Some surgeons obtain an elective upper GI contrast study to exclude malrotation (and to gain some estimate of reflux and gastric emptying). Assessment of reflux may be required with pH/impedance study.

Indications

To facilitate long-term nutrition in children with feeding difficulties. This most commonly includes infants/children with unsafe swallow secondary to cerebral palsy. The gastrostomy tube is then used instead of NG tube feeding.

Preoperative preparation

Explanation to the parents/carers includes discussion and demonstration of the types of gastrostomy. Broadly there are two types available: the PEG (percutaneous endoscopic gastrostomy, e.g. Freka™ device) and balloon-button devices (e.g. Mic-Key™).

Position and theatre set-up

GA, supine.

Procedure

PEG insertion

PEG devices (9Fr or 15Fr Freka™) are inserted using gastroscopy, with or without laparoscopic assistance. The gastroscope is passed into the stomach, which is then partially inflated. The Freka™ insertion kit includes a cannula that is passed through the abdominal wall directly into the anterior body of the stomach. A length of thread is passed down the cannula into the stomach and grasped with either a snare or biopsy forceps and retrieved via the mouth. The Freka™ tube is tied to the thread and pulled down the oesophagus into the stomach with the external portion of the tube now positioned externally. This technique can be combined with laparoscopy to visualize the insertion needle as it passes through the abdominal wall into the stomach.

Button gastrostomy

Alternatively, a laparoscopic-assisted approach allows a balloon-button or (temporary) tube (e.g. Monarch™) to be placed. This can be achieved using a mini-Stamm procedure, where the anterior stomach is withdrawn with a laparoscopic grasper inserted through a left upper quadrant incision, and elevated to the abdominal wall. The stomach is anchored to the posterior sheath with 4/0 absorbable suture. A purse-string is then fashioned on the wall of the stomach again using 4/0 absorbable suture. A gastrotomy is made inside the purse-string suture and the feeding tube inserted directly into the stomach. The purse-string is tied closed and the tube anchored to the abdominal wall (e.g. 3/0 absorbable suture). Tube position can be checked with laparoscopic visualization before closure.

Postoperative care

The tube can be used for feeding or medications within 6–8h of insertion.

Complications

Damage to intra-abdominal contents during insertion, most commonly colon, but also rare reports of liver injury. With the PEG 'pull' technique (if used without laparoscopy), skewering of the colon may go unnoticed at the time of insertion and come to light at the time of tube change.

Tips and tricks

- Over-inflation of the stomach with the gastroscope causes the stomach to rotate exposing the posterior aspect, which may be inadvertently accessed with the insertion cannula/needle.
- A balloon-button device can easily fall out if the balloon bursts. As these devices are difficult to secure in any other way to the abdomen, place a Monarch™ feeding tube at initial insertion and replace this (without GA [general anaesthetic]) with a Mic-Key™ balloon button device 6 weeks later.

Change of gastrostomy

Surgical anatomy

As for 'Gastrostomy insertion—open/lap-assisted' (p. 322).

Indications

Tube needs replacing. PEG tubes (e.g. Freka devices) typically need replacing after 18–24 months. These can be replaced with the same type or changed to balloon-button devices.

Preoperative preparation

Usually non-specific; can be day-case procedure.

Position and theatre set-up

- GA, supine.
- Requires two operators with simultaneous gastrosopy and tube change via abdomen.

Procedure

The tube is visualized via endococoscopy. A long length of '0' silk suture is attached to the base of the external portion of the tube, which is then cut. The stump of the tube is pushed into the stomach leaving the long length of silk suture externally. The tube is grasped by the endoscopist and retrieved via the mouth, leaving the silk suture now passing from the mouth, via the oesophagus out via the gastrostomy site. This allows safe re-insertion of a PEG-type tube, by tying it to the silk and pulling it via the mouth down the oesophagus into the stomach again. Alternatively, the track can be dilated, if necessary, under endoscopic vision, and an appropriate length Mic-Key balloon-button device sited. A balloon-tipped measuring device is inserted first down the track and the balloon inflated. The measuring device is withdrawn so that the balloon within the stomach abuts the abdominal wall. The measuring device has markings that will then indicate the required length of feeding tube to be used.

Postoperative care

The new tube can be used immediately for feeds.

Complications

Trauma to the gastrostomy track. As the PEG technique does not include suturing of the stomach to the abdominal wall, elective replacement is usually deferred for 6 months post-insertion to allow a secure fistula to form.

Tips and tricks

Urethral (rather than Hegar) dilators are tapered and are best to dilate the gastrostomy track.

Chest-drain insertion

Surgical anatomy

5th intercostal space in the mid-axillary line is the standard site for insertion. This site allows safe passage of the drain to the apex or base of the pleural space, as required, avoiding the pectoralis major and intra-thoracic structures. Spaces above and below are occasionally used to drain specific collections.

Indications

- Thoracic empyema or para-pneumonic effusions—the drain is often used to administer thrombolytic agents (e.g. Urokinase™) post-insertion.
- Haemothorax.
- Pneumothorax—spontaneous or traumatic.

Preoperative preparation

For effusions/empyema, it is useful for the site of collection to be marked at the sonographic assessment.

Position and theatre set-up

- Supine, with ipsilateral arm elevated (e.g. behind the head). Bolster under posterior chest to expose site of insertion.
- Radiological imaging should be displayed in the operating theatre.
- In the acute setting, oxygen delivery and IV cannulation are required.

Procedure

- The insertion site is infiltrated with local anaesthetic.
- Size of chest drain: 8–14 Fr according to age. 12Fr is the commonest size used for infants with empyema/effusion.
- Seldinger technique—can be performed with ultrasound guidance.
- The needle/syringe is inserted and position confirmed by aspiration of air or fluid from the pleural space. The guide wire is passed through the needle and the needle is withdrawn. A small incision is made at the site of the guidewire insertion and the dilator is passed carefully into the pleural space and then withdrawn. The chest drain is passed over the guidewire and secured (e.g. 0 silk suture).
- Open insertion technique. A small incision is made parallel to the superior aspect of the 6th rib in the 5th intercostal space. The incision is deepened into the pleural space with a blunt arterial clip while controlling the depth of insertion with the index finger. When the pleural space has been entered the drain is inserted and secured (e.g. 0 silk suture). In children it is not usually possible to perform the 'finger sweep' to confirm that the pleural space has been entered.
- The chest drain is connected to an underwater seal which is placed below the level of the patient's chest at all times.

Postoperative care

- CXR is undertaken when practical.
- Usually no suction is required.
- Low-level suction (e.g. <2.5kPa) may be used to encourage lung expansion following spontaneous pneumothorax. Wall suction is applied until gentle bubbling is seen.
- If large volumes of fluid drain initially, then clamping may be considered if the volume approaches 15ml/kg, to avoid mediastinal shift or pulmonary oedema.

Chest-drain removal

This is planned when:

- There is no further air leak (note 'bubbling' will be present if suction is continued). 'Swinging' will continue in a patent chest-drain system but will reduce as the lung expands fully.
- Minimal fluid drainage.
- Lung re-expansion is confirmed.

After appropriate analgesia, the drain is removed and the skin defect closed with steristrips, gauze, and occlusive dressings. Some surgeons place an untied suture at the time of insertion, which is closed at removal.

Complications

- Drain falls out/partially dislodges (common)—remove the drain. If for unresolved pneumothorax, then place a three-sided dressing. If not for pneumothorax, place an occlusive dressing. Consider whether new drain is required.
- Large air leak—likely cause is partial/complete displacement so that side holes are exteriorized, or disconnection from the underwater seal system.
- Other causes include bronchial injury or leak from lung parenchyma surface.
- Bleeding—from intercostal vessels, from lung surface or intra-thoracic structures.

Tips and tricks

- Seldinger technique—care must be taken when inserting the dilator, ensure this is only passed a short distance. Ideally use ultrasound guidance.
- Clamping a chest drain—never while there is a continuing air leak. Usually not required pre-removal, unless there are concerns about lung expansion. Main indication is changing or re-attaching the underwater seal.

Circumcision

Surgical anatomy

The foreskin is comprised of an inner and outer preputial layer. The superficial dorsal vein lies outside Buck's fascia and drains the prepuce; it generally runs in the midline for most of the length of the prepuce, before veering left or right at the proximal shaft. The frenulum anchors the prepuces to the ventral aspect of the glans penis.

Natural history is of adherence of prepuce to glans in all neonates ('physiological phimosis', no retraction should be attempted) followed by gradual spontaneous separation over the next 5–10 years. Circumcision is not required to treat physiological phimosis.

Indications

Absolute

- Balanitis xerotica obliterans (BXO).

Relative

- Recurrent balano-posthitis.
- In male infants in the presence of a congenital anomaly that predisposes to urinary tract infections (severe vesico-ureteric reflux, posterior urethral valves).
- Cultural/religious request.

Preoperative preparation

Either caudal block or penile block.

Position and theatre set-up

GA, supine.

Procedure

(See Fig. 7.2)

- Retract foreskin and clean inner prepuce and glans. Skin marker to plan incision.
- Protract foreskin, identify where the ridge of the corona sits under the skin—mark this point with a clip dorsally and ventrally.
- Place clips on the dorsal and ventral apices of the foreskin and have an assistant apply vertical traction to the clips.
- Excise the foreskin along a line between the two marks—this should be slightly oblique in favour of the ventral aspect.
- Bipolar diathermy to any large bleeding vessels.
- Place four clips around the inner prepuce and again have an assistant provide vertical traction.
- Make a vertical incision in the dorsum of the inner prepuce to approximately 2mm from the corona.
- Trim inner prepuce from the frenulum, leaving a 2mm margin all the way round ('mucosal cuff').
- Bipolar diathermy haemostasis.
- Place absorbable suture between the dorsal aspect of the inner preputial cuff and the outer prepuce and use as a stay. Place another suture between the frenulum and the outer prepuce and use as a stay.
- Anastomose the outer prepuce to the 2mm cuff of the inner prepuce using a rapidly absorbable suture.

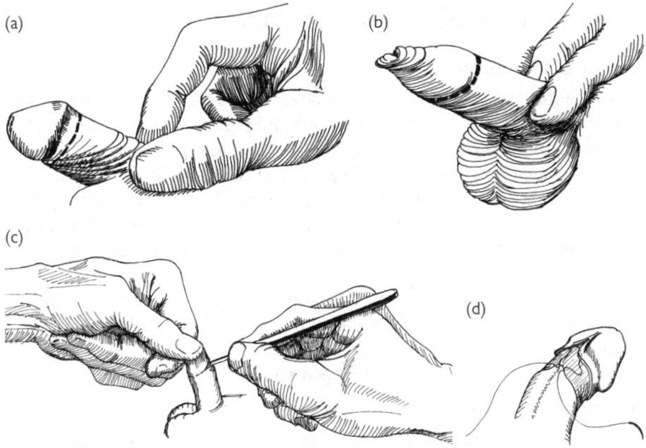
(a)
(b)
(c)
(d)

Fig. 7.2 Circumcision. Reproduced with permission from McLatchie, G, and Leaper, D. Operative Surgery 2nd edition, Oxford University Press: 2006.

Postoperative care

- Topical Chloramphenicol™ or local anaesthetic gel to the glans and wound for 5–7 days—this will mainly prevent the wound from sticking to nappies or pants.
- Advise to bathe/shower daily from 24h postoperative.

Complications

- Bleeding.
- Infection.
- Stitch sinus.
- Inclusion cysts.
- Glans or urethral injury.

Tips and tricks

- Avoid monopolar diathermy.
- Some surgeons use a subcuticular closure or use glue, thus avoiding stitch sinuses or inclusion cysts.
- If there is postoperative bleeding, then an elastic, self-adhesive dressing may be used.
- If bleedings persists, then exploration under GA will often reveal a haematoma with underlying oozing from small vessels; usually the main bleeding point is the frenulum.

Correction of malrotation

Surgical anatomy

Normal intestinal rotation occurs by physiological herniation of the embryonic intestinal loop into the umbilical cord (4th gestational week). The mid-gut returns to the peritoneal cavity by the 8th–10th week and rotates 270° anticlockwise, such that the duodenal-jejunal (DJ) comes to lie on the left of the midline and the caecum in the right iliac fossa. The commonest type of malrotation is that of the caecum lying high in the midline or to the left of the midline, the DJ flexure lying to the right of the midline, narrow small-bowel mesentery, which lacks fixation, and peritoneal (Ladd's) bands passing from the caecum to the right side across the duodenum. This anatomical configuration predisposes to total mid-gut volvulus and rapid infarction (<6h). Bilious vomiting in neonates and infants is a surgical emergency and should be assumed to be secondary to malrotation/volvulus until proved otherwise (Fig. 7.3).

Indications

- Emergency—malrotation/volvulus—bilious vomiting leading to upper GI study confirming malrotation/volvulus; or bilious vomiting/gasless abdomen (often with dilated stomach) on plain XR mandating immediate surgery.
- Semi-elective if malrotation detected incidentally on upper GI contrast study.

Preoperative preparation

- IV fluid resuscitation, NG decompression, IV antibiotics.
- Surgery is time-critical and should not be delayed.

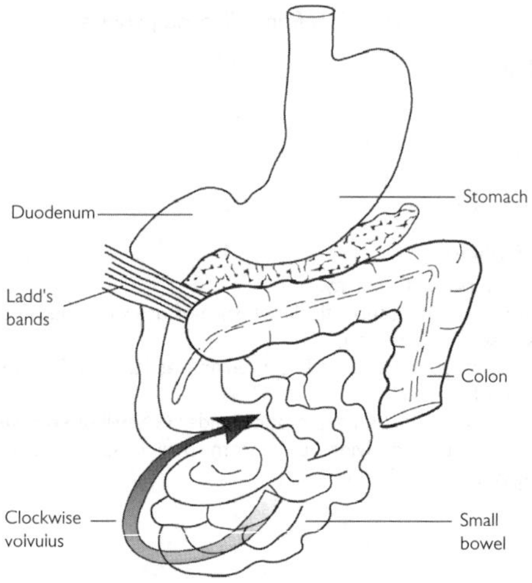
Stomach
Duodenum
Ladd's
bands
Colon
Clockwise
volvulus
Small
bowel

Fig. 7.3 Malrotation predisposing to volvulus of the small bowel. Reproduced with permission from McLatchie, G, and Leaper, D. Operative Surgery 2nd edition, Oxford University Press: 2006.

Position

Supine (open or laparoscopic).

Procedure

- Ladd's procedure: upper transverse incision. If twisted, the bowel should be de-rotated in an anticlockwise direction. The bowel is assessed for compromise and, if necessary, wrapped in warm saline-soaked swabs and re-assessed.
- For an elective case, the position of the DJ flexure is identified (the inferior mesenteric vein is to its left) with respect to the spine to ascertain if it is to the left or right.
- The right colon is mobilized by dividing the lateral peritoneal attachments and then reflected medially. The mesentery of the small bowel is widened by carefully opening the peritoneum overlying the mesenteric vessels. This dissection is continued to the root of the mesentery. The duodenum is straightened by dividing the lateral attachments. Appendicectomy, usually by inversion, is carried out to avoid future diagnostic confusion. The bowel is replaced with the colon (and caecum) on the left and the small bowel on the right.
- If the bowel is necrotic, the authors' preference is to untwist it, replace it in the abdomen, and plan for a re-look laparotomy in 48h. Careful counselling with the family is required, as assuming the bowel remains necrotic, then resection and stoma formation commits to short-gut management and later consideration of small-bowel transplantation.

Laparoscopic Ladd's procedure

- Ladd's procedure can be completed laparoscopically, but it is debatable if this is merited in the emergency situation.
- In cases where it is unclear radiologically whether, if malrotation exists or not, the DJ flexure, position of the caecum, and width of the mesenteric root can be assessed laparoscopically. Mobilization and placement of the intestine in the post-Ladd's position can be achieved laparoscopically.

Postoperative care

- IV antibiotics for at least 24h.
- NG decompression.
- Feed re-started at >24h when gut function has returned.

Complications

- Total mid-gut necrosis (resection, stoma, management of short gut).
- Adhesive small-bowel obstruction.
- Recurrent volvulus.

Tips and tricks

- Never ignore bilious (dark green) vomiting in infants/children. It should be assumed to be secondary to malrotation/volulus until proved otherwise.
- Laparotomy and bowel de-rotation is time-critical and should be performed immediately after the diagnosis is confirmed.
- Systemic thrombolysis for 48h has been reported to salvage apparently necrotic small bowel secondary to malrotation/volvulus at 2nd look laparotomy.

Rigid bronchoscopy

Surgical anatomy

As for 'Oesophageal atresia (OA) and tracheo-oesophageal fistula (TOF)' (p. 348).

Indications

- Prior to repair of oesophageal atresia—confirm diagnosis, assess for upper pouch fistula, tracheomalacia. Diagnose H-type trachea-oesophageal fistula (H-TOF).
- Diagnose recurrent trachea-oesophageal fistula.
- Removal of foreign body.

Preoperative preparation

CXR—inspiratory/expiratory film to assess for foreign body.

Position

Supine, neck extended, roll/pillow under shoulders.

Procedure

Direct laryngoscopy—blade passed into left side of mouth, withdrawn to display vocal cords. Bronchoscope (size 0.5 smaller than endotracheal tube used) passed through cords into trachea. Inhalational anaesthetic gas tubing connected to side hole of scope. Scope advanced to carina and right/left main bronchi inspected. Trachea assessed during withdrawal of scope. Posterior wall can be probed gently with fine ureteric stent to exclude upper pouch trachea-oesophageal fistula, or as initial step of H-TOF repair.

Foreign body can be extracted using graspers.

Complications

Trauma to airway, pharynx, or teeth.

Tips and tricks

Assemble bronchoscope in advance and check laryngoscope and suction are working.

Central venous catheter insertion

Indications

For <4 weeks use, peripherally inserted central catheter (PICC) is used. Long-term catheter for:

- Parenteral nutrition, chemoetherapy, haemodialysis, antibiotic therapy, regular transfusions, intensive blood sampling, or where other peripheral sites have been used.
- Options include a tunnelled catheter (Broviac or Hickman line), or implantable device (Portacath™).

Surgical anatomy

- Internal jugular vein (IJV), subclavian vein (SCV), external jugular vein (EJV) are commonly used.
- Femoral vein (or even aygos vein) are last resorts.

Preoperative preparation

- If multiple previous catheters have been placed, preoperative vein mapping with Doppler ultrasound or MR (magnetic resonance) venography to ensure vein patency.
- Blood tests—platelet count, coagulation.

Position

Supine, shoulder roll to extend neck, tilt head away from intended neck site.

Procedure

Percutaneous insertion is preferred.

Percutaneous access

Internal jugular vein

Position patient with head down. Portable ultrasound (probe placed in sterile cover) to demonstrate IJV. Needle/syringe inserted into IJV whilst aspirating venous blood. Guidewire passed into right atrium (RA) or IVC, confirmed with image intensifier. Small incision is made lateral to needle insertion site. Line is tunnelled from lateral chest to neck incision and cut so that tip will lie in mid-right atrium. Dilator/sheath passed over wire into IJV. Dilator removed and line inserted into sheath. Sheath split while advancing line into RA. Line secured and position confirmed as for open technique.

Subclavian vein

Palpate midpoint of clavicle, insert needle/syringe just proximal to this point under clavicle into SCV, whilst aspirating. Insert guidewire into RA or IVC. Rest of procedure as for Percutaneous access (IJV).

Open technique (jugular veins)

- Transverse neck incision, >one finger breadth above clavicle.
- Divide platysma, split sternomastoid, and expose IJV, which is fully mobilized.
- Right-angled instrument around IJV and two slings placed.
- Chlorhexidine-soaked swabs around operative field.

- Line tunnelled antegradely from lateral chest wall to neck incision; ensure cuff is well-clear of chest incision.
- Line cut so that tip will lie in mid-right atrium.
- Slings elevated by assistant, venotomy made with fine scissors, and line inserted.
- Position checked with image intensifier. Check line aspirates blood and flushes freely.
- Line secured at chest site with two non-absorbable sutures and dressing.
- Sternomastoid re-approximated with absorbable suture.
- Neck incision closed with absorbable suture

Postoperative care

- Line is ready to use when position is checked with image intensifier.
- Line should only be accessed by staff trained/experienced in aseptic technique.

Complications

- Bleeding, pneumothorax/haemothorax, guidewire slips into vein and passes distally, trauma to vein.
- Medium-term—infection, blockage/fracture, line-dislodgement.

Tips and tricks

- Repeat image intensifier use at each step of percutaneous access, to ensure wire remains in situ. Only advance dilator/sheath into IJV/SVC, while checking wire slides in/out, to avoid trauma, e.g. to right ventricle.
- A 'vein pick' can be placed into a small vein venotomy (open insertion) to facilitate line insertion.
- Radio-opaque contrast will be required for small (2.7Fr) catheters to visualize on image intensifier.
- Smaller access kits (e.g. 4, 4.5, 5Fr) are more user-friendly to place needle then wire into small veins.

Epigastric hernia

Surgical anatomy

Epigastric hernias are a defect in the linea alba, allowing a small plug of extra-peritoneal fat to herniate into the preperitoneal space. The defect is superficial to the peritoneum so there is no associated hernia sac. Although these do not close spontaneously, there is no risk of incarceration of abdominal contents.

Indications

Usually cosmesis, rarely cause pain or tenderness.

Preoperative preparation

Careful marking of the skin with the child awake (and supine) is important as the defect in the linea alba is very small and may be difficult to find.

Position

Supine, GA.

Procedure

- Small transverse incision over site as marked.
- The small 'mushroom' of extra-peritoneal fat is isolated and either excised or pushed back through the line alba. The edges of the linea alba are defined and closed with monofilament absorbable sutures.

Postoperative care

Non-specific.

Complications

Recurrence.

Tips and tricks

Careful preoperative skin marking.

External angular dermoid cyst

Surgical anatomy

Usually located at lateral aspect of eyebrow. If midline, preoperative imaging is required to assess for deep extension (Fig. 7.4).

Indications

Usually cosmesis (age >1 year). Very small risk of infection.

Preoperative preparation

None.

Position

Supine, GA, head drape.

Procedure

- Transverse skin crease over cyst, parallel and close to eyebrow if possible.
- The cyst is located deep to the orbicularis oculi muscle and is attached to the periosteum. Careful dissection is undertaken to avoid rupture.
- Once separated from the periosteum, there is usually a small central feeding vessel (use bipolar). The cyst ideally should be removed intact. 4/0 absorbable suture to re-oppose the muscle/fat.
- Fine absorbable suture to close skin + steristrips.

Complications

Recurrence, visible scar.

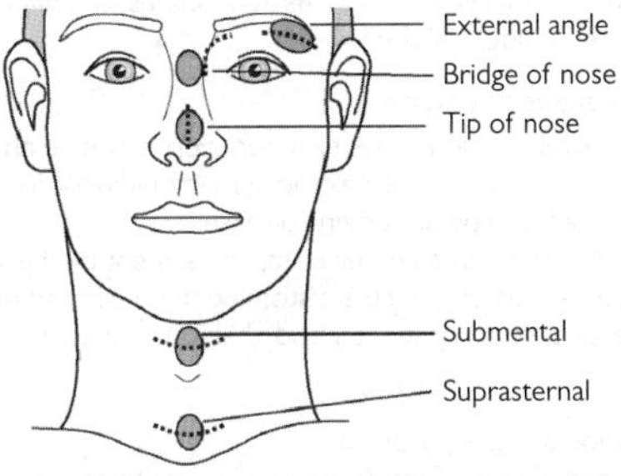
External angle
Bridge of nose
Tip of nose
Submental
Suprasternal

Fig. 7.4 Sites of dermoid cysts. Reproduced with permission from McLatchie, G, and Leaper, D. Operative Surgery 2nd edition, Oxford University Press: 2006.

Formation of neonatal/non-neonatal ileostomy/colostomy

Surgical anatomy

Colostomy are of three types—split, loop, or end. The commonest sites used are transverse colon and sigmoid colon. Small-bowel stoma is usually a terminal ileostomy where the underlying disease is colo-rectal, or maybe elsewhere, depending on disease presentation (e.g. necrotizing enterocolitis).

Split stomas can be placed at opposite ends of an incision for anorectal malformations, which may be of importance in minimizing overflow into the distal limb. Disadvantages are that a longer incision is required to close the stoma. Variations include Hartmann's procedure, where the distal colon is over-sewn and returned to the abdominal cavity, and a proximal end colostomy fashioned.

Loop stomas are quicker and easier to perform, and require a smaller incision to reverse, but may allow spill-over of bowel content.

Confirmation of the correct part of colon is achieved by identifying the *taeniae coli* (to distinguish colon from small bowel), the mesentery (to distinguish sigmoid and transverse colon from descending and ascending colon), and presence or absence of the attached greater omentum (present on transverse colon).

Indications

- Defunction bowel by diverting faecal stream, where a distal anastomosis is present, where resection/anastomosis is not possible, or there is a distal obstruction.
- Examples include congenital anorectal malformations, Hirschsprung disease, and necrotizing enterocolitis in neonates, or inflammatory bowel disease in older children.

Preoperative preparation

- Usually no bowel preparation is required. Perioperative antibiotic cover, e.g. with co-amoxiclav, or cefotaxime + metronidazole for elective stoma, or as dictated by underlying disease.
- For an elective stoma in an older child, assessment by the stoma therapy team is important to demonstrate stoma equipment and mark the best site, with respect to the patient's body habitus and usual clothing.

Position

- Supine position as for laparotomy.
- Consider Lloyd–Davies if intraoperative access to the rectum is required in an older child.

Procedure

- Initial laparoscopy (umbilical port placement) can be performed to assess the status of the bowel, to provide assistance in identifying the correct segment of bowel (e.g. Crohn's disease), and help avoid twisting. Not all surgeons perform this. Either a transverse incision, or a

'V' skin flap, is placed in the left iliac fossa (LIF) (sigmoid colostomy) or right upper quadrant (RUQ) (transverse), right iliac fossa (RIF) (ileostomy), depending on the intended method of supporting the stoma.
- The correct segment of colon or terminal ileum is identified and withdrawn.
- A small window in the mesentery is made (bipolar or ligation with absorbable ties).
- If a catheter (e.g. Jacque's catheter) is used as the stomal bridge, this is passed through the mesenteric window and clips applied to each end to prevent tube displacement.
- Care should be taken to confirm the correct orientation of the proximal and distal limbs of the bowel.
- For a loop stoma, the proximal loop is further exteriorized. The serosa of the bowel is sutured to the external oblique to anchor the stoma and reduce the risk of prolapse (e.g. Vicryl®). For a loop stoma, the bowel is opened longitudinally. Three-point absorbable suture sutures are placed in the proximal limb to create a spout (Brooke stoma)—skin edge, bowel serosa at level of skin edge, and bowel mucosa. The stoma is then spouted.
- Further sutures from skin edge to bowel are placed to complete the stoma.
- The catheter passing under the stoma is sutured to the skin on either side, close to the bowel to allow stoma bag placement.

Postoperative care

- Enteral intake is dictated by underlying disease course and recovery of bowel function (gas and stool via the stoma).
- Application of a clear stoma bag (term neonates and older children) on the operating table to prevent early spillage of contents on to a laparotomy incision and allows early regular observation of the stoma.
- Supporting catheter can be removed at approximately 7 days postoperatively.
- Early involvement of stoma therapy team for older children (in hospital and community).

Complications

- Prolapse—can be managed conservatively if easily reducible and asymptomatic. Rarely may require reduction under sedation or anaesthesia. May require stoma revision (or early closure) if problematic.
- Stenosis—may cause pain around stoma site. May require stoma revision.
- Volvulus of proximal loop internally—presents with severe peri-stomal pain and/or obstruction. Requires re-fashioning.
- Skin excoriation/problems with bags remaining attached—best managed by stoma therapy team with appropriate barriers/adhesives/ stoma appliances.

Tips and tricks

- Use of a more rapidly absorbed suture to suture the stoma to skin may allow easier application of the stoma bags in the early months.
- Pass an appropriately-sized Hegar dilator into the stoma at operation to ensure patency.
- Laparoscopic visualization of the stoma may help with correct orientation and may prevent twisting of the proximal bowel.

Fundoplication

Surgical anatomy

- The oesophageal hiatus is likely to be widely open and need repair.
- Hiatus hernia (sliding or rolling) may be present and require sac excision.
- Gastro-oesophageal reflux is more common in infants with previous oesophageal atresia/tracheo-oesophageal fistula or congenital diaphragmatic hernia.

Indications

In the UK, most children requiring fundoplication are neurologically impaired.

- Gastro-oesophageal reflux disease (GORD) refractory to maximal medical management.
- Respiratory complications of GORD, including aspiration pneumonia, acute life-threatening events.
- Oesophagitis, oesophageal stricture.
- Dental problems.

Preoperative preparation

- IV antibiotic prophylaxis as per local hospital policy.
- NG tube + large bore orogastric tube.

Position and theatre set-up

- Supine, GA. Urinary catheter is usually placed, may be removed at end of procedure if not required postoperatively.
- Once ports are in place, patient positioned head-up. Laparoscopy screen placed at patients head end, facing surgeon and assistant. For older children, surgeon stands between patients legs.
- Patients >20kg vessel sealing device is useful, e.g. Harmonic ACE™, LigaSure™.

Procedure

- Procedure is usually performed laparoscopically.
- Open insertion of umbilical port (5mm), either supra- or infra-umbilical. Use 5mm laparoscope and instruments. Additional ports (5mm) left and right lateral, and epigastric for liver retractor. Additional port can be used in the planned gastrostomy position, if being fashioned during the same operation. Left lobe of liver elevated with Nathanson retractor.
- Thin peritoneum over the caudate lobe is opened to enter lesser sac.
- Peritoneum over anterior oesophagus ('white line') opened while drawing down the body of the stomach.
- Right crus is identified lateral to right side of oesophagus.
- Oesophagus is elevated with atraumatic grasper (right hand), and window behind oesophagus is opened by sweeping membrane away from the posterior oesophagus. Care is taken to open plane in front of left crus rather than superiorly (pleura). When plane is established, some surgeons pass a Nylon tape around the oesophagus.
- The upper short gastric vessels are divided in most cases (hook monopolar or vessel sealing device).

- Curoplasty is fashioned to narrow the oesophageal hiatus—left to right crus—with 3/0 non-absorbable suture. The space is narrowed to the equivalent of allowing the tip of the index finger into the space between crura and oesophagus.
- 360° Nissen fundoplication is fashioned by passing the fundus through the established posterior oesophageal window. The wrap is sutured stomach–oesophagus–stomach with three 3/0 non-absorbable sutures.
- Ports are removed and sites closed under lap vision.

Postoperative care

- Usually no further antibiotics.
- Orogastric tube is removed at the end of the procedure.
- NG tube in situ and on free drainage and 4-hourly aspiration.
- Gastrostomy on free drainage and 4-hourly aspiration.

Complications (procedure-specific)

Gas bloat, dysphagia, recurrent hiatus hernia, failure of wrap, recurrence of reflux.

Tips and tricks

- Marking laparoscopic clips can be placed on the fundoplication sutures to confirm wrap remains below diaphragm if future XRs are undertaken.
- Alternative anterior fundoplications include Thal or Watson.

Inguinal hernia/hydrocele

Surgical anatomy

Subtypes:

- In infants and children, 99% are indirect inguinal hernia. Direct or femoral herniae are rare in children. Anatomy of indirect inguinal hernia and hydrocele are the same in children—failed spontaneous obliteration of the processus vaginalis.
- Hernia—intermittent groin swelling, extending from groin to scrotum, cannot get above the swelling.
- Hydrocele—scrotal swelling, can get above (in neck of scrotum).
- Hydrocele of cord—mobile cystic swelling in upper scrotum or groin (usually non-tender, well child).

Indications

- Hernia—requires emergency manual reduction (IV morphine or sedation) if irreducible.
- Elective repair of hernia—urgent in neonates, routine in infants/older children.
- Hydrocele—80% resolve spontaneously, elective ligation of patent processus vaginalis offered at >2 years if persists.

Preoperative preparation

Screening for complete androgen insensitivity (CAIS, 1% risk) advocated for phenotypic females with inguinal hernia.

Position

Supine.

Procedure

(See Fig. 7.5)

Unilateral groin incision, Scarpa's opened and external oblique (EO) defined. Window in EO made.

Males

- Cremasteric muscle fibres split and spermatic cord delivered.
- Hernia sac separated from vas/testicular vessels. Sac is isolated, divided, and dissected to deep inguinal ring.
- Base of sac transfixed with absorbable suture, and redundant sac excised.
- Ensure vas/vessels isolated and preserved.

Females

- Sac mobilized (distally) and opened.
- Ovary/Fallopian tube, if present, are reduced.
- Round ligament may be adherent to edge of sac and require separation/reduction.
- Sac twisted closed, dissected to deep inguinal ring, and transfixed with absorbable suture.
- Redundant sac excised.

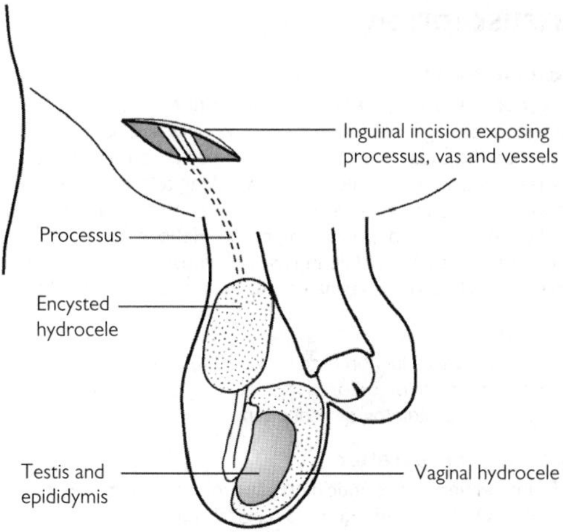
Inguinal incision exposing processus, vas and vessels
Processus
Encysted hydrocele
Testis and epididymis
Vaginal hydrocele

Fig. 7.5 Approach for hydrocele. Reproduced with permission from McLatchie, G, and Leaper, D. Operative Surgery 2nd edition, Oxford University Press: 2006.

Hydrocele

- Operation is same as for male inguinal hernia.
- Additional final step is to drain fluid retrogradely via opened processus vaginalis.

Closure

- EO and Scarpa's closed—4/0 absorbable suture.
- Subcut fat layer 5/0 absorbable suture.
- Skin 5/0 absorbable suture subcuticular.

Postoperative care

- Can feed when awake.
- Day case if age >50 weeks post-conceptual age.

Complications (procedure-specific)

- Recurrence (1%).
- Damage to vas (1%).
- Testicular atrophy.

Tips and tricks

- Identify inferior edge of inguinal ligament to ensure EO window is not made too high.
- Laparoscopic purse string closure of deep inguinal ring—higher recurrence rate, but allows concomitant closure of contralateral deep inguinal ring, resulting in lower rate of metachronous hernia.

Intussusception

Surgical anatomy

Intussusception is usually ileo-colonic in children. The majority can be treated with radiological air reduction. The peak age is 9 months and in this age group the cause is usually non-pathological enlargement of Peyer's patches (secondary to viral infection), provoking telescoping of the bowel. In children >2 years of age a pathological lead point should be considered, e.g. Meckel's diverticulum, polyp, lymphoma, Henoch Schonlein purpura.

The caecum is usually mobile in cases of intussusception. The intussusceptum (proximal bowel) invaginates into the intussuscipiens (distal bowel).

Indications

- Failed radiological reduction (occurs in ~20%).
- Evidence of perforation before/after radiological reduction.
- Peritonitis before radiological reduction.

Preoperative preparation

- Significant dehydration is anticipated and infants require >40ml/kg as fluid boluses before attempted radiological reduction or surgery.
- IV antibiotic cover, e.g. co-amoxiclav or cefotaxime + metronidazole.

Position and theatre set-up

Supine, NG tube, urinary catheter.

Procedure

(See Fig. 7.6)

- Palpate for mass under anaesthetic.
- Usually a right upper quadrant transverse incision is used for open surgery.
- The caecum is delivered, and usually does not require mobilization to do so.
- Manual reduction is performed by squeezing the distal portion of the colon and reducing the small bowel retrogradely back into the ileum. It is preferable not to pull on the proximal ileal end as there is a risk of tearing the serosa.
- If manual reduction cannot be achieved due to serosal tearing, or there is ischaemia/infarction, then an ileo-caecectomy is performed.
- Laparoscopic-assisted reduction is possible, but views may be limited if there is significant distension. 5mm umbilical, RUQ, and LIF ports are used allowing triangulation towards the caecum. Atraumatic graspers are used to squeeze the distal colon while gently drawing the ileum out of the caecum.

Postoperative care

- If manual reduction, no further antibiotic prophylaxis is required.
- If resection/anastomosis, then e.g. 24h antibiotic is sufficient.
- NG tube is left in place for 24h. Feeding can be started once signs of bowel function recovery are present.
- Infants can be discharged if well after 24h observation after radiological reduction, or once tolerating full feeds if resection is required.

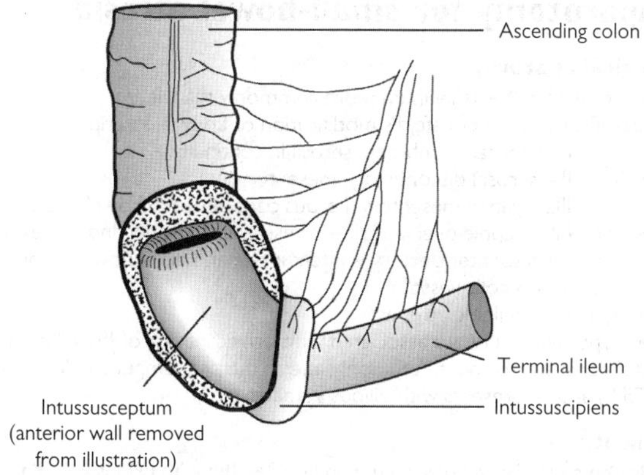
Ascending colon
Terminal ileum
Intussusceptum
(anterior wall removed
from illustration)
Intussuscipiens

Fig. 7.6 Intussusception of terminal ileum. Reproduced with permission from McLatchie, G, and Leaper, D. Operative Surgery 2nd edition, Oxford University Press: 2006.

Complications

- 15% risk recurrence if radiological reduction; lower after manual reduction.
- Risk of perforation with radiological reduction, or leak after anastomosis.

Tips and tricks

Laparoscopic visualization of the ileo-caecum is useful to confirm radiological reduction has been achieved if there is doubt.

Laparotomy for small-bowel atresia

Surgical anatomy

- Bowel atresia affects jejunum more commonly than ileum.
- Classification is by Grosfeld's modification of Louw's description:
  - Type I—internal membrane, serosa in continuity.
  - Type II—serosal discontinuity, mesentery intact.
  - Type IIIa—gap in mesentery, fibrous cord between bowel ends.
  - Type IIIb—'apple peel' atresia—atresia starts just beyond DJ flexure, superior mesenteric artery is interrupted, and distal bowel is coiled around ileo-colic vessel.
  - Type IV—multiple atresias.
  - Types IIIa and IV are associated with significant loss of bowel length.
- Duodenal atresia more commonly affects the post-ampullary duodenum (75%) and so presents with bilious vomiting.

Indications

- Presents with bowel obstruction in first 24–48h with bilious vomiting and distension.
- Antenatal diagnosis occurs in up to half of cases.
- Postnatal diagnosis is confirmed on plain abdominal XR showing a double bubble (duodenal atresia), or several dilated bowel loops (jejunal or ileal atresia), and (usually) no distal bowel gas.

Preoperative preparation

- Usually diagnosed on plain abdominal XR only.
- Cross-match blood as for any neonatal laparotomy.
- NG tube placed.

Position

Supine.

Procedure

(See Fig. 7.7)

- Upper transverse incision. All of small bowel is delivered to identify site of atresia and exclude multiple atresias. The proximal bowel end will be dilated and can be excised to a more normal calibre if there is no overall concern about bowel length. The distal pouch is opened and end–end seromuscular anastomosis is performed (e.g. 5/0 absorbable suture). Multiple anastomoses may be required. Overall length of remaining intestine should be measured.
- Duodeno-duodenostomy—the upper and lower pouches are mobilized laterally, but no attempt at excision is made (risk of damage to common bile duct). Enterotomy is made in each pouch and duodeno-duodenostomy fashioned (see Fig. 7.7), thus 'bypassing' the atresia.

Closure

4/0 absorbable suture muscle, 5/0 absorbable suture subcut fat layer, 5/0 absorbable suture subcuticular to skin.

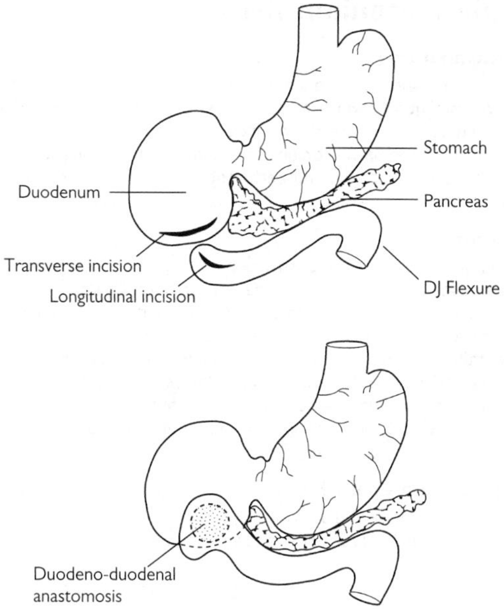
Stomach
Duodenum
Pancreas
Transverse incision
Longitudinal incision
DJ Flexure
Duodeno-duodenal
anastomosis

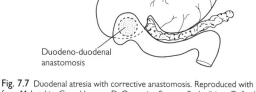

Fig. 7.7 Duodenal atresia with corrective anastomosis. Reproduced with permission from McLatchie, G, and Leaper, D. Operative Surgery 2nd edition, Oxford University Press: 2006.

Postoperative care

- Most patients with jejunal or ileal atresia require short-term parenteral nutrition via long line.
- 24h of IV antibiotic cover is sufficient.
- NG remains on free drainage and at least 4-hourly aspiration with replacement of losses with IV fluid, until signs of recovery of bowel function.
- A trans-anastomotic (naso-jejunal) tube can be placed in the duodenal atresia, allowing early enteral feeding and avoiding parenteral nutrition.

Complications

Leak, stenosis, adhesions, short-gut.

Tips and tricks

Oblique incision or 'fish-mouth' of distal bowel end will allow an easier anastomosis if large size discrepancy. Some surgeons advocate a more minimal access through a small curved supra-umbilical incision.

Simple meconium ileus

Surgical anatomy

Meconium ileus occurs secondary to cystic fibrosis (CF), an autosomal recessive condition in which abnormally viscid intestinal luminal contents are formed due to pancreatic insufficiency. Approximately 15% of neonates with CF develop meconium ileus. Antenatal complications, such as segmental volvulus, atresia, and perforation (with pseudocyst formation), can occur.

Indications

Presents with distal bowel obstruction in the first 24–48h with bilious vomiting, distension, and failure to pass meconium. Obstruction occurs in the terminal ileum secondary to abnormally viscid luminal contents (simple meconium ileus). Radiological decompression may be achieved using Gastrograffin™ or N-Acetyl-Cysteine rectal irrigation. Complicated meconium ileus refers to segmental volvulus, atresia, perforation, meconium peritonitis with pseudo-cyst formation. Complicated meconium ileus, as well as cases that fail to respond to therapeutic enema, require surgical intervention.

Preoperative preparation

- IV fluid resuscitation and antibiotics.
- NG decompression (size 8Fr in a term neonate).

Position

Supine.

Procedure

- Enterotomy and irrigation.
- Upper transverse incision. All of the small bowel is delivered to confirm the diagnosis and site of obstruction. Atresia and other complications are excluded. A purse-string suture is placed in the dilated proximal bowel (5/0 absorbable suture). The bowel is opened and removal/irrigation of inspissated contents undertaken. N-Acetyl-Cysteine (diluted to form a 2% solution) or Gastrograffin (diluted to ¼ strength) are used to irrigate and soften the meconium, thereby allowing direct removal or flushing through the colon. Enterotomy is closed with absorbable suture.
- Alternative procedures include temporary stoma formation, or resection and primary anastomosis (rarely required).

Closure

4/0 absorbable suture muscle, 5/0 absorbable suture subcut fat layer, 5/0 absorbable suture subcuticular to skin.

Postoperative care

- 24h of IV antibiotic cover.
- NG tube on free drainage, at least 4-hourly aspiration with replacement of losses with IV fluid.
- Feed is introduced after signs of recovery of bowel function.
- Enteral administration of dilute N-Acetyl-Cysteine or Gastrograffin™ (via ng and per-rectum) should be started postoperatively to prevent recurrence.

Complications

- Leak, stenosis, adhesions, short-gut (if antenatal volvulus or atresia).
- Re-obstruction with inspissated contents.
- Long-term respiratory management of CF is required.

Tips and tricks

Palpation of the vasa in the upper scrotum of term male neonates with distal bowel obstruction has been reported to aid in the diagnosis of meconium ileus. In cases of CF/meconium ileus, the vasa are atretic.

Oesophageal atresia (OA) and tracheo-oesophageal fistula (TOF)

Surgical anatomy

Subtypes:

- OA + distal TOF (lower oesophagus into distal trachea).
- H-type—TOF only, no atresia (usually approached via right neck incision).
- Isolated long gap OA—no fistula, usually requires delayed primary anastomosis (or oesophageal replacement).
- OA with upper and lower pouch fistulae.

Indications

- Antenatal diagnosis—OA may be suspected with absent (or small) fetal stomach.
- Postnatal presentation—'mucousy' baby, unable to swallow saliva, cannot pass NG tube (size 10Fr arrests at 10cm).

Preoperative preparation

- Cross-match blood.
- Echocardiography—check side of aortic arch, cardiac anomalies.
- Renal USS—not urgent.
- Chest XR—assess cardiac shadow, rib/vertebral anomalies. Confirms NG coiled in upper pouch.
- AXR—exclude concomitant intestinal atresia. Presence of gas in intestine confirms OA + distal TOF. Gasless abdomen suggests isolated OA (without TOF).
- Pass Replogle tube into upper oesophagus and maintain continuous low-pressure suction to prevent aspiration.

Position

- Rigid bronchoscopy may be performed prior to repair—confirms diagnosis (not essential), assess tracheomalacia, exclude concomitant upper pouch fistula (present in 25% of 'long gap' OA).
- Left lateral, right arm elevated and secured above head.

Procedure

(See Fig. 7.8)

- Right postero-lateral muscle-cutting thoracotomy, starting at tip of scapula, extending posteriorly, avoiding long thoracic nerve.
- 5th intercostal space (ICS) is entered. Finichetto retractor is used.
- Extra-pleural approach is favoured by most surgeons—pleura is stripped away from chest wall by inserting (then withdrawing) an opened moist gauze swab in to 5th ICS, then using moist pledgelets to continue posterior dissection. Assistant retracts right lung medially.
- Azygos vein is ligated and divided.
- Vagus nerve allows identification of the distal fistula, which is mobilized away from trachea and slung. Stay suture to distal fistula.
- Junction of distal TOF and trachea is identified and confirmed by occluding while the anaesthetist performs positive pressure ventilation. Fistula is sutured with non-absorbable sutures, and divided. Tracheal stump closure is confirmed by instilling saline and asking the anaesthetist to perform positive pressure ventilation.

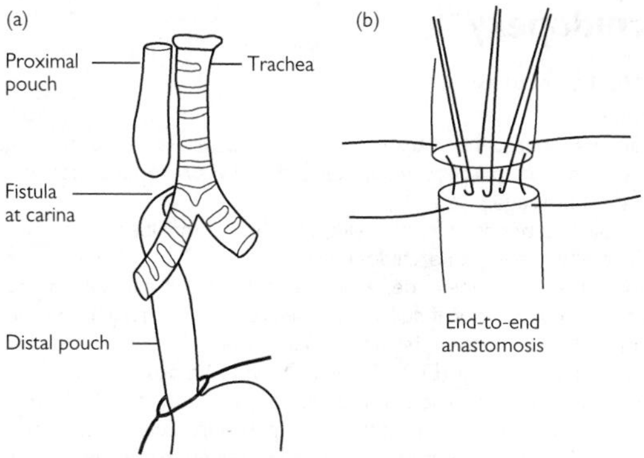
(a)
Proximal pouch
Trachea
Fistula at carina
Distal pouch
(b)
End-to-end anastomosis

Fig. 7.8 Oesophageal atresia. Reproduced with permission from McLatchie, G, and Leaper, D. Operative Surgery 2nd edition, Oxford University Press: 2006.

- Upper pouch is identified by asking the anaesthetist to push carefully on the Replogle tube. Upper pouch is mobilized and stay suture placed. Upper pouch is opened at most dependent point.
- Primary anastomosis is performed with fine absorbable sutures—three to four back wall sutures first (untied), which are then crossed sequentially to apply even tension. Trans-anastomotic tube (TAT) is passed into the stomach (e.g. 6Fr) and front wall anastomosis completed.
- Chest drain is not usually required.

Closure

- Ribs opposed 3/0 absorbable suture.
- Muscle closed in layers 3/0 absorbable suture.
- Subcut fat layer 5/0 absorbable suture.
- Skin 5/0 absorbable suture subcuticular.

Postoperative care

- TAT secured and left on free drainage for 24–48h.
- TAT used for intra-gastric feeds at 24–48h.
- Oral feed commenced ~day 3.
- Contrast study in absence of clinical concerns to assess anastomosis not routinely necessary.
- TAT removed when full oral feed established.

Complications (procedure-specific)

- Anastomostic leak—consider re-exploration if large and identified in 1st 24–48hs postoperative.
- Stricture (25%)—balloon dilatation.
- Tracheal stump leak.
- Chest wall deformity, scoliosis.

Tips and tricks

Nerve hook into oesophageal lumen facilitates front wall anastomosis.

Orchidopexy

Surgical anatomy

Subtypes:

- Unilateral undescended testis occurs in 1% boys. Spontaneous postnatal descent occurs in a proportion. Orchidopexy is recommended at 6–12 months age.
- Approach depends on testis being palpable or impalpable.
- Palpable testis—open orchidopexy.
- Impalpable—examine under anaesthetic (EUA)—if palpable, proceed to open orchidopexy. If still impalpable, proceed to laparoscopy. If intra-abdominal testis—1st stage laparoscopic procedure. Testis close to deep inguinal right (DIR) ('peeping')—may be possible to undertake single stage laparoscopic-assisted orchidopexy. 2nd stage is deferred by >6 months. If vas and vessels passing through deep inguinal ring—ipsilateral groin exploration to find and excise nubbin testis, and fix contralateral testis in Dartos pouch.

Indications

Elective orchidopexy is recommended at 6–12 months age.

Preoperative preparation

Usually no investigations are required. US is of no value in locating an impalpable testis. Consider karyotyping for bilateral impalpable testes (exclude congenital adrenal hyperplasia), or for unilateral undescended testis with hypospadias (possible mixed gonadal dysgenesis).

Position

Supine.

Procedure

Open orchidopexy

- Unilateral groin incision, Scarpa's fascia is opened and external oblique (EO) defined. Testis most commonly is at superficial inguinal pouch. If not, EO opened.
- Testis mobilized and gubernaculum divided. Testis placed out of wound towards anterior superior iliac spine, thus reversing anatomical position of vas/vessels with respect to the patent processus vaginalis (PPV, now posterior). The internal spermatic fascia over the vas/vessels is opened. The edges of the PPV are grasped with a clip and the PPV stretched out. The PPV is carefully separated from the vas/vessels. The PPV is clipped, divided, dissected to the DIR then transfixed with absorbable suture. Full mobilization of the vas/vessels (including retroperitoneal) may be required to gain adequate length. Hydatid cyst (if present) is excised.
- Transverse scrotal incision is made and a Dartos pouch developed with sharp-pointed scissors. A clip is passed retrogradely from the scrotal incision to the inguinal incision and the testis passed down to the Dartos pouch.

1st stage laparoscopic procedure

- Standard diagnostic laparoscopy (5mm instruments). If intra-abdominal testis is present, right and left 5mm ports are placed.
- Patient is positioned head-down.
- The testicular vessels are mobilized by dividing the peritoneum on the medial and lateral sides.
- The vessels are divided (clips or suture) and left in continuity.

2nd stage Fowler–Stephens' orchidopexy

- Laparoscopic approach is repeated.
- The testis is mobilized by dividing the peritoneum lateral to the testis in an arc towards the DIR. Medial mobilization is parallel to the vas. An atraumatic grasper is passed via the DIR to the scrotum and a Dartos pouch fashioned. The grasper is exteriorized into the scrotal incision and a short length of suture grasped, with the other end attached to a clip. The atraumatic grasper is withdrawn back into the abdominal cavity carrying the clip with it, which can then grasp the testis and draw it into the Dartos pouch.

Groin exploration

- If vas/vessels are passing through DIR on laparoscopy, ipsilateral groin incision is made, EO opened, and nubbin testis excised.
- Scrotal fixation of the contralateral testis (Dartos pouch) can be undertaken to reduce risk of later torsion in the single testis.

Closure

- Absorbable sutures to port sites.
- 5/0 absorbable suture to scrotal skin.

Postoperative care

Day-case procedure.

Complications

Recurrence, damage to vas, testicular atrophy.

Tips and tricks

For 1st stage Fowler–Stephen's procedure, leave the testicular vessels in continuity to prevent torsion (around the vas).

Pyloromyotomy

Surgical anatomy

- Pyloric stenosis, peak age 4–6 weeks.
- Presents with non-bilious projectile vomiting.
- Infant likely to have metabolic alkalosis.
- Cause unknown, hypertrophic obstruction of pyloric canal results.

Indications

Pyloric stenosis—confirmed with palpation or ultrasound.

Preoperative preparation

- Adequate fluid resuscitation to correct electrolyte and acid/base imbalance. Surgery is not an emergency.
- NG tube (8Fr) should already be sited.
- If using a supra-umbilical approach, consider chlorhexidine soaked swab dressing for 6h preoperatively.
- IV antibiotic prophylaxis, e.g. co-amoxiclav.

Position

- For open procedures, baby supine in middle of table.
- For laparoscopic procedures either supine at the end of the table or lying sideways across the table.
- For a laparoscopic procedure, place the stack to the patients left, ideally with an extension arm to swing the screen over the patients head.

Procedure

Open technique

- The Ramstedt procedure was previously performed via a midline laparotomy or right upper quadrant incision. A supra-umbilical approach is more commonly used (Fig. 7.9).

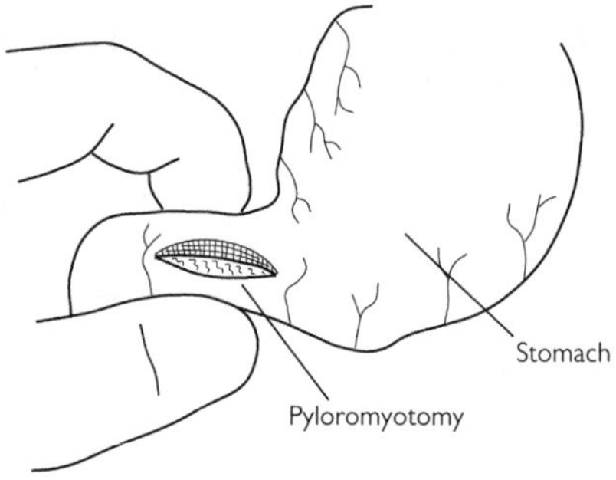
Stomach
Pyloromyotomy

Fig. 7.9 Ramstedt's pyloromyotomy. Reproduced with permission from McLatchie, G, and Leaper, D. Operative Surgery 2nd edition, Oxford University Press: 2006.

- Curved supra-umbilical skin incision. Linea alba opened longitudinally. The stomach is withdrawn with atraumatic forceps and the pylorus delivered. The skin incision can be extended laterally on both sides, creating an Ω shape if it is difficult to deliver the pylorus.
- The serosa of the avascular area of the pylorus (antero-superior aspect) is scored up to the pre-pyloric vein. A blunt instrument, e.g. McDonald dissector, is used to widen the incision.
- The edges are carefully spread with a clip and the mucosa will bulge into view. The two halves (upper and lower) should move independently.
- The anaesthetist can inflate air down the NG tube, which is milked across the pyloric canal to confirm patency and confirm there is no perforation. Return the pylorus to the abdomen.
- Linea alba closed with absorbable suture, e.g. 3/0.

Laparoscopic technique

- 5mm open umbilical port insertion, with 3mm right and left stab incisions.
- Establish pneumoperitoneum to 8mmHg CO_2 and perform a laparoscopy.
- An arthroscopy blade or monopolar hook is used to incise the pyloric muscle.
- An atraumatic grasper or pyloric spreader is used to spread the myotomy incision, and as for the open technique, the mucosa is seen to bulge.
- The final steps of the open technique are performed.
- Umbilicus fascia is closed with 3/0 absorbable suture. Skin glue to oppose the skin.

Postoperative care/instructions

Feed when hungry, warning parents that baby may vomit for 24h postoperatively.

Complications

- Umbilical wounds have a higher risk of wound infection.
- Perforation of duodenum.
- Incomplete pyloromyotomy requiring redo myotomy.
- Port site hernia.

Tips and tricks

2cm myotomy has been demonstrated to be adequate, and can be easily measured intraoperatively.

Scrotal exploration

Surgical anatomy

The testis is covered with tunica vaginalis, internal spermatic fascia, cremasteric fascia, and external spermatic fascia. In ~10% of males, there is a 'bell-clapper' deformity, where the tunica vaginalis does not completely invaginate the testis, allowing it to rotate freely within the scrotum. Small Mullerian remnant structures are often present, the most common of which are the appendix epididymis and the appendix testis (hydatid cyst of Morgagni).

Indications

- Testicular pain, swelling, tenderness—differential diagnosis is torsion, torsion of testicular appendix, epididymo-orchitis.
- Scrotal exploration is a time-critical emergency to excluded/manage torsion.
- Although the majority of explorations in children will not demonstrate torsion, an exploration is mandatory because of the risk of testicular loss.

Preoperative preparation

None.

Position

Supine.

Procedure

- Transverse incision. Fashion Dartos pouch if pre-pubertal child. Incise through layers of the scrotum until reaching the tunica vaginalis. Pick up the tunica with forceps and open with scissors, often there will be reactive fluid present—send for culture if no other obvious abnormality found.
- Deliver the testicle and epididymis.
- Assess the position and viability of the testis and presence of twisted appendix (remove with bipolar).
- If twisted, untwist the testis, and if good viability, replace in the scrotum and perform three-point fixation with non-absorbable suture (or place in Dartos pouch).
- If doubtful viability, place in warm saline-soaked swabs for several minutes and re-examine. If infarcted, high ligation of the spermatic cord is performed and the testis excised. The contralateral testis should then be fixed.

Closure

With absorbable suture, interrupted.

Small-bowel resection and anastomosis

Surgical anatomy

Limited resections are usually required in infants and children. The mesentery and its vessels can be divided close to the bowel wall in paediatric practice.

Indications

Neonates

Necrotizing enterocolitis, atresia.

Infants

- Intussusception—if there is necrosis, a non-reducible mass, or a pathological lead point (Meckel's, polyp, lymphoma).
- Meckel's diverticulum, Crohn's disease.

Preoperative preparation

Antibiotic cover, NG tube, urinary catheter in older children.

Position

Supine.

Procedure

The small bowel is delivered and the limits of resection defined. A window in the mesentery is made at each end of the intended resection. Bipolar can be used to diathermy and divide the mesentery in infants. In older children the mesenteric vessels can be clipped, divided, and ligated with absorbable ties. An alternative is to use a vessel-sealing device if the procedure has been laparoscopic-assisted. The mesentery is divided close to the bowel wall at each of the resection. The edges of the wound are protected with povidone-iodine-soaked swabs. The bowel is divided and any bleeding points on the luminal ends can be addressed with bipolar diathermy. It is not usually necessary to use bowel clamps.

The bowel is anastomosed using a single-layer, interrupted, seromuscular suture. The anastomosis starts at the mesenteric end, and the first suture is held out on a clip. The second suture is at the opposite ante-mesenteric point of the bowel lumen and again is held out on clips. Individual sutures are placed in between. The defect in the mesentery is closed with absorbable sutures.

Postoperative care

24h NBM, two further doses IV antibiotics.

Complications

Leak, stricture, adhesions, recurrence (e.g. NEC, Crohn's).

Tips and tricks

Assistant inverts any protruding mucosa as each suture is tied.

Umbilical hernia

Surgical anatomy

Umbilical hernias occur via a defect through the umbilical scar at the site of the previous attachment of the umbilical cord. There is a small (1 in 1,000) risk of incarceration of abdominal content. Overall, from the newborn period, 80% close spontaneously by age 3–4 years, so initial observation through infancy is usually undertaken.

Indications

Usually cosmesis if present at 3–4 years of age.

Preoperative preparation

None.

Position

Supine, GA.

Procedure (including closure)

Curved skin crease, either supra- or infra-umbilical. The subcutaneous fat is opened. Dissection is made on either side of the umbilicus so that a haemostat clip can be passed from one side of the incision, around the hernia sac, and back into the other side of the incision. The sac is partially opened by incising (monopolar) on to the clip. Once opened, it can be confirmed that the sac is empty. Clips are applied to the edges of the sac. The excess sac is excised and the fascial edges of the defect are clearly defined. The defect is closed with multiple absorbable sutures, left untied sequentially, and tied when all are in place.

The underneath of the umbilicus is tacked onto the now closed defect with absorbable suture so that the umbilical skin sits flat or puckers in.

Postoperative care

Small pressure dressing for 24–48h to allow the umbilical skin to stick flat.

Complications (procedure-specific)

Recurrence.

Tips and tricks

Carefully define the fascial edges to ensure robust closure.

Cystoscopy, endoscopic correction of VUR, endoscopic insertion/removal of JJ stent, and endoscopic puncture—ureterocoele

Surgical anatomy

The interior of the bladder and two ureteric orifices, situated at either end of the trans-trigonal bar, can be visualized using a cystoscope, passed per-urethrally. The triangle between the ureteric orifices and the internal urethral meatus is referred to as the trigone of the bladder.

Indications

Diagnostic

- Recurrent urinary tract infections.
- Urinary incontinence.
- Obstructive uropathy.
- Haematuria.
- Radiological abnormalities.
- Urogenital sinus.
- Epispadias.

Therapeutic

- Posterior urethral valve ablation.
- Ureterocoele puncture.
- Vesico-ureteric reflux—endoscopic correction.
- Urethral stricture—ablation.
- Ureteral access for ureteroscopy and lithotripsy.
- Ureteric stenting/removal.
- Bladder stone.

Preoperative preparation

- Ensure negative urine culture.
- Antibiotic prophylaxis.

Position and theatre set-up

- Lithotomy position (in the infant, frog-legged with a towel roll underneath thighs).
- Monitors for fluoroscopic and video-camera imaging.
- Warm irrigant fluid.
- Appropriate cystoscopes and other equipment, such as bugbee electrodes, guide wires, catheters, stents, baskets, laser fibres, and STING needles.

Procedure

Cystoscopy

- Inspect the external genitalia closely for anomalies.
- The term infant's urethral meatus should accept a 7.5–8Fr cystoscope.
- The male infant's urethral meatus may require dilatation with urethral sounds.
- The cystoscope tip is inserted with lubricant while the irrigant fluid is running.

- Negotiate through the urethra, visualizing the lumen in the centre, at all times.
- In the male urethra, identify the part traversing the external urethral sphincter, verumontanum, and bladder neck.
- Inspect the bladder interior noting the location, number, and configuration of the ureteric orifices.
- Empty the bladder and remove the scope.

Endoscopic correction of vesico-ureteric reflux
- Choose a paediatric cystoscope with an offset lens and carry out cystoscopy.
- The injection needle, commonly called a STING needle, is introduced through the working channel of the cystoscope into the 6 o'clock position, 2–3mm below the ureteric orifice.
- Advance the needle by 0.5cm behind the intra-vesical ureter and inject the bulking agent (0.2–0.5ml, Deflux™) until a mound is created which turns the orifice into a cresentic slit.

Endoscopic insertion/removal of JJ stent
- Choose a cystoscope with a working channel that would allow an appropriate size JJ stent.
- Insert the cystoscope, identify the ureteric orifice, and insert ureteric catheter to perform retrograde ureteropyelogram.
- Insert a guide wire through the ureteric catheter.
- Remove the ureteric catheter, insert the JJ stent over the guide wire, and place the stent in a satisfactory position under fluoroscopy.
- JJ stent can be easily removed using a stent grasper passed through an appropriate cystoscope. Grasp the end of the stent and hold on to it while gently removing the cystoscope.

Endoscopic puncture of ureterocoele
- Carry out cystoscopy, noting the urethral anatomy and ureterocoele with the bladder empty and full.
- Puncture the ureterocoele by either using a bugbee electrode or a laser fibre.
- Ensure ureterocoele is decompressed.

Postoperative care

The majority of the patients can be discharged home on the same day, after voiding urine.

Complications

- Bleeding.
- Infection.
- Ureteric perforation.
- Persistence of VUR and ureteric obstruction following endoscopic correction.
- Increased chance of VUR after puncture of ureterocoele.

Tips and tricks

If difficulties are encountered visualizing the ureterocoele, attempt while bladder is near empty and manually compressing the ipsilateral flank.

Formation/closure of vesicostomy, suprapubic catheterization

Surgical anatomy

The urinary bladder, a hollow viscus organ with strong muscular (detrusor) walls, lies in the pelvis when empty. The superior surface of the bladder is covered by peritoneum. As the bladder fills, it rises out of the true pelvis and separates the peritoneum from the anterior abdominal wall. Hence the distended bladder may be punctured or approached surgically for insertion of suprapubic catheter/vesicostomy, without breaching the peritoneum.

Indications

These are simple forms of incontinent urinary diversion, employed when bladder empties inadequately in conditions like:

- Posterior urethral valves when endoscopic primary valve ablation is not feasible.
- Neuropathic bladders when clean, intermittent catheterization is unable to be established.
- Rarely, in prune belly syndrome and functional voiding disorders.

Preoperative preparation

Appropriate case selection and choice of procedure after having an in-depth discussion with the family.

Position and theatre set-up

- General anaesthesia.
- Supine position.
- Urethral catheter to fill the bladder when required.

Procedure

Formation of vesicostomy (Blocksom)

- Make a 2cm transverse skin incision halfway between the umbilicus and the pubis.
- Incise the rectus fascia transversely.
- Mobilize the peritoneum superiorly, identify and divide the urachal remnant.
- Place a traction suture in the dome of the bladder and mobilize until the posterior wall is level with the skin.
- Secure the rectus fascia to the bladder wall.
- Open the dome of the bladder to form a 24Fr defect and mature the stoma with 5/0 absorbable sutures.

Closure of vesicostomy

- Dissect the vesicostomy off the skin and fascia.
- Close the bladder in two layers using 5/0 and 4/0 absorbable sutures.
- Close the fascia and the skin using absorbable sutures.
- Leave a urethral catheter for 4–5 days.

Suprapubic catheterization

Suprapubic catheter can be placed via an open procedure (which is described here) or percutaneously under cystoscopic guidance.

- Ensure bladder is full.
- Make a small transverse skin incision 1–2cm above the symphysis pubis and expose the rectus fascia.
- Incise the fascia, separate the rectus muscle, and identify the bladder (aspirate the bladder content with a fine needle for confirmation if necessary).
- Place a stay suture through the anterior bladder wall, incise it, and insert an appropriate size catheter (10–14Fr).
- Close the bladder snugly around the catheter and bring the catheter out through a separate stab wound.
- Close the wound in layers using 3/0 and 5/0 absorbable sutures.

Postoperative care

- Feed the baby as tolerated.
- Allow vesicostomy to drain urine freely in to the diapers.
- Following supra-pubic catheter insertion, leave it on free drainage for 48h followed by 2–3-hourly clamp and release.

Complications

- Stomal stenosis.
- Stomal prolapse.
- Peri-stomal dermatitis.
- Bladder spasm following suprapubic catheterization.

Tips and tricks

The risk of prolapse is minimized by securely suturing the dome of the bladder to the rectus fascia.

Nephrectomy, partial nephrectomy, and hemi-nephroureterectomy for duplex kidney

Surgical anatomy

Peri-renal fascia, commonly called Gerota's fascia, encloses the kidney and perinephric fat. The renal vascular pedicle, comprising of a single renal artery and vein, enters the kidney via the renal hilum medially.

Indications

- Non-functioning/poorly functioning kidney (secondary to congenital malformations, such as obstruction at pelvi-ureteric junction, vesico-ureteric junction, vesico-ureteric reflux, and dysplasia).
- Congenital nephrotic syndrome causing intractable protein loss.
- Renal malignancy such as Wilm's tumour.
- Partial necphrectomy is strongly considered for children with bilateral renal malignant tumours or a tumour in a solitary kidney.
- Hemi-nephrectomy is indicated for excision of a complicated upper or lower moiety of duplex kidney.

Preoperative preparation

- Informed consent.
- Availability of blood/blood products.
- Antibiotics along with induction of anaesthesia.
- Urinary catheter—surgeon's discretion.

Position and theatre set-up

Open surgery

Supine position with a folded towel under the ipsilateral flank.

Laparoscopic—transperitoneal

Supine position with flank of the affected kidney elevated using a pillow and patient secured with straps.

Retroperitoneoscopic approach

- Lateral decubitus or prone with appropriate support/padding and patient secured with straps.
- Prep and drape to expose the entire abdomen or back or ipsilateral side of the abdomen/flank, depending upon the approach.
- Monopolar/bipolar diathermy (and vessel-sealing device for laparoscopic procedures).

Procedure

Open simple nephrectomy

- Anterior muscle splitting, extra-peritoneal approach, which is explained here.
- Split the external oblique, internal oblique, and transversus abdominis along the line of their fibres.
- Each muscle layer is undermined to achieve good exposure.

- Identify and preserve the neurovascular bundles.
- Sweep the peritoneum medially.
- Palpate the kidney through Gerota's fascia. Enter Gerota's fascia.
- Dissect the perinephric fat off the kidney using blunt dissection and bipolar diathermy.
- Expose the anterior surface of the kidney.
- Identify the proximal ureter and hilar vessels. Renal vein anteriorly and artery posteriorly, should be individually isolated, ligated in continuity, and divided.
- The kidney is mobilized and the attached ureter traced as far distally as possible and divided. The distal ureteric stump can be left open if vesico-ureteric reflux was not demonstrated on preoperative investigations.

Hemi-nephroureterectomy
- Following dissection of the peri-nephric fat off the lower pole of the duplex kidney, identify both upper and lower moiety ureters.
- The ureter from the affected moiety usually is dilated (in the majority, upper moiety ureteric dilatation is secondary to obstruction, lower moiety ureteric dilatation is secondary to reflux) and can be traced proximally to their respective moieties.
- For upper moiety hemi-nephroureterectomy, encircle the dilated ureter, dissect it off the renal vessels, divide the blood supply to the upper moiety, taking care of the vessels and the collecting system to the lower moiety.
- Excise the upper moiety with monopolar diathermy and approximate the cut surfaces of the renal parenchyma to achieve haemostasis.
- Trace the upper moiety distal ureter as far low as possible in to the pelvis and divide.
- For lower moiety hemi-nephroureterectomy, the procedure is similar and care must be taken to preserve the upper moiety, its ureter, and renal vessels.
- Both these procedures can be performed laparoscopically and these are not described here.

Partial nephrectomy
- Transperitoneal approach.
- Dissect the vascular pedicle and apply a vessel loop around the renal artery.
- Identify the renal artery branches leading to the involved portion of the kidney.
- Place a bull-dog clamp temporarily on the identified artery.
- If the affected segment of the kidney shows a clear line of demarcation, ligate and divide the identified artery.
- Incise the parenchyma and use finger compression to control the bleeding.
- Suture ligate all bleeding vessels and close the capsule of the remnant kidney using mattress sutures.

Postoperative care

- Close monitoring of vital signs.
- Feed enterally as tolerated.
- Urinary catheter can be removed 24–48h later and mobilize.

Complications

- Urine leak.
- Atrophy of the remnant renal moiety.

Tips and tricks

In hemi-nephroureterectomy, if the state of the vesico-ureteric reflux is not known, an in-dwelling urinary catheter is recommended to be left longer, for up to 5 days, to reduce the incidence of urine leak.

Repair of hypospadias

Several procedures are available for the repair of hypospadias. Regardless of the technique used, the principles of repair are:

- Correction of ventral curvature of the penis (chordee).
- Urethroplasty to move the hypospadiac meatus to the terminal glans.
- Meatoplasty/glanuloplasty.
- Adequate skin coverage.

Surgical anatomy

The penis comprises three cylindrical bodies of erectile cavernous tissue: the paired corpora cavernosa and the single corpus spongiosum ventrally. Each cavernous body is enclosed by the tough tunica albuginea. The corpus spongiosum tapers and runs on the underside of the corpora cavernosa and then expands to cap them as the glans penis. The spongiosum is traversed throughout its length by the anterior urethra. Buck's fascia surrounds both cavernosal bodies dorsally and splits to surround the spongiosum ventrally. The neurovascular bundle runs dorsally underneath the Buck's fascia.

Indications

- Moderate and severe hypospadias that are expected to interfere with voiding and sexual function.
- Surgery for hypospadias on the mild end of the spectrum may be considered for cosmetic and psychosocial reasons.

Preoperative preparation

- Informed consent.
- Antibiotic prophylaxis along with induction of anaesthesia.

Position

- Patient supine.
- Prep and drape to expose the genitalia.

Procedure

- Stay suture through the glans penis.
- Release preputial adhesions.
- Mark and make a circumferential incision 5mm proximal to the corona and de-glove the penis to the penoscrotal junction. This corrects the chordee in the majority of cases.
- In severe hypospadias, perform an artificial erection test using saline irrigation. If residual chordee is present, one or two of the following steps may have to be carried out to correct the curvature complete:
  - Dorsal tunica albuginea plication or ventral dermal patch graft.
  - Transection of the hypoplastic urethra and dissect it off the corporeal bodies to recede the meatus further proximally—if this is needed, hypospadias surgery will have to be a staged operation.
- If the urethral plate distal to the hypospadiac meatus is wide, tubularize the plate over a 6 or 8Fr silastic stent, with 6/0 or 7/0, absorbable monofilament sutures. Complete the urethroplasty distally leaving a

vertical neo-meatus. If the plate is narrow, a dorsal relieving incision of the urethral plate (Snodgrass repair) will enable an adequate-calibre urethroplasty.
- Use a vascularized Dartos flap to cover the neo-urethra.
- Meatoplasty and glanuloplasty are then carried out by raising lateral flaps of glans tissue and approximating over the distal neo-urethra.
- Excise the hooded prepuce and re-fashion the penile shaft skin in such a way as to provide adequate ventral skin coverage and circumcised appearance of the penis.
- In severe hypospadias, following correction of chordee, staged repair is carried out by using genital (preputial) skin or extra-genital skin/tissue (such as post-auricular skin or buccal mucosa) graft in the first stage, followed by tubularization of the grafted tissue to form the neo-urethra with reconstruction of the penis, at least 6 months later, as a 2nd stage. Some surgeons perform a one-stage repair, even in severe hypospadias.
- Secure the urethral stent and apply a non-adherent, compressive dressing

Postoperative care
- Allow the patient to go home on the same day in distal hypospadias repair and after 24h in proximal hypospadias repair.
- Anticholinergic medication (such as oxybutynin) until stent/dressing is removed.
- Limited evidence for antibiotic use—surgeon's discretion.
- Remove dressing and stent after 5–7 days on the ward.

Complications
- Complete breakdown of repair.
- Urethro-cutaneous fistula.
- Urethral stricture/meatal stenosis.
- Poor graft take and potential need for revision.
- Urethral diverticulum.

Tips and tricks
- Double diapers for ease of postoperative care—urethral stent drains into the outer nappy.
- Preoperative penile hormonal stimulation could be considered in children with severe hypospadias and very small penis.

Bladder augmentation

The majority of bladder augmentations are performed with gastro-intestinal segments. The ileum is the most popular segment and ileocystoplasty is described here. It often includes the formation of a continent catheterizable abdominal stoma fashioned using appendix—appendicovesicostomy, commonly referred as Mitrofanoff channel.

Surgical anatomy

De-tubularized bowel segments provide capacity at lower pressure. In children, 20–30cm of distal ileum, 20cm from the ileo-caecal valve, will reach for the proposed anastomosis to the bladder.

Indications

Small capacity, poorly compliant bladder—often secondary to neuropathic bladder, posterior urethral valves, or bladder exstrophy.

Preoperative preparation

- Each patient and family must be prepared and they should be committed to performing clean intermittent catheterization (CIC).
- Thorough urodynamic evaluation.
- Bowel preparation—clear fluids only for 24h prior to operation.
- Availability of blood/blood products.

Position and theatre set-up

- General anaesthesia.
- Patient supine.
- Antibiotic prophylaxis.

Procedure

- Make a lower midline or Pfannenstiel incision.
- Mobilize the bladder extra-peritoneally.
- Open the peritoneum and mobilize a 20–30cm loop of distal ileum with its mesentry, 20cm proximal to ileo-caecal junction.
- Divide the chosen ileal segment between bowel clamps and restore the intestinal continuity using 5/0 absorbable sutures.
- If appendicovesicostomy is to be performed concomitantly, mobilize the appendix with its mesentry and detach from the caecum. Close the caecal defect with absorbable sutures.
- De-tubularize the mobilized ileal segment along its ante-mesenteric border.
- Close the peritoneum and extra-peritonealize the de-tubularized segment. Fold this segment in half and anastomose the medial edges to form a U-patch. Fold it further to form a cup.
- Open the bladder sagitally or coronally. You can perform the appendicovesicostomy over a 12Fr Jacque's catheter at this stage, if necessary using the mobilized appendix.

- Perform the ileocystoplasty by anastomosing the ileal cup to the opened bladder using 3/0 continuous absorbable suture. Ensure a 16Fr suprapubic catheter is inserted and secured well before completing the anastomosis.
- Close the abdominal wall wound in layers.

Postoperative care

- Suprapubic catheter on free drainage for 3 weeks and then clamp/release 3-hourly.
- Remove the catheter in the appendicovesicostomy 3 weeks later and commence education on CIC through the stoma.
- When CIC is established, remove the suprapubic catheter.

Complications

- Urine leak.
- Adhesive bowel obstruction.
- Urinary infections.
- Mucus blockage.
- Metabolic and acid based disturbances.
- Bladder calculi.
- Malignancy.

Tips and tricks

Anastomose the bowel segment to the posterior bladder first; this can be performed from within the bladder.

Anderson Hynes dismembered pyeloplasty

Surgical anatomy

Pelvi-ureteric junction obstruction (PUJO).

Indications

Children with PUJO who have either breakthrough urinary tract infections, despite appropriate prophylactic antibiotics, worsening hydronephosis (>50mm), or renal scarring.

Preoperative preparation

- Urethral catheter.
- Intravenous gentamicin.

Position

- Supine with gel roll under flank on side of operation.
- Larger children/adolescents break table.

Procedure

- Muscle-splitting sub-costal incision, care taken to dissect the adventitial tissue between each muscle layer to maximize exposure through the smallest wound possible.
- Peritoneum bluntly dissected medially with finger, exposing Gerota's fascia.
- Open Gerota's fascia with scissors; this should expose kidney. Blunt dissection in this plane will cause the kidney to drop posteriorly and inferiorly, bringing the renal pelvis into view.
- Identify the pelvi-ureteric junction and gently dissect the fascial attachments distal to it, so a sling can be passed around the ureter.
- Place 6/0 stay sutures at the most dependant aspect of the pelvis, the superior pelvis and on the ureter.
- The pelvi-ureteric junction is then excised; a variable amount of pelvis is also taken, depending on the size and thickness of the renal pelvis.
- The end of the ureter is spatulated.
- Place three 7/0 PDS sutures between the apex of the inferior aspect of the spatulated ureter and the inferior aspect of the pelvis.
- Then run a continuous 6/0 PDS to anastomose the back wall between the ureter and pelvis.
- Place an appropriately sized JJ stent or nephron-stent into the distal ureter; a 'give' should be felt as it passes through the vesico-ureteric junction and into the bladder—now wash the pelvis out with saline to remove clots.
- Run a 6/0 continuous PDS suture along the anterior wall of the anastomosis.
- Perform a layered closure with absorbable suture.

Postoperative care

- Allow diet.
- Continue prophylactic antibiotics for as long as stent is in situ.
- If nephron-stent, plan to 'knot' at 24–48h and then remove urethral catheter. If passing urine and no flank pain, then patient can go home for stent removal 5–7 days postoperative.
- If JJ stent, remove cystoscopically between 6 and 12 weeks postoperative.

Complications

- Anastomotic leak.
- Recurrence (due to structuring of anastomosis/inadequate excision of PUJO).

Tips and tricks

- Can remove gel/un-break table to facilitate closure.
- A nephron-stent is most easily sited using a large-bore cannula, passed through the abdominal wall into the renal pelvis, needle removed and stent fed back through cannula to exteriorize it.
- Laparoscopic repair now increasing in popularity.

Chapter 8

Vascular surgery

Carotid endarterectomy

The carotid bifurcation lies deep to the internal jugular vein and the sternocleidomastoid. The bifurcation can be higher in some patients than others, making the endarterectomy more challenging. Patients with a relatively short, broad neck often pose a challenge to the surgeon.

Indications

- TIAs (transient ischaemic attacks) or recent stroke with ^{3}70% stenosis of the internal carotid artery on the symptomatic side.
- Surgery should be carried out as soon as possible following index symptoms, ideally within 48h and certainly within 2 weeks.

Preoperative preparation

- Two different forms of imaging, ideally Duplex scan and MRA (magnetic resonance angiography), should be performed to confirm the degree of stenosis.
- It can be done under local or general anaesthesia.

Position

- Place the patient supine in a head-up position with the neck extended and rotated to the opposite side.
- Place a ring under the patient's head to stabilize it.
- Drape the patient from the angle of the jaw to the chin, so that the endo-tracheal tube is covered.

Procedure

- Make an incision anterior to the sternocleidomastoid muscle.
- Divide the platysma, and retract the internal jugular and sternocleidomastoid laterally to gain access to the carotid sheath.
- The anterior facial vein may need to be ligated and the omohyoid muscle retracted or divided.
- Carefully dissect the common, internal, and external carotid arteries. Be gentle, particularly around the bifurcation as the carotid body lies here and manipulation can lead to blood pressure instability or bradycardia.
- Identify the hypoglossal nerve crossing the carotid bifurcation and protect it
- The ansa cervicalis, which arises from the hypoglossal nerve, may need to be divided to gain better exposure.
- Administer heparin 5,000IU intravenously and apply vascular slings around the common carotid, external carotid, internal carotid, and the superior thyroid branch of the external carotid arteries (Fig. 8.1). Clamp each of these in sequence, starting with the internal carotid artery.
- Make an arteriotomy over the carotid artery bifurcation and extend it cephalad into the internal carotid using a Pott's scissors.
- Insert a Pruitt Inahara shunt with a larger blue balloon in the proximal common carotid artery and the distal white balloon in the internal carotid artery (Fig. 8.2). Alternative shunts like the Javid can be used, depending on the surgeon's preference.
- Once the shunt is in place extend the arteriotomy.

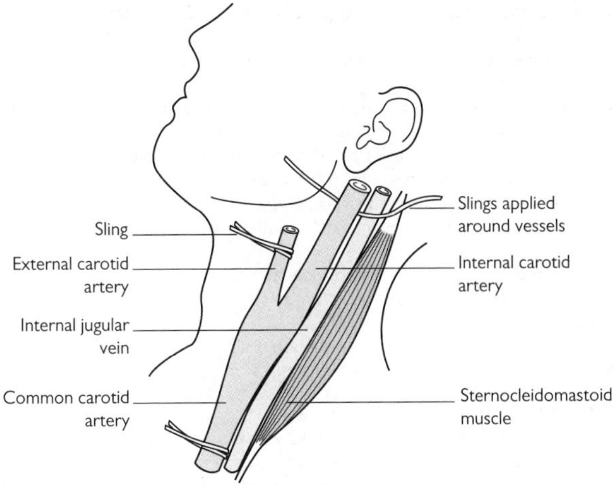
Sling
External carotid artery
Internal jugular vein
Common carotid artery
Slings applied around vessels
Internal carotid artery
Sternocleidomastoid muscle

Fig. 8.1 Exposure of the left carotid vessels. Image created by Vish Bhattacharya.

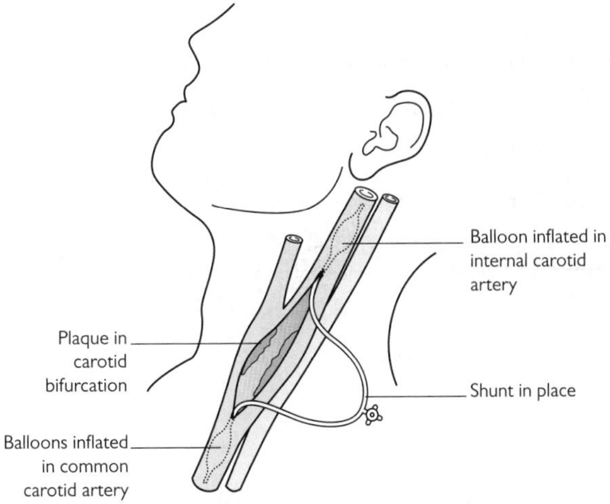
Balloon inflated in internal carotid artery
Plaque in carotid bifurcation
Shunt in place
Balloons inflated in common carotid artery

Fig. 8.2 Left carotid artery opened with shunt in situ. Image created by Vish Bhattacharya.

- Dissect the plaque using a Watson Cheyne dissector and then free and remove it.
- The distal intima in the internal carotid may need to be tacked down using 7-0 Prolene® sutures.
- Irrigate the endarterectomized vessel copiously with heparinized saline and remove any loose fragments of atheroma.
- Close the arteriotomy using 5-0 Prolene® or using a Dacron®, bovine pericardial, or vein patch using 6-0 Prolene® (Fig. 8.3).
- Once the patch closure is nearing completion, remove the shunt sequentially, first from the internal and then from the common carotid artery.
- Once the closure is complete remove the clamps sequentially with first the external carotid, then the common carotid, and finally the internal carotid clamps.
- Secure haemostasis and place a suction drain in the wound if necessary.
- Close the platysma and apply skin sutures or clips.

Postoperative care

- The patient is monitored in the HDU with close monitoring of neurological signs and blood pressure, pulse, and ECG.
- The patient should be commenced on clopidogrel the morning following surgery and continued on this indefinitely.

Complications

- Haematoma can occur, particularly if the patient coughs excessively when rousing from anaesthetic. It may be necessary to re-explore the wound urgently.
- Neuropraxia of the hypoglossal nerve can lead to temporary tongue deviation to the same side.
- Fatal or non-fatal stroke is extremely rare and is seldom seen.

Tips and tricks

- Mark the landmarks with a skin marker prior to making the skin incision.
- Doubly ligate the anterior facial vein as the ligature can come loose when the patient is waking up.
- Dissection of the carotid has to be done very gently as any rough handling can lead to distal embolization of debris.

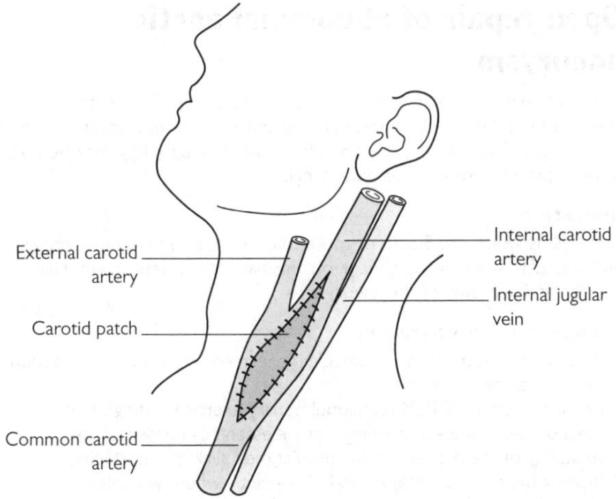
External carotid artery
Carotid patch
Common carotid artery
Internal carotid artery
Internal jugular vein

Fig. 8.3 Completed left carotid endarterectomy with patch closure. Image created by Vish Bhattacharya.

Open repair of abdominal aortic aneurysm

The abdominal aorta is a retroperitoneal structure. The extent of the aneurysm is established by preoperative imaging and may dictate the type of exposure. Most aneurysms are infra-renal, although they may be juxta-renal, suprarenal, or thoraco-abdominal.

Indications

Aneurysms which are 5.5cm or more may be treated with open repair or endovascular stenting dependant on the patient's fitness, co-morbidities, and age and anatomy of the aneurysm.

Preoperative preparation

- Patients should be seen in a vascular anaesthetic clinic and optimization of risk factors carried out.
- Investigations like CPEX (cardiopulmonary exercise testing), lung function tests, and echocardiogram are essential in order to assess suitability of the procedure and predict mortality and morbidity.
- Review the patient's imaging and plan exactly where you intend to clamp the vessels and where you intend to place your anastomoses. Patients with juxta-renal aneurysms will need suprarenal clamping.

Position

The patient should be supine with the abdomen and both groins shaved.

Theatre set-up

As a prosthetic graft is used, ideally the operation should be carried out in a theatre with laminar flow, and the number of people and traffic in the theatre should be minimized.

Procedure

- Perform a midline or transverse incision.
- Reflect the small intestine to the right and dissect the retroperitoneum.
- Dissect and reflect the transverse colon superiorly and place the small intestine in a bowel bag and either retract it laterally or place it outside the abdominal cavity.
- Use an Omni-tract or a similar retractor and dissect the neck of the aortic aneurysm.
- The inferior mesentery vein may need to be retracted laterally or ligated and divided.
- Use a renal vein retractor to retract the renal vein superiorly, but if the neck of the aneurysm is short, the left renal vein may also need to be ligated and divided.
- Then, dissect the iliac arteries.
- Give heparin 5,000IU intravenously and then clamp the aorta and iliac arteries (Fig. 8.4).
- Open the aneurysm and remove any thrombus. Extend the arteriotomy to the neck of the aneurysm and divided sideways for a short distance (Fig. 8.5).

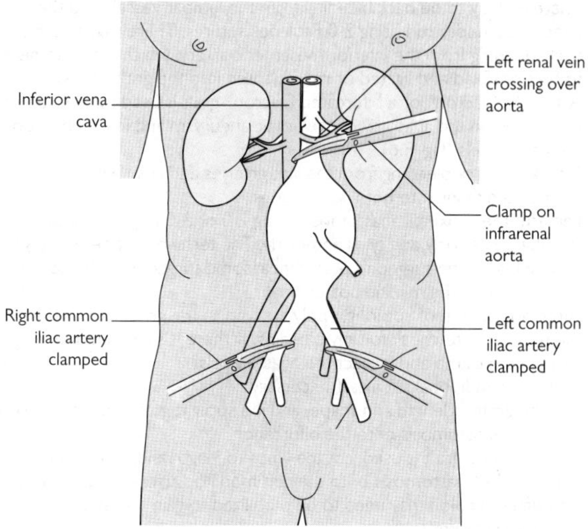
Inferior vena cava
Left renal vein crossing over aorta
Clamp on infrarenal aorta
Right common iliac artery clamped
Left common iliac artery clamped

Fig. 8.4 Infra-renal aortic aneurysm with clamps applied. Image created by Vish Bhattacharya.

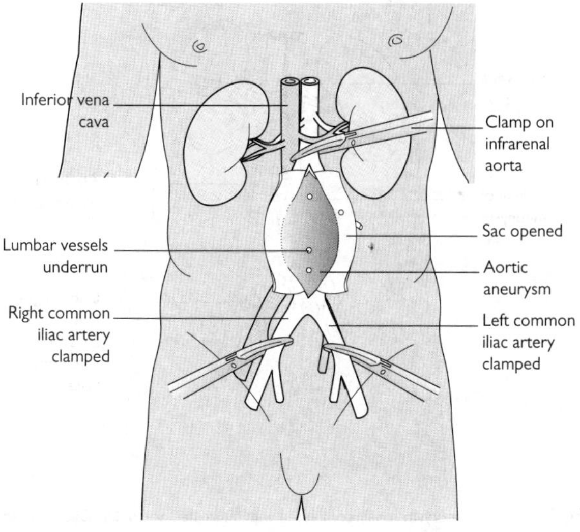
Inferior vena cava
Clamp on infrarenal aorta
Sac opened
Lumbar vessels underrun
Aortic aneurysm
Right common iliac artery clamped
Left common iliac artery clamped

Fig. 8.5 Infra-renal aortic aneurysm with sac opened. Image created by Vish Bhattacharya.

- There is likely to be back bleeding from the lumbar vessels and these need to be under run using 2-0 Prolene® sutures. There may also be back bleeding from the inferior mesenteric artery, which may also need to be transfixed and ligated or re-implanted into the graft later on.
- A straight Dacron® or a bifurcated Dacron® graft is used for the repair, depending on the anatomy of the aortic aneurysm and involvement of the iliac vessels (Fig. 8.6).
- Check for back bleeding from the iliac arteries and flush with heparinized saline into both iliac arteries.
- Perform the proximal anastomosis using 2-0 or 3-0 Prolene® sutures starting posteriorly and tying anteriorly. The technique varies slightly, depending on the surgeon's preference; some surgeons prefer to start on one side of the midline posteriorly.
- After completion of suturing, apply a clamp to the graft, and release the top clamp to check for any bleeding. If there is significant bleeding, reapply the clamp and inspect the anastomosis.
- Insert any additional sutures if necessary.
- Cut the graft to length and shape, and if a straight graft is used, perform the distal anastomosis onto the bifurcation.
- If a bifurcated graft is used, cut the limbs to length and shape, and perform the anastomosis onto the common iliac arteries sequentially. The sigmoid colon may need to be mobilized to gain access to the left external iliac artery.

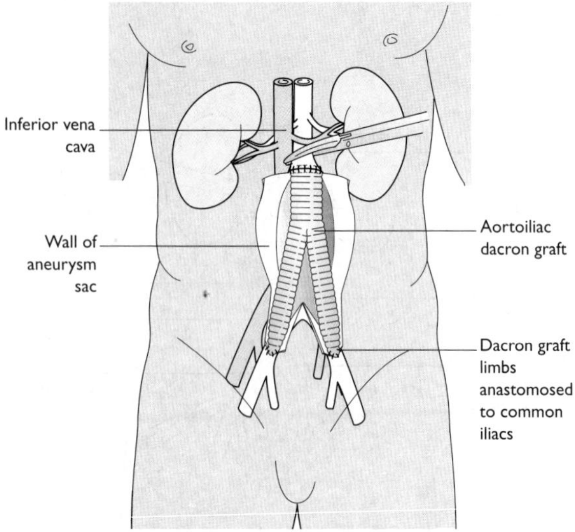
Inferior vena cava
Wall of aneurysm sac
Aortoiliac dacron graft
Dacron graft limbs anastomosed to common iliacs

Fig. 8.6 Aortic aneurysm repair completed with bifurcated aorto-iliac Dacron graft. Image created by Vish Bhattacharya.

- It may occasionally be necessary to tunnel the grafts and anastomose the limbs to the common femoral artery in the groins.
- Prior to completion of the distal anastomoses, establish forward and backward flow to flush out any clots within the graft.
- Release the clamps, one leg at a time, after liaising with the anaesthetist, as there may be a sudden drop in blood pressure following clamp release.
- Close the retroperitoneum with 2-0 Vicryl®. Close the abdomen with loop PDS® or Ethilon®.

Postoperative care

- Intensive care monitoring is required for at least 24–48h.
- Monitor renal function and circulation of the legs.

Complications

- Limb ischaemia can occur either due to graft occlusion or emboli dislodging from the aneurysm. A femoral embolectomy may be required.
- Renal function needs to be monitored closely and a period of temporary haemofiltration may be needed.
- Bowel ischaemia due to lack of blood supply from the inferior mesenteric or sigmoid vessels is a rare but well-recognized complication. This may necessitate a Hartmann's procedure.

Tips and tricks

- Leave the top of the clamp open but still in position after proximal anastomosis in case proximal control is required for any reason.
- Use buttress sutures with Dacron if anastomotic bleeding is difficult to control.
- Check perfusion of limbs on table at the end of the procedure, and perform femoral embolectomies if in any doubt.

Open repair of ruptured abdominal aortic aneurysm

The procedure for a ruptured abdominal aortic aneurysm is essentially the same as an elective procedure, albeit with some changes to the order, priorities, and urgency.

Indications

- Classical clinical features of a palpable mass, hypotension and sudden onset of back pain may be present.
- Often the patient is an arteriopath and has a known aortic aneurysm.
- In these cases a CT scan may not be necessary.
- However, when there is a clinical suspicion of a rupture and the patient is stable, a CT scan should be done urgently.
- A full blood count, serum electrolytes, and a blood cross-match should be done urgently.

Preoperative preparation

- Insert a large-bore cannula in the arms and give crystalloids cautiously.
- Allow permissive hypotension so that the patient remains mentally alert and has an acceptable blood pressure of around 70mmHg systolic.
- Insert a urinary catheter and get emergency help from the anaesthetists for analgesia, central line insertion, arterial line insertion, and possibly intubation.

Differences to elective repair

- Once the diagnosis has been made, contact the relevant staff and transfer the patient to theatre urgently.
- Once on the table, the patient should continue to receive high-flow oxygen whilst the theatre staff prepare for surgery.
- Shave the patient over the abdomen and groins whilst still awake and insert a urinary catheter.
- Paint the abdomen and groins with antiseptic solution and drape the abdomen while the patient is still awake.
- The patient should be anaesthetized only when you are ready to make the first incision.
- Assistant to retract the small intestine laterally, and rapidly dissect the neck of the aneurysm.
- Place the proximal clamp as quickly as possible after identifying the left renal vein and renal arteries.
- If the patient is in extremis, a supra-coeliac clamp can be placed temporarily to gain control.
- Dissect the iliac vessels and clamp them next in succession.
- Once control has been established, take some time to place your retractors adequately and gain good exposure.

Complications

- These are similar to that after an open elective repair, although the frequency of renal, respiratory, or cardiac failure is much higher.
- The risk of bowel ischaemia and limb thrombosis are also higher after repair of ruptured aneurysms.

Tips and tricks

- Close the abdomen using a temporary mesh in order to prevent compartment syndrome, if primary abdominal closure compromises respiratory or renal functions.
- Pack the abdomen and re-explore the following day in case there is persistent oozing and coagulopathy needs to be corrected.

Endovascular repair of abdominal aortic aneurysm

Indications

- Aneurysm size >5.5cm.
- For infra-renal aneurysm, stenting the proximal neck should be at least 1.5cm, the neck angulation less than 60°, and there should be no thrombus or calcification in the neck.
- The iliac vessels should be at least 6mm in diameter and lack extreme tortuosity or calcification. The neck diameter should be <2.5cm. Despite these relative contraindications, more challenging aneurysmal aortas can be stented in experienced hands.
- Juxta- or suprarenal aneurysms can be stented with customized branched or fenestrated grafts.
- Aneurysms that extend into the common iliac arteries may be stented using iliac branch devices.

Procedure

This description is for the Cook Medical Zenith® device, although other devices like the Gore® or AneuRx® devices are also available.

Preoperative preparation

- Meticulous preoperative planning of the stent using a CT scan on a workstation is essential.
- Patients should be seen in a vascular anaesthetic clinic and optimization of risk factors carried out.
- Investigations like CPEX, lung function tests, and echocardiogram are essential.

Surgery

- Transverse incisions are made in both groins and the common femoral arteries are exposed and vascular slings applied.
- A guide wire is inserted using a Seldinger technique under image intensification.
- 7F sheaths are inserted in both groins and an additional 5F catheter is inserted in the left common femoral artery for angiography.
- The main body of the graft is oriented to allow the contralateral limb of the main body to open in the correct position for subsequent catheterization.
- Conventionally, the main body is inserted through the right femoral artery (Fig. 8.7). The guide wires are replaced on the right side by a Lunderquist or Amplatzer stiff wire, which is placed in the thoracic aorta.
- The main body is then deployed over the Lunderquist wire until the 'gold markers' at the top end are noted to be below the renal arteries (Fig. 8.8). These markers appear as opaque dots on the screen and indicate the area between the bare proximal segment of the graft and the covered main body.
- The body of the graft is then deployed and the top two to three stent rings released. This is continued until the contralateral limb opens completely.

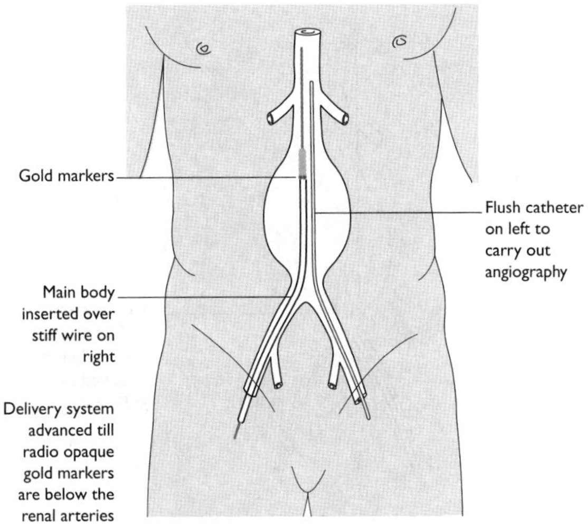
Gold markers
Flush catheter on left to carry out angiography
Main body inserted over stiff wire on right
Delivery system advanced till radio opaque gold markers are below the renal arteries

Fig. 8.7 Stenting of abdominal aortic aneurysm with main body inserted via right groin. Image created by Vish Bhattacharya.

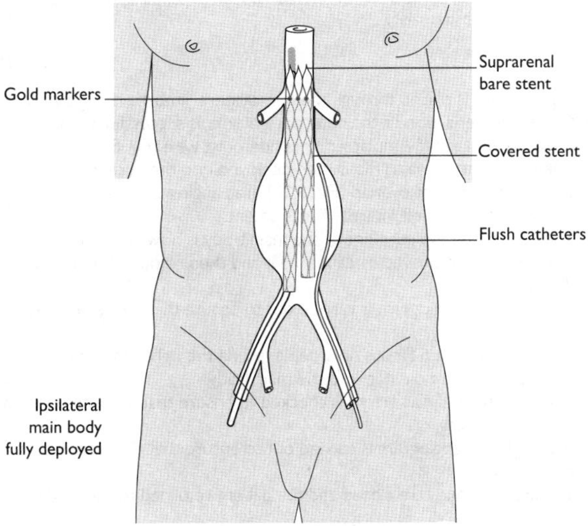
Suprarenal bare stent
Gold markers
Covered stent
Flush catheters
Ipsilateral main body fully deployed

Fig. 8.8 Stenting of aortic aneurysm with main body deployed. Image created by Vish Bhattacharya.

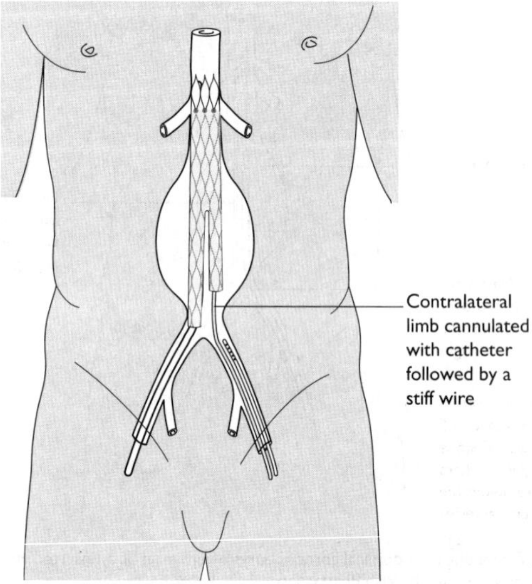
Contralateral
limb cannulated
with catheter
followed by a
stiff wire

Fig. 8.9 Stenting of aortic aneurysm with cannulation of contralateral limb. Image created by Vish Bhattacharya.

- A guide wire is placed through the contralateral limb via the left groin.
- Once catheterization of the contralateral limb is successful, the wire is replaced with a stiff Amplatzer or Lunderquist wire (Fig. 8.9).
- The contralateral main limb is then deployed into the body of the graft with a two-segment overlap (Fig. 8.10). Iliac angiography is carried out to ensure that the left internal iliac is patent.
- The bare metal top segment of the main body is now released and the nose cone retrieved by capturing it and then retracting it into the delivery sheath.
- A completion angiogram is carried out to ensure that the renal vessels are patent.
- The ipsilateral main limb is now deployed via the right groin, ensuring at least two segment overlap into the main body.
- The right internal iliac artery is checked to ensure that the limb does not cover its opening.
- A completion angiogram is carried out to ensure that there are no endoleaks.
- The arteriotomies are closed and the patient returned to the HDU.

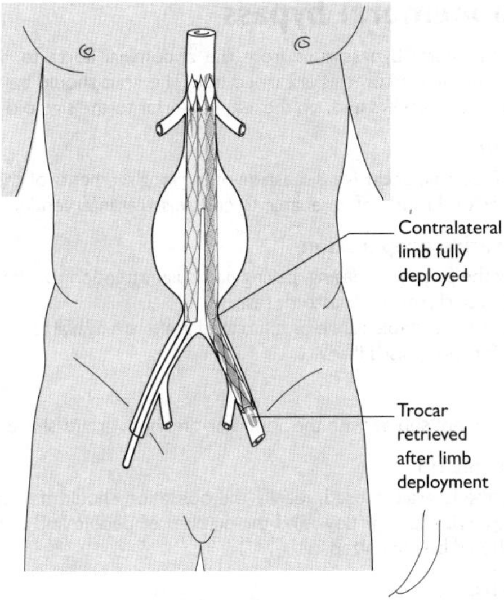
Contralateral limb fully deployed
Trocar retrieved after limb deployment

Fig. 8.10 Stenting of abdominal aortic aneurysm with contralateral limb deployment. Image created by Vish Bhattacharya.

Endoleaks

There are four types of endoleaks:

- Type 1 is when there is contrast seen to leak at the attachment sites. This needs to be treated before patient leaves theatre.
- Type 2 endoleaks are due to back bleeds from the lumbar vessels or inferior mesenteric artery and these can be monitored closely and treated only if the sac expands.
- Type 3 endoleaks are due to damage to the main fabric of the graft or junctions between the main body and limbs.
- Type 4 endoleaks are due to the porosity of the graft material.

The latter two types are very rare.

Aortobifemoral bypass

An aortobifemoral bypass runs from the abdominal aorta to the groin, where the distal anastomosis is carried out. The graft should be tunnelled posterior to the ureters and, on the left, posterior to the sigmoid colon.

Indications

Severe diffuse iliac occlusive disease involving long segments of the iliacs or distal aortic occlusion not amenable to endovascular intervention.

Preoperative preparation

- Review the patient's imaging, paying particular attention to where you intend to perform the anastomoses.
- Ensure that a suitable range of bifurcated grafts are available.
- Check for foot pulses if any.

Position

Place the patient supine with the abdomen and both groins shaved.

Theatre set-up

As a prosthetic graft is used, ideally the operation should be carried out in a theatre with laminar flow, and the number of people and traffic in the theatre should be minimized.

Procedure

Exposure

- Expose the femoral vessels prior to opening the abdomen to minimize intra-abdominal fluid loss and ensure the femoral vessels are suitable for the distal anastomosis.
- Make vertical incisions over both femoral arteries.
- Dissect the common femoral artery, superficial femoral artery, and profunda arteries carefully and then apply vascular slings to each. Dissect up to the inguinal ligament.
- You may need to divide the lower part of the inguinal ligament in order to gain exposure of the external iliac arteries proximally.

Proximal anastomosis

- Make a midline incision and reflect the small intestine to the patient's right.
- Consider opening the abdomen using a transverse incision This has the advantage of potentially reducing postoperative pain as the incision will traverse through fewer dermatomes.
- Open and dissect the retroperitoneum.
- Reflect the transverse colon superiorly and pack it away.
- Wrap the small intestine in a bowel bag and apply packs around the abdominal wound.
- Apply a self-retaining retractor like the Omni-tract.
- Retract the inferior mesenteric vein to the left or doubly ligate it and divide it if necessary.

- Dissect the aorta, avoiding dissection near the bifurcation in order to prevent damage to the pelvic parasympathetic nerves.
- Give 5,000IU of heparin intravenously and then clamp the aorta infra-renally.
- Clamp the distal aorta or the iliac vessels in order to gain distal control.
- Make an incision in the aorta and if necessary perform an endarterectomy at the site of the planned anastomosis. Clamp the inferior mesenteric artery if there is back bleeding.
- Trim the main body of an aortobifemoral Dacron® graft to size in order to prevent any angulation.
- An end–side anastamosis preserves existing pelvic circulation especially if there is extensive external iliac disease preventing retrograde flow into the pelvis.
- Perform the proximal anastamosis using 3-0 or 4-0 Prolene® sutures.
- Clamp the graft, release the iliac clamps, then slowly release the proximal aortic clamp to check for any bleeding. Apply extra sutures if required.
- Now tunnel the limbs using blunt forceps and blunt finger dissection. Perform the tunnelling behind the ureters on both sides.
- Retrieve the limbs of the graft into the femoral wounds.

Distal anastomosis

- Clamp the femoral vessels and perform an arteriotomy in the common femoral artery. Avoid heavily calcified plaques if possible.
- Carry out an endarterectomy if necessary.
- Divide the limbs of the graft to length and shape, and carry out the distal anastomoses using 5-0 Prolene®.
- Check forward flow from the graft and back bleeding from the superficial and profunda vessels prior to placing the final suture (Fig. 8.11).
- Carry out a similar procedure on the contralateral side.
- Release the clamps on the superficial artery and profunda, one leg at a time, after checking with the anaesthetist, as there may be a sudden drop in the blood pressure when the limbs are reperfused.
- Close the retroperitoneum using 2-0 Vicryl®.
- Replace the small intestine and remove the packs. Do a mass abdominal closure using loop PDS®.
- Close the groin with Vicryl® sutures and skin with clips or Monocryl®. You may wish to leave a drain.

Postoperative care

- The patient will require at least high-dependency care, most likely intensive care.
- Routine limb observations should be carried out, including checking Doppler signals distally.

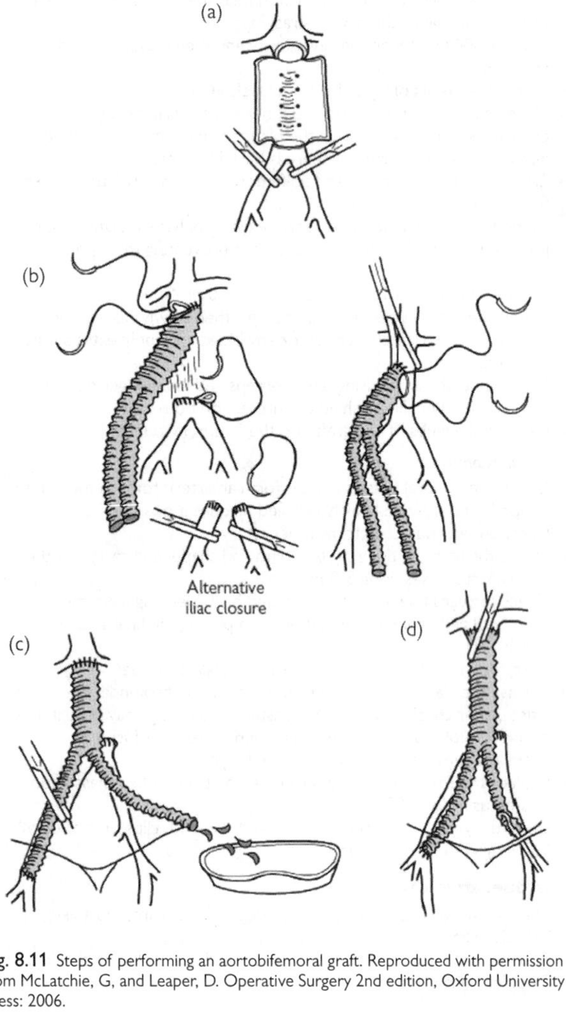
(a)
(b)
Alternative
iliac closure
(c)
(d)

Fig. 8.11 Steps of performing an aortobifemoral graft. Reproduced with permission from McLatchie, G, and Leaper, D. Operative Surgery 2nd edition, Oxford University Press: 2006.

Complications

Observe the patient for any signs of graft occlusion. If this should occur, urgent re-exploration improves the chances of successful revascularisation.

Tips and tricks

- You may only be able to fully retract the small intestine to the right once the retroperitoneum has been opened. You may need to re-adjust your exposure once this has been performed to avoid tractional injury.
- Ensure that the graft is lying in a suitable position with no sharp bends or kinks. Ensure that there is enough space under the inguinal ligament so that the graft is not compressed.
- If the origin of the superficial femoral artery (SFA) is heavily diseased, the distal arteriotomy can be extended down the profunda femoris to primarily perfuse this rather than the SFA.

Femoral popliteal above knee bypass graft

The femoral bifurcation can be easily accessed and dissected in the groin. The graft is then tunnelled under the sartorius muscle or subcutaneously to the popliteal fossa.

Indications

- Short distance intermittent claudication.
- Critical limb ischaemia causing rest pain.

Types of grafts

- Native, long saphenous vein, which may be reversed or in situ.
- Prosthetic grafts, which may be made of Dacron® or PTFE.

Preoperative preparation

- Review imaging and plan the point of proximal and distal anastomoses.
- Consent and mark the patient.
- If the patient has a suitable long saphenous vein, scan and mark this preoperatively or on the table.
- Ensure that a variety of graft sizes is available if the vein is unsuitable.

Position

Place patient supine with the knee rested on a sterile saline bag to allow slight flexion of the hip and knee joint.

Procedure

Exposure of the femoral artery

- Make a vertical incision over the femoral vessels.
- Dissect the common femoral, superficial, and profunda arteries, and apply vascular slings around them.
- Give 5,000IU of heparin and then clamp the vessels.
- Perform an arteriotomy and extend it for a couple of cm.
- Check that the inflow is adequate.
- Perform an endarterectomy of the common femoral artery if necessary.
- Check to see if there is good back flow from the profunda.

Exposure of the popliteal artery above the knee joint

- Make an incision longitudinally above the medial femoral condyle over the medial aspect of the leg.
- Deepen the incision in order to expose the adductor muscles anteriorly and the sartorius posteriorly.
- Incise the fascia and dissect the popliteal fossa.
- Identify the popliteal vessels in the roof of the fossa.
- Dissect the neurovascular bundle in order to separate the popliteal artery from the vein and nerve lying adjacent to it.
- The long saphenous vein may be used either reversed or in situ.
- Make an incision along the pre-marked long saphenous vein and then harvest the vein.
- Ligate and divide the branches of the long saphenous vein.

- Flush the vein with heparinized saline and keep it aside while the vessels are being prepared.
- Create a tunnel in the sub-sartorial space using a tunneller.
- Pass a Dacron® or PTFE graft through the tunneller.
- A subcutaneous tunnel is sufficient if the long saphenous vein is used for the bypass.
- Give 5,000IU of heparin intravenously and then clamp the common femoral, profunda, and superficial vessels.
- Make an arteriotomy over the common femoral artery using a 10 or 15 Bard Parker blade and extend the arteriotomy using Pott's scissors.
- Carry out an endarterectomy of the common femoral artery using a Watson Cheyne dissector.
- Cut the end of the graft in a lazy S-shape.
- Carry out the proximal anastamosis using 5-0 Prolene®.
- Commence the anastamosis in the heel of the graft and continue suturing in a continuous fashion over the side and toe of the anastomosis.
- Commence suturing the opposite side and tie the final knot on the side of the anastamosis and not at the heel or toe (Fig. 8.12).

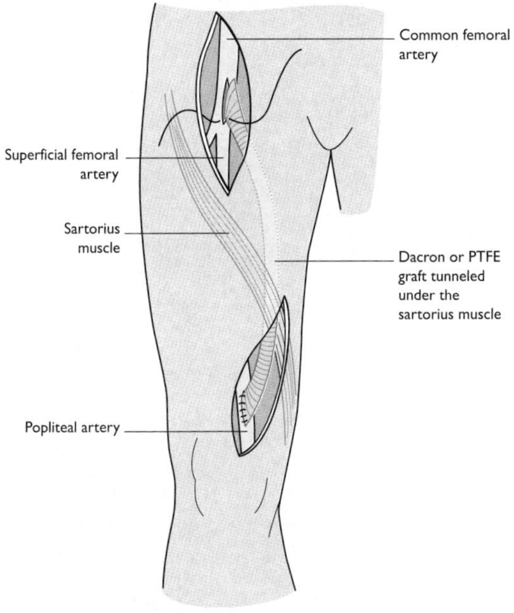
Common femoral artery
Superficial femoral artery
Sartorius muscle
Dacron or PTFE graft tunneled under the sartorius muscle
Popliteal artery

Fig. 8.12 Right femoropopliteal above knee prosthetic graft. Image created by Vish Bhattacharya.

Using in situ vein graft

- Insert a Le Maître valvulotome or a Hall's valvulotome if you are using an in situ vein graft, through the distal end of the graft.
- Withdraw the valvulotome with the blades open in order the divide the valves.
- Carry out the popliteal anastamosis using 5-0 or 6-0 Prolene® sutures.
- Remove the clamps and then secure haemostasis using extra sutures and Surgicel if needed.
- Close the subcutaneous tissue with Vicryl® and close the skin using skin clips or sutures.

Femoral popliteal below knee bypass graft

Femoral popliteal below knee bypass graft

Indications

Rest pain or critical ischaemia of the foot where the superficial artery has a long occlusion till the level of the knee.

Procedure

(See Fig. 8.13)
Femoral arteries are dissected as described on p. 392.

Popliteal dissection

- Make a 10cm incision from the knee joint distally.
- Divide the intramuscular fascia and enter the popliteal space between the soleus muscle anteriorly and the gastrocnemius muscle posteriorly.
- Identify the tendons of the semi-membranosus and the semi-tendinosus muscles and divide them if necessary to gain better exposure.
- The popliteal vein lies in front of the artery at this level.
- Dissect the popliteal vein away from the artery using careful blunt and sharp dissection.
- Clear the artery and apply silastic vascular slings.
- Place the vein graft in the subcutaneous tunnel and carry out the distal anastomosis using 6-0 Prolene®.

Complications

- Immediate complications like bleeding and graft thrombosis and delayed complications like graft occlusion and infection.
- Graft occlusion occurring within 30 days of a bypass is usually due to technical errors. Therefore make sure that inflow and outflow of the bypass are satisfactory and that there is no narrowing or twisting of the graft during the bypass.
- Perform a completion angiogram or Duplex scan at the end of the procedure.
- Serial Duplex scans at 3, 6, and 12 months should be requested to detect stenosis due to intimal hyperplasia, which occurs within the first 2 years. Early detection and treatment of these lesions or narrowing in the outflow or inflow vessels by angioplasty or surgery prevents graft occlusion.

Femoral to anterior tibial artery bypass

Lateral approach

- Make an incision 10cm long over the lateral part of the leg between the tibia and fibula running parallel to the tibia.
- Dissect the space between the tibialis anterior in front and the extensor digitorum muscle behind.
- The tibial artery and vein will be identified in the space between these muscles.
- The long saphenous vein graft is tunnelled subcutaneously and the distal anastomosis to the anterior tibial artery carried out using 6-0 Prolene®.

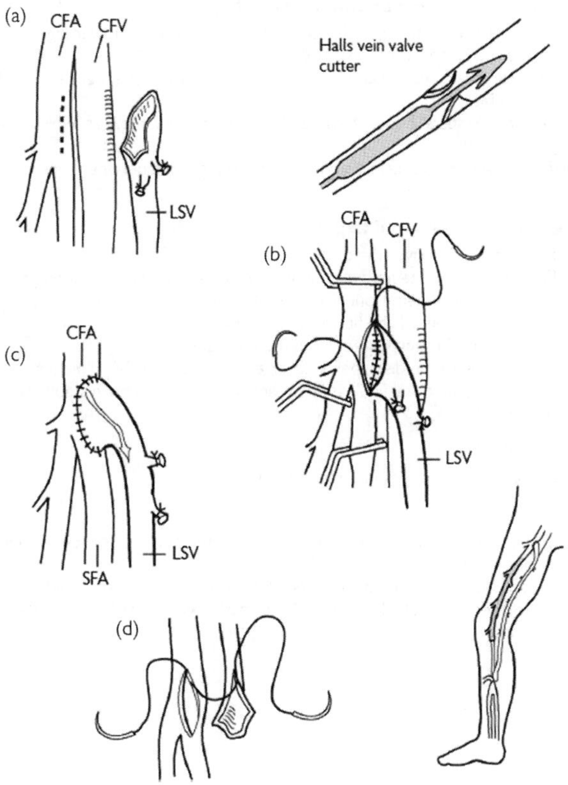
(a)
CFA
CFV
LSV
Halls vein valve cutter
CFA
CFV
(b)
LSV
CFA
(c)
LSV
SFA
(d)

Fig. 8.13 Steps of a femoropopliteal in situ vein bypass graft. Reproduced with permission from McLatchie, G, and Leaper, D. Operative Surgery 2nd edition, Oxford University Press: 2006.

Femoral to posterior tibial artery bypass

- Make a 10cm incision parallel to the tibia over the distal lower leg.
- Divide the fascia over the soleus muscles.
- Split the soleus muscle and identify the flexor digitorum longus attached to the tibia.
- Dissect the space between this and the flexor hallucis longus, which lies posteriorly.
- The posterior tibial artery and vein lie in the groove between these muscles.

Femoral to peroneal bypass

- Make an incision over the distal fibula.
- Elevate the periosteum over the fibula and clear muscles attached to avoid damaging the peroneal artery, which lies immediately below this.
- Resect a segment of the fibula using a Gigli saw or a power saw.
- Tunnel the vein subcutaneously in the thigh and lower leg and anastomose to the distal peroneal artery using 6-0 or 7-0 Prolene®.
- Ensure that the distal fibula is left intact in order to maintain stability of the ankle joint.

Complications

These are similar to the ones mentioned on p. 396.

Tips and tricks

- Distal bypasses below the knee are best performed with conduits using long saphenous vein.
- Prosthetic bypasses below the knee have poor results and should be performed using a Miller cuff or Taylor patch, which may improve the outcome.

Femoral embolectomy

An acutely ischaemic leg is a surgical emergency and rapid restoration of blood flow reduces the haemodynamic and renal consequences of reperfusion and therefore should be dealt with promptly.

Anatomy

- Emboli most commonly preferentially travel down the superficial femoral artery.
- The arteriotomy should be performed over the femoral bifurcation so the profunda femoris can also be cleared.

Indications

- Acute onset of signs and symptoms of an acutely ischaemic leg in the absence of a history suggestive of pre-existing peripheral vascular disease.
- The vast majority of acutely ischaemic legs due to embolic phenomena are of cardiac origin secondary to atrial fibrillation. Consider also the possibility of emboli from an undiagnosed abdominal aortic aneurysm (AAA) or an acutely thrombosed popliteal aneurysm.

Preoperative assessment

- If the history is highly indicative of an embolic cause for limb ischaemia without cause for concern that one may encounter long-standing arterial disease, it would be appropriate to transfer the patient to theatre for embolectomy without further imaging.
- If, however, one suspects that there could be pre-existing disease it would be wise to perform enhanced cross-sectional imaging to evaluate the cause for sudden ischaemia and assess whether more complex revascularization would be required.
- Time is of the essence and the patient should be operated on urgently if the patient starts developing motor or sensory symptoms.

Theatre set-up

Ensure a variety of sizes of Fogarty catheter are available, including multiples of the most commonly used sizes as balloon rupture is common.

Procedure

- Administer a bolus of heparin 5,000IU as soon as the diagnosis is made.
- Place the patient supine and prepare the abdomen in order to allow access to the aorta and iliac vessels if necessary.
- Make an incision over the common femoral artery, which is located midway between the anterior superior iliac spine and pubic symphysis.
- Dissect the common femoral (CFA), SFA, and profunda arteries and pass vascular slings around all three to achieve control.
- Place De Bakey clamps on the CFA, profunda femoris artery (PFA), and SFA, and make a longitudinal arteriotomy just proximal to femoral bifurcation.
- Release the proximal clamp momentarily to verify adequacy of inflow and then release the distal clamps individually to check for back bleeding.

- Pass a Fogarty balloon catheter proximally into the iliac vessels in case the inflow is inadequate and there are clots in the iliac vessels that need to be cleared.
- Pass a Fogarty catheter appropriate to the calibre of the vessel selectively down the SFA and PFA.
- The catheter is inserted gently into the lumen of the vessels.
- Inflate the balloon and then trawl the catheter up the artery extracting any blood clots (Fig. 8.14).
- Repeat this until no further clots are retrieved, being mindful of intimal trauma inflicted with each pass.

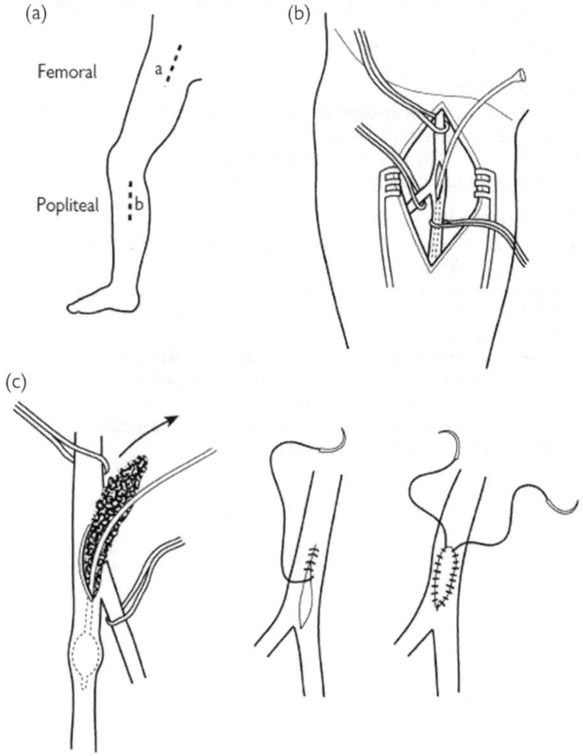
(a)
Femoral
a
Popliteal
b
(b)
(c)

Fig. 8.14 Steps of performing a femoral embolectomy. Reproduced with permission from McLatchie, G, and Leaper, D. Operative Surgery 2nd edition, Oxford University Press: 2006.

- Carry out a completion on table angiography to ensure adequate patency of the vessels.
- Flush the branches of the SFA and profunda with heparinized saline.
- Close the arteriotomy with interrupted 5-0 Prolene® taking each bite from inside the artery to ensure that no intimal flaps are raised. If the vessel has a risk of becoming narrowed, use a vein or pericardial patch.
- Release the proximal and then distal clamps.
- Place a drain if there are any concerns over possibility of haematoma formation.
- Close the groin wound with Vicryl® followed by interrupted or subcuticular skin closure.

Postoperative care

- Continue heparin infusion for 24–48h until adequate anticoagulation is established.
- Check limb perfusion and Doppler signals in the foot.

Complications

- Inability to successfully clear an embolus or developing 'trash' emboli can lead to a threatened limb.
- The patient will be fully anticoagulated so observe the groin for signs of haematoma formation.

Tips and tricks

- Place the Fogarty catheter alongside the leg to give you an idea of how far you are inserting the catheter.
- Remember that the size of the Fogarty catheter becomes larger as its number increases, unlike a vascular suture where the higher the number, the smaller the needle.
- Insert the Fogarty catheter for about 10cm and withdraw and remove the clots, and then gradually increase the length of insertion, instead of trying to insert it all the way at one go.
- Do not attempt an excessive number of runs with the catheter as you risk causing unnecessary intimal damage.

Brachial embolectomy

- Acutely ischaemic upper limbs are far less common than lower limbs. However, much like in the lower limb, an acutely ischaemic arm is a surgical emergency.
- The brachial artery bifurcation lies deep to the bicipital aponeurosis.
- The brachial artery usually has accompanying deep veins, with communicating branches that may need to be divided.
- The brachial bifurcation is usually at the level of the intersection of the brachioradialis and pronator teres muscles.

Indications

- Acute onset of signs and symptoms of an acutely ischaemic arm in the absence of a history suggestive of pre-existing peripheral vascular disease.
- The causative factor is almost exclusively cardiac in origin with the vast majority of patients in atrial fibrillation and sub-optimally anticoagulated.
- In the very elderly, collateralization is sometimes sufficient to render an arm viable, even in the presence of an embolus. It is therefore occasionally appropriate to manage such patients conservatively if the operative risks are prohibitively high.

Position and theatre set-up

- Place the patient supine with the affected arm placed on an arm-board.
- Ensure a variety of sizes of Fogarty catheter are available, including a couple of the most commonly used sizes as balloon rupture is common.

Procedure

- Administer a bolus of heparin 5,000IU intravenously as soon as the diagnosis is made.
- Prepare the skin circumferentially from neck down, including the hand, allowing for access to subclavian artery in case of uncontrolled bleeding and need for proximal control.
- Make an 8–10cm 'lazy-S' incision from the medial aspect of biceps muscle, curving laterally over the antecubital fossa and proceeding distally in the groove between brachioradialis and the flexor musculature.
- Dissect the brachial artery and its bifurcation into radial and ulnar arteries and pass slings around all three for control.
- The bicipital aponeurosis may be partially or completely divided for access.
- Place clamps on brachial, radial, and ulnar arteries, and perform a transverse arteriotomy just proximal to the bifurcation. A longitudinal arteriotomy may be made and closed with a vein patch later if necessary.
- Release the proximal clamp is to verify adequacy of inflow.
- Release the distal clamps individually to check for back bleeding. If inflow is poor, pass a Fogarty catheter appropriate to the calibre of the artery (usually size 4 or 5) proximally, inflate the balloon, and trawl the catheter down the artery.
- Pass a Fogarty catheter appropriate to the calibre of the vessel (usually size 3 or 4) selectively down radial and ulnar arteries.
- Pass the catheter as far as it goes without force, inflate the balloon, and trawl the catheter up the artery extracting any blood clots present.

- Repeat this until no further clots are retrieved, being mindful of intimal trauma inflicted with each pass.
- Verify that inflow remains unchanged and then flush each artery with heparinized saline.
- Close the arteriotomy with interrupted 5-0 Prolene®, taking each bite from inside the artery to ensure that no intimal flaps are raised. Use a vein patch if there is any risk of narrowing of the artery (Fig. 8.15).

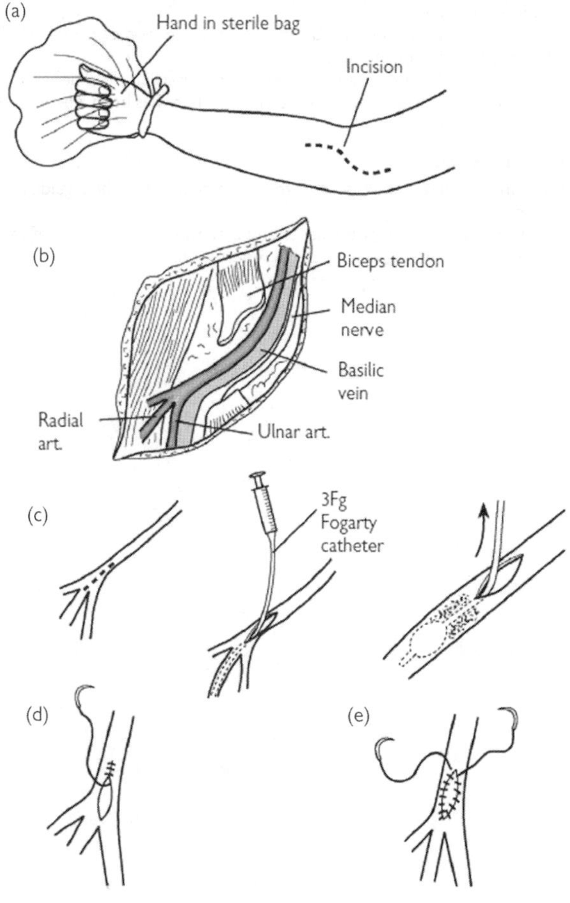
(a)
Hand in sterile bag
Incision
(b)
Biceps tendon
Median nerve
Basilic vein
Radial art.
Ulnar art.
(c)
3Fg Fogarty catheter
(d)
(e)

Fig. 8.15 Steps of performing a brachial embolectomy. Reproduced with permission from McLatchie, G, and Leaper, D. Operative Surgery 2nd edition, Oxford University Press: 2006s.

- Release the clamps sequentially.
- The distal flow is checked with intraoperative Doppler or confirmation of palpable pulses.
- Consider placing a drain if there is any concern over possibility of haematoma formation. Close the subcutaneous layer with Vicryl® followed by interrupted or subcuticular skin closure.

Postoperative care

- Commence the patient on intravenous heparin provided there are no contraindications.
- Commence the patient on Warfarin, ensuring a period of overlap till the INR reaches therapeutic range.
- Request an echocardiogram to rule out structural abnormalities and mural thrombi. Seek a cardiology opinion if there has been a new onset of atrial fibrillation.

Tips and tricks

- You may need to bend the tip of the catheter slightly to help guide it down the ulnar artery.
- Perform a fasciotomy of the flexor and extensor compartments of the forearm if there has been a delay in reperfusion.

Lower limb fasciotomy

Anatomy

- The lower limb is separated into four compartments each with distinct neurovascular supply.
- The four compartments are:
  - Anterior compartment.
  - Lateral compartment.
  - Deep posterior compartment.
  - Superficial posterior compartment.
- The four compartments are separated from each other by the interosseous membrane of the leg, the anterior intermuscular septum, and the posterior intermuscular septum.

Indications

- To prevent compartment syndrome or to treat this if it has already occurred after peripheral revascularization in an ischaemic limb or after trauma to the leg.
- Compartment syndrome occurs when there is build-up of interstitial pressure within a muscle compartment, which is confined within a fascial compartment and bone.
- Typically the diagnosis is clinical and includes pain out of proportion to clinical findings, pain on passive stretching, and pain on palpation of the compartment.
- The peripheral pulses may be present.

Position

Place the patient supine with a saline bag support under the knee joint.

Procedure

- Make two longitudinal incisions over the anterolateral and posteromedial aspect of the leg (Fig. 8.16).
- The anterolateral incision should start midway between the tibial tuberosity and the fibula, and extended to the lateral malleolus.
- Make an incision over the skin and subcutaneous tissue and expose the fascia covering the anterior and lateral compartments.
- You will notice the intermuscular septum in between.
- Release the anterior compartment by making an incision over the anterior muscle fascia and extend this with scissors to the ankle.
- Release the lateral compartment by incising the fascia parallel to the fibula, taking care not to injure the superficial peroneal nerve.
- For the posteromedial compartment, make an incision 2cm behind the posteromedial border of the tibia.
- Release the superficial medial compartment by making an incision over the fascia covering the gastrocnemius and soleus muscles.
- Release the deep medial compartment by incising the fascia over the flexor digitorum longus.
- Avoid damage to the posterior tibial artery and vein lying in this compartment between the flexor digitorum longus and flexor hallucis longus.

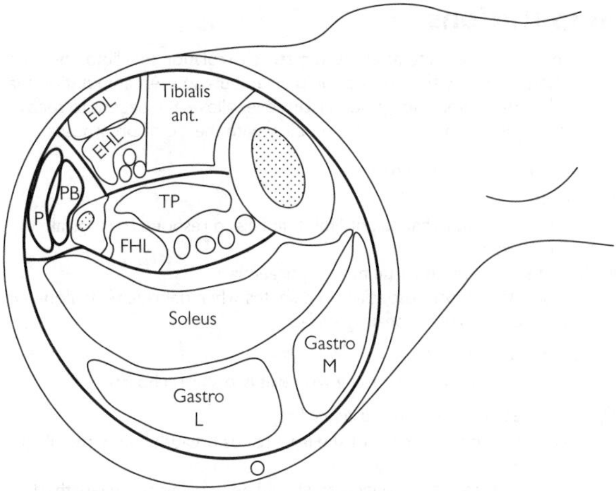
Tibialis
ant.
EDL
EHL
PB
P
TP
FHL
Soleus
Gastro
M
Gastro
L

Fig. 8.16 Compartments in the lower leg for fasciotomy. Reproduced from Hands, L., Murphy, M., et al. Vascular Surgery, 2007, with permission from Oxford University Press.

Postoperative care

- Leave the wounds open and cover with Kaltostat or Mepitel dressings.
- They can be closed at a second stage once the leg swelling has subsided using primary sutures or skin grafts.
- A semi-closed fasciotomy may be carried out through small skin incisions but with complete division of the fascial covering, by sliding a pair of scissors along the fascial planes. This avoids the need for extensive skin closure at a later date.

Complications

- Avoid injury to the saphenous vein and nerve while performing the medial compartment fasciotomy.
- Avoid injury to the superficial peroneal nerve while extending the anterior or lateral fascial compartment proximally.
- Avoid incomplete fasciotomy by ensuring that the incisions are generous.

Amputations

Despite various means to attempt to restore circulation to a limb, there are circumstances where the only option is an amputation. An amputation that yields a healthy stump with good muscle cover allows the patient to recover quicker and, if appropriate, regain mobility with the aid of prostheses.

Below knee amputation

Indications

- Chronic or acute ischaemia of limb that fails to respond to surgical revascularization.
- Gross tissue necrosis resulting in septicaemia.
- Extensive foot sepsis, especially in diabetes when debridement alone will result in loss of weight-bearing surface.

Preoperative assessment

The most distal site where healing will reliably occur is chosen.

Operative steps (Burgess long posterior flap)

- Measure the circumference of the leg a hands breadth below the tibial tuberosity.
- The length of the anterior incision should be two-thirds the length of the circumference at this level.
- The length of the posterior flap should be one-third of this circumferential length.
- Divide the fibula 2cm proximal to the tibial division.
- Divide the tibia 12cm below the tibial tuberosity.
- The tibia should be bevelled at an angle of about 45° halfway through the bone.
- After this the bone should be divided transversely to make the end of the stump more rounded.
- The division of the bone should be at least 1cm above the skin incision.
- Ligate the posterior tibial and peroneal vessels and nerves.
- Fashion a myocutaneous flap and bring it forward to stitch it to the anterior tibial fascia using Vicryl® (Fig. 8.17).
- Close the skin with interrupted Ethilon® or skin clips.

Skew flap technique

- Draw a circumferential line, a hands breadth below the tibial tuberosity.
- Mark the anterior point of the flap 2cm lateral to the tibial crest.
- The posterior end of the flap should be at a point that is diametrically opposite this point in the back of the leg.
- Draw equal semicircular flaps over the anteromedial and posterolateral aspects of the calf.
- Incise the skin and subcutaneous tissue and divide the muscles of the anterior and peroneal compartment.
- Raise the periosteum using periosteal elevators.
- Ligate the anterior tibial vessels.
- Divide the peroneal nerve as high as possible to avoid formation of a neuroma.
- Now divide the tibialis posterior muscles and ligate and divide the posterior tibial vessels.

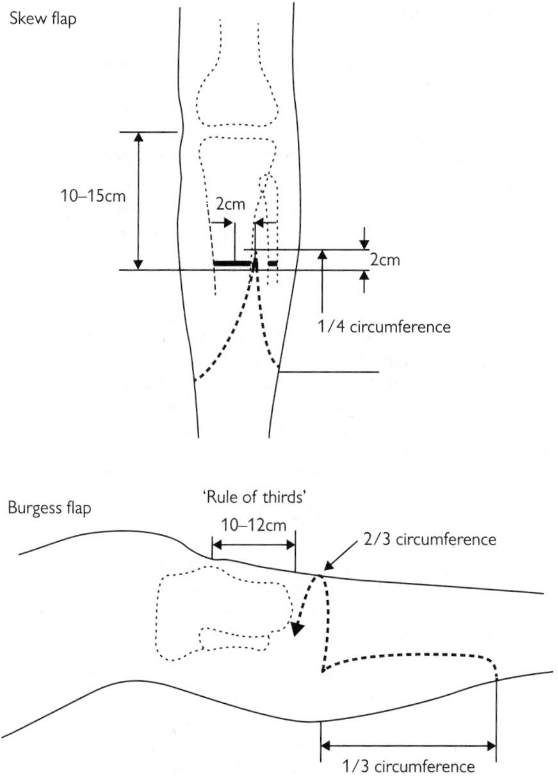
Skew flap
10–15cm
2cm
2cm
1/4 circumference
Burgess flap
'Rule of thirds'
10–12cm
2/3 circumference
1/3 circumference

Fig. 8.17 Steps of performing a Skew flap and Burgess flap. Reproduced from McLatchie, G. and Leaper, D., Operative Surgery 2nd edition, 2006, with permission from Oxford University Press.

- Divide the posterior tibial nerve high up.
- Divide the fibula 2cms proximally and then divide the tibia at a 45-degree angle.
- Fashion a myocutaneous closure by bringing the muscles over the anteromedial aspect of the incision.

Postoperative care

Start physiotherapy as soon as possible after the surgery to allow for knee extension. This will prevent a knee-flexion deformity, which can interfere with wearing a leg prosthesis.

Above knee amputation

Indications

- Unsalvageable limb due to non-reconstructable peripheral vascular disease or extensive trauma.
- Life-saving where ischaemic leg is causing sepsis but patient is not fit for major revascularization.
- Failed below knee amputation where the stump has broken down.

Anaesthesia

This is most commonly performed under general anaesthesia, but can be performed under spinal anaesthesia and sedation if patient fitness precludes a general anaesthetic.

Procedure

- Mark the level of amputation and skin flaps preoperatively on table.
- Make 'fish-mouth 'shaped flaps, conventionally with anterior flap slightly longer than posterior flap. The distal edge of the anterior flap should be three to four fingerbreadths proximal to superior border of patella. The level of bone transection should be 5–7cm proximal to the flap edges.
- A tourniquet may be used, depending on indication for amputation and expected blood loss.
- Transect the anterior thigh muscles sharply in line with anterior flap skin edge.
- Transect the femur early in order to provide easy access to the neurovascular bundle.
- Use a periosteal elevator prior to transection with either a hand or an electric saw. The SFA and associated bundle lies posterior to the vastus medialis and profunda femoris immediately posterior to the transected femur. Dissect out the respective arteries and veins, and ligate individually.
- Identify the sciatic nerve and apply gentle traction distally. A sciatic nerve block with or without an infusion catheter can be performed at this stage prior to transecting the nerve as proximally as possible.
- The sciatic nerve should be ligated as high as possible to avoid a neuroma formation. There is a large artery supplying the sciatic nerve and this should be ligated along with the nerve.
- Approximate the flaps without tension ensuring adequate coverage of transected femur.
- Approximate the anterior and posterior deep fascia using Vicryl®.
- Place a drain deep to musculature.
- Close the skin with interrupted or subcuticular sutures.

Postoperative care

- Ensure good analgesia with the help of nerve blocks.
- Start early physiotherapy and mobilization.

Complications

- Phantom limb pain is very common and can be quite resistant to treatment. Simple opiates or gabapentin and amitriptyline may help ameliorate some of the symptoms.
- Non-healing of stump may lead to revision to a more proximal level.
- Stump haematoma or superficial wound collections can be treated by removing some of the skin clips or sutures and draining the collection.
- Avoid hip or knee flexion contracture by starting physiotherapy early.
- Revision to a more proximal level may be necessary in case of non-healing.

Surgery for varicose veins

High tie and stripping of long saphenous vein

Indications

- Prevention of leg ulceration, thrombophlebitis, lipodermatosclerosis, and varicose eczema.
- Relief of symptoms like swelling, itching, and aching.
- Current NICE guidelines suggest that open surgery should be considered only if endothermal ablation or foam sclerotherapy is not indicated.

Preoperative preparations

- All patients with varicose veins should have a Duplex scan first. This will delineate whether the veins are in the long or short saphenous areas and whether there is any perforator incompetence.
- This is also useful to check whether there is any deep venous incompetence or scarring of deep veins from previous DVT.
- Duplex also help to inform whether the veins are suitable for radiofrequency ablation.
- The veins are marked on the day of surgery with the patient standing up, using a skin marker.
- In case of saphenopopliteal incompetence, the saphenopopliteal junction has to be marked on the day of surgery in the vascular laboratory under ultrasound guidance.

Position and theatre set-up

- For high tie and stripping, place the patient supine in a Trendelenberg position.
- Paint the groin and the entire leg using an antiseptic solution and drape the patient with the groin exposed.
- For saphenopopliteal ligation, the patient will need to be placed in a prone position with the back of the knee and the lower leg exposed.

Procedure

- Make a transverse incision in the groin just medial to the femoral pulse.
- Identify the saphenofemoral junction and the tributaries.
- Ligate and divide the tributaries at the junction, typically the superficial and deep pudendal veins, anterolateral thigh vein, superficial epigastric vein, and the superficial circumflex iliac vein (Fig. 8.18).
- Clearly identify the femoral vein and the junction with the long saphenous vein.
- Ligate and divide the saphenofemoral junction and disconnect the long saphenous vein completely.
- Strip the long saphenous vein using an inversion stripper, an olive head stripper, or a PIN (perforate invaginate) stripper.
- Insert the inversion stripper, which is a firm plastic tube, into the open end of the long saphenous vein and thread it down the vein till the level of the lower thigh or upper calf.
- Feel for the tip of the stripper over the skin and make an incision over it.
- Retrieve the tip of the stripper using artery forceps.

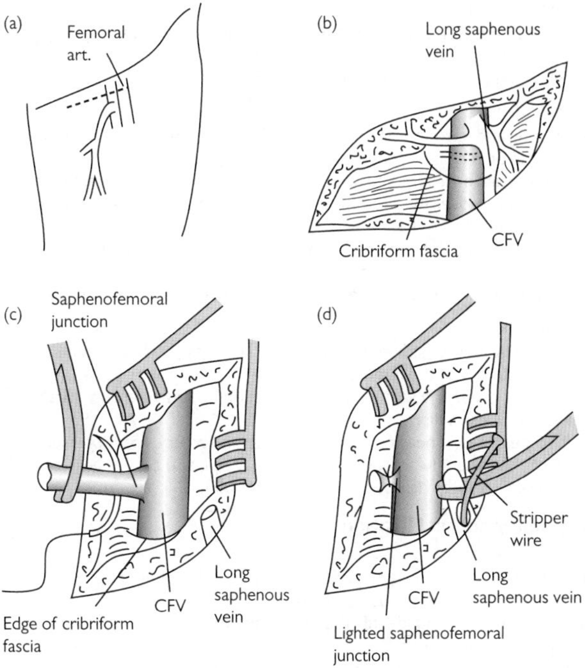
(a)
Femoral art.
(b)
Long saphenous vein
Cribriform fascia
CFV
(c)
Saphenofemoral junction
Edge of cribriform fascia
CFV
Long saphenous vein
(d)
Stripper wire
CFV
Long saphenous vein
Lighted saphenofemoral junction

Fig. 8.18 Steps of performing a saphenofemoral ligation for varicose veins. Reproduced from McLatchie, G. and Leaper, D., Operative Surgery 2nd edition, 2006, with permission from Oxford University Press.

- Ligate the other end of the stripper to the proximal end of the vein using a long silk suture or attach the small plastic olive that comes with the kit.
- Strip the vein out from the thigh or calf incision you had made.
- As the stripper is pulled down the leg, the branches in the thigh will be torn and you should therefore apply firm pressure over the medial aspect of the thigh when the vein is stripped, in order to prevent a haematoma.
- Remove the superficial varies using a hook phlebectomy instrument.
- Close the groin with with Vicryl® for the subcutaneous layer and use subcuticular sutures for the skin. The stab incisions can be closed with steristrips.
- Apply rolled up surgipads over the tract of the stripped vein and areas of avulsions and apply firm crepe bandages from the ankle to the groin.

Postoperative care

- Remove the crepe bandages after 24h and ask the patient to wear TED stockings for a week.
- Allow the patient to mobilize as soon as possible.

Complications

- Bruising and haematoma formation are well-recognized complications and can be managed conservatively in most cases.
- Groin infection is rare and can be treated with antibiotics or drainage.
- Paraesthesia over the site of the stripped vein or avulsions is common and most of this will settle with time.
- Damage to the deep femoral vein is a dreaded but extremely rare complication of this surgery.
- Recurrent veins have been reported in up to 40% of patients at 5 years.

Tips and tricks

- Do not ligate the saphenofemoral junction unless you have clearly seen the junction with the femoral vein.
- You may divide the saphenofemoral junction doubly to ensure that the ligature doesn't slip.
- If you encounter heavy bleeding during groin surgery, apply pressure, place the patient head down (if not already so), and ask for help instead of trying to apply clamps or artery forceps blindly.

Saphenopopliteal ligation

Procedure

- Make a transverse incision just below the site of saphenopopliteal junction marked previously by Duplex.
- Incise the fascia and identify the saphenous vein and follow it to the saphenopopliteal junction.
- Dissect this carefully avoiding damage to the sural nerve, which lies in close proximity.
- The common peroneal nerve lies laterally and you should avoid excessive retraction or inadvertent dissection of this nerve as it can lead to the alarming complication of a foot drop.
- Ligate the junction and divide it completely.

Postoperative care

- Apply a compression bandage for 24h.
- Remove this the following day and advise the patient to wear Grade 2 TED stockings for a week.

Complications

- Postoperative morbidities include bruising and haematoma, which usually settle with conservative management.
- Damage to the cutaneous nerves, especially the sural nerve, can cause numbness in the back of the calf or lateral aspect of the foot.
- Recurrence is reportedly 20–28% at 5 years.

Tips and tricks

Avoid excessive lateral retraction during short saphenous surgery as this can lead to common peroneal nerve damage and temporary foot drop.

Radiofrequency ablation of varicose veins (RFA)

Indications

Position

Procedure

Radio-frequency ablation of varicose veins (RFA)

Indications

- This is undertaken for patients with superficial venous insufficiency and symptoms of aching, swelling, or itching of legs with signs of varicose eczema, lipodermatosclerosis, or non-healing venous leg ulcers.
- NICE guidelines now state that radio-frequency or laser ablation should be the first line of treatment for incompetent suitable long saphenous veins.

Preoperative preparations

- All patients should have a Duplex scan in order to identify the anatomy and check for suitability for RFA.
- Relative contraindications for RFA include previous thrombophlebitis or vein diameter greater than 15mm or extreme venous tortuosity.

Position

- For RFA of the long saphenous vein, place the patient supine in an anti-Trendelenberg position to allow for easy cannulation of the vein.
- Once the vein has been cannulated and a catheter placed in the long saphenous vein, place the patient in a Trendelenberg position in order for the vein to collapse.
- This will also prevent inadvertent injection of tumescent fluid inside the lumen of the vein.

Procedure

- The procedure is done under local or general anaesthesia.
- Place the patient in an anti-Trendelenberg position and map the incompetent long saphenous vein using a Duplex scan.
- Inject a local anaesthetic at the site of the proposed catheter insertion, usually in the upper calf.
- Under US guidance puncture the long saphenous vein and insert the guide wire within the vein.
- Pass a 7F introducer sheath over the guide wire using Seldinger technique.
- Now insert the radio-frequency catheter over the guide wire through the sheath and advance the tip under US guidance to a point 2cm distal to the saphenofemoral junction.
- This is done in order to prevent inadvertent damage to the deep veins when the catheter is heated.
- Place the patient in a Trendelenberg position to collapse the vein and inject tumescent local anaesthetic (usually 0.1% Lidocaine with sodium bicarbonate) into the tissue surrounding the long saphenous vein within its fascia.
- Inject this along the entire course of the vein from the saphenofemoral junction down to the point of entry of the catheter.

- This is useful for analgesia and also creates a heat sump that prevents damage to the adjacent nerves and tissues. It also helps compress the vein to allow adequate heat transmission to the wall.
- Ensure that the injection of tumescent fluid pushes the vein at least 1cm away from the skin to avoid any skin burns.
- Once enough tumescent fluid is injected around the catheter tip, a probe at the tip shows a drop in temperature.
- A temperature drop below 30° is reassuring as this ensures that the tip has not been inadvertently inserted into the deep vein.
- Switch the radio-frequency catheter on and treat first segment of vein.
- In the ClosureFast® device the instrument shows the probe temperature rising to 120°C. This is sustained for 20s after which the safety system has an automatic cutoff mechanism that prevents overheating of the vein.
- The top end is treated twice to ensure complete closure.
- Withdraw the catheter sequentially until the long saphenous vein is treated along its entire length (Fig. 8.19).
- The remaining varicosities in the calf are treated at the same time with foam sclerotherapy or multiple phlebectomies.
- Some surgeons prefer to treat these 6 weeks later by which time some of these veins would have collapsed and there is less need for phlebectomies.

Postoperative care

- A compression stocking is applied to the treated leg, which can be applied for 48h to 1 week, depending on the practice of the surgeon.
- Recovery is very quick and most patients are able to resume normal activities in a couple of days.

Complications

- A phlebitis reaction can occur along the vein treated by RFA. This can be treated with anti-inflammatory medication.
- Sensory changes along the course of the vein are usually transient.
- A tugging sensation along the course of the treated vein can be felt for several weeks following this procedure. This usually settles with time.
- Successful closure of the saphenous vein is seen in about 90% of cases at 1 year.
- DVT is extremely rare and is due to extension of the thrombus from the treated vein into the deep vein. Start anticoagulation therapy if this occurs. A small extension usually settles down spontaneously and a repeat US scan should be done in a week. Continue anticoagulation if the deep vein thrombus persists.

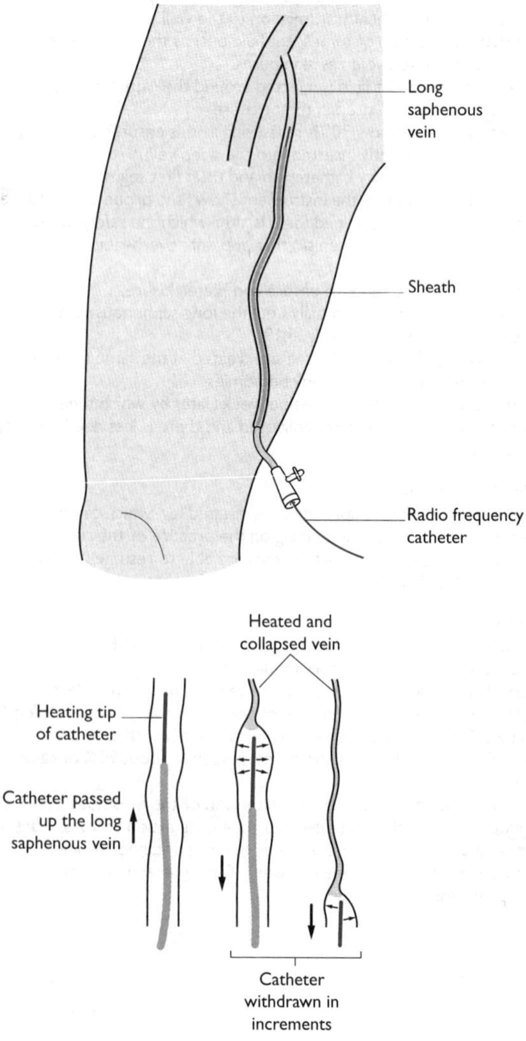
Long saphenous vein
Sheath
Radio frequency catheter
Heated and collapsed vein
Heating tip of catheter
Catheter passed up the long saphenous vein
Catheter withdrawn in increments

Fig. 8.19 Radiofrequency ablation of right long saphenous vein. Image created by Vish Bhattacharya.

Foam sclerotherapy

Indications

In addition to the indications on p. 418, foam sclerotherapy can be used for treatment of telangiectasias and reticular veins

Preoperative preparations

- All patients should have a Duplex scan, as mentioned on p. 418.
- It is done under local anaesthesia and so is suitable for patients who are otherwise unfit for general anaesthesia.
- The foam is made using a Tessari technique. In this method sodium tetradecyl sulphate is mixed with air in a 1:4 ratio using two syringes and a three-way tap.
- The foam has to be prepared immediately prior to injection to avoid it from dispersing.

Procedure

- Cannulate the long saphenous vein under US guidance and place Venflons along the course of the vein.
- Place a butterfly needle in the smaller branches of the vein.
- Once the cannulas and butterfly needles have been inserted, place the patient in a Trendelenberg position to empty the veins.
- The foam can now be injected under US guidance into the veins.
- A 3% solution of sodium tetradecyl sulphate is used for the main truncal veins. A 1% or 0.5% solution can be used for the calf veins or smaller branches.
- The foam causes an inflammatory reaction in the vein wall, thus causing an occlusion.
- Compression bandages are then applied and typically worm for a week.

Complications

- Skin pigmentation at site of injection and along course of veins injected is seen in almost 30% of patients.
- Thrombus formation in the vein can cause an inflammatory reaction and postoperative pain. This can easily be drained under a local anaesthetic.
- Rarer complications include visual disturbances with transient scotomas and chest tightness due to micro bubbles.
- Extravasation of the sclerosant outside the vein can cause skin damage and ulceration.
- Successful saphenous closure is seen in about 70% of cases and can be repeated easily in those with recanalization.

Vascular access

Indications

Dialysis access for end-stage renal disease for patients waiting to have a renal transplantation.

Procedure

- Allen's test must be performed to ensure that the radial and ulnar arteries are patent.
- Cephalic vein patency should be assessed clinically or with Duplex scan.
- The preferred site is in the distal forearm in the non-dominant arm.
- The patient is placed supine with the arm on an arm board or side table.

Radiocephalic fistula

- Make a longitudinal incision between the radial artery and cephalic vein at the wrist.
- Mobilize the radial artery and ligate the branches with Vicryl®.
- Apply clamps to the ends of the radial artery and distal cephalic vein.
- Make an arteriotomy over the radial artery over the lateral aspect and a venotomy over the medial aspect to allow the vessels to lie side by side.
- Carry out a side–side anastamosis using 5-0 Prolene®. An end–side anastamosis can also be done after ligating the distal cephalic artery with 3-0 Vicryl® or silk.
- After successful completion, a thrill or bruit should be confirmed in the cephalic vein.

Brachiocephalic fistula

- Expose the brachial artery in the antecubital fossa.
- Divide the bicipital aponeurosis.
- Pass vascular slings around the vessels, then apply bull-dog clamps.
- Ligate the cephalic vein proximal to the origin of the antecubital vein to allow basilic vein drainage.
- Fashion an end–side anastomosis using 5-0 Prolene® (Fig. 8.20).
- A thrill in the proximal cephalic vein confirms good flow.
- If the veins are unsuitable, a PTFE graft may be used and a graft loop tunnelled subcutaneously with anastamosis to the cephalic vein and brachial artery.
- An AV vein fistula may need up to 6–8 weeks to mature to be used for dialysis and a PTFE fistula can be used in a day following the procedure.
- However longevity of a PTFE graft is much lower than that of a vein fistula.

Complications

- Graft stenosis can be treated by angioplasty to prevent thrombosis and eventual graft occlusion.
- A thrombosed graft can be treated with thrombectomy or thrombolysis.

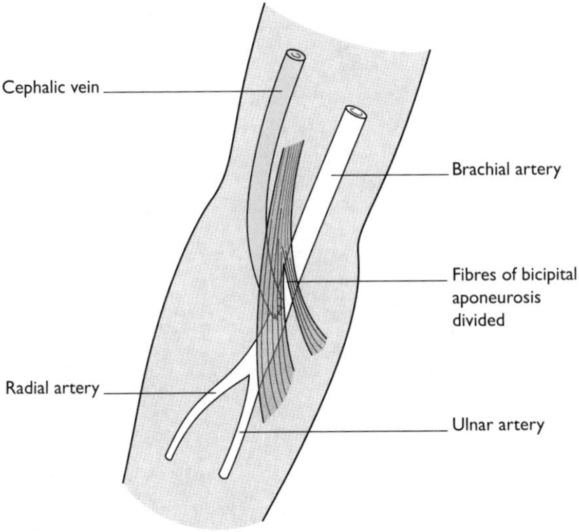
Cephalic vein
Brachial artery
Fibres of bicipital aponeurosis divided
Radial artery
Ulnar artery

Fig. 8.20 Right brachiocephalic fistula for vascular access. Image created by Vish Bhattacharya.

- A pseudoaneurysm of the fistula can lead to rupture, infection or bleeding and will need revision if there are signs of expansion or infection. It can be avoided by rotating the sites of venepuncture during dialysis
- Infection due to frequent puncture can lead to vascular access loss.
- Arm oedema can be due to venous hypertension either due to proximal vein stenosis and can be treated with venoplasty.

Chapter 9

Transplantation

Introduction

- Kidney transplantation is heterotopic—graft placed in a non-anatomical site.
- Liver transplantation is orthotopic—native liver is explanted and the dual blood supply reconnected.
- Kidneys in most developed countries are allocated to an individual on the basis of the blood group human leucocyte antigen (HLA) match between donor and recipient with algorithms also emphasizing other factors like age, geography, and waiting time.
- Livers are allocated in the UK to a centre and the centre then chooses the most appropriate recipient taking into account how ill their recipient is (MELD or UKELD score), the underlying diagnosis (HCC or cirrhosis), size match, and blood group.

Definitions

- Donor after brain-stem death (DBD): deceased donor certified dead on the basis of brain-stem criteria.
- Donor after circulatory death: deceased donor certified dead on the basis of circulatory criteria (absence of breath/heart sounds).
- Live related donor (LRD): genetic relationship between donor and recipient.
- Live unrelated donor (LURD): emotional relationship between donor and recipient.
- Non-directed altruistic donor (NDAD): organ donation by an individual to the pool of potential recipients.
- First warm ischaemia time: time from cessation of circulation to perfusion with cold preservation solution.
- Cold ischaemia time: time from cold perfusion to start of anastomoses in the recipient.
- Second warm ischaemia time: time from start of anastomoses to re-establishing circulation in the recipient.
- Delayed graft function: absence of urine/bile production in the early postoperative period may progress to either return of function or graft failure (primary non function).
- Model for end-stage liver disease (MELD): score predicts mortality on the waiting list and takes into account bilirubin, prothrombin time, and renal function.
- UK model for end-stage liver disease (UKELD): score adds serum Na to UKELD and has been optimized for the UK population.

Kidney transplantation

- Landmarks for the right iliac fossa incision are the symphysis pubis and anterior superior iliac spine (ASIS).
- The choice of incisions includes Rutherford Morrison, 'J', Hockey stick (Fig. 9.1).
- Depending on the length of the renal vessels and the condition of the recipient vessels, either the external or common or internal iliac arteries need to be exposed.
- In the case of multiple previous operations, spina bifida, or the presence of ileal conduit—midline laparotomy and anastomosis to the IVC or aorta may be appropriate.
- Most surgeons prefer to place a kidney graft in the right iliac fossa. Traditionally a left kidney would then have the renal pelvis anterior and be easier for radiological nephrostomy, if required.

Indications

- End-stage renal failure.
- Pre-emptive transplantation, before dialysis is preferred, potentially offers a long-term survival advantage.

Preoperative preparation

- Exclude active infection/malignancy.
- Check potential recipient fitness for surgery when called in; ECG, CXR, and bloods, including serum K^+.
- Review donor details (cadaveric/live).
- Check blood group compatibility.
- Review cytotoxic cross-match results.
- Final consent and check femoral pulses.
- Check the paperwork enclosed with the organs for donor details, organ perfusion times, reported damages, pathology, and reported vascular anatomy.

Back table preparation

- Prepare iced container and remove kidney from packaging in aseptic conditions.
- Identify and confirm integrity of renal artery, vein, and ureter.
- In the case of multiple vessels, decide on reconstruction technique.
- Send for recipient to start anaesthetic preparations.

Recipient preparation

- WHO checks and DVT protection measures.
- Urinary catheterization.
- Give induction antibiotics.
- Give antibody medication (basiliximab or alemtuzumab).
- Patient supine with arms out.
- Expose abdomen from symphysis to pubis.

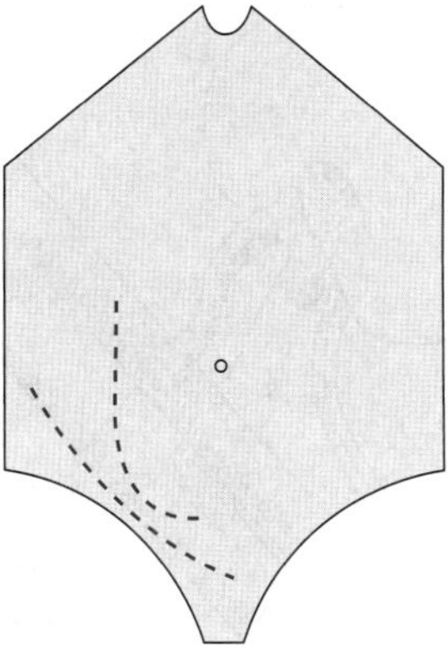

Fig. 9.1 Kidney transplantation incision choices.

Procedure

- Dissection depends on the type of incision (Fig. 9.1). Begin through the skin, Scarpa's fascia, and then abdominal wall muscles, which may be divided, split in the line of the fibres, or retracted according to surgeon preference and type of incision.
- Push the peritoneum away from the vessels.
- ♀ divide the round ligament between clips.
- Retract the cord from the operative field.
- Expose and sling the vessels for anastomosis.
- Ligate the lymphatic channels with a non-absorbable suture to prevent lymphocoele formation.
- Clamp artery and vein in preparation for the anastomosis and make longitudinal venotomy and arteriotomy in the anterior wall.
- Do the typical anastomotic technique of end–side on both artery and vein using a running 5/0 Prolene® suture (Fig. 9.2) when a Carrel patch is present and 6/0 in live donors when the patch is absent.
- Give before reperfusion steroids (methylprednisone) ± mannitol to reduce reperfusion injury.
- Once the kidney is reperfused and haemostasis is confirmed, complete the ureteric anastomosis. Fill the bladder with warm saline ± methylene blue before cystostomy and ureteric anastomosis for easy identification and to avoid opening the peritoneum. Follow the standard re-implantation Lich–Gregoir technique (extravesical neocystostomy) using a ureteric stent.

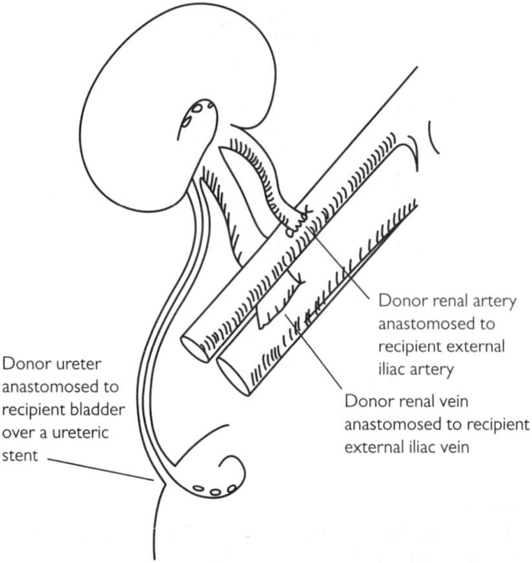
Donor renal artery anastomosed to recipient external iliac artery
Donor ureter anastomosed to recipient bladder over a ureteric stent
Donor renal vein anastomosed to recipient external iliac vein

Fig. 9.2 Arterial anastomosis end–side on external iliac artery with a donor arterial patch.

Closure

- Place suction drains in retroperitoneal space.
- Monofilament (PDS® or nylon) running suture single-layer fascia.
- Continuous absorbable subcuticular or surgical clips.
- Local anaesthetic infusion techniques may aid postoperative pain control.

Postoperative care

- Start immunosuppression (this may be started in the preoperative period for recipients of live donor grafts).
- Maintain central venous pressure (CVP) between +6 and +10cm H_2O with saline or Hartmann's electrolyte solution.
- Check U&E; consider dialysis if high K^+.
- Doppler US or renal radioisotope scan of the kidney graft, if urine output not satisfactory (delayed graft function).
- If US satisfactory consider graft biopsy to diagnose acute rejection, acute tubular necrosis, or other rarer causes of graft dysfunction.

Complications

- Renal artery thrombosis presents with delayed graft function and no flow on US or perfusion on radioisotope scan (Day 0–3).
  - Urgent re-exploration with nephrectomy is required.
- Renal vein thrombosis (Day 0–5) can present dramatically with haematuria, graft tenderness, and hypotensive shock from graft rupture.
  - Emergency transplant nephrectomy is indicated.
- Ureteric stenosis (Day 3–10) diagnosed with hydronephrosis on US.
  - Radiological nephrostomy and antegrade stent is preferred.
  - Definitive surgical management requires revision of the ureterocystostomy or in long strictures uretero-ureterostomy—re-implantation on the native ureter.
- Ureteric leak (Day 3–10) is evident by high urea in drain or wound fluid.
  - As for ureteric stenosis, although ureteric re-implantation is required more often. In cases of ureteric necrosis, a Boari flap or uretero-ureterostomy may be required.
- Lymphocoele (Day 10 onwards) presents with a palpable mass, deteriorating urine output, and hydronephrosis on US scan.
  - Immediate management requires percutaneous drainage and sampling of fluid to rule out urine leak.
  - Persistent drainage mandates a definitive procedure typically laparoscopic fenestration or marsupialization.

Tips and tricks

- Cold ischaemia time should be minimized for donors after cardiac death (cadaveric donors exposed to warm ischaemia)—best results are achieved with times less than 12h.
- Second warm ischaemic time should be 30–40min.
- Attaching the catheter bag to a saline drip allows the bladder to be distended to aid in identification.
- Delayed graft function is rare from a live donor (<5%), re-exploration should not be delayed.

Live donor nephrectomy

- More and more kidneys for transplantation are being recovered from live donors using laparoscopic techniques.
- Pure laparoscopic and hand-assisted donor nephrectomy are associated with less pain, fewer hernias, and reduced recovery time when compared with open donor nephrectomy.
- The commonest approach is via a transperitoneal route, although the retroperitoneal route is now well established and may offer advantages in terms of reduced intraperitoneal complications (splenic and bowel injury).
- Open donor nephrectomy is reserved for centres without laparoscopic experience or for right-sided kidneys with multiple vessels.
- Robotic donor nephrectomy is being pioneered in a few centres and may gain popularity.
- In cases of different split renal function, the kidney with the greatest function stays with the donor.

Anatomy

The left kidney has a longer renal vein and is potentially easier to remove if there is one artery.

Indications

Related, unrelated, and altruistic kidney donation.

Preoperative preparation

- Confirm cross-match suitability with recipient and laterality of procedure.
- Mark side for donation.
- DVT prophylaxis pre- and perioperatively.

Position and theatre setup

Dependent on kidney side, up to five working ports may be needed with an 8cm Pfannensteil incision premarked on the side to be extracted.

Donor preparation

- WHO checklist.
- Urinary catheterization.
- Give induction antibiotics.
- Patient position is dependent on the approach with the side for donation elevated and the table angulated to open the space between the ribs and the pelvis. In the retroperitoneal approach the patient is positioned in full lateral.
- Expose abdomen from xiphisternum to pubis.

Procedure (laparoscopic anterior approach)

- Insert laparoscopic ports under direct vision (Fig. 9.3).
- Mobilize colon away from kidney.
- Identify and sling gonadal vein, ureter, renal artery, and renal vein.
- Dissect adrenal free from upper pole and divide venous tributaries.
- Prepare the extraction site for quick delivery of kidney after devascularization.

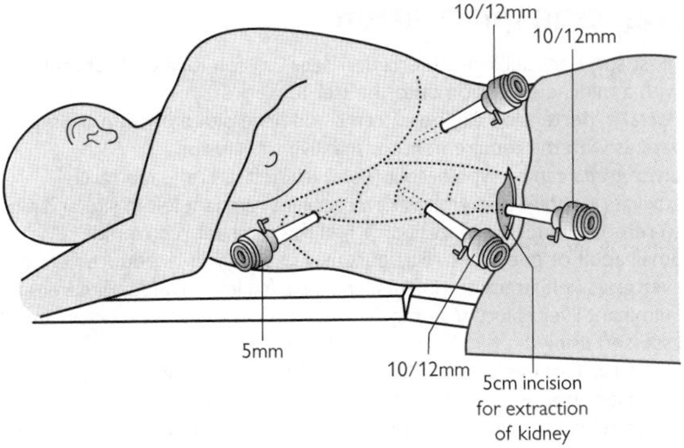
10/12mm
10/12mm
5mm
10/12mm
5cm incision
for extraction
of kidney

Fig. 9.3 Position of patient and port placement for laparoscopic donor nephrectomy for living donor renal transplantation.

- Clamp (staple) and cut in sequence ureter, then artery, and finally vein.
- Remove kidney and perfuse with chilled preservation solution until renal vein effluent is clear.
- Transfer to recipient operating theatre for implantation.

Closure

- Monofilament (PDS® or nylon) running suture single layer fascia for the extraction site.
- Continuous absorbable subcuticular or surgical clips.

Postoperative care

Remove catheter and drain on Day 1.

Complications

- Bleeding from staple/clip misapplication.
  - Emergency conversion to open nephrectomy and rapid control of the renal pedicle.
- Splenic/bowel injury.
  - May initially be subtle with the only indication being pain.
- Most common serious complication is venous thromboembolism.
- Donor serum creatinine will rise immediately after nephrectomy but contralateral hypertrophy (25%) over the first year will compensate.
- Some registries report an increased incidence of hypertension over long-term follow-up.

Tips and tricks

A second surgeon is required on the 'back bench' to perfuse the kidney whilst the operative team ensures haemostasis and close the Pfannenstiel incision.

Liver transplantation

- Most surgeons still use a Mercedes-Benz incision (bilateral subcostal with a midline extension onto the sternum).
- Portal hypertension can be extreme and necessitate division of multiple varices with the requirement for massive transfusion.
- Liver grafts can be whole, split (right, left, left lateral), and rarely auxiliary (whole/split graft with a recipient remnant left in situ and a plan to remove immunosuppression when the remnant recovers).
- Small adult or paediatric recipients may need a split or reduced adult liver graft (left lateral for infants/children, full left for older children).
- Fulminant liver failure may require 'super urgent' transplantation and is assessed using the King's College Criteria (1).
- In the Far East live donation is well established, and laparoscopic or robotic donor hepatectomy is being pioneered in France.
- Acute rejection is less common than in kidney transplantation and lower doses of tacrolimus are required.

Indications

Adult

- Cirrhosis.
  - Virus (Hep B/C/D/E).
  - Alcohol, non-alcoholic fatty liver disease.
  - Primary biliary cirrhosis.
  - Primary sclerosing cholangitis.
  - Secondary biliary cirrhosis.
  - Autoimmune hepatitis.
  - 'Vanishing bile duct' syndrome (chronic rejection).
- Hepatocellular carcinoma (Milan criteria):
  - One lesion <5cm.
  - Up to three lesions <3cm.
  - No extrahepatic manifestations.
  - No vascular invasion.
- Metabolic dysfunction (e.g. primary hyperoxaluria).
  - Haemochromatosis.
  - Wilson's disease.
  - Alpha 1 antitrypsin deficiency.
- Fulminant liver failure.
  - Drug-induced (e.g. paracetamol).
  - Virus (Hep B/C/D/E).
  - Non-A/non-B hepatitis (idiopathic).
  - Primary non-function or hepatic artery thrombosis after primary liver transplant.

Paediatric

- Extra hepatic biliary atresia.
- Intrahepatic cholestasis (Alagille's syndrome, progressive familial intrahepatic cholestasis).
- Metabolic and viral causes.

Preoperative preparation

- Exclude active infection/malignancy.
- Check PT, platelet count.
- Review donor details (cadaveric/live).
- Check blood group compatibility (no requirement to wait for crossmatch with donor, cf. kidney).
- Cross-match multiple blood products if portal hypertension, varices.

Position and theatre set-up

Back table preparation

- Check the paperwork enclosed with the organs for donor details, organ perfusion times, reported damages, pathology, and reported vascular anatomy.
    - Prepare iced container and remove liver from packaging in aseptic conditions.
    - Identify and confirm integrity of IVC, portal vein (PV), hepatic artery (HA), and general state of the graft (steatosis, quality of the graft).
    - Split the liver if required.
    - Send for recipient to start anaesthetic preparations.

Recipient preparation

- WHO checks and DVT protection measures.
- Urinary catheterization.
- Give induction antibiotics.
- Patient supine with arms out on boards.
- Expose abdomen from symphysis to pubis.
- In some patients where the IVC is replaced (or where there is no established portosystemic shunts) portosystemic bypass may be required.
    - Cannula inserted into the femoral vein and SVC or axillary vein by Seldinger technique or direct cutdown.

Procedure

- Hepatectomy proceeds by identifying and dividing the bile duct, HA, and PV in sequence close to the liver.
- If portosystemic bypass is being used, a further cannula is then inserted into the PV and an extracorporeal circuit established linking blood from the femoral and PVs back to the SVC.
- The IVC is then clamped and divided above and below the liver or the liver dissected free from the IVC and the PVs divided leaving the IVC in continuity.
- Native liver removed and haemostasis established.
- Implantation commences IVC 'top' cava anastomosis (3/0 Prolene® running suture) and IVC 'bottom' cava anastomosis (3/0 Prolene® running suture) or if the IVC is in continuity with a cavo/cavostomy (Fig. 9.4).
- PV clamped and cannula removed (if on bypass).
- PV anastomosis 5/0 running suture.
- Before reperfusion the liver is 'rinsed' to remove the large volume of high K^+ preservation solution, which can cause cardiac arrthymia on reperfusion. Steroids (methylprednisone) ± mannitol are given.
- Clamps are released on the IVC then PV and HA anastomosis 6/0 or 7/0 Prolene®.

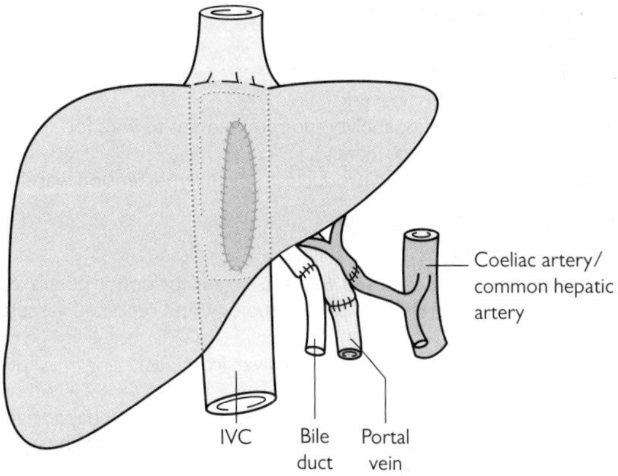
Coeliac artery/
common hepatic
artery
IVC
Bile
duct
Portal
vein

Fig. 9.4 Diagram showing the standard reconstruction post liver transplantation.

- Cholecystectomy.
- Bile duct then either anastomosed to the recipient duct (interrupted 5/0 PDS®) or a Roux-en-Y hepaticojejunostomy if the recipient bile duct is diseased (Fig. 9.5).
- Hepaticojejunostomy.
  - Small bowel divided distal to the ligament of Treitz using a linear stapler.
  - Distal limb brought up to bile duct and small enterotomy fashioned in anti-mesenteric border.
  - Interrupted 5/0 PDS® hepaticojejunostomy.
  - Proximal limb anastomsed using stapler or sutured 3/0 to distal limb 70cm downstream from biliary anastomosis.

Closure

- Ensure haemostasis, place large-bore drains around the liver and next to the biliary anastomosis. Monofilament (PDS® or nylon) running suture single layer fascia.
- Continuous absorbable subcuticular or surgical clips.

Postoperative care

- Transfer to the intensive care department.
- Start immunosuppression.
- Doppler US, if PT or lactate not improving (delayed graft function).
- If US satisfactory consider graft biopsy to diagnose acute rejection or disease recurrence.
- Check liver enzymes daily. Day 1 ALT/AST (alanine/aspartate transaminase) is a marker of ischaemia reperfusion injury. Rising transaminases on Day 5 suggests rejection. Rising alkaline phosphatase suggests bile leak or obstruction.

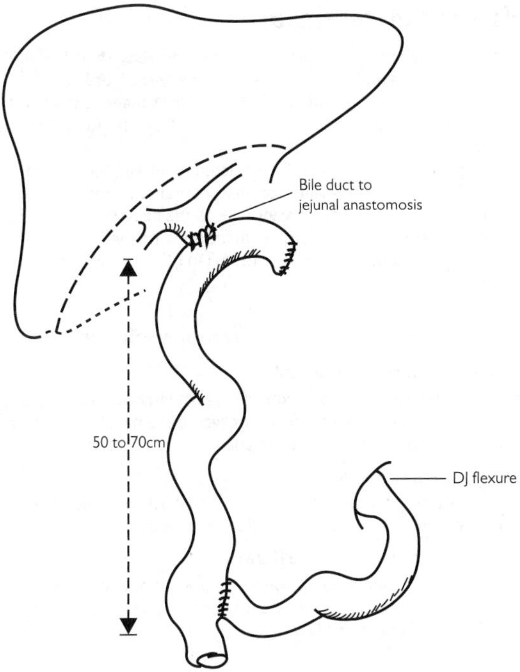
Bile duct to
jejunal anastomosis
50 to 70cm
DJ flexure

Fig. 9.5 Standard Roux-en-Y reconstruction for biliary enteric anastomosis.

Complications

- Hepatic artery thrombosis (2–5%) presents with failure of PT and lactate to normalize post-implantation, graft dysfunction in the first week, and bile leak in the first 2–3 weeks.
    - CT or contrast angiography to confirm.
    - Thrombectomy is rarely successful and retransplantation is indicated.
    - Bile in the drain suggests biliary anastomotic leak requiring ERCP and stent or formal conversion to Roux-en-Y hepaticojejunostomy.

Multi-organ retrieval

- DBD donors can provide heart, lungs, liver, pancreas, small bowel, and kidneys for transplantation. Organ recovery is co-ordinated with recipient availability and condition. In most situations the heart transplant dictates the time of 'cross clamp' (donor perfusion) as the ischaemic tolerance is the shortest.
- DCD organ donors are generally restricted to lungs, liver, pancreas, and kidneys. The aim of the organ-recovery procedure in both situations is to flush, cool, and remove organs with all the necessary vessels/ conduits/ patches to ensure successful transplantation.
- The principle is to replace blood with chilled (4°C) preservation solution (Box 9.1).

Box 9.1 Abdominal organ preservation solutions

University of Wisconsin solution (UW)

The 'gold standard' and most expensive, high viscosity, sodium lactobionate with a colloid starch to prevent organ oedema, also contains free radical scavengers. Suitable for all organs.

Marshall's hypertonic citrate

Hyperosmolar to prevent cellular oedema; cheap, low viscosity, only suitable for live donor, and DBD kidney flush and storage.

Histidine tryptophan ketoglutarate (HTK)

Cheap, low-viscosity solution favoured by some units to flush and store the liver. Utilizes amino acids to prevent oedema and to provide cellular energy. Not as effective as UW.

- Abdominal perfusion is performed via cannulas placed in the aorta just proximal to the bifurcation or via the right iliac artery having tied off the left.
- A cannula placed in the portal circulation can improve the liver flush and is mandatory when the liver is being considered for splitting or in the DCD setting.
- Portal perfusion should be above the pancreas when this is being retrieved for solid organ transplantation or islet isolation.

Indications

- *Either* (DBD): death diagnosed by brain-stem criteria.
  - *Preconditions*: known cause of death leading to ventilator dependence, no depressant drugs, hypothermia.
  - *Exclusions*: circulatory, metabolic, endocrine causes; cervical injury, muscle relaxants.
  - *Tests*: fixed, dilated pupils; no corneal, oculovestibular, or cough reflexes, no response to supraorbital pressure; no respiratory effort in response to hypercarbia on disconnecting ventilator (apnea test).

- *Or* (DCD): futility decision in conjunction with family, plan to 'withdraw' life-sustaining care, and diagnose death on the basis of cardiorespiratory criteria (cardiac asystole with absent breath and heart sounds).
- Appropriate assent from donor's family/partner.
- Satisfactory organ function on relevant criteria.
- Absence of contraindications (infectious/malignant history).

Preoperative preparation (DBD and DCD)

- Review necessary documentation with Specialist Organ Donation Nurse.
- Confirm donor consent, virology, blood group.
- WHO checklist with team in theatre.

Position and theatre setup (DBD)

- Patient supine with arms in by the side.
- Chest and abdomen exposed (symphysis to symphysis).

Procedure (DBD)

- Midline laparotomy.
- Right colon and duodenum mobilized.
- Abdominal aorta slung just proximal to bifurcation to provide rapid access if required.
- Median sternotomy.
- Full inspection of organs to ensure suitability for transplantation and absence of pathology.
- Gallbladder and bile duct opened and flushed.
- Discussion with cardiothoracic team about placement of aortic clamp either in chest (descending aorta) or abdomen (supracoeliac) and venting of blood (chest or abdomen).
- Heparin given (350IU/kg) intravenously.
- Distal aorta tied and cannula inserted proximal to level of renal arteries.
- Thoracic/supra-coeliac aortic clamp placed, vena cava opened.
- Pressurized organ preservation flush begun.
- Abdominal sequence of removal: liver/pancreas/kidneys.
- Organs placed in ice/cool (4–8°C) preservation solution on back bench.

Positioning and theatre set-up (DCD)

- Confirm with intensive care team site of treatment withdrawal (intensive care or anaesthetic room).
- Confirm with implanting surgeons acceptable periods of 'functional' warm ischaemia (time from treatment withdrawal to retrieval).
- Await cardiac asystole or declaration of 'non-proceeding' donor (50% of DCD donors do not proceed to asystole within 3–4h of treatment withdrawal).
- After declaration of death, transfer patient to operating theatre.
- Patient supine with arms in by the side.
- Chest and abdomen exposed (symphysis to symphysis).
- Knife to skin only after appropriate 'stand off' period to confirm asystole has been observed.

Procedure (DCD)

- Rapid midline laparotomy.
- Aorta identified, slung, and cannulated.
- Median sternotomy and placement of proximal aortic clamp.
- IVC opened in chest and/or abdomen.
- Pressurized organ-preservation flush starts (4–6min from start).
- Portal vein cannula placed and liver flushed.
- Gallbladder and bile duct opened and flushed.
- Full inspection of organs to ensure suitability for transplantation and absence of pathology.
- Abdominal sequence of removal: liver/pancreas/kidneys.
- Organs placed in ice/cool (4–8°C) preservation solution on back bench.

Closure

Midline wound closed with cadaveric silk suture.

Postoperative care

- Organs flushed to ensure microcirculation clear, anatomy and vessel integrity confirmed.
- Each organ 'triple' bagged with copious preservation solution; then handed off for packing in appropriate containers.
- Appropriate documentation completed for each organ.
- Discussion with implanting surgeon as appropriate.
- Relevant documentation complete with each organ.

Complications

- Common injuries include liver capsular tears on mobilization, cuts to the arterial, venous patches, division of accessory vessels (polar renal arteries, accessory left and right hepatic arteries), and parenchymal injury (pancreas).
- Most vessel injuries can be repaired by the implanting surgeon.

Tips and tricks

Organ damage is more common in the DCD situation when the procedure is rapid and there are no pulses to help identify arteries. In this situation retrieving the liver and pancreas together 'en bloc' and separating them on the back table can reduce the risk of damage to portal structures.

References

1. O'Grady JG, Alexander GJ, Hayllar KM, Williams R. Early indicators of prognosis in fulminant hepatic failure. Gastroenterology (1989) 97, 439–45.

Chapter 10

Urology

Circumcision

Anatomy

The 'foreskin' is the skin at the end of the penis. It is a double-layered fold of smooth muscle tissue, blood vessels, neurones, skin, and mucous membrane that covers the glans penis and protects the urinary meatus. The external meatus is a highly innervated mucocutaneous zone of the penis near the tip of the foreskin. The foreskin is mobile, fairly stretchable, and acts as a natural lubricant. The smegma is a whitish pollution of the glans and prepuce, and arises due to bacterial colonization of the desquamated epithelium.

The nerve supply to the penis is important to understand as circumcision can be performed with a local anaesthetic penile ring block. The sensory innervation of the penis is via the dorsal nerve of the penis, which arises from the first branch of the pudendal nerve in the Alcock's canal.

Indications

- Phimosis—non-retractile foreskin.
- Balanitis xerotica oblitrans (BXO).
- Recurrent balanitis/infections of the foreskin.
- Reduction of recurrent urinary tract infection in paediatric/neonatal patients.
- Penile carcinoma (carcinoma in situ of the penis).
- Obstructed voiding.
- Reduction of risk of transmission of HIV.
- Religious/cultural.

Contraindications

- Epispadias.
- Hypospadias.

Preoperative preparation

Patient consented for circumcision; discuss the following specific side-effects (marked with an asterisk throughout this chapter) on the basis of the British Association of Urological Surgeons procedure specific consent form*:

- *Common side-effects* (>1 in 10): swelling of the penis lasting several days.
- *Occasional side-effects* (between 1 in 10 and 1 in 50): bleeding requiring emergency re-surgery/exploration wound infection; alteration at the head of penis/altered sexual sensation during intercourse; presence of absorbable stitches after 3–4 weeks, requiring removal.
- *Rare side-effects* (<1 in 50): tenderness at surgical scar site; unsatisfactory cosmetic outcome requiring further surgery for cosmetic reasons, i.e. excessive removal of foreskin and need for biopsy of abnormal area.

Theatre set-up

- The World Health Organization (WHO) safety checklist is implemented in theatre.
- The patient can be offered a circumcision under general anaesthesia, spinal anaesthesia, or local anaesthesia with a penile ring block. The penile ring block is given to anesthetize the dorsal nerve of the penis. The block is given either by the surgeon or the anaesthetist. After checking the local anaesthetic (drug, expiry date, and ensure that the patients is not allergic or has any contraindications for local anaesthetic injection), it is important to ensure that the local anaesthetic contains *no adrenaline*. Clean and drape the patient. The anatomical landmark to inject the penile ring block is into the triangular space between the inferior border of the symphysis pubis, the corpora inferiorly, and Buck's fascia anteriorly.

Procedure

- Clean and drape patient.
- Give local anaesthetic penile ring block, as described.
- Dilate the phimosis and separate the prepucio-glandular adhesions using a blunt instrument (blunt probe/artery forceps).
- Use a marker pen to mark the external incision on the outer foreskin at the level of the coronal sulcus. Make a V-shaped extension ventrally on the foreskin (Fig. 10.1).
- Retract the foreskin back after releasing all the adhesions.
- Mark the inner incision with the marker pen below the foreskin proximal to the fusion of the Colles' and Buck's fascia.
- Open both external and internal markings.
- Secure haemostasis with bipolar diathermy.

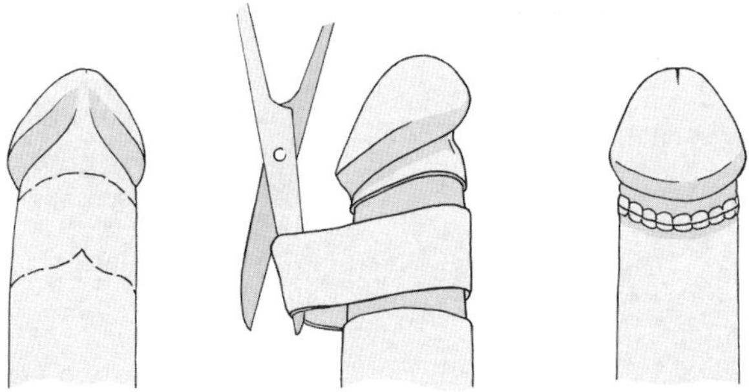
C

Fig. 10.1 Circumcision being performed after marking the inner and outer cuff of the foreskin.

- Dissect the Colles' fascia and divide and excise the skin between the internal and external incisions.
- After securing haemostasis, close the circumcision incision using interrupted absorbable sutures.
- Place a sterile dressing.

In certain situations when there is a severe degree of phimosis, the foreskin cannot be retracted to make the inner incision. In this situation a dorsal slit incision is made through the outer and inner skin layers at the same time in the midline.

Postoperative care

- Wound care.
- No intercourse for 6 weeks.

Complications

- Wound infection.
- Wound dehiscence.
- Acute urinary retention.
- Immediate/delayed meatal stenosis.
- Unsatisfactory cosmetic outcome.
- Alternation in normal sexual sensation.
- Urethrocutaneous fistula.

Tips and tricks

- Ensure *no adrenaline* in local anaesthetic agent for penile ring block.
- Ensure only bipolar diathermy is used.
- Use absorbable sutures.

Excision of epididymal cyst

Anatomy

The epididymis is an integral part of the male reproductive system and connects the efferent ducts from the testis to the vas deferens. The epididymis is 'comma shaped' and is composed of a single, fine, tubular structure that is approximately 6m long. The epididymis is highly compressed and convoluted. It is solid in consistency. The three parts of the epididymis are the head, body, and tail.

The blood supply of the epididymis is shared in common with the testis. The venous drainage occurs through the Pampiniform plexus, which eventually becomes reduced to a single vein known as the testicular vein. There is a small risk of injury to the testicular artery during surgery on the epididymis.

Indications

Symptomatic epididymal cyst (confirmed preoperatively on US testis).

Preoperative preparation

- Consent patient*; discuss the following complications:
  - *Common* (>1 in 10): swelling of the testis lasting several days and seepage of yellowish discharge from the surgical wound.
  - *Occasional* (between 1 in 10 and 1 in 50): recurrence of the cyst; blood collection around the testis, which resolves slowly or requires surgical removal; wound infection or infection of the epididymis requiring further surgery or antibiotics.
  - *Rare* (<1 in 50): scarring of the epididymis causing impaired fertility and chronic pain in the testicle or scrotum.
- Mark the side of the surgery.

Theatre set-up

- Implement the WHO checklist.
- Confirm the side at the time of consent check.

Procedure

- Make either a midline raphe incision or a transverse incision in the hemi-scrotum.
- Open scrotum in layers and create a sub-Dartos space to expose the epididymal cyst. There is normally no need to open the tunica vaginalis.
- Use a combination of blunt and sharp dissection to develop a plane between the epididymis and the epididymal cyst.
- Excise the cyst.
- Secure haemostasis with bipolar diathermy.
- Return testis to the scrotum.
- Close Dartos with a running 3-0 absorbable suture and skin with 4-0 absorbable suture.
- Apply scrotal support.

Postoperative care

- Wound care.
- Postoperative scrotal support.

Complications

- Wound infection.
- Wound dehiscence.
- Postoperative haematoma.
- Scarring of the epididymis causing pain and infertility.
- Recurrent epididymal cyst.

Tips and tricks

- Ensure patient has had a preoperative US scan.
- Only use bipolar diathermy for haemostasis on testis and epididymis.

Cystoscopy—flexible/rigid + biopsy, insertion JJ stent

Anatomy

The adult urinary bladder is lined with transitional epithelium. The bladder is located in the anterior pelvis and is surrounded by extraperitoneal fat and connective tissue. The bladder is separated from the pubic symphysis by a space called the 'space of Retzius'. The surrounding structures of the urinary bladder include the peritoneum anteriorly at the dome of the bladder and structures formed by the reflection of the pelvic fascia and true ligaments of the pelvis.

Indications

- Haematuria (visible and non-visible).
- Lower urinary tract symptoms with suspicion of pathology in the urinary bladder (carcinoma in situ, bladder cancer).
- Surveillance of bladder cancer.
- Part of urological surgical procedures (e.g. stent insertion/pre-bladder tumour resection).
- Cystoscopic removal of bladder stones.
- Cystoscopic injections of therapeutic agents (e.g. botulinum toxin injection).

Contraindications

Active UTI.

Preoperative preparation

- Patient can either undergo a flexible or rigid cystoscopy (see Figs. 10.2 and 10.3). The advantage of a flexible cystoscopy is that the procedure can be performed using local anaesthesia. The commonest local anaesthesia used for a flexible cystoscopy is Instillagel®, which contains lidocaine hydrochloride (local anaesthetic) 2.000g, chlorhexidine gluconate solution (antiseptic) 0.250g, methyl hydroxybenzoate (E218) (antiseptic) 0.060g, and propyl hydroxybenzoate (E216) (antiseptic) 0.025g. The flexible cystoscope can be manipulated at the tip, which makes visualization of the bladder at different angles possible (i.e. 70°). Rigid cystoscopy has the advantage of better views during the procedure due to superior optics and irrigation volume. Instruments such as biopsy forceps and injection devices for intravesicle injections are more easily passed via a rigid cystoscope.
- Preoperatively all patient should have a urine dipstick analysis performed to ensure that the patient does not have an active urinary tract infection (UTI). Once a UTI is excluded, obtain consent using the British Association of Urological Surgeons procedure-specific consent form, highlighting the potential side-effects of the procedure.

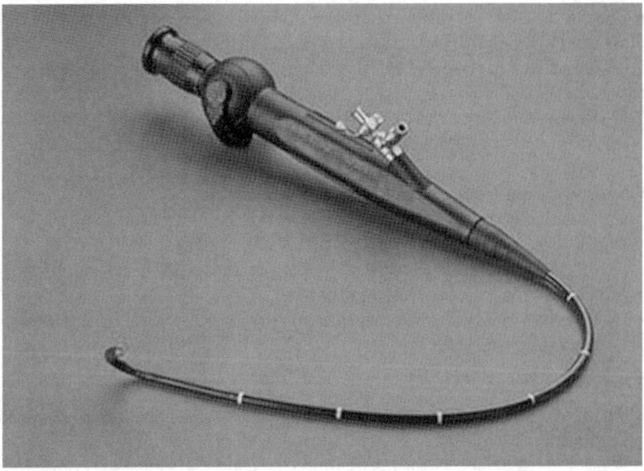

Fig. 10.2 Flexible cystoscope.

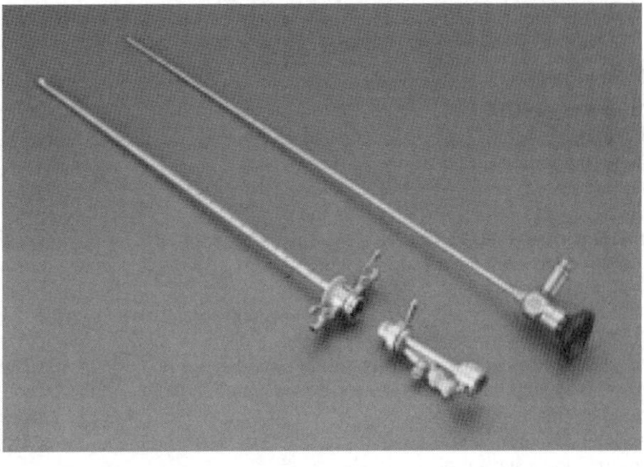

Fig. 10.3 Rigid cystoscope.

- Specific side-effects of flexible cystoscopy include*:
  - *Common* (>1 in 10): dysuria and need for biopsy.
  - *Occasional* (between 1 in 10 and 1 in 50): infection requiring oral antibiotics.
  - *Rare* (<1 in 50): post-procedure catheterization, delayed haematuria, and injury to the urethra resulting in the formation of urethral stricture.
- Specific side-effects of a rigid cystoscopy include:
  - *Common* (>1 in 10): dysuria and insertion of a catheter.
  - *Occasional* (between 1 in 10 and 1 in 50): urinary tract infection requiring antibiotics, incidental finding of cancer, or need to perform a telescopic removal/bladder biopsy.
  - *Rare* (<1 in 50): delayed haematuria, urethral stricture, or small risk of bladder perforation.

Theatre set-up

- The World Health Organization (WHO) safety checklist is implemented in theatre.
- A urine dipstick analysis is performed to exclude an active UTI prior to the procedure.
- In female patients it is important to document the last menstrual cycle date and to perform a urinary pregnancy test if required preoperatively.
- For patients who are immunosuppressed and those who have prosthetic heart valves or artificial joints, intravenous antibiotics must be given pre-procedure as per local guidelines.

Procedure

Clean and drape patient

When a patient is undergoing a flexible cystoscopy, the procedure can be performed using local anaesthesia. The patient is always in the supine position. Most patients experience a minimal amount of discomfort when the flexible cystoscope is introduced as the diameter of a normal flexible cystoscope is between 15 and 18Fr. Most patients complain of a sensation of wanting to void during these procedure, but the procedure is generally very well tolerated.

In patients undergoing a rigid cystoscopy, a general/spinal anaesthetic is required. The normal rigid cystoscope has a diameter of 22Fr. During the procedure an irrigant is used to fill the bladder and this allows superior views in comparison to the flexible cystoscope due to the option of continuous irrigation. The advantage of a rigid cystoscope is the versatility of additional treatments that can be performed, which includes biopsy, diathermy, and insertion of stents.

When a biopsy of the bladder needs to be performed, this can be done with either a flexible cystoscope or rigid cystoscope. The advantage of flexible cystoscopy biopsies is that the procedure can be performed without a general anaesthetic. The disadvantage is the small biopsies performed due to the biopsy forceps and the risk of an inability to control haemostasis in the event of bleeding, as the irrigation is not on a continuous flow. The advantage of rigid cystoscopy and biopsy is that the biopsy volume is larger and haemostasis is better controlled due to continuous irrigation systems.

A double JJ stent is inserted when a patient has a ureteric obstruction. The stent is deployed over a guide wire into the kidney using a cystoscope. The commonest cause of acute ureteric obstruction is renal calculi and chronic obstruction is benign/malignant pelvic or retroperitoneal pathology.

Postoperative care

- Ensure the patient has voided prior to discharge.
- Advise patient to watch for symptoms of UTI post-procedure.

Complications

- UTI.
- Haematuria.
- Acute urinary retention.
- Immediate/delayed bleeding.
- Urethral stricture.
- Bladder perforation.

Indications for ureteric stent insertion

- Urinary sepsis secondary to acute ureteric obstruction.
- Failure of medical therapy to counter symptoms of acute ureteric obstruction (e.g. obstructing ureteric calculus).

Hydrocele repair

Anatomy

A hydrocele is a fluid-filled sac surrounding a testicle that results in swelling of the scrotum.

The testicle is situated in a special sac called the 'processus vaginalis'. The sac and its fluid have nothing to do with testes' performance and are merely a result of the development of the testicle. There are different types of hydroceles: primary hydrocele, secondary hydrocele, infantile hydrocele, congenital hydrocele, and encysted hydrocele of the cord. Normally the processus vaginalis becomes obliterated along the entire length apart from where the process vaginalis surrounds the testis itself. When the central part of the processus vaginalis remains patent, fluid secreted by the peritoneum accumulates and forms a hydrocele around the testis.

Indications

- Symptomatic.
- In the case of infantile hydrocele, most will resolve by the age of 1 year and therefore no surgery is required. The indication to operate is if the hydrocele persists after the age of 2 years. The recommended procedure is ligation and division of the processes vaginalis.

Contraindications

Pyocele.

Preoperative preparation

Patient is consented for hydrocele repair after discussing the following specific side-effects on the basis of the British Association of Urological Surgeons procedure specific consent form*:

- *Common* (>1 in 10): swelling of the scrotum lasting several days.
- *Occasional* (between 1 in 10 and 1 in 50): blood collection around testis that resolves slowly or requires surgical removal. Possible infection of the incision or the testis requiring further treatment with antibiotics or surgical drainage.
- *Rare* (<1 in 50): recurrence of fluid collection, chronic pain in the testicle or scrotum, scarring of the epididymis causing impaired fertility, and chronic pain in the testicle or scrotum.

Theatre set-up

The World Health Organization (WHO) safety checklist is implemented in theatre. The side of surgery must be marked and confirmed at the time of consent check.

Procedure

- Clean and drape patient.
- Make either a midline raphe or a transverse incision in the hemi-scrotum.
- Open scrotum in layers.
- The two main surgical operations are either a Lord's procedure or a Jaboulay procedure.

Jaboulay procedure

- Dissect the tunica vaginalis off the Dartos muscle and deliver the entire hydrocele sac. The best method to separate the hydrocele sac from the surrounding Dartos is via blunt-finger dissection, ensuring haemostasis as there can be prominent veins in this layer.
- Open the tunica vaginalis and drain the hydrocele. During opening of the hydrocele sac care must be taken not to damage the spermatic cord posteriorly.
- Evert the hydrocele sac with a 3-0 absorbable suture. It is important to ensure that the eversion suture is not made too tight in order to prevent strangulation of the spermatic cord.
- When the tunica vaginalis is closed and everted, place the testis back into the Dartos pouch.
- Close the Dartos and skin with a 2-0 or 3-0 absorbable suture.

Lord's procedure

In the event of the hydrocele being large, perform a Lord's procedure:

- Create a sub-dartos space.
- Open the tunica vaginalis and drain the fluid from the hydrocele.
- Secure haemostasis with bipolar diathermy.
- Evert the tunica vaginalis. Commence the eversion from the free edge of the tuniva vaginalis with 3-0 absorbable sutures at 1cm intervals. It is important not make this suture too tight.
- Once haemostasis is confirmed, the tunica vaginalis is everted and placed in a sub-Dartos pouch.
- Close in layers using 3-0 absorbable sutures.

Postoperative care

Scrotal support and wound care.

Complications

Occasional (between 1 in 10 and 1 in 50)

- Blood collection around testis, which resolves slowly or requires surgical removal.
- Possible infection of the incision or the testis requiring further treatment with antibiotics or surgical drainage.
- Recurrence of fluid collection.
- Chronic pain in the testicle or scrotum.

Tips and tricks

- Place a drain postoperatively in large hydrocele to prevent the risk of a postoperative haematoma.

Suprapubic catheter insertion

Indications

- Failed/unsuccessful urethral catheter insertion in a patient with urinary retention.
- Replacement from urethral catheter to a long-term catheter.

Contraindications

- Patient in clot retention.
- Patient with abdominal/pelvic midline incisions from previous surgery.
- Pelvic fracture where there is risk of the haematoma expanding with insertion of suprapubic catheter.
- Uncorrected coagulopathy.
- Uncooperative patient (when procedure is being attempted under local anaesthetic).

Preoperative preparation

Prior to insertion of the suprapubic catheter it is important to ensure that the patient is in acute retention both clinically and with an US scan. In patients with previous lower abdominal surgery/scars there is a risk of the bowel being adhered to the abdominal wall and bladder, risking injury to both these structures during catheter insertion.

Patient is consented for suprapubic catheter insertion after discussing the following complications*:

- *Common* (>1 in 10): temporary mild burning or bleeding during urination.
- *Occasional* (between 1 in 10 and 1 in 50): infection of the bladder needing antibiotics (occasionally, recurrent infections); blocking of the catheter; bladder discomfort and pain; persistent leakage from the water pipe (urethra) that may need a further operation to close the bladder neck; development of stones and debris in the bladder causing catheter blockage and requiring removal or crushing by a further procedure.
- *Rare* (<1 in 50): bleeding requiring irrigation or additional catheterization to remove blood clot; damage to surrounding structures such as bowel or blood vessels with serious consequences, possibly needing additional surgery.

Theatre set-up

The World Health Organization (WHO) safety checklist is implemented in theatre.

Procedure

- Infiltrate local anaesthesia into the planned site of insertion.
- Make a puncture of the full bladder using an 18-gauge needle. The anatomical location of the puncture site is two to three finger-breadths above the pubic symphysis.
- Confirm by aspiration.
- Insert a floppy-tip 0.035in guide wire through the needle into the bladder and withdraw the needle (Fig. 10.4).
- Make a 1cm incision along the guide wire in the rectus sheath.
- Dilate the track over the guide wire, remove the guide wire and dilator, and pass a 14Fr Foley catheter (standard length of 43cm) through the peel-away sheath, which is part of the dilator assembly (Fig. 10.5). The catheter is then secured to the skin with a silk suture.

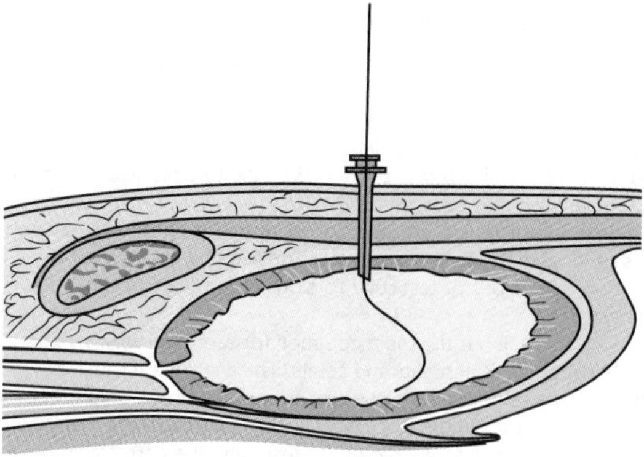

Fig. 10.4 The 0.035in floppy-tip guide wire being passed through an 18-gauge needle into the bladder.

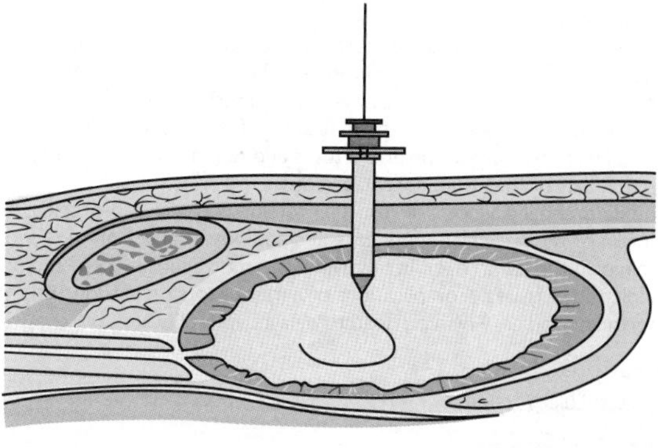

Fig. 10.5 Dilatation of the established tract over the 0.035in floppy-tip using the Seldinger technique.

Postoperative care

Catheter care.

Complications

- Bowel perforation.
- Persistent haematuria.
- Recurrent UTI.
- Catheter dislodgment.

Tips and tricks

In the event of previous abdominal surgery/lower midline incisions, use US to localize the bladder and to exclude any interposing bowel.

Torsion of testis

- Torsion of testis is an acute urological emergency. Testicular torsion results from a twist of the spermatic cord, resulting in strangulation of the blood supply of the testis, including the epididymis.
- Testicular torsion is a clinical diagnosis. The main aim is quick diagnosis and urgent surgical exploration. An US of the testis is usually normal and a Doppler scan may be equivocal.
- The peak age of clinical presentation of testicular torsion is between the ages of 12 and 18 years with a smaller peak in the first year of life.
- The two main types of testicular torsion are intravaginal and extravaginal.
- Intravaginal torsion is the most common form of testicular torsion, which is seen in adolescents and adults. The anatomical cause of intravaginal torsion is a high investment of the tunica vaginalis on the cord, which results in the testis lying horizontally causing a 'bell clapper' abnormality. This anomaly allows the testis and the cord to rotate. It is common for the 'bell clapper' deformity to be bilateral, which results in the risk of torsion of the contralateral testis. It is hence important to perform an orchidopexy of the opposite side in order to prevent a further torsion.
- An extravaginal torsion is the most common type of torsion in the first year of life. This type of torsion can be either pre- or postnatal. The attachment between the tunica vaginalis and scrotum is mal-developed whereupon there is an incomplete fixation of the gubernaculum to the scrotal wall, resulting in the entire testis and tunica vaginalis twisting in a vertical axis of the entire spermatic cord.
- The differential diagnosis of testicular torsion is epididymo-orchitis, torsion of the testicular appendage and additional causes of loin/groin pain (ureteric colic). In the event of a misdiagnosis, there can be medico-legal issues. Complications of a missed torsion include anti-sperm antibodies, which can lead to delayed infertility.

Indications

Acute testicular torsion.

Contraindications

Nil.

Preoperative preparation

Consent for torsion of testis after discussing the following complications*:

- *Common* (>1 in 10): it may be necessary to remove the affected testis if it is too damaged to recover.
- *Occasional* (between 1 in 10 and 1 in 50): it may be possible for patients to feel the stitch used to fix the testis through the skin, blood clot around the testicles which resolves slowly, or may require surgical removal, infection of the incision or the testis needing further treatment.
- *Rare* (<1 in 50): later shrinkage of the testicle; even if the testis is preserved, there is no guarantee of fertility.

Theatre set-up

- Implement the World Health Organization (WHO) safety checklist.
- The side of surgery must be marked and confirmed at the time of consent check.

Procedure

- The patient normally has an emergency general anaesthetic following rapid induction.
- It is best to perform a midline raphe incision in view of performing a contralateral orchidopexy.
- Open the layers of the scrotum from the skin, dartos muscle, external spermatic fascia, cremasteric fascia, internal spermatic fascia, and tunica vaginalis.
- Examine the testis looking at the degree of torsion and de-tort the testis.
- Place the testis in warm saline and request the anaesthetist to give the patient 100% oxygen.
- Examine the testis regularly and if the testis is viable, perform an ordchidopexy using a three-point fixation. Prior to the fixation evert the tunica vaginalis. Do the fixation with 3-0 non-absorbable sutures at medial, lateral, and infero-anterior positions. In the event of there being a question as to whether the testis is viable or not, open the tunica albugenia to assess if the seminiferous tubules are viable. If the testis is ischaemic, perform an orchiectomy.
- Once the three-point orchidopexy/orchiectomy is performed on the side of the torsion, expose the contralateral testis, evert the tunica vaginalis, and perform orchidopexy, as described above.
- Place the testis in a sub-dartos pouch.
- Close the layers of the dartos and skin using absorbable sutures.

Postoperative care

- Wound care.
- Postoperative scrotal support.

Complications

- Wound infection.
- Wound dehiscence.
- Postoperative haematoma.
- Scarring of the epididymis causing pain and infertility.

Tips and tricks

- An US is not reliable for diagnosis of a testicular torsion.
- Only use bipolar diathermy for haemostasis on testis and epididymis.

Transrectal ultrasound/biopsy of prostate

Anatomy

Prostate is easily accessible for clinical examination and radiological assessment using a transrectal US. It is the most commonly used modality for assessing the prostate and is the commonest method used to biopsy the prostate. The prostate is an extraperitoneal structure, lying anterior to the rectum and at the bladder neck. The prostate encircles the urethra and it empties its secretions into the urethra. It comprises of glands that are surrounded by smooth muscle and connective tissue. The prostate has three glandular regions: the central, the peripheral, and the transition zones. There is a further non-glandular area called the anterior fibromuscular stroma.

The peripheral zone accounts for 75% of the prostate tissue in young men but with age the transition zone increases in size due to benign prostate enlargement (BPE), whilst the central zone atrophies, the peripheral zone stays static. Thus, for clinical purposes the important regions are the peripheral and transition zones. It is the peripheral zone in which the majority of prostate cancers occur, whereas BPE arises in the transition zone.

A transrectal US of the prostate and seminal vesicles is normally performed using a 7.5Hz piezoelectric transducer. The probe is 1.5cm in diameter. Most patients find the procedure uncomfortable. The options are to perform the procedure with local anaesthetic, sedation, or in some cases general anaesthetic. A transrectal US of the prostate is not only diagnostic but also therapeutic in certain circumstances, such as a prostate abscess that requires aspiration/drainage via the transrectal route.

Indications

- Prostate volume assessment (no biopsies).
- Male infertility patients with azoospermia (no biopsies).
- Clinically suspected prostate abscess- drainage (no biopsies).
- Abnormal digital rectal examination (biopsies).
- Elevated PSA (biopsies).
- Regular interval biopsies on patients on active surveillance for low-risk prostate cancer (biopsies).

Contraindications

- Active infection.
- Abnormal clotting (must be corrected and optimized pre-procedure).

Preoperative preparation

Consent after discussing the following complications*:

- *Common* (>1 in 10): patients may experience blood in urine, blood in the semen for up to 6 weeks post biopsy, blood in stools, urinary infection (10% risk), discomfort from the prostate due to bruising, haemorrhage (bleeding) causing inability to pass urine (2% risk).
- *Occasional* (between 1 in 10 and 1 in 50): blood infection (septicaemia) needing admission (2% risk), haemorrhage (bleeding) needing admission (1% risk), failure to detect a significant cancer of the prostate, the procedure may need to be repeated if the biopsies are inconclusive or PSA level rises further.
- *Rare* (<1 in 50): inability to pass urine (retention of urine).

Theatre set-up

- Implement WHO safety checklist.
- Give a dose of antibiotics prior to transrectal US of the prostate and biopsy.

Procedure

- Place patient in lateral position and perform a digital rectal examination.
- Administer a single dose of an injectable antibiotic, ensuring the patient's drug allergy profile (commonly Gentamycin single dose).
- Place the transrectal US probe and perform a detailed US of the prostate, calculating the prostate volume, looking for any abnormal focus, assessing capsular breech, and seminal vesicle involvement.
- Use an 18-gauge trucut needle to biopsy the prostate, targeting any particular areas of abnormality either on digital rectal examination or sonographically. Biopsy the apex, mid, and basal regions of the prostate.
- In the UK, a metronidazole suppository is placed per rectally. Some surgeons also place either a paracetamol or diclofenac suppository at the end of the procedure.

Postoperative care

- Post-procedure antibiotics.
- Ensure patient voids before discharge.

Complications

- 0.5% risk of sepsis post-biopsy.
- 0.5% risk of per rectal bleeding.
- 0.5% risk of clot retention.
- Post-procedure haematuria and haematospermia.

Tips and tricks

- Ensure patient is aware that negative transrectal biopsy does not exclude prostate cancer.
- A patient with a rising PSA, despite negative prostate biopsies, may require further biopsies using the transperineal route and newer MRI-guided fusion biopsies.

Vasectomy

Anatomy

The vas deferens is where the sperm from the epididymis are transported to the ejaculatory ducts. Vasectomy involves surgical division of both vas deferens to allow permanent contraception.

Indications

Permanent contraception.

Contraindications

In a patient with no partner and no children it is important to counsel with documented written consent and discuss the case with their GP, highlighting that the patient does not want children in the future.

Preoperative preparation

- Take a thorough history from the patient and ensure that both the patient and partner are aware of the operative methodology and potential side-effects of the procedure, as there are significant medico-legal issues. It is very important to counsel patients thoroughly preoperatively.
- Evaluate how co-operative a patient is to having the vasectomy under local anaesthetic.
- Do a clinical examination to ensure that bilateral vas deferens are palpable
- Consent after discussing the following complications*:
  - *Common* (>1 in 10): a small amount of bruising and scrotal swelling for several days; seepage of a small amount of clear, yellow fluid several days later; blood in the semen for the first few ejaculations; the procedure should be regarded as irreversible (although vasectomy may be reversed this is not always effective in restoring fertility, especially if more than 7 years have lapsed since the vasectomy); semen must be examined after the operation until shown to contain no motile sperms on two consecutive specimens; contraception must be continued until no motile sperms are present in two consecutive semen samples; chronic testicular pain (10–30%) or sperm granuloma (tender nodule at the site of surgery).
  - *Occasional* (between 1 in 10 and 1 in 50): significant bleeding or bruising needing further surgery; inflammation or infection of the testes or epididymis needing antibiotic treatment.
  - *Rare* (<1 in 50): early failure of the procedure to produce sterility (1 in 250–500), re-joining of vas ends after negative sperm counts resulting in fertility and pregnancy at a later stage (1 in 4,000).
- No evidence that vasectomy causes any long-term health risks (e.g. testicular cancer, prostate cancer).

Theatre set-up

Implement the WHO safety checklist

Procedure

- There are many methods described in the literature for performing a vasectomy either under local anaesthesia or general anaesthesia.
- The patient is cleaned and draped.
- Infiltrate local anaesthetic into the skin and peri-vas deferens tissue.
- The surgical incisions can be either single or bilateral, or no incision technique. Once made, dissect each vas deferens and isolate it from the spermatic cord and bring it to the level of the skin.
- Inject the vas deferens further with local anaesthetic.
- Make a 1cm transverse incision through the sheath of the vas deferens until the vas deferens is exposed.
- Deliver the vas deferens with the accompanying vasal artery, veins, and accompanying nerves.
- Excise 1cm segment of the vas deferens and send for histological analysis. Diathermise the ends of the vas deferens with bipolar diathermy and suture ligate with a 3-0 absorbable suture.
- The ends of the vas deferens can be buried using a fascial interposition technique, which provides a protective barrier to prevent the risk of re-cannulization of the vas deferens. This technique involves the suturing of the vas–spermatic fascia. Carry out haemostasis meticulously
- Close the dartos and skin in layers with a 3-0 absorbable suture.

Postoperative care

- Patients are instructed to continue with contraceptives methods till two consecutive semen analyses are negative.
- The British Andrological Society (BAS) has recommended that patients should be instructed to ensure that they have had at least 24 ejaculations and waited for 16 weeks before the submission of the first sample for semen analysis.
- The Royal College of Obstetricians and Gynaecologist and the Family Planning Association guidelines, UK have recommended the analysis of two semen analysis at least 2–4 weeks apart (normally deposited at weeks 12–14 and weeks 16–18 post-vasectomy).

Complications

- Wound infection.
- Wound dehiscence.
- Postoperative haematoma.
- Chronic scrotal/testicular pain.
- Pregnancy/fertility.

Surgical management of scrotal abscess

A scrotal abscess is an acute urological emergency. The scrotal abscess may be either superficial or deep. The commonest aetiology of scrotal abscess is an infected hair follicle or infections on the scrotum related to either scrotal lacerations or postoperative wound infections. Deeper abscesses that form within the scrotum are normally secondary to progressive acute epididymitis. The infection produces ischaemia and necrosis of the tunica albugnia and surrounding tissue. This leads to an acute perforation and rupture of the tunical albugenia. Very rarely a perforated appendix can lead to pus within the scrotum due to a patent processes vaginalis. In patients with diabetes or colo-rectal pathology a deeper infection may be present at the time of presentation called Fournier's gangrene (necrotizing fasciitis) that involves the external genitalia.

Indications

- Acute abscess confirmed clinically and on US.
- Fournier's gangrene.

Preoperative preparation

Consent highlighting the risks of bleeding, infection, wound dehiscence, need for second look, orchidectomy, and drain placement.

Theatre set-up

- Implement WHO safety checklist.
- The side of surgery must be marked and confirmed at the time of consent check.

Procedure

- The options of incision are either transverse or vertical in the hemi-scrotum. Incise skin and dartos, and drain the abscess.
- Send microbiology swab for culture and sensitivity.
- Confirm viability of the testis.
- Use normal saline to wash the abscess cavity.
- Secure haemostasis.
- Place a corrugated drain within the abscess cavity and bring it through the scrotum via a different incision. Secure the drain with 1/0 silk.
- Close the dartos with interrupted 2/0 Vicryl® as this wound has a high risk of dehiscence. Close skin with interrupted 3/0 absorbable suture.

Postoperative care

- Wound care.
- Postoperative scrotal support.
- Antibiotics.

Complications

- Wound infection.
- Wound dehiscence.
- Recurrent abscess requiring second surgery.

Tips and tricks

Ensure there is no evidence of Fournier's gangrene—examine the perineum thoroughly.

Inguinal orchidectomy

Inguinal orchidectomy involves the removal of the testis with the spermatic cord. A radical inguinal orchidectomy involves the high ligation of the spermatic cord at the level of the internal ring and is the procedure of choice for suspected testicular cancer.

Indications

Testicular tumour.

Contraindications

Nil.

Preoperative preparation

- The decision to proceed with a radical inguinal orchiectomy in suspected testicular cancer is made after careful consideration of all available data, including clinical findings, imaging studies, and serum tumour markers. It is frequently performed to support a clinical suspicion of testicular cancer, as US scan of a testicular mass cannot replace surgical and histologic examination of the testis.
- Evaluate patient's fertility status as preoperative sperm banking may be required.
- Discuss the role of a testicular prosthesis with the patient.
- Consent after discussing the following complications*:
  - *Common* (>1 in 10): cancer if found may not be cured by removal of the testis alone. Additional treatment such as surgery, radiotherapy or chemotherapy may be needed. Permission is needed to biopsy the other testis if it is small, abnormal, or has not descended properly.
  - *Occasional* (between 1 in 10 and 1 in 50): microscopic examination of the removed testicle may not give a definite result; infection of the incision needing further treatment and possible removal of the implant; bleeding needing further surgery and possible removal of implant, loss of fertility.
  - *Rare* (<1 in 50): pain, infection, or leaking needing removal of implant; cosmetic appearance of the implant may not be acceptable; implant often lies higher in the scrotum than normal testis; it may be possible to feel a stitch at one end of the implant; long-term risks from use of silicone products are not known.

Theatre set-up

- The World Health Organization (WHO) safety checklist is implemented in theatre.
- The patient side of surgery must be marked and confirmed at the time of consent checked.

Procedure

- Make an incision on the side of the tumour-bearing testis similar to an inguinal herniorrhaphy.
- Use diathermy to divide the subcutaneous fat and to expose the external oblique fascia.

- Clean fat bluntly off the fascia for better exposure using a sponge and/or retractors.
- Use scalpel to make a small incision in the external oblique fascia in line with the muscle fibres.
- Extend the incision towards the external ring.
- Identify the ilioinguinal nerve and dissect it carefully off the inner layer of the external oblique fascia.
- Encircle and lift off the spermatic cord using either a swab or penrose drain. Apply a clamp across the spermatic cord at the level of the internal ring to prevent haematogenous dissemination of micrometastases during tumour manipulation.
- By pulling the spermatic cord gently, bring up and deliver the testis from the scrotum. Ligate and divide the gubernaculum. Take care not to divide the scrotal skin. Use blunt dissection to free the scrotum from the testis.
- On delivering the testis, clamp the cord with two more artery forceps and divide near the internal ring. Ligate the cord with 1/0 absorbable suture.
- Close the external oblique fascia followed by the subcutaneous fat and the skin.
- Apply a scrotal support.

Postoperative care

- Wound care.
- Postoperative scrotal support.

Complications

- Wound infection.
- Wound dehiscence.
- Postoperative haematoma.
- Complications of prosthesis insertion (extrusion from scrotum, scrotal contraction and migration, chronic pain, haematoma, and infection).

Tips and tricks

Avoid breach of scrotum.

Transurethral resection of prostate (TURP)

Anatomy

The prostate consists of three zones: peripheral zone, central zone, and transition zone, as described by McNeal (Fig. 10.6).

The transition zone is usually the smallest of the three and occupies only 5% of the prostate volume in men younger than 30 years. This is the zone thought to be the origin of benign prostatic hyperplasia (BPH). The transition zone consists of two separate lobes on either side of the urethra. It usually involves a small grouping of ductal tissue near the central portion of the prostatic urethra near the internal sphincter.

As the transition zone expands, it can comprise up to 95% of the prostate volume, compressing the other zones. During a TURP, the two enlarged lobes of the transition zone can be seen obstructing the prostatic urethra on either side. Thus, the term lateral lobe is often used intraoperatively for this tissue to distinguish it from any hyperplastic periurethral gland tissue.

When a patient undergoes a TURP there is a small risk of post-TURP incontinence. The anatomy and physiology of continence in the male has not been fully elucidated, and there exists varied opinions on neurovascular supply and exact anatomical elements contributing to the maintenance of continence. Continence is thought to be controlled by four main structures: the detrusor muscle, lissosphincter, ureterotrigonal muscles, and rhabdosphincter. The male urethral sphincter complex consists of a smooth muscle and skeletal muscle component. The smooth muscle component

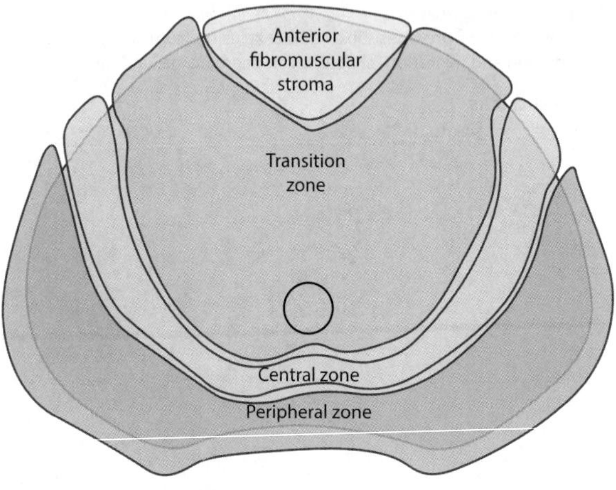
Anterior fibromuscular stroma
Transition zone
Central zone
Peripheral zone

Fig. 10.6 McNeal's prostate zones.

forms the internal or lissosphincter, as a separate entity to the bladder musculature, and is instead derived from the musculature of the urethra. The smooth muscle sphincter surrounds the urethra and lies between the mucosa and the skeletal urethral muscle, and along with connective tissue makes up the bulk of the urethral wall. There is a distinct layer of longitudinal smooth muscle surrounded by circular smooth muscle, whereby contraction of the circular fibres results in urethral narrowing providing continence, while contraction of the longitudinal fibres widens the urethra for urination. The lissosphincter controls passive continence, and holds urine at the level of the vesical orifice; a minimal length is crucial to maintain this.

The skeletal muscle sphincter or rhabdosphincter surrounds the membranous urethra from the apex of the prostate to the corpus spongiosum, in the shape of an inverted horseshoe. It then continues proximally over the anterolateral surface of the prostate as the semilunar cap. The caudal part of the muscle is attached to the posterior median raphe, causing movement of the anterior urethral wall toward the posterior wall when contracted. The rectourethralis muscle, together with Denonvillier's fascia, forms a rigid plate posteriorly, and thus compression of the anterior urethral wall against this produces a transversely flattened urethral lumen. This large surface area results in higher urethral resistance compared with the lissosphincter and hence produces active continence. This urethral occlusion occurs in the membranous urethra for rapid and forceful closure, as demonstrated by increased maximum urethral pressure during urethral pressure profilometry and contrast arrest under fluoroscopy. The nervous supply maintaining continence is complex, and not fully determined. The cavernous nerve, which was originally thought to form a bundle structure, has been found to be in this formation in only 30% of patients, whilst 70% have been shown to have plate formation. The branches provide innervation to the ipsilateral side of the bladder and urethra, but also have some midline extension to supply the contralateral side. The nervous supply of the vesicourethral smooth muscle is from the hypogastric and pelvic nerves for sympathetic and parasympathetic supply, respectively, while the external sphincter receives somatomotor innervation from the pudendal and pelvic nerves.

Indications

- Refractory urinary retention.
- Recurrent urinary tract infections due to prostatic hypertrophy.
- Recurrent gross haematuria.
- Renal insufficiency secondary to bladder outlet obstruction.
- Bladder calculi.
- Permanently damaged or weakened bladder.
- Large bladder diverticula that do not empty well secondary to an enlarged prostate.
- High pressure chronic retention.

Contraindications

- Active urinary tract infection/sepsis.
- Uncontrolled coagulopathy.
- Prostate volume >100g and where resection time is beyond 60min in view of risk of TURP syndrome.

Preoperative preparation

- Preoperative urine culture, clotting profile, and group, and save.
- Consent after discussing the following complications*:
  - *Common* (>1 in 10): temporary mild burning, bleeding, and frequency of urination after the procedure. No semen is produced during an orgasm in approximately 75%. Treatment may not stop all symptoms. Poor erections (impotence in approximately 14%). Infection of the bladder, testicles, or kidneys, which needs antibiotics. Bleeding that may require a return to theatre or a blood transfusion (5%). Possible need to repeat treatment later due to re-obstruction (~10%). Injury to the urethra causing delayed scar formation.
  - *Occasional* (between 1 in 10 and 1 in 50): finding of unsuspected cancer in the removed tissue, which may need further treatment. May need self-catheterization to empty bladder fully if the bladder is weak. Failure to pass urine after surgery, requiring a new catheter. Incontinence, which may be temporary or permanent (2–4%).
  - *Rare* (<1 in 50): irrigating fluids getting into the bloodstream causing confusion and heart failure (TUR syndrome) and, very rarely, perforation of the bladder requiring a temporary urinary catheter or open surgical repair.

Position and theatre set-up

- Implement WHO safety checklist.
- Administer antibiotics at induction as per policy.
- Place in Lloyd–Davis position.
- Clean and drape. A TURP drape is placed that allows the examination of the prostate.

Procedure

- Perform an initial cystoscopy using 22Fr cystoscope to exclude any other pathology, such as urethral stricture or any additional intravesicle pathology.
- Introduce a 26Fr or 28Fr resectoscope and resect the median lobe down to the circular fibres of the bladder neck. Then resect the lateral lobes creating a satisfactory channel. Commence the initial resection at 10 o'clock and 2 o'clock.
- Remove tissue using an Ellik evacuator.
- Secure haemostasis with a rollerball diathermy.
- Place a 22Fr irrigating catheter.

Postoperative care

- Irrigation to continue.
- Watch for symptoms of TURP syndrome.
- Check haemoglobin and sodium as per postoperative progress.

Complications

- Intraoperative and postoperative haemorrhage.
- Bladder perforation.
- TURP syndrome—arises from the absorption of irrigation fluid (1.5% glycine). The fluid is hypotonic in comparison to plasma and this results in dilutional hyponatremia and fluid overload. The clinical manifestations include tachycardia, bradycardia, cardiac dysrhythmias, hypotension, headache, and convulsion. The glycine itself can be metabolized into the GABA pathway to produce neurotransmiter that produces visual disturbances and convulsions.
- Urinary tract infection/chest infection.
- Retrograde ejaculation/erectile dysfunction.
- Urinary incontinence.
- Bladder neck stenosis/urethral stricture.

Tips and tricks

- Always ensure that there is no active infection and that blood is available.
- Identify patients with a high risk of TURP syndrome (>45g resected tissue, >90min resection time).

Transurethral resection of bladder tumour (TURBT)

Anatomy

The urinary bladder is the most anterior organ in the pelvis, located behind the pelvic bone. During transurethral resection of a bladder tumour there is a risk of bladder perforation. Bladder rupture is divided into three broad types: extraperitoneal, intraperitoneal, or combined.

Extraperitoneal rupture is the most common type of bladder injury, accounting for ~85% of cases. It is usually the result of pelvic fractures or penetrating trauma. Cystography reveals a variable path of extravasated contrast material. Intraperitoneal bladder rupture occurs in approximately ~15% of major bladder injuries and typically is the result of a direct blow to the already distended bladder. Cystography demonstrates intraperitoneal contrast material around bowel loops, between mesenteric folds, and in paracolic gutters.

A combined bladder rupture results from simultaneous intraperitoneal and extraperitoneal injury. Cystography usually demonstrates extravasation patterns that are typical for both types of injury. If an intraperitoneal perforation occurs during a TURBT, the patient will require an urgent laparotomy and bladder repair. An extraperitoneal rupture can be managed conservatively with a catheter.

The urinary bladder has four layers that include the epithelium, lamina propria, muscularis propria or detrusor muscle, and perivesical soft tissue.

Indications

- To provide accurate bladder tumour staging and grading.
- Non-muscle invasive bladder tumours.
- Histology for muscle invasive bladder cancer and debulking of tumour pre-chemotherapy.
- To control bleeding from tumour for palliation.

Contraindications

- Active urinary tract infection/sepsis.
- Uncontrolled coagulopathy.

Preoperative preparation

- Preoperative urine culture, clotting profile, and group and save.
- Consent for TURBT discussing the following side-effects*:
  - *Common* (>1 in 10): mild burning or bleeding on passing urine for short period after operation. Need for additional treatments to the bladder to prevent later recurrence of tumours.
  - *Occasional* (between 1 in 10 and 1 in 50): infection of bladder needing antibiotics. No guarantee of cure of cancer by this operation alone. Recurrence of the bladder tumour and/or incomplete removal.
  - *Rare* (<1 in 50): delayed bleeding needing removal of clots or further surgery. Damage to drainage tubes from kidney (ureters) needing additional therapy. Injury to the urethra causing delayed scar formation. Perforation of the bladder needing a temporary urinary catheter or open surgical repair.

Position and theatre set-up

- Implement the WHO safety checklist.
- Administer antibiotics at anaesthetic induction.
- Place patient in Lloyd–Davis position.
- Clean and drape.

Procedure

- Perform a bimanual examination.
- Perform an initial cystoscopy using a 22Fr cystoscope to assess the urethra and bladder.
- Introduce a 26Fr or 28Fr resectoscope.
- Plan the resection of the tumour depending on its location. If the tumour is postero-lateral there is a risk of an 'obturator jerk' during the operation that can result in a perforation (Fig. 10.7).
- Use monopolar diathermy loop to resect the exophytic part of the tumour. Then take deeper resection biopsies for evaluation of invasion of the muscle.
- Use rollerball diathermy for haemostasis and to potentially destroy any atypical cells around the site of the TURBT.
- Introduce a 22Fr three-way catheter.

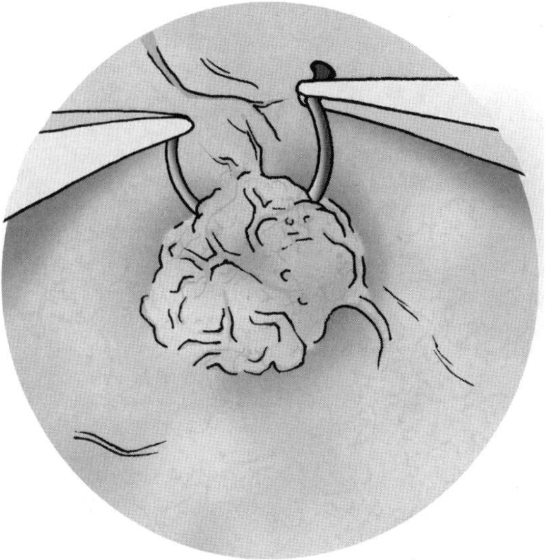

Fig. 10.7 Bladder tumour being resected via the transurethral route using a resectoscope with a loop.

Postoperative care

- Irrigation to continue.
- Postoperative intravesical agent if indicated (mitomycin C).
- Haemoglobin and sodium estimation as per postoperative progress.

Complications

- Intraoperative and postoperative haemorrhage.
- Bladder perforation.
- Urinary tract infection.
- Chest infection.
- Delayed urethral stricture.

Tips and tricks

- If the patient has an 'obturator kick', reduce the diathermy setting and request the anaesthetist to give the patient a muscle relaxant.
- Assess the use of newer TURBT techniques such as photodynamic diagnosis (PDD).

Nephrectomy

Anatomy

The left kidney is located slightly more superior than the right kidney due to the liver. Unlike the other abdominal organs, the kidneys lie behind the peritoneum that lines the abdominal cavity and are thus considered to be retroperitoneal organs. The ribs and muscles of the back protect the kidneys from external damage. Adipose tissue, known as perirenal fat, surrounds the kidneys and acts as a protective padding. Anterior to both kidneys lie the stomach, spleen, tail of pancreas, and descending colon. The blood supply to the kidney is via the renal arteries, which are branches of the aorta.

Nephrectomy is done via an open, laparoscopic, or robotic approach.

Indications

- Malignant neoplasm of the kidney.
- Symptomatic non-functioning kidney.
- As a part of a nephroureterectomy for transitional cell carcinoma of the renal pelvis/ureter.

Contraindications

- Uncontrolled clotting.
- Anaesthetically unfit patient.

Preoperative preparation

- Staging and renal function of the patient must be available.
- Consent patient after discussing the following complications*:
  - *Common* (>1 in 10): bulging of the wound due to damage to the nerves innervating the abdominal wall muscles.
  - *Occasional* (between 1 in 10 and 1 in 50): bleeding needing further surgery or transfusions; infection, pain, or bulging of the incision site needing further treatment; entry into the lung cavity needing insertion of a temporary drainage tube; need of further therapy for cancer.
  - *Rare* (<1 in 50): anaesthetic or cardiovascular problems possibly requiring intensive care admission (including chest infection, pulmonary embolus, stroke, deep vein thrombosis, heart attack, and death); involvement or injury to nearby local structures (blood vessels, spleen, liver, lung, pancreas, and bowel) needing more extensive surgery; the pathology of the kidney may subsequently be shown not to be cancer; dialysis may be needed to improve kidney function if other kidney functions poorly.

Theatre set-up

- Implement the WHO safety checklist.
- Side of surgery must be marked, confirm at the time of consent check.

Procedure

- The commonest approach used for an open nephrectomy is either transabdominal or thoracoabdominal. The laparoscopic or robotic nephrectomy approach can be either transperitoneal or reteroperitoneal.
- For left nephrectomy, reflect the colon and dissect up to Gerota's fascia. Divide the lino-renal and spleno-renal ligaments.
- Carefully dissect the spleen off the kidney and mobilize the upper pole.
- For right nephrectomy, divide the hepatorenal ligaments.
- Expose the renal hilum and divide the renal artery initially followed by the renal vein.
- For tumours that are large and involve the IVC, expose the IVC further.
- When a tumour thrombus is high and extends into the heart, then surgery must be performed with an additional specialist.
- Whilst performing a radical nephrectomy, divide the ureter at a point of view; however, in patients undergoing a nephreoureterectomy, divide the ureter at the level of the ureteric orifice. The ureteric orifice can also be resected with a cystoscope in certain patients
- Close all port sites in patients undergoing laparoscopic and robotic nephrectomy
- Place a drain, if indicated, at the level of the renal bed.

Postoperative care

- Test postoperative haemoglobin and renal function.
- Low molecular weight heparin prophylaxis.

Complications

- Injury to spleen/liver/colon/pancreas/superior mesenteric artery.
- Urinoma (in patients undergoing a nephroureterctomy).

Prostatectomy

A radical prostatectomy is the surgical removal of the prostate with the seminal vesicles. During a radical prostatectomy there is risk of nerve damage and damage to different mechanisms responsible for urinary continence. The prostate itself has a degree of control of continence as part of the proximal sphincteric unit and this is lost with the removal of the prostate. In addition to this, the proximal urethral sphincter itself is lost. Therefore, continence depends largely on the rhabdosphincter postoperatively. Furthermore, the proximity of the neurovascular supply and rhabdosphincter to the prostate puts these structures at high risk of damage intraoperatively. The bladder is also affected by radical prostatectomy with effects on detrusor innervation and function.

Indications

- Organ-confined prostate cancer.
- Salvage prostatectomy (post-radiotherapy/post-brachytherapy).

Contraindications

Uncontrolled clotting or anaesthetically unfit patient.

Preoperative preparation

- Preoperative enema.
- Consent after discussing the following complications*:
    - *Common* (>1 in 10): impotence due to unavoidable nerve damage (60–90%); the risk will depend on whether the surgeon removes one or both nerves because of tumour involvement; inability to ejaculate or father children because the structures that produce seminal fluid have been removed (occurs in all patients); urinary incontinence (temporary or permanent) needing pads or further surgery (3–30%); minor problems with urinary leakage.
    - *Occasional* (between 1 in 10 and 1 in 50): scarring at the bladder exit resulting in weakening of the urinary stream and needing further surgery (~14%); serious urinary incontinence (temporary or permanent) needing pads or further surgery (2–5%); blood loss needing transfusion or repeat surgery; discovery that cancer cells have already spread outside the prostate needing further treatment; apparent shortening of the penis; further treatment at a later date, if required this may include radiotherapy or hormone treatment; lymph fluid collection in the pelvis if node sampling has been performed; development of a hernia in the groin at least 6 months after the operation.

Theatre set-up

- Implement WHO safety checklist.
- Position patient either in the supine position for open prostatectomy or steep Trendelenburg position for robotic prostatectomy.

Procedure

- The commonest approach currently in USA and Europe is robotic radical prostatectomy.
- Patient is placed in supine position and pnemoperiteum created using open Hasson technique.

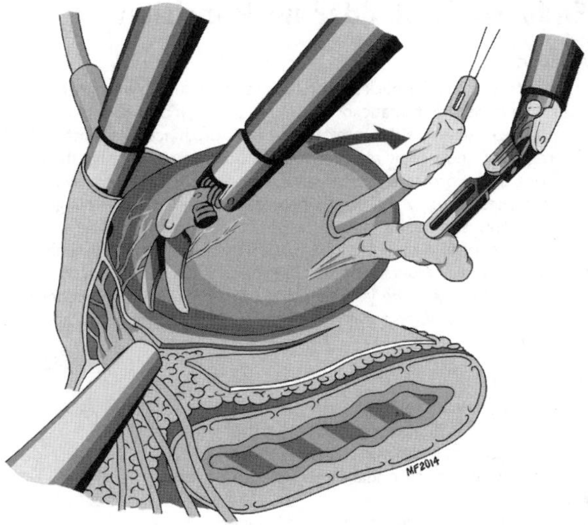
MF2014

Fig. 10.8 Robotic radical prostatectomy.

- Additional robotic and laparoscopic ports are placed under vision.
- The endopelvic fascia is incised and the dorsal venous complex is exposed. The bladder neck is opened and preserved if possible (Fig. 10.8).
- A plane is developed between the prostate and bladder followed by dissection of the seminal vesicles and vas deferens.
- The prostatic pedicles are divided with Weck clips or ligated with 2/0 absorbable sutures.
- A nerve spare is then performed followed by opening the Denonvilliers' fascia. The dorsal vein complex is divided followed by division of urethra and rectourethralis.
- An urethrovescile anastomosis is performed with a 3/0 absorbable suture.

Postoperative care

- Postoperative haemoglobin and renal function test.
- Low molecular weight heparin prophylaxis.

Complications

- Injury to rectum.
- Urine leak.
- Erectile dysfunction.
- Urinary incontinence.

Tips and tricks

Ensure nerve sparing, if appropriate, without compromising oncological outcome.

Endoscopic bladder neck incision

Anatomy

In patients with bladder neck stenosis or in those patients with smaller prostates who have symptomatic lower urinary tract symptoms, an endoscopic bladder neck incision is the surgical treatment of choice as against a TURP. The region of endoscopic bladder neck incision surgery is within the transition zone of the prostate. The transition zone is usually the smallest of the three: it occupies only 5% of the prostate volume in men younger than 30 years. This is the zone thought to be the origin of BPH. The transition zone consists of two separate lobes on either side of the urethra and usually involves a small grouping of ductal tissue near the central portion of the prostatic urethra near the internal sphincter. An endoscopic bladder neck incision can either be performed with the use of monopolar diathermy or Holmium laser.

Indications

- Refractory urinary retention.
- Recurrent UTIs due to prostatic hypertrophy.
- Recurrent gross haematuria.
- Renal insufficiency secondary to bladder outlet obstruction.
- Bladder calculi.
- Permanently damaged or weakened bladders.
- Large bladder diverticula that do not empty well secondary to an enlarged prostate.
- High pressure chronic retention.
- Post-radical prostatectomy anastomotic stricture.

Contraindications

Active urinary tract infection/sepsis.

Preoperative preparation

- Preoperative urine culture, clotting profile, and group and save.
- Patient consented for bladder neck incision after discussing the following specific side-effects on the basis of the British Association of Urological Surgeons procedure-specific consent form*:
  - *Common* (>1 in 10): temporary mild burning, bleeding, and frequency when passing urine; no semen is produced during an orgasm in approximately 20%; treatment may not relieve all the urinary symptoms and poor erections (impotence) in approximately 14%; infection of the bladder, testicles, or kidney requiring antibiotic treatment; need to repeat the treatment later due to further blockage (~10%) and injury to the urethra (water pipe) causing delayed scar formation.
  - *Occasional* (between 1 in 10 and 1 in 50): need to self-catheterize to empty bladder fully; failure to pass urine needing bladder catheter.
  - *Rare* (<1 in 50): bleeding requiring either a return to theatre or blood transfusion (<2%).

Theatre set-up

- The World Health Organization (WHO) safety checklist is implemented in theatre.
- Patient receives antibiotics at anaesthetic induction.

Procedure

- Patient is placed in the Lloyd–Davies position.
- Place a TURP drape that allows the examination of the prostate.
- Perform cystoscopy to exclude any other pathology, such as urethral stricture or any additional intravesicle pathology.
- Introduce a 26Fr or 28Fr resectoscope. Make a bladder neck incision with a Collin's knife at 5 and 7 0'clock positions. Avoid incision at 6 o'clock to prevent injury to the rectum.
- Remove tissue via an Ellik evacuator.
- Secure haemostasis with a rollerball diathermy.
- Irrigate using a 22Fr catheter.

Postoperative care

- Irrigation to continue.
- Watch for symptoms of TURP syndrome.
- Haemoglobin and sodium check as per postoperative progress.

Complications

- Intraoperative and postoperative bleeding.
- Bladder perforation.
- TURP syndrome—arises from absorption of irrigation fluid (1.5% glycine). The fluid is hypotonic in comparison to plasma and this results in dilutional hyponatremia and fluid overload. The clinical manifestations include tachycardia, bradycardia, cardiac dyshrythmias, hypotension, headache, and convulsion. The glycine itself can be metabolized into the GABA pathway to produce a neurotransmitter that produces visual disturbances and convulsions.
- Retrograde ejaculation/erectile dysfunction.
- Urinary incontinence.
- Bladder neck stenosis/urethral stricture.

Pyeloplasty

A pelvi-ureteric junction (PUJ) obstruction is a narrowing at the PUJ that obstructs the flow of urine from the renal pelvis to the proximal ureter. The condition affects both children and adults. A PUJ obstruction is the commonest congenital cause of urinary tract obstruction. A pyeloplasty can be performed using robotic, laparoscopic, or open methods.

Indications

- Paediatric patients:
  - Reduced function of affected kidney.
  - Symptoms of pain or UTI.
  - Deterioration in renal function.
  - Concern that renal function will decline if the kidney is left untreated.
- Adult patients:
  - Symptoms of pain or recurrent UTI.
  - Deterioration in renal function.

Contraindications

Active urinary tract infection/sepsis.

Preoperative preparation

- Preoperative imaging confirming PUJ obstruction, urine culture.
- Consent for pyeloplasty discussing the following complications*:
  - *Common* (>1 in 10): further procedure to remove ureteric stent usually under a local anaesthetic; bulging of the wound due to damage to the nerves in the abdominal wall muscles.
  - *Occasional* (between 1 in 10 and 1 in 50): bleeding needing further surgery or transfusions; entry into the pleural cavity needing insertion of a temporary drainage tube.
  - *Rare* (<1 in 50): recurrent kidney or bladder infections, which may need further surgery; anaesthetic or cardiovascular problems possibly requiring intensive care admission (including chest infection, pulmonary embolus, stroke, deep vein thrombosis, heart attack); need to remove kidney at a later time because of damage caused by recurrent obstruction or infection; pain or hernia of incision site needing further treatment.

Theatre set-up

- Implement the WHO safety checklist.
- Confirm the side of the surgery.
- Administer antibiotics at induction.

Procedure

- All patients have a cystoscopic JJ stent insertion either on table during the time of pyeloplasty or the stent can be placed a few days prior to pyeloplasty.
- The patient is placed in the supine position with a rolled-up towel underneath. Use transverse 12th rib incision.
- Expose the kidney and dissect anteromedially to the PUJ region. Identify vessel crossing at PUJ.

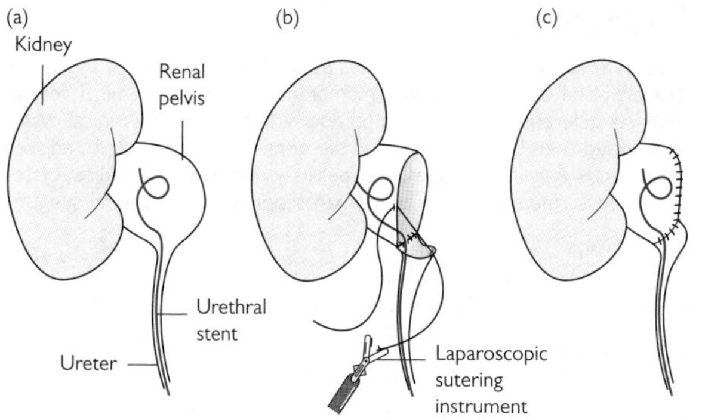
(a)
(b)
(c)
Kidney
Renal pelvis
Urethral stent
Ureter
Laparoscopic sutering instrument

Fig. 10.9 Insertion of urethral stent (a); laparoscopic Anderson–Hynes pyeloplasty (b/c).

- Place stay sutures on the renal pelvis and on the proximal ureter.
- Divide the PUJ at the point of maximum narrowing.
- Spatulate the ureter.
- Reduce the excessive renal pelvis and perform anastomosis between the ureter and pelvis over the JJ stent using absorbable 3/0 or 4/0 sutures.
- Laparoscopic pyeloplasty is shown in Fig. 10.9. The pneumoperitoneum is created either in the transperitoneal or retroperitoneal space. The PUJ is identified and a 3/0 absorbable suture is placed through the renal pelvis. The PUJ is mobilized and the abnormal narrowed region is excised. Similar to open pyeloplasty, excessive pelvis is excised and anastomosis between the pelvis and ureter is performed in a tension-free manner over the JJ stent.

Postoperative care

JJ Stent removal in 4–6 weeks postoperatively.

Complications

- Urine leak.
- Recurrent obstruction requiring redo-pyeloplasty or nephrectomy.

Cystectomy

In males a radical cystectomy includes the en bloc dissection of the urinary bladder, distal ureters, prostate, membraneous urethra, seminal vesicles, distal vas deferens, and pelvic lymph nodes. In the female a radical cystectomy includes en bloc dissection of the urinary bladder, urethra, adjacent vagina, uterus, Fallopian tubes, and pelvic lymph nodes. A radical cystectomy is performed using the open, laparoscopic or robotic technique.

Indications

- Muscle invasive bladder cancer.
- Non-muscle invasive bladder cancer (high-grade disease, BCG failures).

Contraindications

Active urinary tract infection/sepsis.

Preoperative preparation

- Appropriately well-counselled and selected patient.
- Consent for cystectomy discussing the following complications*:
  - *Common* (>1 in 10): cancer may not be cured with removal of bladder alone.
  - *Occasional* (between 1 in 10 and 1 in 50): anaesthetic or cardiovascular problems possibly requiring intensive care admission (including chest infection, pulmonary embolus, stroke, DVT, heart attack); infection or hernia of the incision requiring further treatment; need to remove the penile urethra as part of the procedure; blood loss requiring repeat surgery; decreased kidney function with time; diarrhoea/vitamin deficiency due to shortened bowel requiring treatment.
  - *Rare* (<1 in 50): bowel and urine leakage from anastomosis requiring reoperation; scarring to the bowel or ureters requiring operation in future; scarring, narrowing, or hernia formation around stomal opening requiring revision; intraoperative rectal injury requiring colostomy.

Theatre setup

- Implement the WHO safety checklist.
- Administer antibiotics at induction.

Procedure

- Make a lower midline incision through the skin, subcutaneous fat, superficial and deep fascia, anterior rectus sheath, transversalis fascia. Open the peritoneum.
- Divide the urachus at the level of the umbilicus and carry the dissection down to the level of the bladder, dividing both the median umbilical ligaments.
- During the lateral mobilization of the bladder, divide the ovarian and round ligaments. The initial dissection of the lateral margin of the bladder is the vas deferens in males.
- Divide and ligate the ureters individually at the level of the superior vesicle pedicles.

- Lateral dissection is completed on the division of the endopelvic fascia and division of the inferior vesicle pedicles.
- Commence the anterior dissection by entering the space of Retzius. Divide the dorsal venous complex.
- Commence the dissection by creating the perivesicle space between the rectum and the bladder up to the tips of both seminal vesicles by opening the Denovillier's fascia. In female patients the posterior fornix is opened. The incisions in the vagina are extended on either side inferiorly to join the dissected urethra anteriorly.
- Carry out an extended pelvic lymph node dissection.
- Patients can have a urinary diversion (continent reservoir or non-continent technique).
- Close the wound in layers.

Postoperative care

Follow enhanced recovery protocol.

Complications

- Wound infection.
- Wound dehiscence.
- Urine leak.
- Anastomotic bowel leak.
- Postoperative complications (DVT, PE, UTI).
- Local/distal recurrence.

Ileal conduit diversion

When a radical cystectomy is performed, an ileal conduit is created for a urinary diversion. There is risk of hyperchloraemic acidosis associated with obstruction of the stoma at its distal end or with infrequent emptying of the stoma bag. When urine is in contact with the bowel wall, ammonia, hydrogen, and chloride are also reabsorbed. This results in a chronic acid load. A large-bowel surface area, prolonged contact time, patient co-morbidities, and pre-existing renal failure contribute to the development of metabolic complications. Patients with reservoirs are at increased risk than those with simple conduits due to the prolonged contact time with urine and the larger surface area. Patients may present with weakness, anorexia, and vomiting.

Indications

Urinary diversion.

Contraindications

- Active UTI/sepsis.
- Severe renal/liver dysfunction.

Preoperative preparation

- Preoperatively counsel patient with regard to application/details of stoma bag.
- Ileal conduit site marked and bowel preparation given.
- Consent for ileal conduit formation discussing the following complications*:
  - *Common* (>1 in 10): high risk of impotence in men; inability to ejaculate or father children; cancer may not be cured with removal of bladder alone.
  - *Occasional* (between 1 in 10 and 1 in 50): anaesthetic or cardiovascular problems possibly requiring intensive care admission (including chest infection, pulmonary embolus, stroke, DVT, heart attack and death); infection or hernia of the incision requiring further treatment; need to remove the penile urethra as part of the procedure; bleeding requiring repeat surgery; decreased kidney function with time; diarrhoea/vitamin deficiency due to shortened bowel requiring treatment.
  - *Rare* (<1 in 50): recurrent kidney or bladder infections; need to remove kidney at later time because of damage caused by recurrent obstruction; bowel and urine leakage from anastomosis requiring reoperation; narrowing or hernia formation around stomal opening requiring revision.

Theatre set-up

- Implement WHO safety checklist.
- Administer antibiotics at induction.

Procedure

- Make a midline incision and open the peritoneum.
- Identify both the ureters. Transpose left ureter to the right side below the sigmoid mesocolon.

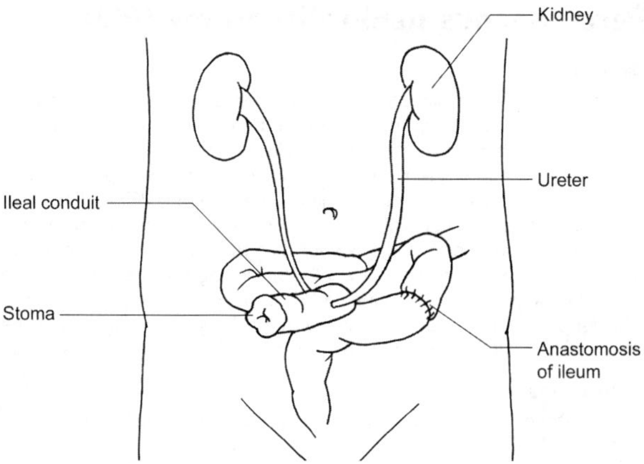
Kidney
Ureter
Ileal conduit
Stoma
Anastomosis of ileum

Fig. 10.10 Ileal conduit formation using Brickers anastomosis.

- Chose a segment of ileum approximately 15–20cm from the ileo-caecal junction.
- Both ureteric segments are either anastomosed together using the Wallace plate or are anastomosed individually using the Bricker's technique over stents (Fig. 10.10).
- Complete the ileo-ureteric anastomosis.
- Form a stoma and bring it up to the anterior abdominal wall.

Postoperative care

Removal of conduit stents.

Complications

- Urine leak.
- UTIs.
- Parastomal hernia.
- Stenosis.
- Metabolic complications.

Percutaneous nephrolithotomy (PCNL)

Anatomy

A percutaneous nephrolithotomy (PCNL) is an endourological procedure that aims to remove stones from the kidney by a small puncture wound (up to ~1cm) through the skin. The kidneys lie in the retroperitoneum, although a significant portion of each is actually supracostal, the lower pole is nearly always subcostal. There is a risk of pneumothorax during PCNL. The longitudinal axis of each kidney is oblique and dorsally inclined, making the upper pole calyces more medial and posterior than the inferior pole. The posterior calyces of the kidney are at a 30° oblique angle to the vertical plane when the patient is prone. During a PCNL direct puncture of the infundibulum is associated with risk of injury to renal vessels or branches of the renal artery resulting in bleeding and formation of an arterio-venous fistula.

Indications

- Renal stones >3cm in size, renal pelvis stones >2cm, and lower pole stones >1cm.
- Stone position and anatomical abnormality that will prevent stone clearance using extracorporeal shockwave lithotripsy (ESWL) or ureteroscopic techniques.
- Failed ESWL/failed ureteroscopy.
- Stones associated with foreign bodies (stent).
- Patient choice.
- Paediatric patients with large stones.
- Stones in horseshoe kidneys.

Contraindications

- Active UTI/sepsis.
- Pregnancy.

Preoperative preparation

- Preoperative imaging indicating side.
- Consent for PCNL discussing the following complications*:
  - *Common* (>1 in 10): blood in the urine (temporary); Raised temperature (temporary).
  - *Occasional* (between 1 in 10 and 1 in 50): occasionally the surgeon will need to make more than one puncture, there is no guarantee all the stones will be removed, further operations may be required; new stone-formation; inability to get access to the kidney and need for further surgery.
  - *Rare* (<1 in 50): severe kidney bleeding requiring transfusion, embolization, or as a last resort removal of kidney; damage to the lung, bowel, spleen, liver, which may need surgery; kidney damage or infection needing further treatment; irrigating fluids may get into the blood system and cause a strain on the heart.

Theatre set-up

- Implement the WHO safety checklist.
- Confirm side of the surgery.
- Administer antibiotics at induction.

Procedure

- The patient is placed in prone or supine position.
- Kidney is localized using US and/or fluoroscopic guidance.
- A reterograde catheter is used to opacify and identify the pelvicalycael system. The appropriate calyx is identified and punctured.
- A guide wire is advanced into the pelvicalyceal system and into the ureter.
- Serial dilation of the tract is performed using dilators.
- A large sheath is placed into the main tract and a rigid nephroscope is passed through the sheath along the guidewire into the pelvicalyceal system (Fig. 10.11).
- Ultrasonic, electrohydraulic, laser, or pneumatic lithotripsy is used to fragment the stones. Stone fragments are extracted.
- Additional fragments can be removed by passing a flexible cystoscope or flexible ureteroscope.
- On completion of stone extraction the sheath is removed and a pigtail ureteric stent is attached to a large-bore nephrostomy catheter.
- In certain situations an antegrade stent is inserted without the insertion of nephrostomy catheter.

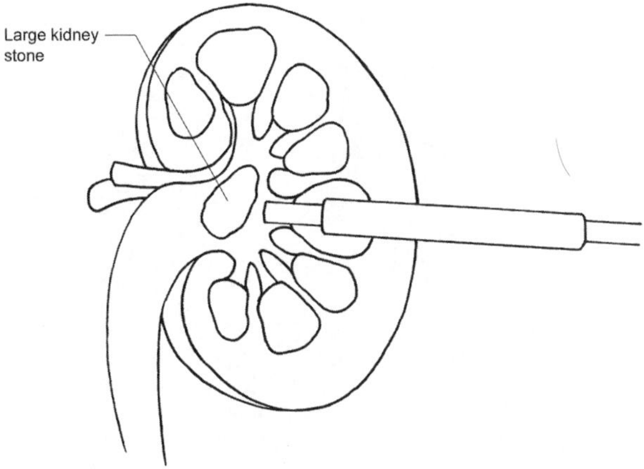
Large kidney
stone

Fig. 10.11 Nephroscope being used during PCNL.

Postoperative care

- Antibiotics.
- Postoperative radiological imaging to ensure stone clearance if indicated.

Complications

- Bleeding.
- Perforation of bowel.
- Access failure.
- Infection
- TUR syndrome.
- Extravasation.
- Pneumothorax/pleural effusion.
- Residual stones.

Rigid ureteroscopy

Anatomy

In adults, the ureters are usually 25–30cm (10–12in) long and ~3–4mm in diameter. The ureter contains transitional epithelium and an additional smooth muscle layer in the distal one-third. The blood supply of the upper ureteric is by renal arteries, the mid-ureter by the common iliac artery, the abdominal aorta, and the gonadal artery, and the lower ureter is supplied by branches from the internal iliac artery. A kidney stone has a high chance of getting obstructed at the level of the pelvi-ureteric junction, at the level of the ureter crossing the iliac vessels. and at vesicoureteric junction.

Indications

- Stone extraction.
- Endoscopic management of ureteric lesions.
- Diagnostic procedure for ureteric lesions.
- Biopsy.

Contraindications

Active UTI/sepsis.

Preoperative preparation

- Preoperative imaging indicating side.
- Consent for ureteroscopy discussing the following complications*:
  - *Common* (>1 in 10): mild burning or bleeding on passing urine for a short period after operation; insertion of a stent with a further procedure to remove it; the stent may cause pain, urinary frequency, and blood in urine.
  - *Occasional* (between 1 in 10 and 1 in 50): it may not be possible to retrieve the stone; displacement of the stone into an inaccessible site in the kidney; kidney damage or infection needing further treatment; failure to pass the telescope if the ureter is narrow; recurrence of stones.
  - *Rare* (<1 in 50): damage to the ureter with need for open operation or tube placed into kidney directly from back to allow any leak to heal; scarring or stricture of the ureter needing further procedures.

Theatre set-up

- Implement WHO safety checklist.
- Confirm side.
- Administer antibiotics at induction.

Procedure

- Place patient in lithotomy or Lloyd–Davis position.
- Perform a rigid cystoscopy.
- Cannulate the ureteric orifice on the side of surgery and advance into the upper ureter and pelvi-ureteric junction.
- Dilate the ureteric orifice with a balloon dilator if required.
- Introduce a rigid ureteroscope and identify the stone/lesion.

- If a stone is found, use an energy source such as electrohydraulic, laser (pulse-dye or holmium YAG) to fragment the stone. An ultrasonic energy source should not be used in the ureter due the high temperature leading to ureteric damage.
- If the lesion being investigated is thought to be malignant, take a ureteric biopsy with a cold-cup forceps.
- At the end of the rigid ureteroscopy, place a stent,

Postoperative care

- Antibiotics.
- Postoperative radiological imaging to ensure stone clearance if indicated.

Complications

- Bleeding.
- Perforation of ureter.
- Urinary extravasation.
- Infection.
- Stricture.

Tips and tricks

Never force a ureteroscope into the ureter; in the event of any resistance, place a JJ stent and return for a further procedure in a few weeks (4–6 weeks).

Optical urethrotomy

Anatomy

Optical urethrotomy is an endoscopic incision of a urethral stricture. The male urethra is a narrow fibromuscular tube. It is a single structure composed of a heterogeneous series of segments: prostatic, membranous, and spongy. The blood supply of the male urethra is derived from the internal pudendal branch of the internal iliac artery. This artery enters the perineum via the pudedal cancal and terminates into the common penile artery. Additional blood supply to the urethra is from the bulbourethral and dorsal penile branches. The generous blood supply is the reason why further surgery, such as urethroplasty, is an option for recurrent/dense strictures.

Indications

- Short urethral stricture (<1.5cm).
- Strictures located at the bulbar urethra.
- Strictures associated with minimal spongiofibrosis.
- Primary strictures not previously treated.

Contraindications

Active urinary tract infection/sepsis.

Preoperative preparation

Consent for optical urethrotomy discussing the following complications:

- *Common* (>1 in 10): mild burning or bleeding on passing urine for a short period after the operation; need for self-catheterization to keep the narrowing from closing down again; recurrence of narrowing needing further procedures or repeat incision.
- *Occasional* (between 1 in 10 and 1 in 50): infection of the bladder needing antibiotics; permission for telescopic removal or biopsy of any bladder abnormality or stone, if found.
- *Rare* (<1 in 50): decrease in the quality of erections.

Theatre set-up

- Implement the WHO safety checklist.
- Administer antibiotics induction.

Procedure

- Place patient in lithotomy or Lloyd–Davis position.
- Perform a rigid cystoscopy.
- Identify the stricture and pass a guide wire through the stricture into the bladder. Introduce an optical urethrotome and incise the stricture with knife.
- Advance the optical urethrotome into the bladder.
- Introduce a catheter over the guide wire.

Postoperative care

Need for commencement of intermittent self-catheterization/dilatation.

Complications

- Bleeding.
- Perforation of the urethra requiring a suprapubic catheter insertion.

Tips and tricks

In the event of a very narrow stricture, a rigid ureteroscope can be introduced to evaluate the stricture and to pass a wire through the stricture.

Penile implant

Anatomy

A penile implant is inserted for severe erectile dysfunction. A penile implant is a device that is either malleable (bendable) or inflatable. The simplest type of prosthesis consists of a pair of malleable rods surgically implanted within the erection chambers of the penis. With this type of implant the penis is always semi-rigid and merely needs to be lifted or adjusted into the erect position to initiate sex.

Indications

- Medically refractory severe erectile dysfunction.
- Emergency insertion in post-priapism.

Contraindications

Active urinary tract infection/sepsis.

Preoperative preparation

Consent for penile implant by discussing the following complications:

- *Common* (>1 in 10): temporary swelling and bruising of the penis lasting several days.
- *Occasional* (between 1 in 10 and 1 in 50): significant bleeding or infection needing further treatment (including removal of all or part of the prosthesis in 2–3%); nerve injury with temporary or permanent numbness of the head of the penis; drooping of the glans penis needing correction; mechanical failure needing revision at a later stage, this may involve replacement of all or part of the device and can happen at any stage from a few month to several years later; self-inflation due to mechanical failure.
- *Rare* (<1 in 50): injury to the bowel or bladder during insertion of the balloon component within the abdomen; erosion of the prosthesis where a part of the device may break out of its normal position and appear at another site.

Theatre set-up

- Implement WHO safety checklist.
- Administer antibiotics at induction.

Procedure

- Patient is placed in supine position.
- Insert Foley catheter and drain bladder.
- The initial incision can be infrapubic, scrotal, or subcoronal.
- Identify the corpora cavernosa. Make a corporotomy measuring 2–3cm from the edge of the glans and extend proximally.
- Dilate the corpora cavernosa using serial Heger or Rossello dilators. The final dilation has to be up to the ischial tuberosity.
- Insert the prosthesis. This can be either malleable or inflatable. An inflatable penile implant consists of a three-piece implant: a reservoir that is implanted into the abdomen, a pump that is placed in the scrotum, and pair of cylinders that are placed in the penis.

Postoperative care

Antibiotics.

Complications

- Infection.
- Erosion.
- Mechanical failure requiring reoperation.

Trans-obturator/trans-vaginal tape

Anatomy

Stress urinary incontinence is a devastating condition that afflicts 20% of the women. Although many therapeutic options are available, surgical treatment remains the most effective. In tension-free vaginal tape (TVT) surgery, a mesh tape is placed under the urethra like a sling or hammock to keep it in its normal position. The tape is inserted through tiny incisions in the abdomen and vaginal wall. No sutures are required to hold the tape in place. Other sling procedures are done in a way that is similar to TVT surgery.

Indications

Stress incontinence secondary to detrusor areflexia and low pressure sphincter.

Contraindications

Active urinary tract infection/sepsis.

Preoperative preparation

Consent for synthetic vaginal tape for stress incontinence after discussing the following complications:

- *Common* (>1 in 10): need to go to the toilet frequently and urgently, and sometimes with urine leakage due to the urgency; failure so patient continues to have bad leakage; some women will have mild leakage; inability to empty the bladder completely needing either to keep a catheter in all the time or to insert a catheter several times a day (intermittent self-catheterization); infection; slow urine flow; recurrence of stress incontinence can happen years after the tape has been inserted; some discomfort/pain for a while, usually where the skin was cut during the operation; TOT can cause thigh or groin pain but this can be relieved by simple painkillers in most patients. There are occasions when more powerful painkillers may be needed.
- *Occasional* (between 1 in 10 and 1 in 50): injury to the bladder during the TVT operation (the risk is much less for TOT surgery); misplacement of the tape, this should be discovered at the time of surgery and the tape re-positioned correctly; pain or discomfort during sexual intercourse for either patient or sexual partner (9%, 1 in 11); bleeding, injury to surrounding tissues (e.g. bladder, rectum, and blood vessels); erosion of the tape into the vagina;, bladder, or urethra—this can occur years after the operation. The estimated risk is in 5 out of every 100 operations.
- *Rare* (<1 in 50): migration of the tape into the vagina, bladder, or urethra, which can happen several years after the tape was inserted. Symptoms such as recurrent UTI, change in urinary symptoms, vaginal discharge, and discomfort during intercourse may occur.

Theatre set-up

- Implement WHO safety checklist.
- Administer antibiotics at induction.

Procedure

- The patient is placed in the gynaecological position with thighs in hyperflexion. Insert a urethral catheter.
- Make a 1cm incision on anterior vaginal wall 1cm proximal to urethral meatus.
- Introduce fine dissection scissors through the incision towards the upper part of the ischio-pubic ramus in a horizontal plane to the urethra.
- Once the upper part of the ischio-pubic ramus is reached, perforate the obturator membrane with tip of scissors.
- Push an introducer, with the open side of its gutter facing you, along the preformed dissection canal until it reaches and perforates the obturator membrane. Gently slip the distal end of the tube mounted onto the spiral segment of the needle along the gutter of the introducer in order to pass through the obturator foramen. Remove the introducer. (See Fig. 10.12.)
- After the tube has appeared at the previously determined skin exit point, pull it off from the supporting needle. Remove needle.
- Apply same technique on the other side.
- Cut the ends of both tapes. Align the tape without any tension under the middle of the urethra by creating a space using a blunt clamp. Bury the ends of both tapes subcutaneously.

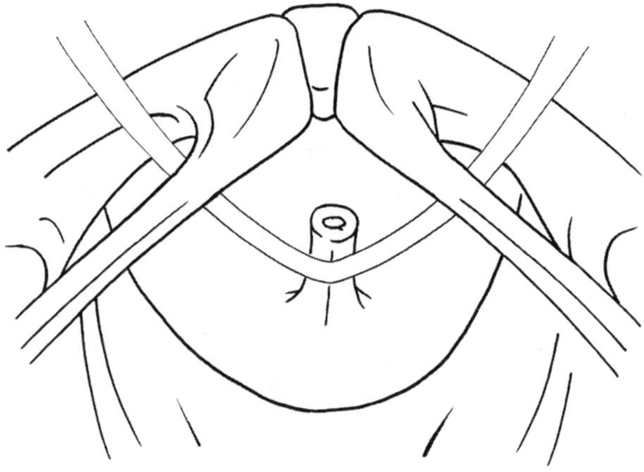

Fig. 10.12 Final position of the tape under the urethra.

Postoperative care

- Antibiotics.
- Removal of catheter.

Complications

- Bladder perforation.
- Bleeding.
- Urethral laceration.
- Bowel injury/neural injury.
- Erosion of tape.
- Urinary tract infection.
- Postoperative voiding dysfunction.
- Urinary retention and need for intermittent self-catheterization.

Tips and tricks

- Always ensure patient catheterized and bladder is empty prior to commencing procedure.
- A cystoscope should be available in theatre in case an on-table cystoscopy is required at the time of tape insertion.

Cystoplasty

Cystoplasty is a surgical technique used to increase bladder capacity by augmentation of the bladder using a segment of bowel. The principal is to bi-valve the bladder coronally and patch the defect with small bowel, which is generally ileum. The technique impairs bladder contraction, lowers the detrusor pressure, and increases bladder capacity.

Indications

Refractory overactive bladder.

Contraindications

- Severe inflammatory bowel disease (i.e. Crohn's disease).
- Previous pelvic radiotherapy.
- Critical short bowel.
- Inability to self-catheterize.
- Significant renal and hepatic impairment.

Preoperative preparation

Consent patient for augmentation cystoplasty discussing the following complications:

- *Common* (>1 in 10): infection or hernia in the incision requiring further treatment; diarrhoea/vitamin deficiency due to shortened bowel requiring treatment; anastomotic leak; urine leak; recurrent infections; temporary or long-term tendency for the blood to be more acidic than normal; need for self-catheterization; passing mucus in the urine.
- *Occasional* (between 1 in 10 and 1 in 50): blood loss requiring further surgery; scarring of the bowel or ureter; anaesthetic or cardiovascular problems requiring intensive care admissions.
- *Rare* (<1 in 50): tumour formation where the bowel patch is joined to the bladder and need for follow-up.

Theatre set-up

- Implement WHO safety checklist.
- Administer antibiotics at anaesthetic induction.

Procedure

- The patient is placed in the supine position.
- Make lower midline incision and open peritoneum.
- Identify 20–25cm segment of ileum, which reaches the pelvis. Avoid 20cm of ileum from the ileo-caecal junction.
- Mobilize the mesenteric pedicle.
- Restore ileal continuity.
- Incise the anti-mesenteric border of the isolated segment.
- Bivalve bladder using midline sagittal incision.
- Configure the opened segment of the bowel like an inverted U and suture on to the bladder.
- Place urinary catheter.
- Close in layers.

Postoperative care

- Antibiotics.
- Removal of catheter after cystogram.

Complications

- Bladder perforation.
- Bleeding.
- Chronic bacteriuria.
- Metabolic alterations (acidosis/bone demineralization).
- Need for intermittent self-catheterization.
- Malignancy.

Tips and tricks

Ensure that renal function and liver function are optimized prior to surgery.

Chapter 11

Plastic and reconstructive surgery

The specialty of plastic and reconstructive surgery

Plastic surgery is a diverse, responsive, ever-evolving specialty, which interlinks with and is frequently involved in the undertaking of joint procedures with other specialties for some of the more demanding surgical procedures.

In reconstruction, the plastic surgeon follows the 'reconstructive ladder' (Fig. 11.1), which sets out the principles to cover any wound starting from the simplest techniques and gradually progressing in complexity: from healing by secondary intention, through direct closure, skin grafting, flaps, and variants thereof.

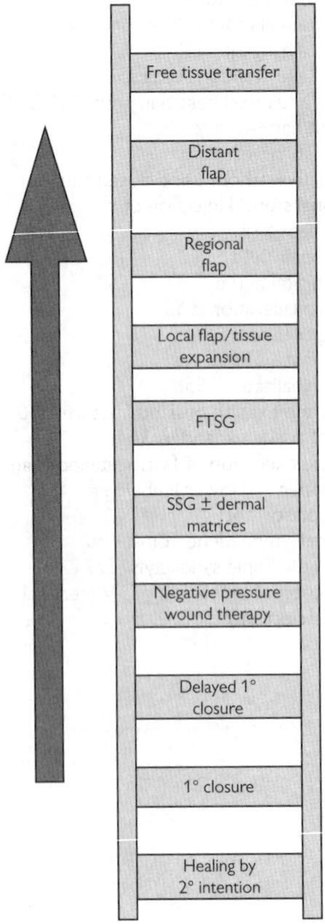

Free tissue transfer
Distant flap
Regional flap
Local flap/tissue expansion
FTSG
SSG ± dermal matrices
Negative pressure wound therapy
Delayed 1° closure
1° closure
Healing by 2° intention

Fig. 11.1 The reconstructive ladder.

The word 'plastic' comes from the Greek '*plastikos*', which means 'to mould' or 'to form', and indeed a primary aim is for the *restoration of normal form and function*. The specialty is defined as 'the combination of various surgical skills and techniques to attempt to restore normal, functional anatomy from the abnormal, whether the abnormality is congenital, traumatic or as a result of a disease process such as cancer or infection'. It is indeed far more diverse and innovative a specialty than lay people or even those medically qualified often realize (1). It is our intention that this chapter will be of aid in grasping the basics of the craft and we hope that you may have the opportunity at some point in your career to work alongside some of the modern-day pioneers of the specialty.

Useful websites

British Association for Surgery of the Hand: www.bssh.ac.uk
British Association of Plastic Surgery: www.bapras.org.uk
British Burns Association: www.britishburnassociation.org Note, both BAPRAS and the BSSH run a series of affordable all-encompassing 'Instructional courses', endorsed by the SAC.
Hand Surgery Orthopaedics: www.wheelessonline.com
Microsurgery: www.buncke.org
Oncoplastic Breast Surgery: www.orbsweb.com
PLASTA: Plastic Surgery Trainees Association: www.plasta.org.uk
RSTN: Reconstructive Trials Network: www.reconstructivesurgerytrials.net
Skin Cancer Guidelines: www.bad.org.uk/search?search=guidelines

Reference

1 AJ Reid, PSC Malone. Plastic surgery in the press. JPRAS (2008) 61, 866–9.

Debridement of a complex wound

Indications

'Debridement' means to 'lay open' and not per se to remove tissue, although this is often undertaken at the same time in a contaminated wound. Generally, a 'complex wound' is considered one that specifically requires plastic surgery techniques in order to restore normal form and function due to wound location/proximity to critical structures or persistent non-healing.

Preoperative preparation

Consideration should be given to patient factors that may have impaired healing, such as poor nutrition, diabetes, use of steroids, etc. All patient factors must be optimized.

Position

Standard theatre positioning as per wound location.

Procedure

- Adequately expose the area.
- Remove all devitalized necrotic areas; use blade for sharp debridement to healthy, bleeding tissues.
- Take careful consideration of proximity to nearby important structures such as nerves, tendons, muscles, etc. Judicious debridement is required in these areas.
- Ensure adequate haemostasis.
- Lavage. Lavage. Lavage. 'The solution to pollution is dilution'!
- Dress with non-adherent antiseptic dressing.
- Consider reconstruction at the same operation or in subsequent procedures, following the principles of the 'reconstructive ladder'.

Postoperative care

- Early and regular wound review.
- Continue to optimize systemic patient factors.
- Plan definitive management to cover/reconstruct defect.

Complications

- Persistent non-healing wound.
- Failure of subsequent reconstructive procedures.
- Scarring and deformity.

Tips and tricks

Negative-pressure wound therapy (NPWT)/vacuum-assisted dressings, can be an excellent choice of dressing to temporize complex wounds and can occasionally permit sufficient wound shrinkage to convert a complex wound into a 'simple' wound. The dressing consists of a base-layer (sponge or guaze) that is cut to fit the wound contours, with an airtight dressing applied over the top, connected to a vacuum air-suction pump. It can be left in place for up to 5 days before needing changing. A typical setting is at '125mmHg continuous therapy' for the first 48 hours, which is then ideally adjusted to '5 minutes on, 2 minutes off' for increased speed of healing and granulation tissue formation. The precise settings are modified to the situation. When the wound cavity is lined with a non-adherent silicon dressing or similar, it can be more easily changed in the outpatient setting or even in the community by district nurses or tissue viability nurses. More recent modifications include incorporated irrigation systems, which wash the wound bed within the dressings at regular (e.g. 2-hourly) periods, and which can even flush the wound surface with antibiotics.

Debridement of a burn and split skin grafting

Anatomy

(See Fig. 11.2)

- SPT (superficial partial thickness): epidermal or superficial layer of dermis, characterized by blisters, which when debrided have pink tissue underneath that blanches on pressure, is sensate, and painful.

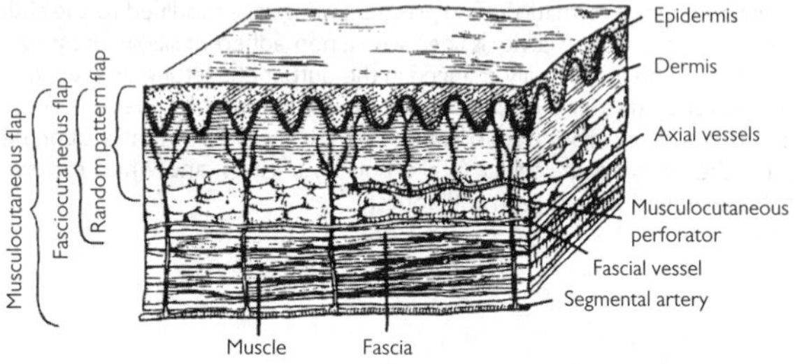
Epidermis
Dermis
Axial vessels
Musculocutaneous perforator
Fascial vessel
Segmental artery
Muscle
Fascia
Musculocutaneous flap
Fasciocutaneous flap
Random pattern flap

Fig. 11.2 Layers of skin. Reproduced from McLatchie, G. and Leaper, D., Operative Surgery 2nd edition, 2006, with permission from Oxford University Press.

Depth of burn

(See Table 11.1)

Table 11.1 Depth of burn

Depth of burn		Usual history	Appearance	Blister formation	Sensation	Results
Superficial		Sunburn	Red, bloated	Absent	Painful	Heals in 7days
Partial thickness	Superficial Dermal	Scalds of limited duration	Red or pink with a capillary return	Present	Painful	Heals in 14 days
	Deep dermal	Scalds of long duration Contact with high temperature	Red without capillary return	Absent Wet or waxy surface	Painless	Heals in months
Full thickness		Contact with high temperature Chemicals Electrical injury	Charred black-brown or white, dry, thrombosed vessels	Absent	Painless	Granulates

Reproduced from McLatchie, G. and Leaper, D., Operative Surgery 2nd edition, 2006, with permission from Oxford University Press.

- DPT (deep partial thickness): deep layer of dermis, characterized by some fixed red staining, which does not blanche with pressure and could be insensate.
- FT (full thickness): through dermis onto subcutaneous tissue ± underlying fat, fascia, and muscle. Characterized by a leathery solid eschar, which has no capillary refill and is insensate.

Assessment of burn area and possible inhalation injury

- History.
  - Explosion in confined space.
  - Smoke inhalation.
  - Consider electrical injury entry and exit wound as well as cardiac involvement.
  - Chemical injury—acid/alkali.
  - Assess, is burn secondary to:
    —Stroke.
    —MI.
    —Seizure.
    —Non-accidental injury (child abuse).
- Assess area of burn.
  - Wallace's rule of nines is the simplest means for a rough assessment (Fig. 11.3).
  - Lund and Browder chart is a more precise and age-adjusted means by which to estimate the size of a burn as a percentage of body surface area (Fig.11.4).

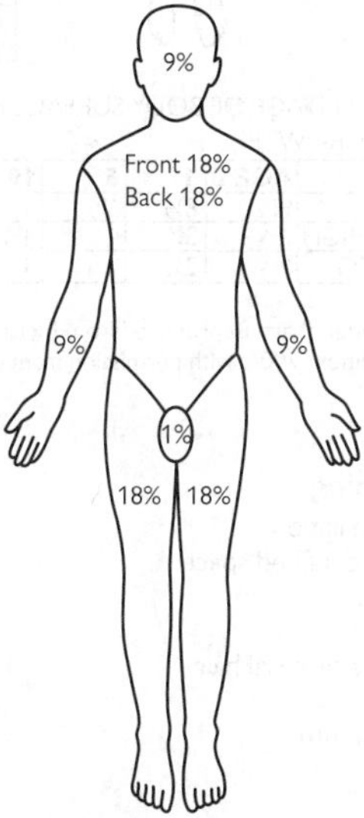
9%
Front 18%
Back 18%
9%
9%
1%
18%
18%

Fig. 11.3 Wallace's rule of nines. Reproduced from McLatchie, G. and Leaper, D., Operative Surgery 2nd edition, 2006, with permission from Oxford University Press.

CHART FOR ESTIMATING SEVERITY OF BURN WOUND

NAME__________WARD________NUMBER_____ DATE___
AGE__________ADMISSION WEIGHT________

LUND AND BROWDER CHARTS

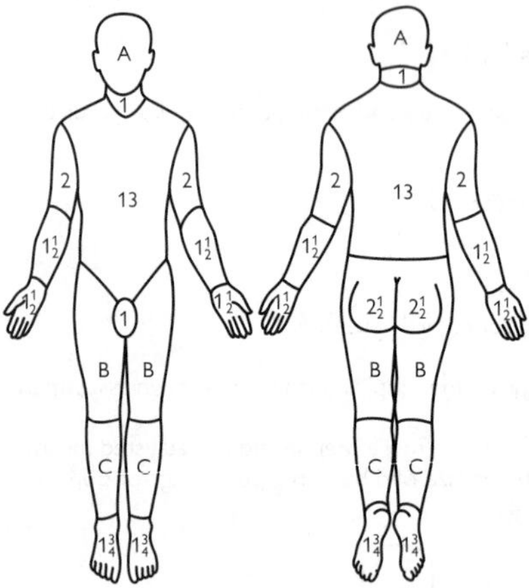
A
1
2
13
1½
1
2½
B
C
1¾

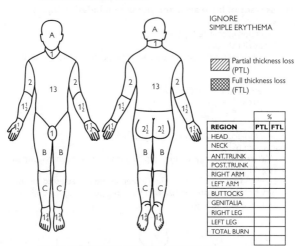

IGNORE
SIMPLE ERYTHEMA

Partial thickness loss (PTL)

Full thickness loss (FTL)

	%	
REGION	**PTL**	**FTL**
HEAD		
NECK		
ANT.TRUNK		
POST.TRUNK		
RIGHT ARM		
LEFT ARM		
BUTTOCKS		
GENITALIA		
RIGHT LEG		
LEFT LEG		
TOTAL BURN		

RELATIVE PERCENTAGE OF BODY SURFACE AREA
AFFECTED BY GROWTH

AREA	**AGE 0**	**1**	**5**	**10**	**15**	**ADULT**
A = ½ OF HEAD	9½	8½	6½	5½	4½	3½
B = ½ OF ONE THIGH	2¾	3¼	4	4½	4½	4¾
C = ½ OF ONE LEG	2½	2½	2¾	3	3¼	3½

Fig. 11.4 Lund and Browder chart. Reproduced from McLatchie, G. and Leaper, D., Operative Surgery 2nd edition, 2006, with permission from Oxford University Press.

Airway and breathing

Indication of smoke inhalation:

- History of burn in a confined space.
- Confusion, agitation.
- Burns to face.
- Singeing of eyebrows or nasal hair.
- Soot in the sputum.
- Burning within the mouth.
- Hoarseness or stridor.

Circulation

- Burns involving >15% TBSA in adults, or >10% TBSA in children, will require circulatory support—set up two large-bore intravenous cannulas.
- Choice of fluids—in the A&E Department the choice of fluid is secondary to the need for urgent and adequate fluid replacement. Any fluid is adequate so long as it contains sodium in a concentration between 130 and 150mmol/l.
- Fluid resuscitation.
  - Oral fluids:
    —<10% TBSA in children or <15% TBSA in adults.
    —Dioralyte or dextrolyte.
    —Moyer's solution.
    —4g NaCl/l and 1.5g NaHCO3.
  - IV fluids:
    —Crystalloid (e.g. Hartmann's): 'The Parkland Formula' = 4ml/kg/% burn TBSA: 50% in first 8h; 25% in next 8h; 25% in next 8h; routine daily maintenance fluids need to be added to the regime.
    —Colloid/4.5% HAS (human albumin solution): Muir and Barclay Formula: 1st 36h is divided into 6 periods of: 4, 4, 4, 6, 6, 12h. Volume HAS (in ml) given in each time period = %TBSA × patient weight (kg).

Indications for burn debridement & SSG (split thickness skin graft)

DPT and FT burns that will not heal on their own within 2 weeks of injury.

Preoperative preparation

Measure dimensions of wound and then mark adequate donor site for SSG.

Position and theatre set-up

- Warm theatre in advance.
- Infiltrate wound and SSG donor site with adrenaline (±LA) solution.
- Swab all wounds individually for MC&S.

Procedure

- Consider use of preoperative infiltration with adrenaline solution, or use of adrenaline soaks intraoperatively.
- Apply and inflate tourniquet if burn is on extremity.
- Excise burn using suitable handheld knife of personal preference (e.g. scalpel/Watson/Humby knife).
- Undertake adequate debridement down to healthy bleeding tissue.
- For larger FT burns, initial incision down to fasica and subsequent excision along fascial plane may be preferable in order to minimize blood loss.
- Ensure meticulous haemostasis, especially with concomitant use of adrenaline solution.
- Calculate size of defect requiring grafting—paper templates may aid, especially for deep wounds with contour deformity at edges.
- Harvest SSG and mesh, as appropriate (see Fig. 11.8).
- Apply SSG to wound with Vicryl Rapide™/tissue glue as desired.

- Dress grafted area with:
  - Non-adherent layer.
  - Damp gauze, which can be tightly imprinted into defect cavities to ensure close contact of SSG to wound bed is maintained throughout.
  - Dry gauze.
  - Velband/crepe.
  - POP may be indicated for extremities.
- Dress donor site with Kaltostat/gauze/velband/crepe, or as per local preferences.

Postoperative care

- Observe dressings for any bleeding through from wound bed (as well as donor site).
- Graft check in 5 days.
- Leave donor site dressings intact until 14 days, by which time they should have fully healed.
- Refer to physiotherapy as appropriate for mobilization.
- Refer to occupational therapy for scar management and pressure garments.
- Follow-up in Multidisciplinary Burns Clinic.

Complications

- Inadequate debridement of burn requiring return to theatre.
- Bleeding and haematoma (requiring reoperation).
- Infection.
- Graft failure.
- Burn contracture.
- Itching and dryness.
- Unfavourable scarring.
- Donor site complications including scarring and delayed healing.

Tips and tricks

Recent wound swabs preoperatively can prove very helpful, especially, e.g. to exclude β-haemolytic streptococcus group, which is a specific contraindication to skin grafting because it will consume the graft.

Debridement of an infected collection in the hand

Anatomy

The hand contains a number of 'spaces' and 'potential spaces' that do not benefit from a blood supply and thus infection that moves into one of these areas can rapidly progress unchecked with devastating consequences. This is why such infections must be prioritized (Figs 11.5 and 11.6).

Spaces include:

- The superficial pulp spaces of the digits, infections within which cause a 'Felon'.
- The synovial flexor tendon sheaths of the 2nd to 4th digits (flexor sheath washout described separately).
- The radial and ulnar bursae, which communicate in the proximal hand and extend up the thumb and little finger, respectively.
- The thenar space, deep to the thumb and index flexor tendons and 1st lumbrical muscles, which may be broached from the associated flexor sheaths.
- The middle palmar space, which may be broached from the middle or ring finger flexor sheaths.
- The hypothenar space, around the hypothenar muscles.

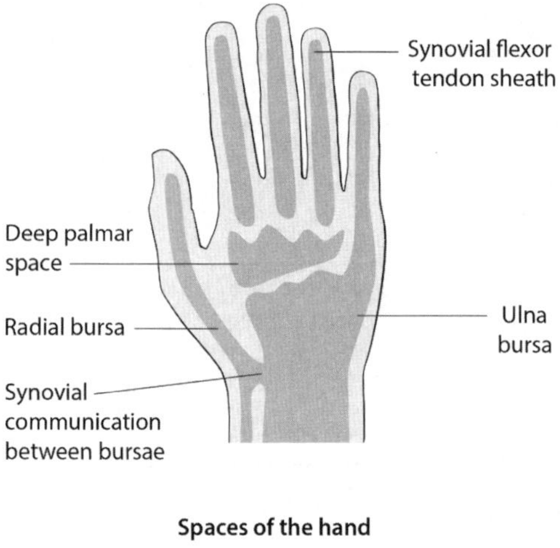
Synovial flexor tendon sheath
Deep palmar space
Radial bursa
Ulna bursa
Synovial communication between bursae
Spaces of the hand

Fig. 11.5 Spaces of the hand. Medical illustrations produced by Helen Day, Medical Artist, Oxford, www.medicalartist.org.uk, reproduced with permission.

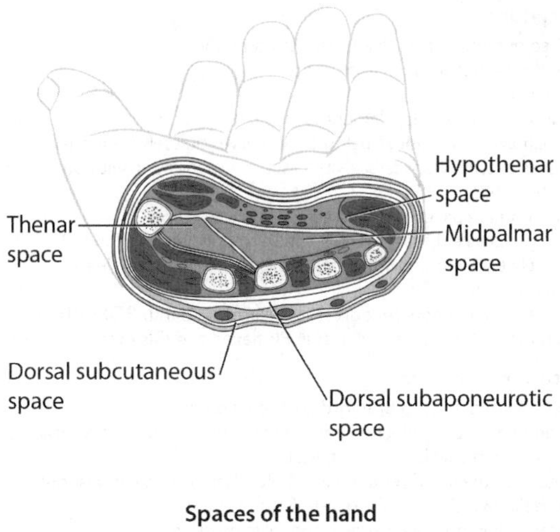
Hypothenar space
Thenar space
Midpalmar space
Dorsal subcutaneous space
Dorsal subaponeurotic space
Spaces of the hand

Fig. 11.6 Hand cross-section. Medical illustrations produced by Helen Day, Medical Artist, Oxford, www.medicalartist.org.uk, reproduced with permission.

- The dorsal subcutaneous space, overlying the entire dorsum of the hand.
- The dorsal subaponeurotic space, lying deep to the aponeurosis of the extensor tendons.

Indications for surgical drainage

- Localized signs of an infected hand as typified by the markers of inflammation, classified by Celsus and then Galen to include Rubor/ Calor/Dolor/tumour/functio laesa ('loss of function').
- Generalized systemic signs of infection, including specifically: ascending lymphangitis, pyrexia, rigors, raised WBC and CRP.

Preoperative preparation

- Treat as an emergency.
- IV antibiotics mandatory.
- Hand elevation in Bradford sling/equivalent.
- Resuscitation as appropriate.

Position and theatre set-up

- Hand table.
- Arm tourniquet (elevate hand for 3min before inflation: *do not* use esmarch or similar to exsanguinate, as this would push infection more proximally!).
- Lead hand.
- Mark incision lines prior to tourniquet inflation.

Procedure

- Incise over most prominent part of collection.
- MC&S swab ± fluid for microscopy.
- Drain abscess.
- Judicious wound debridement of dead/necrotic tissues, taking care not to damage important structures (i.e. nerves/vessels/tendons).
- Assess extent of abscess cavity—is it communicating with other spaces of the hand?
- Open other spaces as indicated.
- Lavage. Lavage. Lavage. 'The solution to pollution is dilution'!
- Loosely pack wound with a betadene-soaked wick and leave wound open.
- Dress with non-adherent dressings/gauze/velband/POP slab for comfort in the 'safe' position (MCPJs flexed and IPJs extended)/crepe.

Postoperative care

- Elevate continually in Bradford sling/equivalent.
- IV antibiotics until infection improved enough to convert to orals.
- *Daily* wound check, initially at least.
- Return to theatre if required at 24/48/72h for further washout (or definitive closure of wounds if appropriate).
- Early review post-discharge in specialist dressing clinic.
- Refer for rehabilitative physiotherapy as needed.

Complications

- Persistent infection necessitating repeated theatre washouts.
- Resistant/atypical bacteria (e.g. mycobacterium) requiring prolonged course of antibiotics.
- Progression to osteomyelitis.
- Stiffness/reduced range of movement.
- CRPS.

Tips and tricks

Mycobacterium marinum can be a persistent infection acquired from fish requiring close liaison with microbiology to guide on optimal antibiotic regimen.

Taking a split skin graft

Anatomy

(See Fig. 11.7)

For SSG harvest, see Fig. 11.8a–d.

Indication

As part of the reconstructive ladder to cover a FT defect such as following burns' excisional surgery, post-excision of a malignant skin lesion or a traumatic wound.

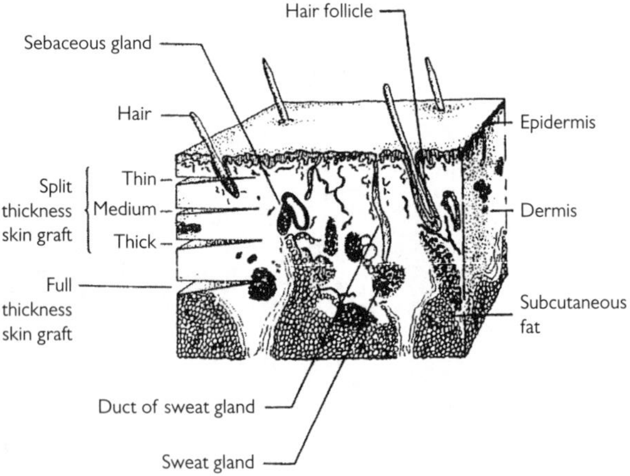
Hair follicle
Sebaceous gland
Hair
Epidermis
Split thickness skin graft
Thin
Medium
Thick
Dermis
Full thickness skin graft
Subcutaneous fat
Duct of sweat gland
Sweat gland

Fig. 11.7 Depth of skin grafts. Reproduced from McLatchie, G. and Leaper, D., Operative Surgery 2nd edition, 2006, with permission from Oxford University Press.

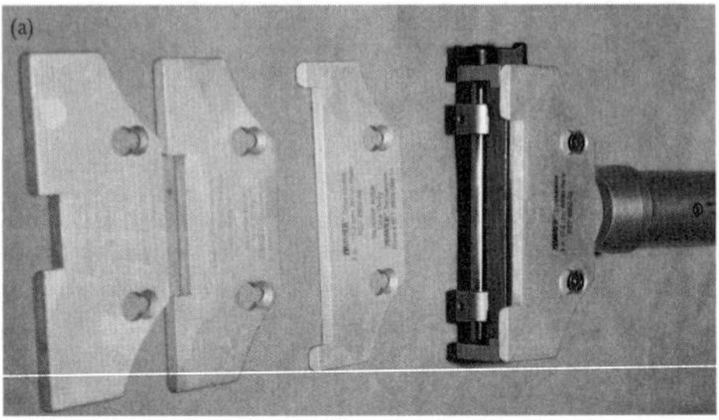
(a)

Fig. 11.8 (a) The electric dermatome and different width guards.(b) Taking the split skin graft. (c) Meshing the skin (here a 1:1.5 ratio meshing board is being used). (d) Meshed SSG is inset.

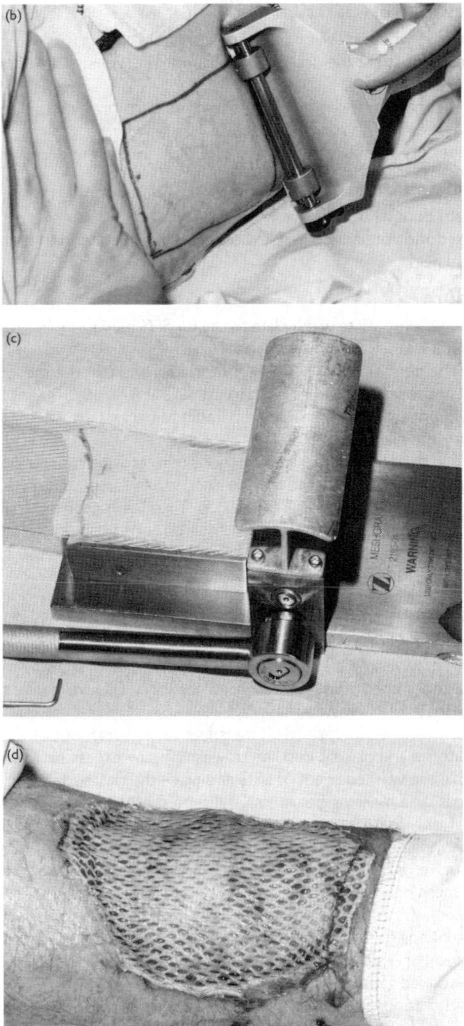
(b)
(c)
WARNING
(d)

Fig. 11.8 (*Contd.*)

Preoperative preparation

- Determine whether LA or GA is most suitable.
- Agree with patient the optimal/ideal donor site(s)—usually upper thigh areas.
- Using a surgical marker, mark the size of area from which to harvest skin after measuring the size of the defect.
- Consider preoperative application of EMLA cream if under LA.

Position and theatre set-up

- Infiltrate donor site using LA with adrenaline.
- Ensure donor site adequately exposed and prepped with the rest of the surgical field.

Procedure

- Select the appropriate width plate to use for SSG harvest (1, 2, 3, or 4in) (see Fig. 11.8a).
- Verify the dermatome is set-up appropriately and test the motor.
- Select appropriate thickness to harvest SSG at (e.g. 10/1000in).
- Apply lubricant of saline or liquid paraffin to harvest area and dermatome blade.
- Place one hand firmly distal to the donor site to provide counter-traction during skin graft harvest. This may be aided with an assistant's help.
- Hold the dermatome at 45° to the skin. Turn the motor on. Using an even pressure apply it to the start of the donor site and progress along the marked region (see Fig. 11.8b). The other hand can be used to steady the blade if not using it for counter-traction.
- Be careful to maintain pressure in-balance with counter-traction and not to 'jump' the dermatome along the donor site.
- When the end of the marked area has been reached, whilst keeping the motor going, lift the blade-end of the dermatome up, bringing it parallel to the donor site, whilst still advancing forward. This will divide the end of the sheet of harvested skin graft.
- Use non-toothed forceps to lift the sheet of skin graft out of the dermatome and place it in saline to wash off any excess paraffin.
- Remove the washed sheet of SSG and place the raw surface facing upwards on a meshing board (e.g. 1:1.5 meshing board) or a wooden block if only fenestration is required.
- Use a syringe of saline and non-toothed forceps to spread the sheet of skin out.
- Insert mesh board into mesher and advance it through slowly (see Fig. 11.8c). Watch as it comes out because you may need to prevent it from adhering to the roller.
- Prepared harvested skin should be kept cool, wrapped in a saline-soaked gauze.
- Dress the donor site with materials of your choice, such as Kaltostat/dry gauze/mefix/crepe/velband.

Postoperative care

Ideally, donor site dressings should be left intact for 14 days. By that time, the dressings will no longer be adherent and will easily peel off, atraumatically.

Complications

- Wound infection/bleeding.
- Delayed healing.
- Hypertrophic/keloid/hypersensitive scar.
- Altered pigmentation in scar.

Tips and tricks

- Although the scrub nurse will often hand you the dermatome ready prepared and loaded, it is the surgeon's responsibility to ensure that it is set up correctly. The following checklist should be adhered to each and every time:
  - Ensure the blade has been inserted into the dermatome the correct way around.
  - Look along the blade to verify no defect.
  - Use the provided screwdriver to check the blade plate is securely held in place.
  - Check that the appropriate thickness of skin harvest is selected—depending upon how hard you press and the thickness of the patient's donor site skin, typically you might select between 8/1,000 and 10/1,000in.
  - Press on the paddle to test the motor is of even tone prior to commencing.
- Ensure you give enough time between donor site infiltration and SSG harvest to ensure that the LA has adequately dispersed and that the skin is not lumpy when harvesting, which would otherwise adversely affect the quality of the harvested skin.
- If the skin does not fully cut-through to detach at the end of harvest, keep the dermatome suspended in mid-air and use tenotomy or MacIndoe scissors to cut through the attached skin. Pull the skin out from the dermatome in the normal manner.
- Always double check that you have the prepared skin graft the right way around: this should be 'sunny side up' on the mesher board whereby the raw side of the harvested skin is shiny and the edges can be seen to furl inwards on this raw underside. If the graft is placed the wrong way round, it will fail. The raw side of the graft is then easily placed onto the raw wound simply by placing the mesher board over the wound.
- Confirm onto which side of the mesher board the sheet of graft is to be placed. If advertently put on the wrong side, the graft will come out like 'spaghetti strips' instead of being meshed.
- SSG is meshed to both increase its surface area and to allow exudate to easily discharge. Fenestrated skin graft (where it is merely pierced with a blade) is used over joints and sometimes other regions, such as in the head and neck, should a meshed appearance be considered less ideal.
- Once dry Kaltostat has been applied to donor site, soak it with LA to minimize post-procedure discomfort.
- Extra top layers of dressings to a thigh donor site (e.g. an extra layer of velband and crepe on top of the base dressing layer) may be more comfortable for the patient and may prevent the deeper layers of dressings from unfurling ahead of time—ideally the base layer dressings should remain intact for 2 weeks.

Excision and direct suture of skin lesion

Anatomy
(See Figs 11.9 and 11.10)

Indications
- For lesions that are:
  - Unsightly.
  - Painful or suffer from other issues such as repeated infections (e.g. infected sebaceous cyst).
- For biopsy of a suspicious lesion.

Preoperative preparation
Mark lesion as an ellipse along RSTLs with a 1–2mm margin.

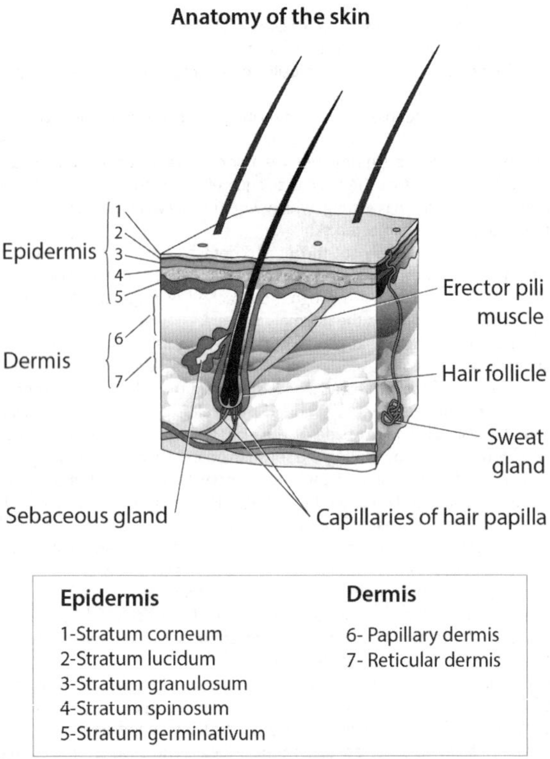
Anatomy of the skin
Epidermis
1
2
3
4
5
Dermis
6
7
Erector pili muscle
Hair follicle
Sweat gland
Sebaceous gland
Capillaries of hair papilla
Epidermis
1-Stratum corneum
2-Stratum lucidum
3-Stratum granulosum
4-Stratum spinosum
5-Stratum germinativum
Dermis
6- Papillary dermis
7- Reticular dermis

Fig. 11.9 Anatomy of the skin. Medical illustrations produced by Helen Day, Medical Artist, Oxford, www.medicalartist.org.uk, reproduced with permission.

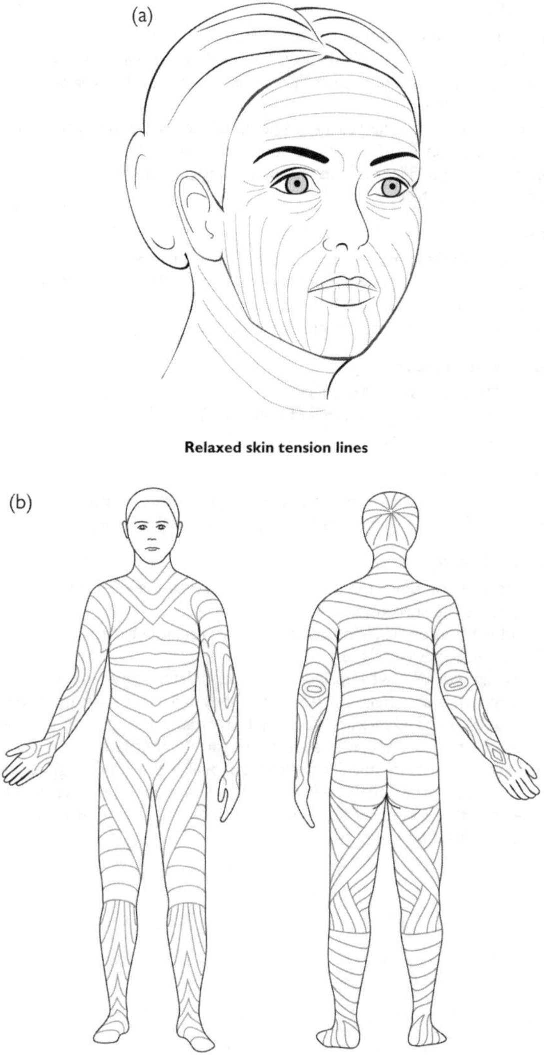
(a)
Relaxed skin tension lines
(b)

Fig. 11.10 Relaxed skin tension lines (RSTLs) of (a) the face and (b) the body: aim to place incisions along these lines. Medical illustrations produced by Helen Day, Medical Artist, Oxford, www.medicalartist.org.uk, reproduced with permission.

Procedure

- Infiltration with LA containing adrenaline (except for digits).
- 15-blade used to incise FT through entire ellipse of skin markings, taking care to incise perpendicular to skin and not undermine the surrounding areas.
- Once subcutaneous fat reached, orientate blade horizontally to excise lesion, including a cuff of subcutaneous adipose tissue.
- Specimen to go in formalin for histopathological analysis.
- Bipolar haemostasis.

Closure

- Suture choice depends on site and personal preference and size of defect, e.g. 5/0 Monocryl® deep dermal and 6/0 Prolene® interrupted simple sutures for tension-free skin closure if lesion excised from face.
- Dressings: ½in steristrips/mepore/tegaderm dressings.

Postoperative care

- Keep dry until first wound check.
- Wound check and r/o sutures (if applicable): face 5–7 days; trunk and extremities 10–14 days.

Complications

- Scarring, including hypertrophic/keloid/hypersensitive scar.
- Need for further procedures if indicated by histopathology.

Tips and tricks

- Ensure that you bevel the blade perpendicular to the lesion and do not undermine the surrounding skin.
- Must be a tension-free closure for optimal wound healing.
- General scar advice to give:
  - When wound is well healed (e.g. 1 month later) patients should commence scar massage. To do this they can use any cream or oil (e.g. 'E45') as a lubricant, applying firm pressure to the scar in concentric circles, enough to blanch the scar. An alternate method is to maintain pressure in a linear direction, pulling along the length of the scar. This should be done for 5min four times per day, preferably for a couple of months if not longer. Scar massage also helps with scar desensitization.

Excision of a malignant skin lesion

[illegible]

Indications

[illegible]

Preoperative preparation

[illegible]

Position and theatre set-up

[illegible]

Procedure

[illegible]

Excision of a malignant skin lesion

Anatomy

(See Figs 11.9 and 11.10)

Indications

- For complete excision of biopsy-proven skin malignancy.
- Clinically highly suspicious lesion, e.g. as outlined by the ABCDE rule for melanoma:
  - Asymmetry.
  - Borders uneven.
  - Colour changes.
  - Diameter larger than ~0.6cm.
  - Evolving changes, including any new change in appearance such as elevation, bleeding, itch, etc.

Preoperative preparation

- Mark periphery of skin lesion under adequate lighting (± use of magnifying 'Loupes' glasses).
- Mark appropriate excision margins. Rule of thumb: BCCs should have 3–5mm margins; SCCs 4–10mm margins; malignant melanoma as per current national BAPRAS/BAD guidelines, currently 0.5–3cm margins.
- Determine whether excision, including margins, would allow direct closure of defect or require reconstruction using a flap or skin graft.
- If direct apposition of wound edges achievable, mark out in an elliptical fashion along RSTLs; otherwise plan closure method.

Position and theatre set-up

- Dependent on site of lesion.
- (NB: Remember to expose area for skin grafting if applicable.)

Procedure

- Infiltration using LA with adrenaline (except for digits).
- 15-blade to incise FT through skin markings, taking utmost care to incise perpendicular to skin and not to undermine surrounding structures.
- Deep margin: for BCCs, a cuff of subcutaneous adipose tissue is normally adequate; however, if SCC or melanoma, then deep margin should extend to the next layer, i.e. down to (but not including) fascia.
- Inspect underside of excised specimen to be certain that deep margins are not involved—if they are, a deeper excision margin will be required.
- Orientate specimen(s) with marker suture (e.g. 4/0 silk).
- Specimen to go in formalin for histopathological analysis.
- Haemostasis.

Closure

- Suture choice depends on site and personal preference and size of defect, e.g. 5/0 Monocryl® deep dermal and 6/0 Prolene® interrupted simple sutures for tension-free skin closure if lesion excised from face.
- Inset skin graft/flap if appropriate.
- Dressings: ½in steristrips/mepore/tegaderm dressings or as dictated by method of closure.

Postoperative care

- Keep dry until first wound check.
- Direct closure: wound check and r/o sutures (if applicable) from face 5–7 days; trunk and extremities 10–14 days.
- Skin graft/flap: check wound in specialist nurse-led clinic at 5–7 days.

Complications

- Scarring, including hypertrophic/keloid/hypersensitive.
- Incomplete excision/recurrence.
- Need for further procedures if indicated by histopathology.

Tips and tricks

- It is crucial that your incision for skin cancers is perpendicular to the skin. Do not undermine surrounding structures.
- The most important matter is for cancer clearance: do not compromise margins to make the wound closure 'easier'. Likewise, structures such as superficial nerves or vessels that might run through the lesion will most certainly have to be sacrificed and excised with the lesion.
- Must be tension-free closure for optimal wound healing.
- 2010 BAPRAS/BAD guidelines for excision margins for malignant melanoma in relation to Breslow thickness of melanoma (2):
  - In situ = 0.5cm margins.
  - <1.0mm thick = 1cm.
  - 1.01–2mm thick = 1–2cm.
  - 2.01–4mm thick = 2–3cm.
  - >4mm thick = 3cm.

Reference

2 British Association of Dermatologists 2010 Guidelines: (http://www.bad.org.uk/search?search=melanoma+guidelines).

Excision of a ganglion

Definition

A ganglion is a fluid-filled cyst, which typically arises from a joint or a tendon sheath. In hand surgery, the most common locations are of dorsal and volar wrist ganglions, flexor sheath ganglions, and mucous cyst ganglions, which typically present from the DIPJ.

Indications

- Enlarging size and discomfort.
- Repeated infection.
- Recurrence after percutaneous aspiration.
- Patient choice.

Preoperative preparation

Arm table and tourniquet.

Position and theatre set-up

- Delineate peripheries of ganglion cyst *before* infiltration with local anaesthetic.
- Mark incision line (see Fig. 11.11).

Procedure

- Skin incision.
- Dissect out cyst, including stalk.
- Excise ganglion in toto from its point of origin as identified at the base of the stalk.
- Leave joint space open.
- Deflate tourniquet.
- Haemostasis.

Closure

- With suture of choice, depending on site.
- Dressing.

Postoperative care

- Wound check at 7–10 days.
- R/o sutures 10–14 days as appropriate.
- Full mobilization usually appropriate from day of surgery.

Complications

- Recurrence (40–60%).
- Nailbed damage/deformity post mucous cyst.

Tips and tricks

- Take care not to rupture the ganglion either during LA infiltration or during dissection, or its course and outline will become less clear to follow.
- Mucous cysts excised from the DIPJ may not close directly but instead leave a defect that requires closure with either an FTSG or a local skin flap.

Extensor/flexor tendon repair

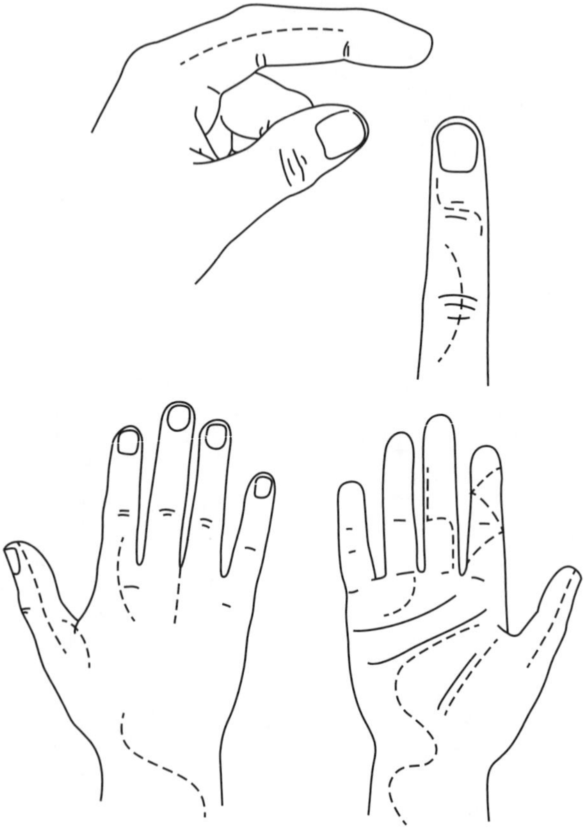

Correct incisions

Fig. 11.11 Optimal incision lines for use in the hand. Reproduced from McLatchie, G. and Leaper, D., Oxford Handbook of Operative Surgery, 1996, with permission from Oxford University Press.

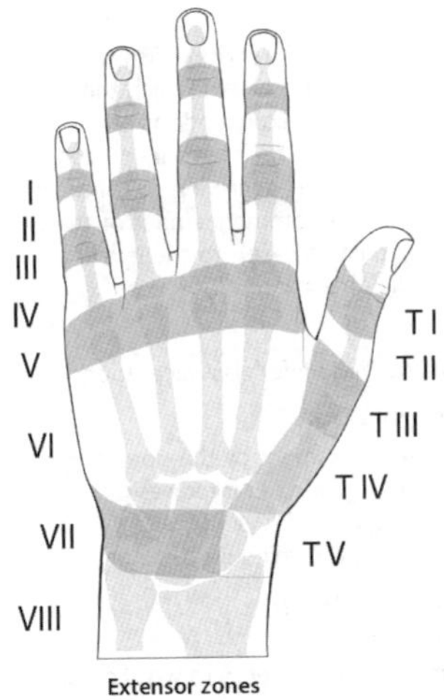
I
II
III
IV
V
VI
VII
VIII
T I
T II
T III
T IV
T V
Extensor zones

Fig. 11.12 Extensor zones of the digits of the hand. Medical illustrations produced by Helen Day, Medical Artist, Oxford, www.medicalartist.org.uk, reproduced with permission.

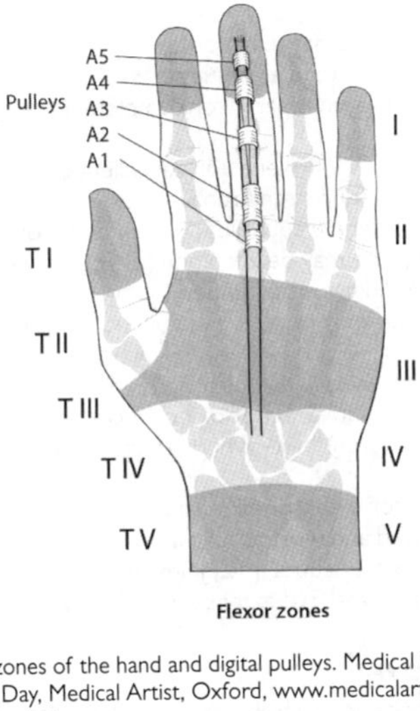
Pulleys
A5
A4
A3
A2
A1
I
II
III
IV
V
T I
T II
T III
T IV
T V
Flexor zones

Fig. 11.13 Flexor zones of the hand and digital pulleys. Medical illustrations produced by Helen Day, Medical Artist, Oxford, www.medicalartist.org.uk, reproduced with permission.

Anatomy

When describing lacerations and tendon injuries, it is important to be specific about the zone of the hand within which the injury lies. Figures 11.12 and 11.13 detail extensor and flexor tendon zones.

Flexor zone 2 is also called 'no man's land' due to the complexity of undertaking surgical repair and achieving an optimal outcome for injury within it. It extends from the commencement of the flexor sheath (around the level of the distal palmar crease), to the level of FDS insertion, around the centre of the middle phalanx.

Indications

Usually open trauma such as knife/glass lacerations, etc.

Preoperative preparation

- Clinical preoperative assessment by the operating surgeon is mandatory.
- Look for concomitant injuries, i.e. fractures or nerve damage.
- Mark appropriate digit(s).
- Tetanus and antibiotic cover is required.

Position and theatre set-up

- IV antibiotics on induction.
- Arm table. Upper arm tourniquet with wool bandage cushioning.
- Lead hand.
- An assistant will be of benefit.

Procedure

- Mark out Brunner's incision lines to extend wounds if required (see Fig. 11.11).
- Raise tourniquet after exsanguination.
- Explore wounds and extend as required.
- Identify if tendon division is partial or complete. Identify both ends of divided tendon.
- Repair tendon using 3/0 Prolene® or equivalent core suture using a two- or preferably a four-strand repair
- Use 5/0 or 6/0 Prolene®/equivalent for epitendonous repair.
- A small partial rupture may be left alone (or require debridement only if it prevents free gliding of the tendon). Larger partial tears may need either epitendonous only or core and epitendonous repair, depending on size of injury.
- Deflate tourniquet; achieve haemostasis.
- Closure of skin, e.g. with 5/0 Ethilon® or Vicryl Rapide™.
- Dress with non-adherent base layer + gauze, velband, POP backslab, and crepe.
- POP placed volar for extensor injuries; dorsal for flexors.
- Immobilize the hand and wrist as follows:
  - Flexor repair: wrist neutral, MCPJ flexion to 70°; IPJs fully extended.
  - Extensor repair: wrist 30° extension, MCPJ 40° flexion; IPJs fully extended.

Postoperative care

- Elevate hand at bedside and high arm sling when ambulant.
- Antibiotics and analgesia as indicated.
- Wound check in specialist clinic 5–7 days.

- Referral to hand therapy at time of surgery for tailored rehabilitation regime, depending on local preferences.
- R/o sutures 10–14 days.
- Patient will need intensive rehabilitation over 8–12 weeks following surgery and will need a 'sick note' to cover them for this period.
- Follow-up in combined MDT Hand Clinic.

Complications

- Tendon adhesions.
- Tendon rupture.
- Non-compliance with rehabilitation regime.
- Stiffness/reduced range of movement.
- Cold intolerance.
- CRPS.

Tips and tricks

- Always rule out pre-existing injuries, e.g. an old fracture that had healed in a suboptimal position or a neglected tendon injury.
- Always stress importance of physiotherapy rehabilitation to the patient preoperative to improve compliance.
- Current evidence suggests that four-strand flexor tendon repair, where achievable, is superior to two-strand repair.
- There are multiple different popular techniques in current use by which to weave the core suture and epitendonous repair. Techniques include: Cruciate, Kessler, Savage, Strickland, Indiana and epitendonous Silfverskiöld.
- Preservation of the A2 and A4 pulleys in flexor tendon repair (and the oblique pulley of the thumb) is preferable. Loss of both the A2 and A4 pulley will cause 'bowstringing' of the flexor tendons. Resist temptation to 'vent the pulleys'. If the A2 and A4 pulleys do both need to be divided, this can be done with either a stepped or an oblique incision, which allows pulley reconstruction afterwards.
- A double-tendon injury in zone 2 will likely cause excessive bulkiness, reduced motion, and glide through the pulley system, and ultimately have a poor long-term outcome. It is therefore indicated to only repair the FDP tendon in these circumstances, thereby 'sacrificing' a damaged FDS for the sake of a better overall functional result.
- When undertaking partial repair, take care not to cause excessive bunching of the intact remaining tendon, which would adversely affect the tendon's biomechanics.
- There are many different regimes for postoperative rehabilitation post-tendon repair for specific tendons injured, and because preferences vary throughout the world, it is important to become most familiar with those in current use in your own unit. Regimes include: Belfast, Capener, Kleinert, Leicester, and Norwich, amongst others. Typically, any tendon repair would do best with EAM (early active mobilization).
- The 'Wide Awake Technique' allows e.g. flexor tendon repairs to be done under LA, through infiltration of lignocaine with adrenaline into the hand/digits: resultant vasoconstriction negates the need for tourniquet. Phentolamine, a potent vasodilator, counteracts adrenaline in case of emergency (3).

Reference

3 DH Lalonde, A Wong. Dosage of local anesthesia in wide awake hand surgery. JHS(Am) (2013) 38:10, 2025–8..

Harvesting a full-thickness skin graft (FTSG)

A FTSG can be harvested from any site that can be directly closed. Generally the site chosen is one that has the closest colour match to the recipient site, e.g. a head and neck donor site will be selected for a recipient site to the face.

It is preferable to leave the donor scar relatively 'hidden'. Common donor sites therefore include:

- Post-auricular.
- Supraclavicular.
- Pre-auricular.
- Medial upper arm.
- Inguinal creases.
- Antecubital fossa.

Indications

- To cover a small defect when direct closure cannot be reliably achieved and when local flap options are less preferable.
- The size of the FTSG required must permit direct closure of the donor site.
- FTSG is often used in preference to SSG in cosmetically sensitive areas, such as the face, because it gives a better end cosmetic result.

Preoperative preparation

- Calculate size of defect and determine ideal donor site with adequate skin of optimal colour match.
- Draw shape of required skin inside donor site (e.g. a circle), then convert donor site into an ellipse to permit direct closure.
- Verify that direct closure will be attainable.
- Infiltrate with LA containing adrenaline.

Position and theatre set-up

This is partly dependent on site of defect. It should be possible to prepare for access both donor and recipient sites without needing to reposition the patient intraoperatively.

Procedure

- Incise full thickness through elliptical skin marking.
- Elevate one apex of the ellipse with a skin hook or Adson's toothed forceps.
- Using a 15-blade, dissect the skin off from underlying subcutaneous tissues, trying not to raise any fat with the skin.
- Counter-traction from an assistant is useful and may expedite the procedure.
- Defat the harvested skin using tenotomy scissors as required.
- Attain haemostasis to donor site and close with suture of choice, e.g. 4/0 Monocryl® deep dermal interrupted and then continuous.

- Dress with ½in steristrips/mepore/glue/local preferences.
- FTSG can be inset with Vicryl Rapide™, including quilting sutures. Frequently a sponge tie-over is also used, lined with Jelonet and affixed with silk or Prolene® sutures.

Postoperative care

Donor site wound can be checked at same time as FTSG graft is assessed for take (5–7 days post procedure).

Complications

- Graft failure.
- Donor site scar problems, including hypertrophy.

Tips and tricks

- Use of an assistant working simultaneously can significantly speed up the operating time: one undertakes resection, whilst the other harvests the FTSG.
- Meticulous haemostasis is required for the recipient site to ensure graft take: FTSGs are not usually intentionally fenestrated, which would otherwise allow small fluid collections to drain out.
- Quilting sutures may be required when suturing the FTSG in place to ensure that it doesn't 'tent up' over the wound.

Nerve graft harvest

Anatomy

Expendable, commonly-used nerves include:

- *Sural nerve*: this superficial cutaneous nerve is initially located 1cm posterior and superior to the lateral malleolus; moving proximally it roughly follows the route of the short saphenous vein and can be traced towards the mid-calf. A long length (upto 30cm) can be easily harvested.
- *Posterior interosseous nerve*: this is located within the IVth extensor compartment of the wrist, just proximal to Lister's tubercle at the level of the DRUJ (distal radioulnar joint). Ideal match for digital nerves.
- *Medial antebrachial cutaneous nerve*: this travels superficial to FCU muscle belly in the proximal forearm.
- *Lateral antebrachial cutaneous nerve*: this travels deep to the cephalic vein on the lateral proximal border of the forearm

Indications

When direct, tension-free nerve apposition is not possible for a primary nerve repair.

Preoperative preparation

- Inform patient about resultant sensory loss from nerve harvest.
- Arm table and tourniquet.
- Lower limb tourniquet if sural nerve is to be harvested.

Position and theatre set-up

- Arm board/tourniquet as indicated.
- For sural nerve: using leg tourniquet expose lower leg; hip adducted to expose lateral malleolus of the ankle and entire lower leg.

Procedure

- Measure length of nerve deficit.
- Nerve 'cabling' (aligning multiple nerve grafts side-by-side) will be required for larger proximal nerves.
- Make an incision directly atop site of nerve to be harvested as described above.
- Locate relevant nerve and extend incision as required along the course of the nerve in order to harvest the required length.
- NB: In sural nerve grafting, this can also be harvested with multiple smaller incisions, tracing the nerve up the leg.
- Tag one end of the nerve as either distal or proximal for later reverse orientation.
- Once adequate length attained, retrieve the nerve after dividing at both ends.
- Store the harvested nerve in a moist gauze.
- Skin closure as per personal preferences for donor site (e.g. 4/0 Monocryl®).
- Dressings with non-adherent dressing, gauze, and compression bandages (e.g. wool + crepe) for the entire region dissected.
- Deflate tourniquet post application of dressings.

Postoperative care

- Elevate.
- Analgesia.
- Wound check 1 week.

Complications

- Haematoma.
- Neuroma formation.
- Sensory loss is a sequelae of nerve harvest.

Tips and tricks

- Ensure that when nerve is inset as graft, it is reversed to prevent aberrant neural regeneration.
- Nerve grafts should be sutured-in-place in a tension free manner using suitable epineural micro sutures (e.g. 8/0, 9/0 Ethilon®).

Tendon graft harvest

Anatomy

- Palmaris longus (PL) and plantaris are most commonly used as 'disposable' tendon grafts. As relics of our evolution, each is variably present.
- PL originates from the medial epicondyle of the humerus and inserts into the palmar aponeurosis.
- Plantaris tendon's origin is the lateral supracondylar ridge of the femur and it inserts into the tendocalcaneum. It is most readily located on the medial side of the tendocalcaneum deep to the gastrocnemius muscle.

Indications

- To reconstruct a flexor/extensor tendon.
- Harvest for static sling for facial reanimation techniques.

Preoperative preparation

- Assess presence of PL by asking patient to pincer-grip by opposing thumb to little finger whilst flexing the wrist.
- If no PL detected, plantaris is the next choice—this requires preoperative radiological imaging (e.g. MRI) to ascertain its presence.

Position and theatre set-up

- Supine with arm board, upper arm tourniquet and lead hand.
- For plantaris: using leg tourniquet expose lower leg; hip abducted to expose medial condyle of the ankle.

Procedure

PL

- Identify tendon at the wrist.
- Small transverse incision.
- Locate tendon and distinguish from FCR.
- Identify and protect median nerve.
- Dissect PL free from all underlying structures.
- Lift PL using tendon hook, thereby tenting the overlying skin proximally up the forearm over the course of the tendon.
- Make multiple small transverse incisions up the proximal forearm over the tented PL. Through these incisions dissect the tendon free from surrounding structures.
- Once adequate length of PL tendon attained, apply a mosquito clip to the distal end of the tendon and divide distal to the clip.
- Start to deliver the tendon through each incision, moving proximally up the arm.
- Once adequate length of tendon harvested/musculotendinous junction reached, divide the proximal end with a blade.
- Store the tendon in moist gauze.
- Skin closure as per personal preferences (e.g. 4/0 Monocryl®).
- Dressings with steristrips, gauze, and compression bandages (e.g. wool + crepe) for the entire forearm and hand.
- Deflate tourniquet post dressings.

Plantaris

Plantaris tendon harvested as per PL, except that its location cannot be assessed clinically preoperatively, so requires an initial localizing transverse incision near the medial end of the tendoachilles, just behind the medial malleolus.

Postoperative care

- Elevate.
- Analgesia.
- Monitor for symptoms and signs of compartment syndrome.

Complications

- Haematoma.
- Compartment syndrome.

Tips and tricks

- If neither PL nor plantaris present, the 2nd and 3rd toe extensors are frequently identified as the next choices of preference.
- Plantaris appears as a very small tendon but its strength can still be relied upon for tendon reconstruction.

Flexor sheath washout using closed catheter irrigation

Anatomy

(See Fig. 11.14)

Indications

- Local signs as decreed by Kanavel's 'four cardinal signs of flexor tenosynovitis':
  - Pain on passive extension of finger.
  - Fusiform swelling of digit.
  - Tenderness on palpation along the flexor sheath.
  - Partially flexed position of digit.
- Systemic signs include pyrexia, ascending lymphangitis, raised WBC, CRP.

Preoperative preparation

- IV antibiotics.
- Hand elevation.
- Treat as an emergency.
- Mark affected digit.

Position and theatre set-up

Arm table/tourniquet (do not use esmarch—elevate only to drain blood)/ 'lead hand'.

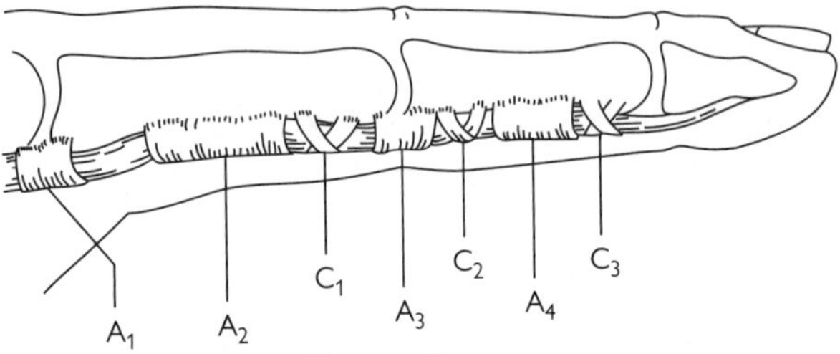
A1
A2
C1
A3
C2
A4
C3
Flexor pulleys

Fig. 11.14 Flexor pulleys of the finger. Reproduced from McLatchie, G. and Leaper, D., Oxford Handbook of Operative Surgery, 1996, with permission from Oxford University Press.

Procedure

- Palmar incision at the origin of A1 pulley (at the level of MCPJ around the distal palmar crease) and open A1 pulley and flexor sheath at its origin.
- Incision at DIPJ level and identify tendon at the end of A5 pulley and end of flexor sheath, to enable washout of the entire sheath.
- Additional incision over PIPJ if point of tenderness is around that area as identified preoperatively.
- Take MC&S swab ± fluid for microscopy.
- Through the proximal-most incision, insert a 6Fr-gauge paediatric feeding tube or an 18G venflon (needle removed) attached to a syringe.
- Use skin hooks as an unobtrusive manner by which to elevate the edge of the pulley for ease of cannulating the flexor sheath.
- Using 20cc syringes, wash out the flexor sheath with copious amounts of normal saline (only from proximal to distal) ensuring free flow from the distal incision.
- If applicable, give further washout proximal to distal through PIPJ incision.
- Ideally aim for ~300cc irrigation through the flexor sheath, but be cautious to watch for compartment pressure effects of injected fluid which may extravasate from the flexor tunnel into the soft tissues of the digit.
- If more extensive infection, e.g. around PIPJ, will require Brunner's incisions to permit adequate washout of infected tissues.
- Leave wounds open/with a loosely-packed wick to permit easy drainage.
- Non-adherent and antiseptic dressings with gauze/wool/POP backslab (for comfort) in safe position/crepe.

Postoperative care

- Continue IV antibiotics and liaise with microbiology as appropriate.
- Elevation.
- Daily wound review ± return to theatre if necessary for further washout (or closure).
- Refer to hand therapy for mobilization *once infection has settled.*

Complications

- Persistent infection.
- Stiffness/loss of range of movement.

Tips and tricks

- Early flexor tenosynovitis may occasionally settle with IV antibiotics and hand elevation alone.
- A fulminant flexor sheath infection is a hand surgery emergency due to both infective and local pressure effects of an expanding collection of pus within the 'closed' restricted confines of the flexor sheath.
- Even in expert hands, this operation can sometimes be extremely fiddly! Having an assistant is ideal: once the irrigation catheter is successfully placed and easily permitting flushing through the flexor sheath, the lead surgeon should then keep their hands dedicated to ensuring the catheter is not dislodged until sufficient irrigation has been undertaken. The assistant should undertake the flushing of fluid.

Intra-lesional steroid injection of scar

Definitions

- *Hypertrophic scar*: overgrowth—confined to borders of original wound.
- *Keloid*: overgrowth extending outwith original wound borders.

Indications

For scar overgrowth.

Preoperative preparation

- Can be done in the outpatient setting.
- Consider use of topical anaesthetic, e.g. EMLA or a 'field block'.
- Use triamcinolone (10mg/ml) drawn-up in an insulin syringe.

Procedure

- Aseptic technique.
- Insert needle within substance of lesion and inject against pressure in tiny aliquots until lesion blanches.
- Reposition needle to inject and blanche the entire lesion.
- Beware of injecting outwith or underneath lesion as this will cause atrophic scarring.
- Light dressings only required.

Postoperative care

- Repeat injections every 2–4 weeks.
- Combine treatment with occupational therapy input for silicone ± compression dressings.

Complications

- Ulceration (more common with greater concentration steroid, e.g. 40mg/ml).
- Atrophic scarring.
- Altered pigmentation.

Local skin flap

Types of local skin flaps

- A local skin flap is a unit of tissue that survives on its original blood supply when moved from a donor to a recipient site.
- Classification is based according to the movement of the flap. There are three principal types: R–A–T: Rotation, Advancement, and Transposition (see Figs 11.15–11.18).

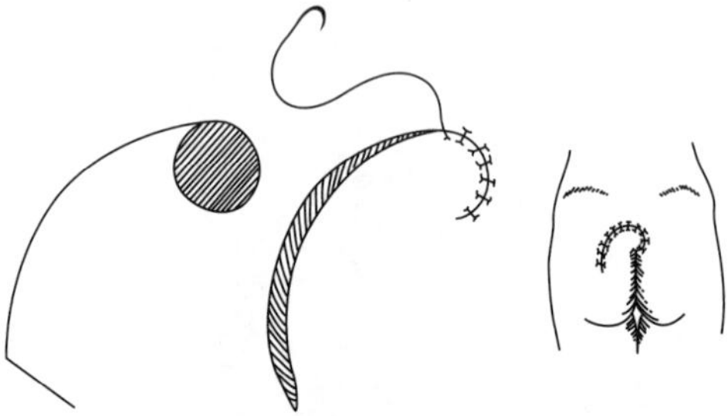

Fig. 11.15 Rotation flap. Reproduced from McLatchie, G. and Leaper, D., Operative Surgery 2nd edition, 2006, with permission from Oxford University Press.

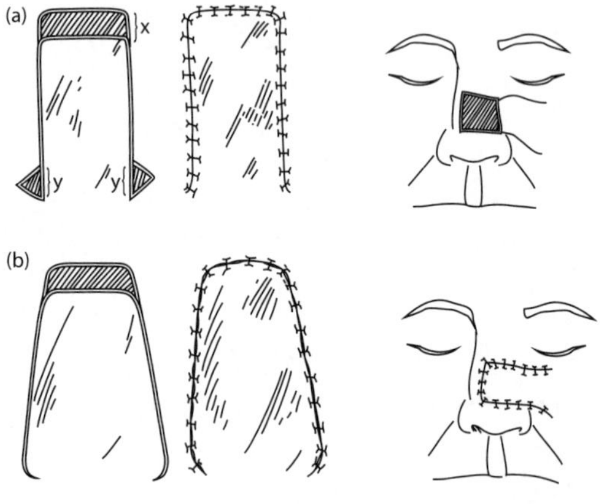
(a)
x
y
y
(b)

Fig. 11.16 Advancement flap. Reproduced from McLatchie, G. and Leaper, D., Operative Surgery 2nd edition, 2006, with permission from Oxford University Press.

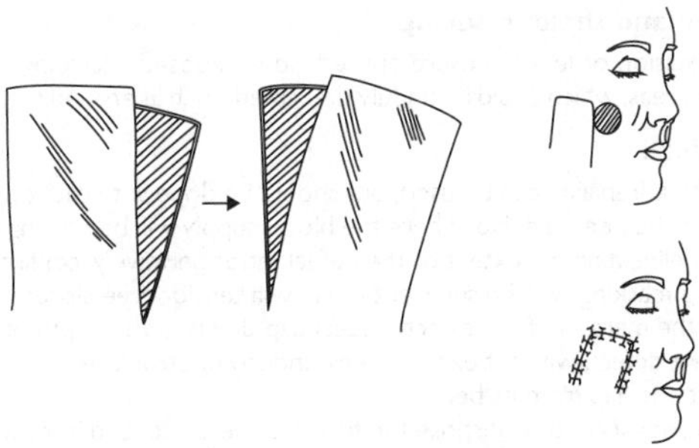

Fig. 11.17 Transposition flap. Reproduced from McLatchie, G. and Leaper, D., Operative Surgery 2nd edition, 2006, with permission from Oxford University Press.

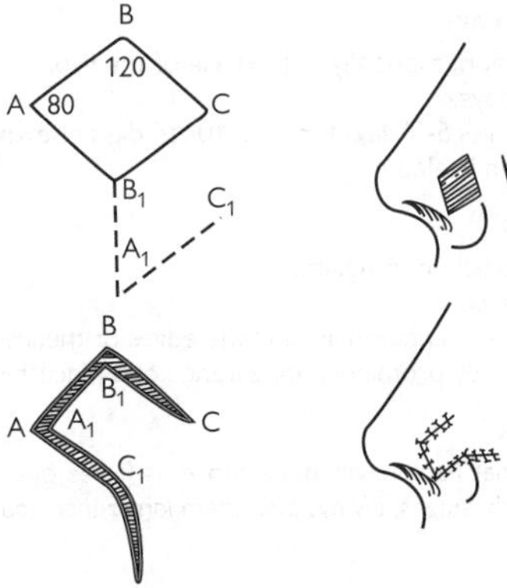
B
120
A
80
C
B1
C1
A1
B
B1
A
A1
C
C1

Fig. 11.18 Limberg flap (a type of transposition flap). Reproduced from McLatchie, G. and Leaper, D., Operative Surgery 2nd edition, 2006, with permission from Oxford University Press.

Indications

A local flap is one of the rungs of the reconstructive ladder. It should be considered when direct closure is not achievable and when the wound is either not suitable for skin grafting or when a local flap will give a cosmetically superior result.

Preoperative preparation

- Mark and measure margins of defect.
- Plan the flap with consideration to leave the final scar lying along relaxed skin tension lines (RSTLs—see Fig. 11.10).

Position and theatre set-up

As for excision of lesion: ensure entire field is exposed, including adjacent sensitive areas, which could be unduly deformed, such as around the eyelids.

Procedure

- LA with adrenaline can be used, but should be done with caution to the base of the intended flap, where the blood supply will be coming from.
- After delineating the extent of the defect intraoperatively, confirm that the flap markings will be sufficient to allow a tension-free closure.
- Incise the margins of the selected local flap down to the depth of the adjacent defect, without exposing key underlying structures.
- Elevate the flap from its bed.
- Rotate, advance, or transpose the flap into the defect and inset with sutures of preference to give a two-layer tension-free closure.
- Closure of donor defect should be achievable directly or for a transposition flap, through utilization of a skin graft.
- Non-compressive dressings as required.

Postoperative care

- Avoid compression, especially at the base of the flap.
- Review at 5–7 days.
- Removal of sutures 5–7 days for face; 10–14 days elsewhere.
- Scar advice when healed.

Complications

- Flap failure—partial or complete.
- Wound dehiscence.
- 'Pincushioning'—indentation around the edges of the inset flap, which gives it the unsightly prominent appearance of a pincushion.

Tips and tricks

Experience tells that flaps never quite move as far as one may first anticipate, so in the early stages, *always plan them larger than you might otherwise expect.*

Nail bed repair

Anatomy

(See Fig. 11.19)

- The *hyponychium* refers to the fingertip, just distal to the nailplate.
- The *paronychium* refers to the lateral borders of the nailbed.
- The *eponychium* refers to the 'cuticle' or tissue abutting the base of the visible nailplate.
- The *germinal matrix* (from where the nailplate grows) is located just distal to the insertion of the extensor tendon and extends to the distal border of the *lunula*, the visible semilunar pale area at the base of each nailplate.
- The *sterile matrix* is the visible portion of the nailbed distal to the lunula up to the fingertip, which enables 'glide' of the nailplate.

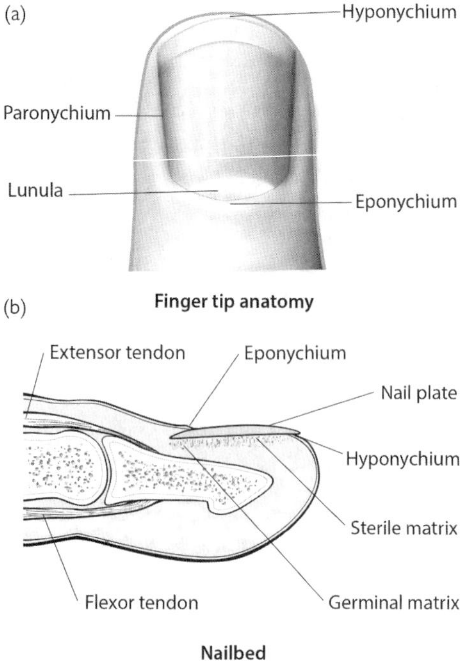
(a)
Hyponychium
Paronychium
Lunula
Eponychium
(b)
Finger tip anatomy
Extensor tendon
Eponychium
Nail plate
Hyponychium
Sterile matrix
Flexor tendon
Germinal matrix
Nailbed

Fig. 11.19 (a) Fingertip anatomy. (b) Nailbed. Medical illustrations produced by Helen Day, Medical Artist, Oxford, www.medicalartist.org.uk, reproduced with permission.

Indications

Trauma.

Preoperative preparation

- Determine level of injury and whether or not there is concomitant bony injury (e.g. 'tuft' fracture) or fingertip amputation.
- Tetanus and antibiotic cover is required.

Position and theatre set-up

Arm table and digital tourniquet.

Procedure

- Apply tourniquet using a clip.
- Remove nailplate in atraumatic manner using suitable instrumentation, such as the flat end of a Mitchell's trimmer.
- Directly visualize extent and location of underlying laceration.
- Lavage.
- Judicious debridement may be required but this should be minimal, if at all, over the sterile matrix.
- Repair pulp and paronychial area first to enable good re-approximation of wound with, e.g. 5/0 Vicryl Rapide™ absorbable sutures.
- Repair nailbed matrix using dissolvable, e.g. interrupted 6/0 Vicryl Rapide™ sutures, or a continuous 6/0 Monocryl® suture with its knots placed on the paronychium/outwith the sterile matrix.
- Clean nailplate/trim if required, and reinsert.
- Stabilize nailplate using same dissolvable suture in figure-of-eight, to splint nailbed repair into place.
- Dress with non-adherent dressings, such as 'Mepitel' silicone dressing, gauze and finger dressing.
- Remove clip and tourniquet.
- Zimmer splinting may be required if underlying fracture.

Postoperative care

- Complete course of antibiotics.
- Wound check 5–7 days.
- Advise patient that old nail will fall out of its own accord once new nail grows through.
- Refer to hand therapy for desensitization if needed.

Complications

- Abnormal/absent nail growth.
- Formation of synechia with subsequent aberrant nail growth.
- Hypersensitivity.
- Cold/heat intolerance.

Tips and tricks

- Splinting the nailfold by reinserting the removed (cleaned) nailplate is believed to reduce the formation of synechiae.
- When there is no nailplate remaining, foil from suture packs or a plastic disposable ruler can be fashioned as a substitute insert in order to splint the nailfold open.

Repair of digital nerve

Anatomy

The digital nerves are contained within the radial and ulnar neurovascular bundles, the nerves being more volar than the arteries

Indication

Trauma.

Preoperative preparation

- Clinical assessment by the operating surgeon is mandatory.
- Look for concomitant injuries, i.e. fractures or tendon damage.
- Mark appropriate digit(s) and side injured.
- Tetanus and antibiotic cover is required.
- Explain to patient that nerve recovery is very slow with a lag-time of 1 month and progression then at ~1mm/day in ideal favourable circumstances.

Position and theatre set-up

- Perioperative antibiotics.
- Arm table. Upper arm tourniquet with wool bandage cushioning.
- Lead hand and assistant to be considered.
- Microsurgical instrumentation should be requested in advance.
- Repair should be either under high-magnification Loupe vision (3.5× or greater), or with the microscope.

Procedure

- Mark out Brunner's incision lines to extend wounds if required.
- Raise tourniquet after exsanguination.
- Explore wounds and extend as required.
- Identify cut ends of digital nerve(s).
- Under magnification, with microsurgical instruments use 9/0 Ethilon® to achieve an epineural tension-free repair whilst endeavouring to align axons, burying their free ends within the epineurium.
- Skin closure by preferred technique, e.g. 5/0 Ethilon®/Vicryl Rapide™ interrupted.
- Non-adherent dressing/gauze/wool/crepe (POP if indicated if a tight repair).

Postoperative care

- Wound check 7 days.
- Removal of sutures at 10–14 days.
- Refer for hand therapy if required, e.g. for desensitization.

Complications

- Delayed/absent nerve recovery.
- Hypersensitivity.
- Hot/cold intolerance.
- Neuroma.
- CRPS.

Tips and tricks

- If there are concomitant injuries, it is often easier to repair these before the digital nerve, although it may be worthwhile 'tagging' the cut nerve ends with a suture as they are identified to make it easier to find them again later.
- Be wary of rolling a pale glove down a digit to use as a digital tourniquet: there are reported instances of surgeons omitting to remove digital tourniquets, with disastrous outcomes. If you elect to use a digital tourniquet, only use a coloured glove (i.e. green underglove) for which a clip should also always be used to secure it around the digit and, most importantly, as a failsafe reminder for removal!
- Nerve repairs should be with minimal tension—nerves do not regrow otherwise. If it is a 'tight' repair, tension can be released by mobilizing the nerve proximally and distally, but if there is still a tense gap despite this, best consideration would be to a nerve graft—e.g. the posterior interosseous nerve, located in the IVth extensor compartment (see p. 536).

Repair of lip laceration

Anatomy

(See Fig. 11.20)

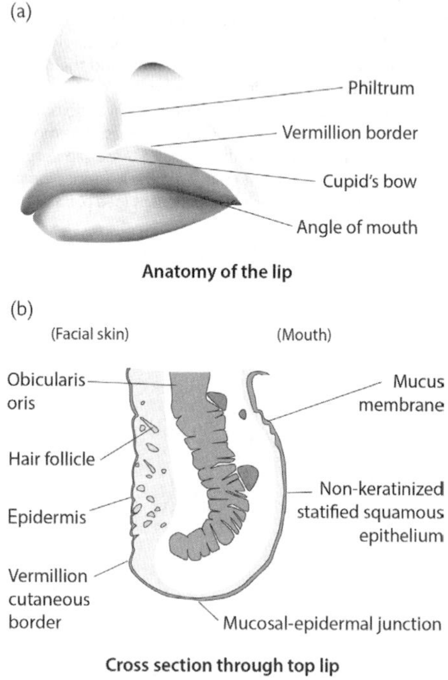
(a)
Philtrum
Vermillion border
Cupid's bow
Angle of mouth
Anatomy of the lip
(b)
(Facial skin)
(Mouth)
Obicularis oris
Hair follicle
Epidermis
Vermillion cutaneous border
Mucus membrane
Non-keratinized statified squamous epithelium
Mucosal-epidermal junction
Cross section through top lip

Fig. 11.20 (a) Anatomy of the lip. (b) Cross-section through top lip. Medical illustrations produced by Helen Day, Medical Artist, Oxford, www.medicalartist.org.uk, reproduced with permission.

Indications

Trauma.

Preoperative preparation

It is likely that the laceration was sustained on the patient's own teeth, therefore, a thorough washout under LA is required *early* in the A&E setting, as well as commencing on broad spectrum antibiotics for a bite injury (e.g. co-amoxiclav).

Position and theatre set-up

This can often be repaired in A&E under LA with the patient supine.

Procedure

- Aseptic technique.
- Ideally magnifying surgical loupes should be worn.
- Thoroughly lavage the wound, assessing in particular if any apparently innocuous minor lacerations are actually 'through and through'.
- Test all the teeth to ensure that none are loose/missing (part or all of a tooth). Complete or partially missing (broken) teeth, which were not found at the time of injury, are an indication for a CXR in order to exclude inhalation.
- Appropriately-sized interrupted Vicryl® sutures (e.g. 4/0) should be used to approximate any underlying split muscle.
- The first superficial suture should be accurately placed directly about the vermillion border, taking care to ensure that it is precisely aligned: a 1mm step in the vermillion border is easily identifiable from 1m away.
- Dissolvable interrupted sutures (e.g. 5/0 Vicryl Rapide™) are preferable on the mucosa.
- Non-absorbable sutures can ideally be used to approximate the skin (e.g. 5/0 or 6/0 Ethilon®).
- Dressings: none required.

Postoperative care

- Skin and dry mucosa sutures should be removed at 5–7 days.
- Advise to keep scar out of direct sunlight and wear factor 50 sunblock, ideally for 12–24 months to reduce scar prominence.

Complications

- Infection.
- Malalignment of the vermillion border.
- Poor, prominent scarring.

Tips and tricks

A lip laceration in a child does not automatically necessitate a GA repair: Treat each child individually, e.g. a 6-year-old has been known to be brave and willing enough to have a full repair under LA without complication.

Trigger digit release

Anatomy

A 'trigger' digit is defined by stenosing flexor tenosynovitis, in turn caused by a thickening of the A1 pulley (MCPJ level), often palpable as a flexor nodule (Notta's nodule).

Triggering is caused by inability of the flexor tendon and nodule to glide freely through the pulley, causing it to 'lock' or 'trigger' in a flexed position after flexion has pulled the thickened area through.

Indications

Persistent problematic locking or 'triggering' of the digit.

Preoperative preparation

- Mark digit.
- Aim to undertake under LA.
- Arm table. Upper arm tourniquet with wool bandage cushioning.
- Lead hand.

Procedure

- Mark incision line overlying A1 pulley/distal palmar crease.
- Under tourniquet control, incise under direct vision, taking care to preserve neurovascular bundles.
- Identify A1 pulley and divide longitudinally with tenotomy scissors, ensuring entire pulley is released.
- Confirm good flexor tendon glide with patient's co-operation, asking them to move digit through its full excursion.
- Haemostasis after release of tourniquet.
- Closure with suture of choice.
- Non-adherent dressings.

Postoperative care

- Immediate mobilization.
- Wound check 5–7 days.

Complications

- Recurrence.
- Inadvertent injury to neurovascular bundle(s) or tendon.

Tips and tricks

Steroid injection in the outpatient setting may improve symptoms without surgery in selected cases.

Use of Z-plasty

Anatomy

A Z-plasty is defined as a double opposition flap, which is a variation of a transposition flap (see Fig. 11.21 and Table 11.2).

Indications

- To lengthen a scar.
- To re-orientate a scar.

Preoperative preparation

- Mark the scar outline.
- Mark the flaps from either end of the scar with the ideal angle of 60°.
- All three limbs of the Z should be of equal length.

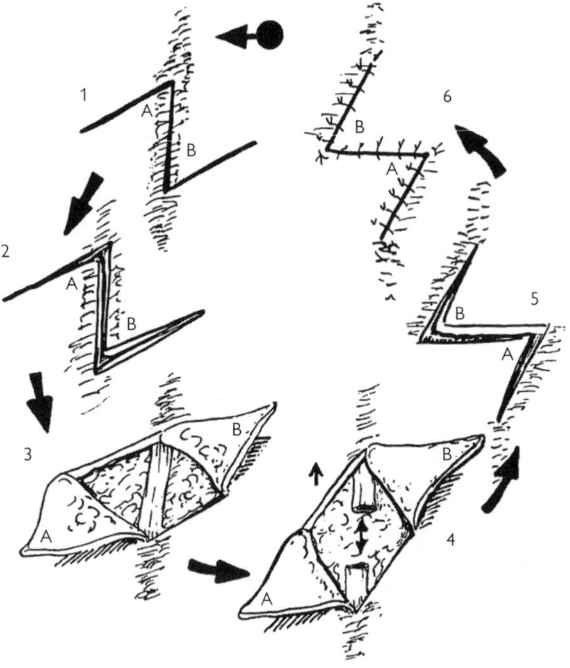
1
A
B
6
B
A
2
A
B
5
B
A
3
B
A
B
4
A

Fig. 11.21 Z-plasty flap. Reproduced from McLatchie, G. and Leaper, D., Operative Surgery 2nd edition, 2006, with permission from Oxford University Press.

Table 11.2 Angles of Z-plasty

Angles of Z-plasty	Theoretical gain in length (%)
30°	25
45°	50
60°	75
75°	100
90°	120

Procedure

- Incise FT through the skin along the predetermined skin markings.
- Elevate the flaps with subcutaneous tissue.
- Excise scar tissue.
- Haemostasis.
- Transpose and inset the flaps (see Fig. 11.21).
- Closure as per preference, e.g. 5/0 Ethilon®.

Postoperative care

- Avoid external pressure to flaps.
- Flap check at 5–7 days.
- Removal of sutures at timing dependent on site and suture material used.

Complications

- Partial or complete flap necrosis.
- Inadequate lengthening.

Tips and tricks

- A Z-plasty only works in an area that has surrounding tissue laxity.
- Multiple Z-plasties may be required in a long scar.
- 60° angulation of Z-plasty flaps lengthens the scar by an additional 75% (a 2cm scar will become 3.5cm long).
- Beware that inadequate planning can easily give an unfavourable outcome.

Digital terminalization

Indications
- Trauma.
- Malignancy.

Preoperative preparation
- Determine level of terminalization required in conjunction with radiographic findings.
- Counsel the patient accordingly.
- Antibiotic ± tetanus cover is required.

Position and theatre set-up
Arm table; upper arm or digital tourniquet required.

Procedure
- Mark out fishmouth incision to stump end.
- Apply tourniquet (avoid esmarch exsanguination in malignancy).
- Dissect out soft tissues from bony stump.
- Dissect out ends of neurovascular bundles.
- Stretch neurovascular bundles and use diathermy cautery as proximal as possible to minimize risk of neuroma formation.
- Divide flexor and extensor tendons as proximal as possible and allow them to retract.
- Use bone cutters/nibblers/saw to trim bone end to desired level, ensuring there is sufficient soft tissue to cover exposed bone.
- If terminalization is at the level of a joint, the cartilage should be removed with the aid of nibblers.
- Use rasp to file the bone end and make it smooth.
- Bipolar haemostasis.
- Tension-free closure using interrupted skin sutures alone is sufficient.
- Dress with non-adherent dressings such as 'Mepitel' or 'Silflex' silicone dressings, gauze, and fingertip dressing.

Postoperative care
- Complete course of antibiotics.
- Wound check 5–7 days.
- Removal sutures 10–14 days.
- Refer to hand therapy for rehabilitation and desensitization.
- Consider referring patient for psychological support if required.
- Consider referring patient for prosthesis.

Complications
- Bone infection/osteomyelitis.
- Hypersensitivity.
- Neuroma formation.
- Cold/heat intolerance.
- Loss of overall hand function, depending on digit amputated; this more pronounced if the loss is to the border digits.
- CRPS.

Tips and tricks

- *Never* suture tendon ends together over the end of the bony stump!* *This adversely affects biomechanical functioning of the remnant tendons.*
- Suture the wound closed with the digit in a flexed position. Check that the wound does not come under undue tension through the full excursion of flexion and extension of the digit.
- Be careful not to leave the refashioned stump too bulky. There is often only minimal soft tissue resorption in the healing process.

Reduction and fixation of hand fracture

Anatomy

There are 27 bones in the hand (excluding sesamoids):
- 8 carpal bones.
- 5 metacarpals.
- 14 phalanges.

Indications

Bony malalignment post-trauma, for which closed manipulation and plaster cast is inadequate to maintain a good fracture reduction.

Preoperative preparation

- Ensure adequate AP and true lateral X-rays have been obtained.
- Exclude concomitant injury.

Position and theatre set-up

- Arm table.
- Upper-arm tourniquet is often used for open reduction and internal fixation (ORIF) but not usually for Kirschner-wiring ('K-wiring').

Procedure

- For placement of any metal work, antibiotic cover is required on induction and before the tourniquet is applied.
- Under image intensifier ('II') guidance:
  - Use counter-traction and direct pressure over the fracture site to reduce the fracture back to the original shape of the bone.
  - Assess stability and verify need for bony fixation as opposed to external splinting alone.

Percutaneous approach for K-wiring

- Determine best direction of approach: either from proximal to distal or distal to proximal.
- On the dorsum of the hand, use the II to locate the exact position of the fracture and use a skin marker pen to draw this in place, together with the full outline of the affected bone.
- Select the most suitable size of K-wire (e.g. 0.9 or 1.1mm) to use.
- Place the K-wire on the skin on top of the fracture to correspond to the exact position required to maintain reduction. Use the II to confirm the accuracy of its position and mark this position on with a pen.
- Determine from the II where the entry point into the bone is to be and trace down the axis of the K-wire to determine where the wire should enter the skin.
- Puncture the skin with the K-wire to locate it on the bone at the determined point of entry.
- Check the position in the AP and lateral planes using the II.
- Activate the K-wire driver and progress it through the bone up to the fracture site.
- Drip saline along the K-wire to keep the tip cool.
- Check progression of the K-wire at intervals using the II in both AP and lateral planes.

- Ensure that the fracture remains well reduced and aligned at all times; re-manipulate as the K-wire nears the fracture site, if appropriate.
- Once the K-wire has reached the outer cortex of the bone at the other side of the fracture, remove the drill.
- Insert second K-wire if desired.
- If burying the wire, cut it flush with the skin; close with suitable suture.
- If leaving wire long, bend the tip over at the desired length prior to cutting and then use pliers to crimp the bent end.
- A POP splint is often used as additional protection following K-wiring.

Open reduction internal fixation

- Identify plate of choice in advance.
- Mark skin incision lines directly atop the bone and fracture site.
- Using a dorsal approach, incise FT through the skin and retract any extensor tendons out to one side/split longitudinally through the centre of the extensor (e.g. over P1) as appropriate.
- Incise longitudinally through the periosteum and use a Mitchell's trimmer to carefully elevate the periosteum to each side.
- Use bone pincers if required to maintain the position of the fracture reduction.
- Lie the selected plate atop the fracture and determine if any plate bending is required.
- Mark the desired location of the most proximal screw hole and select the appropriate sized drill piece.
- Under irrigation, drill through both cortices of the bone, perpendicular to the long axis of the bone.
- Use the depth gauge to determine the correct screw to select.
- Hold the plate in place using the first screw.
- Repeat the same procedure for subsequent screws, using direct vision to ensure that the fracture reduction position is well maintained.
- Once plate and screws are in place, use II to verify that the selected screws are of the correct length on a true lateral view.
- Close the periosteum over the top of the metalwork using Vicryl® (e.g. 4/0).
- Repair any tendon that was divided for access.
- Suture the skin with a continuous suture, e.g. Monocryl® or Ethilon®.

Following any method of fracture reduction, ensure that adequate radiographs are saved ± printed for the patient's file, demonstrating the position of all metalwork at the end of the procedure.

Postoperative care

- Elevate hand at rest.
- Avoid NSAIDs as these impair bony healing.
- Antibiotics and tetanus cover are indicated in open injuries.
- For ORIF, encourage early mobilization; for K-wiring keep splinted until the K-wire is to be removed (between 3–6 weeks postoperative, depending on injury and age of patient).
- Protect the hand from further impact for at least 4–6 weeks.
- Early follow-up in clinic with check X-rays if required.
- Refer to hand physiotherapy for rehabilitation.

Complications

- Bony non-union/Malunion.
- Infection.
- Wound breakdown with subsequent exposure of metalwork.

Tips and tricks

- For K-wiring, take your time with the II to identify the ideal insertion point and correct orientation, before you start. This will better ensure ideal placement with the first pass.
- K-wires blunt after the first use, so should only be used once from each end. If more attempts are needed to attain the correct position, use a fresh K-wire to prevent heat from causing bone damage.
- If using two 'cross K-wires', never cross these at the fracture site.
- When bending the K-wire end to leave long, be cautious not to cause a shift in the fracture reduction.
- The black plastic bung of a 0.5mm syringe can be used to protect the sharp exposed end of the K-wire.
- Avoid over-bending ORIF metal plates.
- Do not place screws closer than one screw head to a fracture site.
- Don't fully tighten all the screws as you go—come back to tighten these after all screws inserted.
- Lag screw may also be used in combination with either K-wires or ORIF plating.

Insertion of tissue expander

The principles of tissue expansion are: biological creep and stress relaxation:

- Creep is elongation of skin and subcutaneous tissue by stretching. It causes the collagen fibres to re-orientate.
- Stress relaxation is a permanent elongation once the stretch has dissipated over time.

Indications

When optimal reconstruction of a defect requires increased volume of tissue with the same characteristics specific to that region of the body but sufficient tissue cannot be found locally, a tissue expander is often employed. This allows gradual acquisition of local soft tissues and skin with the desired properties.

The most commonly used areas of tissue expansion are:

- Breast reconstruction.
- Scalp scar alopecia.

Preoperative preparation

- Select ideal expander; base diameter should be 2–2.5× the size of the defect.
- Determine the desired number of expanders to allow adequate tissue to be produced.
- Shape of expander: round expanders are ideal for breast; semilunar shape for scalp.

Position and theatre set-up

- Position to ensure adequate exposure of operating site.
- Verify the expander's integrity pre-procedure by inflating with saline, before completely emptying it of both air and saline.

Procedure

- Incise along edge of scar (or inframammary fold for breast reconstruction).
- The pocket is created in a sub-galeal plane (scalp) or submuscular plane (breast).
- Ensure the pocket is of adequate size to accommodate the expander.
- Develop a communicating smaller pocket to inset the port.
- Achieve haemostasis.
- Insert expander using a minimal-touch technique whilst ensuring correct orientation.
- Inset the port and ensure that it is the correct way round for easy inflation (the large metal back plate should be against a rigid surface).
- Careful closure in layers taking care not to puncture the expander.
- Expand on-table with e.g. 50–100ml saline, watching to ensure adequate expansion without compromising capillary refill of the tissues.
- Non-compressive dressings only.

Postoperative care

- Wound review 1 week postoperation.
- Start inflation in 3–4 weeks at weekly intervals.
- Inflation volumes should be guided by what the patient can tolerate without undue discomfort whilst ensuring good capillary refill maintained.
- Once the desired inflation volume is achieved, patient will need second-stage reconstruction with advancement of flaps (scalp reconstruction) or possible exchange of expander for permanent prosthesis (breast reconstruction).

Complications

- Infection.
- Expander extrusion.
- Expander displacement/expansion of the wrong area.
- Inadvertent expander rupture.
- Overlying skin necrosis and wound dehiscence.

Tips and tricks

Tissue expanders should be placed distant to the incision site to avoid additional tension upon would edges: tunnel under the adjacent tissues to ensure optimal placement underneath healthy tissues.

Planning and execution of fasciocutaneous and muscle flaps in the upper and lower limbs

Common fasciocutaneous flaps include:

- Radial forearm and reverse radial forearm flaps for upper limb.
- Transposition fasciocutaneous flaps of the lower limb.

Common muscle flaps include:

- Gastrocnemius.
- Soleus/hemisoleus.
- Gracilis.

Indications

These flaps are commonly used to cover exposed bone, joint, or tendon following trauma or surgical resection for other reason, such as local cancer (see Table 11.3 for treatment options).

Preoperative preparation

- In-depth knowledge of the anatomy and vascular supply and location of vascular pedicles is mandatory before undertaking any flap reconstruction.
- Doppler can be used as an adjunct to flap planning in order to locate the position of the vascular pedicle or perforators.
- Ensure that in the planning stage, the flap is of sufficient size to adequately cover the defect, with a tension-free closure.

Table 11.3 Summary of treatment options for lower limb trauma

Region of defect	Flap
• Proximal third	• Gastrocenemius • Proximal fasciocutaneous • Free flap
• Middle third	• Soleus • Anterior compartment muscles • Proximal fasciocutaneous • Free flap
• Distal third	• Distally based fasciocutaneous • Free flap
• Anke	• Distally based fasciocutaneous • Free flap

Reproduced from McLatchie, G. and Leaper, D., Operative Surgery 2nd edition, 2006, with permission from Oxford University Press.

Procedure

- Elevate the flap as per its specific anatomy, ensuring the pedicle is protected at all times.
- The secondary defect may require coverage with a split-thickness skin graft.

Postoperative care

- Ensure that no pressure is applied to the pedicle.
- POP backslab splinting may be required.
- A window may be cut in the dressings in order to enable flap monitoring.
- Early wound check will be required

Complications

- Failure of procedure with partial or complete flap loss.
- Wound dehiscence.
- Graft failure.

Tips and tricks

- Always plan the flap to be larger than you expect.
- Use a template to plan the size of the flap.

Abdominoplasty

An abdominoplasty is the excision of loose/excess skin and subcutaneous tissue from the lower abdomen, usually following weight loss or post-partum.

Indication

Excess skin to the lower abdomen.

Preoperative preparation

- Full history and examination, including to assess for abdominal wall herniae and divarication of the recti.
- The patient will require a full anaesthetic assessment and work-up.
- Mark patient whilst supine and then erect to determine amount of tissue to be excised whilst ensuring that wound healing is not compromised by leaving inadequate tissue for tension-free wound closure.
- The most inferior skin marking is pan-abdominal, in the typical plane of an Pfannenstiel incision.

Position and theatre set-up

- The patient should be supine.
- Consider catheterization.
- Advise patient about repositioning of umbilicus.

Procedure

- Consider infiltration with adrenaline-containing solution along skin incision line.
- Dissect out the umbilicus on its stalk.
- Incise predetermined excision markings down to deep fascia using monopolar cautery, obtaining haemostasis as you proceed.
- Elevate skin flaps taking care to protect the dissected umbilicus.
- Undermine the abdominal flaps by dissecting upwards along the deep fascia until the lower costal margins/xiphisternum.
- 'Break the table'.
- Pull the excess skin inferiorly and excise at a level which will allow tension free closure.
- Insert two drains.
- Close in layers with deep dissolvable sutures and then Monocryl® or other suture of choice to skin.
- Ensure the umbilicus is reinset in an anatomical position in the midline.
- Dressings as per preference.

Postoperative care

- DVT prophylaxis mandatory.
- Drains out when minimal.
- Mobilize in a stooped position gradually increasing to stand straight over the course of a week.
- Wound check at 1 week.

Complications

- Wound dehiscence and flap necrosis, especially centrally.
- Seroma.
- Abnormal sensation.

Tips and tricks

- Beware of the smoker! Preferably insist your patient quits smoking preoperatively given the high incidence of wound necrosis and breakdown in that cohort.
- Rectus plication may be required if there is significant divarication.
- Leaving a thin layer of adipose tissue on the deep muscle fascia is thought to reduce seroma formation.

Infra-inguinal lymphadenectomy

Anatomy

The boundaries of the femoral triangle (see Fig. 11.22) are:

- The inguinal ligament (superiorly).
- The medial border of the adductor longus (medially).
- The medial border of Sartorius (laterally).
- The floor is formed by the pectineus and adductor longus muscles medially and iliopsoas laterally. Its roof is formed by the fascia lata.

Indications

Lymph node involvement with metastases.

Position and theatre set-up,

Supine with leg abducted and knee slightly flexed.

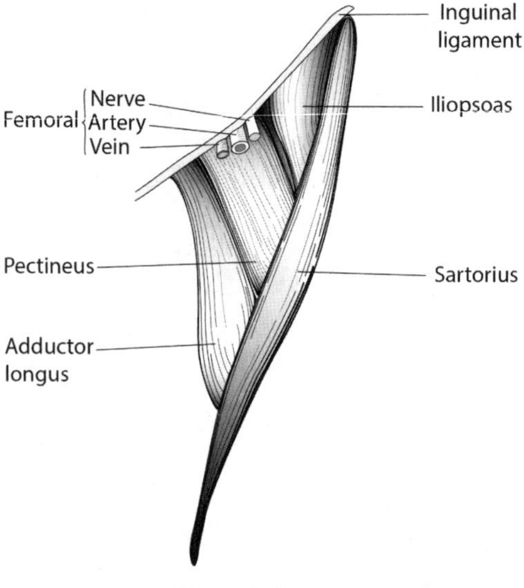
Inguinal ligament
Femoral
Nerve
Artery
Vein
Iliopsoas
Pectineus
Sartorius
Adductor longus
Femoral triangle

Fig. 11.22 The femoral triangle. Medical illustrations produced by Helen Day, Medical Artist, Oxford, www.medicalartist.org.uk, reproduced with permission.

Procedure

- Different incisions are chosen; typical incisions are longitudinal or curvilinear, although some surgeons also use a horizontal incision parallel to the inguinal ligament.
- Remove all the lymph nodes from the femoral triangle 'en bloc', whilst preserving the femoral nerve and artery.
- Orientate specimen with a marker stitch.
- Subcutaneous and skin closure over two drains.

Postoperative care

- Mobilize as able.
- DVT prophylaxis.
- Removal of drains as per output.
- Monitor for signs of seroma, infection, and wound dehiscence.
- Early and regular postoperative wound checks.

Complications

On average, worldwide, 4 out of 5 of patients develop 'complications' following this procedure, despite many different variations on the technique used. Common complications include:

- Seroma.
- Haematoma.
- Infection.
- Wound breakdown.
- Nerve damage and altered sensation distally.
- Lymphoedema.

Tips and tricks

- The orientation of the structures in the femoral triangle can be remembered by the mnemonics 'NAVY' (nerve, artery, vein, and y-fronts) and 'NAVAL' (nerve, artery, vein, empty space, lymphatics).
- Monitor for seroma and consider regular drainage when relevant, to prevent excessive pressure upon the surgical wound, which may otherwise expedite wound breakdown.
- Aim to have clear postoperative policies agreed within your unit for the desired management of the common complications.

Correction of simple syndactyly

This is a failure of separation of adjacent digits.

Classification

- Simple—only skin is involved.
- Complex—skin and bone are involved.
- Complicated—associated with other congenital hand anomalies.
- Complete—the whole lengths of the digits are fused.
- Incomplete—only parts of the digits (at the proximal end) are fused.

Indications

- To separate the digits of the hand.
- Separation of the toes is normally not prioritized as it is deemed a 'cosmetic' procedure.

Preoperative preparation

- Obtain X-rays.
- Careful preoperative counselling together with parents.
- Border digits are separated first; central digits are done in subsequent stages.
- Initial operation is typically from 6 months of age.

Position and theatre set-up

Arm table and upper arm tourniquet.

Procedure

- Mark and incise volarly and dorsally as per preference, separating digit: typically zigzag incisions are combined with skin grafting.
- Haemostasis.
- Closure with 5/0 or 6/0 Vicryl Rapide™.
- Non-adherent dressings and boxing-glove wrapping.

Postoperative care

- Advise parents to keep the dressings intact and dry.
- Wound check 7–10 days.

Complications

- Graft failure.
- Wound breakdown/flap tip necrosis.
- Web creep/recurrence.

Reconstruction of nipple using C-V (cervical-visor) local flap

Anatomy

(See Fig. 11.23)

Indications

Nipple reconstruction is often seen as the final stage of reconstructive breast surgery. Local FT skin flaps are often used to wrap around a central dermal fat pedicle in order to create a nipple prominence. This is usually done in combination with pigment tattooing.

Simple alternatives to a C-V flap include:

- Tattooing on its own.
- 'Stick-on' silicone prostheses.

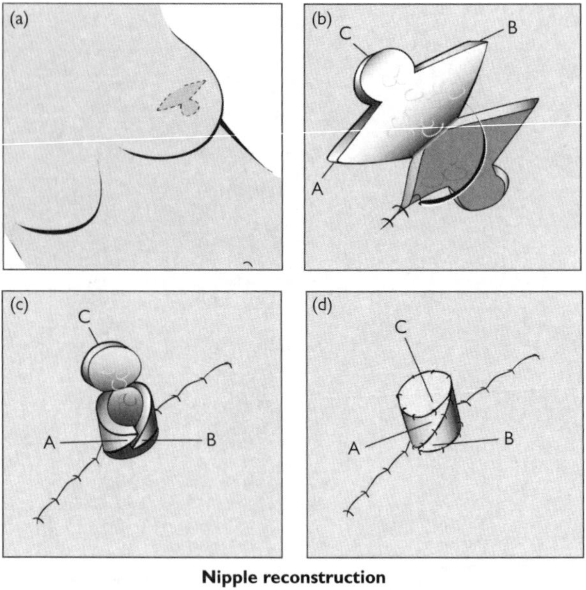
(a)
(b)
C
B
A
(c)
C
A
B
(d)
C
A
B
Nipple reconstruction

Fig. 11.23 (a) Skin markings for C-V flap. (b) Flaps are raised with a small amount of fat still attached whilst leaving pedicle intact for blood supply. (c) The two triangle 'V' flaps (A and B) are wrapped around each other. (d) The constructed nipple: the C-flap has been folded over on top. Medical illustrations produced by Helen Day, Medical Artist, Oxford, www.medicalartist.org.uk, reproduced with permission.

Other surgical alternatives to reconstruct a prominence include:

- Nipple sharing.
- Skate flap.
- Fishtail flap.
- Star flap.
- Top hat flap.

Preoperative preparation

Determine with the patient in advance the ideal nipple location. They can be guided by the surgeon, but ultimately they themselves should decide exactly where they wish the permanent nipple reconstruction to be placed. Full frontal and side views in a mirror, together with the patient, are invaluable for this purpose.

Position and theatre set-up

- The procedure is undertaken under LA, although patients are often insensate at the operative site.
- The patient is supine with both breasts fully exposed.
- Mark the C-V flap, focusing on the final location of the nipple prominence. As it is drawn, the new nipple will be roughly centred halfway between the two 'V's, although it is necessary to also accommodate for local skin movement as the flap 'V' donor sites are directly closed.

Procedure

- Infiltrate with LA.
- Incise FT through the skin and raise the two 'V' and the 'C' flaps as skin with a small amount of adherent adipose tissue.
- Take a slightly larger amount of adipose tissue centrally, being certain not to undermine the pedicle base.
- Bipolar haemostasis.
- Close the 'V' donor sites first using, e.g. 5/0 Monocryl® dermal sutures.
- Wrap the two V-flaps around the central dermal fat pedicle, first anchoring each tip to the base of the opposite flap using dermal sutures. Use more interrupted sutures to join the remainder of the wrapping V-flaps together.
- Inset the base of the reconstructed nipple with dermal and then interrupted skin sutures.
- Fold the 'C' flap into place atop the wrapped central dermal fat pedicle and inset with dermal sutures and then interrupted skin sutures.
- Dress with jelonet/equivalent and a piece of sponge just thicker than the new nipple prominence with a hole cut out of the centre to easily accommodate the reconstructed nipple without applying any pressure to it. The sponge can be held-in-place with tegaderm dressings or equivalent.

Postoperative care

- Ensure there is no compression to the nipple prominence.
- Flap check in plastic surgery nurse-led clinic at 1 week.
- Refer for nipple areolar tattooing to colour match contralateral side, which can be undertaken after a couple of months.

Complications

- Flap failure and breakdown.
- Nipple flattening with time.
- Asymmetry with contralateral side.

Tips and tricks

- It can be helpful if the patient has experimented at home to determine their ideal location for nipple placement prior to the day of surgery, and attends on the day with this marked in advance by them. Round ECG stickers with central metal studs make good aids for them to experiment with as a 'pretend nipple'.
- Reconstructed nipples will shrink by as much as 50% in the first year and slightly more longer term thereafter. Therefore, you should plan to overcorrect and advise the patient of nipple shrinkage with time.
- Different skin behaves differently. Beware the patient who has a DIEP breast reconstruction on one side and an LD reconstruction on the other. Identical templates will not produce identical nipples and must be tailored according to skin turgidity/thickness, etc.

Selective fasciectomy

Anatomy

- This is undertaken for Dupuytren's disease of the hand.
- Dupuytren's is a benign fibroproliferative disorder of the fascia of the palm and digits.

Indications

- Hueston's table-top test: when the patient can no longer place all their fingers flat on the table.
- MCPJ contracture >30°.
- PIPJ contracture.

Preoperative preparation

Careful history and examination including family history.

Position and theatre set-up,

Arm table/upper arm tourniquet/lead hand.

Procedure

- Mark straight line incision directly over cord (as defined by Skoog).
- Separate the skin from the underlying cord taking care not to button-hole.
- Dissect out, identify, and preserve neurovascular bundles, bilaterally.
- Remove diseased fascia of affected digit—send for histopathological examination.
- Ascertain deformity correction on table.
- Plan and undertake Z-plasties for skin closure, especially over joint lines in order to lengthen the scar whilst permitting a tension-free closure.
- Release tourniquet.
- Meticulous bipolar haemostasis.
- Closure as per preference.
- Non-adherent dressings/gauze/velband/POP volar slab/ulnar gutter splint to immobilize in extended position/crepe.

Postoperative care

- Elevate hand.
- Wound check at 1 week ± removal of sutures at 10–14 days.
- Refer to hand therapy for mobilization and splintage.
- Patient will occasionally need a splint to correct residual deformity.
- Patients require night-splinting for 3–6 months.

Complications

- Haematoma.
- Skin necrosis/wound breakdown.
- Neurovascular damage.
- Inability to completely correct deformity.
- Recurrence.
- Cold/heat intolerance.
- CRPS.

Tips and tricks

Some types of Dupuytren's may be considered suitable for trial with collagenase in the clinic setting, avoiding the need for surgery.

Chapter 12

Cardiothoracic surgery

Median sternotomy

The median sternotomy provides safe, reliable and optimal access to the heart, great vessels, and most other structures in the anterior, middle, and superior mediastina.

Anatomy

The landmarks of the sternal notch, xiphoid process, and lateral sternal edges are important to note to stay in the midline.

Indications

- Most cardiac operations.
- Tracheobronchial and some pulmonary surgery.
- Mediastinal tumours and retrosternal goitres.

Contraindications

None absolute but great caution is required in redo-sternotomy.

Preoperative preparation

- Nil by mouth for 6h preoperative and cross-matched blood—usually 2 units.
- Urinary catheter, central line, and arterial line.
- Withhold anticoagulants/anti-platelets (and vasodilators in bypass cases) according to unit protocol.

Position and theatre set-up

- Supine.
- Ensure legs and groins are clipped and prepped as appropriate to allow access to femoral vessels and long saphenous vein (LSV) if needed.

Procedure

- Make a vertical skin incision from below the sternal notch to the xiphoid process (Fig. 12.1).
- Continue incising with diathermy through the deeper tissues.
- Divide the interclavicular ligament and rectus aponeurosis.
- Mark out the midline on the sternal periosteum with the diathermy to guide the osteotomy.
- Bluntly dissect the pericardium off the back of the sternum with a finger and divide the xiphisterum with heavy scissors.
- Notify anaesthetic team and divide the sternum with a saw.
- Attain haemostasis (diathermy and bone wax may be used).
- Cover the wounds edges with towels, position sternal retractor in the lower half of the sternotomy, and progressively open.
- Divide sterno-pericardial ligaments and open the pericardium in an inverted T-shaped incision.
- Hitch up the pericardial edges to the wound towels or periosteum to create a pericardial well.

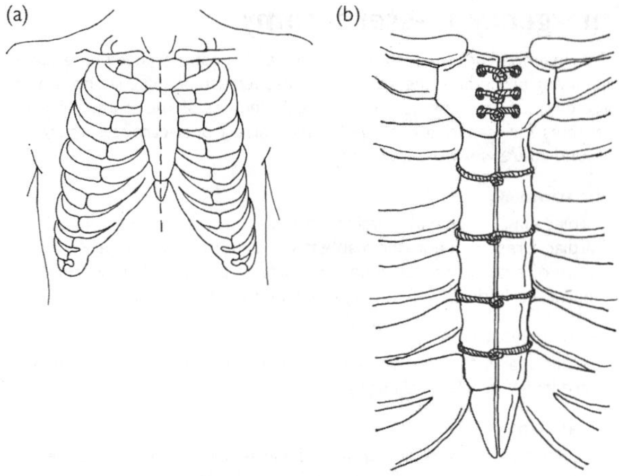
(a)
(b)

Fig. 12.1 Anatomy of the creation and closure of a median sternotomy.

Closure

- Perform haemostasis and site drains—pericardial, mediastinal, and pleural, as appropriate.
- Use six to nine sternal sutures to securely approximate the sternal edges, burying the wire ends in the periosteum (Fig. 12.1).
- Absorbable sutures to close pectoral fascia, fat, and skin.

Complications

- Visceral injury, particularly at redo-sternotomy.
- Superficial and deep wound infection.
- Sternal non-union or dehiscence.
- Brachial plexus injury.
- Epigastric hernia.

Tips and tricks

- To stay in the midline, reassess your landmarks frequently.
- If you inadvertently open the peritoneum, document this so that a subsequent CXR is not misinterpreted as a perforated abdominal viscus.
- Apply upwards pressure to the oscillating saw in order to reduce risk of injury to deeper structures.
- When re-approximating the bone, be sure to get the tension right—don't 'cheese-wire' the bone, but make sure it is secure.

Emergency re-sternotomy

Although emergency re-sternotomy in the early postoperative phase can be a life-saving procedure, the decision to re-open can be difficult and is often made by a junior trainee or non-surgical member of the team. Published algorithms for managing cardiopulmonary arrest post-cardiac surgery can be found at (www.csu-als.com).

Indications

- Cardiac tamponade with imminent arrest.
- Cardiac arrest with non-shockable rhythm after cardiac surgery.
- Failure of external cardioversion to restore a cardiac output in VF/VT (ventricular fibrillation or tachycardia) after cardiac surgery.

Contraindications

None, although if the patient is more than a couple of weeks post-surgery, re-sternotomy may be challenging.

Preparation

- Most cardiac intensive care areas and wards will have pre-packed re-sternotomy sets and an all-in-one adhesive drape.
- Don gown and gloves whilst other team members continue external cardiac massage and life support.

Procedure

- Suspend external massage, remove dressings, and apply adhesive drape.
- Re-open incision with scalpel, cut, and remove sternal wires.
- Gently separate the sternal edges and insert sternal retractor.
- Evacuate clot from mediastinum and pleural cavities.
- Control sources of catastrophic haemorrhage, commence internal massage, cardiovert with internal paddles, or site/use epicardial pacing wires as appropriate.
- If you are unable to re-establish a cardiac output with resuscitation drugs, internal massage, pacing, or cardioversion, prepare to re-institute bypass.

Closure

As for 'Median sternotomy' (p. 583).

Complications

- Injury to cardiac chambers.
- Injury to patent bypass grafts.

Tips and tricks

- Practice and revise the protocol before starting work at a cardiac surgery unit.
- Communicate clearly and work as a team, quickly but carefully.
- Do not avulse the mammary graft from the left anterior descending coronary graft.

Long saphenous vein harvest

The long saphenous vein (LSV) remains the most commonly employed bypass conduit. The short saphenous vein and cephalic veins can also be used, but are associated with poorer patency. The LSV may be procured as an open technique (as described) or minimally invasively using a vein stripper or endoscopic system.

Anatomy

The LSV arises from the dorsal venous arch of the foot and travels up the medial aspect of the lower limb. Key landmarks include immediately anterior to the medial malleolus, 4cm posterior to the medial edge of the patella at the knee, and 1–2cm infero-lateral to the pubic tubercle at the groin (location of the saphenofemoral junction; Fig. 12.2).

Indications

Coronary artery bypass surgery (CABG).

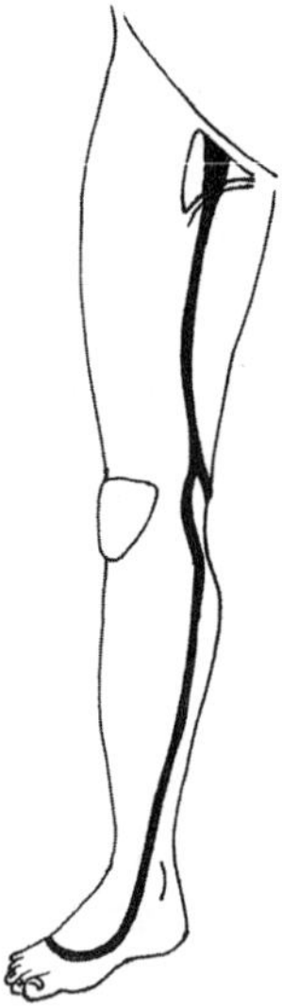

Fig. 12.2 Long saphenous vein anatomy.

Contraindications

- Small calibre or poor-quality vein.
- Varicose LSV, prior varicose vein surgery, or chronic venous insufficiency.
- Severe peripheral arterial disease.
- Cutaneous sepsis of the lower limb.

Position and theatre set-up

- Clip limb and pubic hair prior to surgery.
- Sterile field with both lower limbs (excluding feet) and groins exposed. Ensure the medial malleolus is visible.

Procedure

- Make an incision over the LSV at the ankle.
- Find the plane on the surface of the vein and develop it.
- Extend the incision superiorly, following the course of the LSV.
- Incisions may be bridged to reduce incision length (Figs. 12.3 and 12.4).

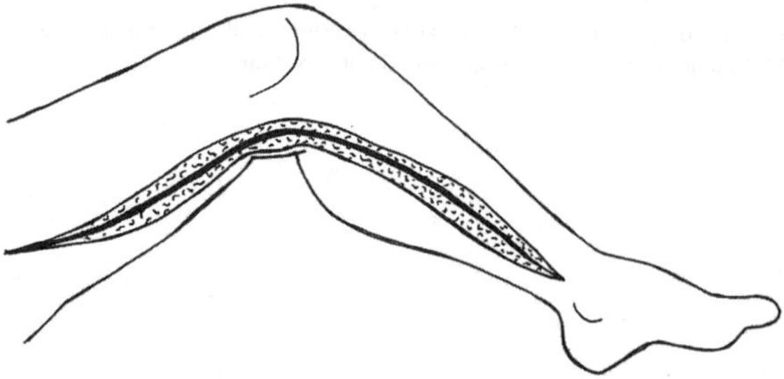

Fig. 12.3 Completely open LSV harvest incision.

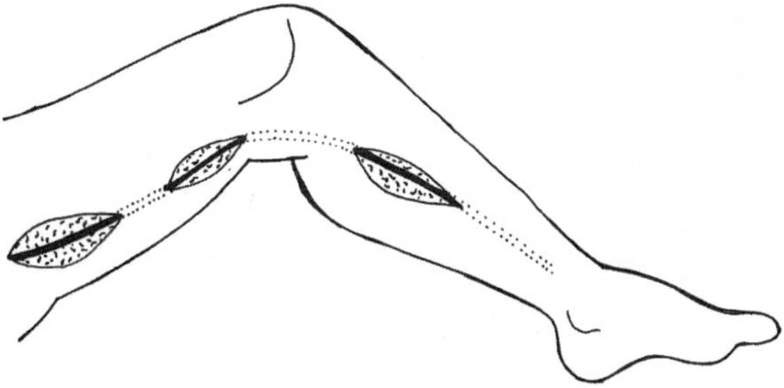

Fig. 12.4 Bridged incisions.

- Once the LSV is fully dissected and shown to be of a suitable diameter and length, ligate branches flush with the LSV and divide them.
- Clip both ends with a haemostat, divide the LSV, and secure a Luer compatible tester to the distal end.
- Gently inflate the LSV with heparinized blood or saline and ligate any missed side branches with clips or fine suture material before placing the vein in a pot of heparinized blood or saline.
- Ligate the cut ends of the LSV and obtain haemostasis.

Closure

- Absorbable suture to fascia and skin.
- A suction drain may occasionally be required.
- Apply a crepe bandage to minimize bruising.

Complications

- Bleeding.
- Infection.
- Saphenous nerve injury.

Tips and tricks

Handle the vein gently and try to avoid avulsing small side branches by minimizing blunt dissection; use scissors to cut, not tear.

Internal mammary artery harvest

Arterial conduits may improve upon the long-term graft patency of venous grafts. Increasingly, total arterial revascularization is being used to extend the durability of CABG. The left internal mammary artery (LIMA) has excellent long-term patency, particularly when anastomosed to the left anterior descending (LAD) coronary artery. Other arterial grafts used include the right internal mammary artery (RIMA), radial artery (RA), and the right gastro-epiploic artery.

Anatomy

The IMA is a descending branch of the subclavian artery that gives rise to the anterior intercostal arteries. It travels down the inner aspect of the anterior thoracic wall over the costal cartilages. As the IMA emerges from underneath the costal margin it gives off the musculo-phrenic artery and continues inferiorly as the superior epigastric artery. It is accompanied along its course by two internal mammary veins. The IMA is usually harvested as a pedicled graft with the veins and thoracic fascia attached or as a skeletonized graft. The vessel can be harvested using a minimally invasive technique as well. The more commonly used open technique is described here.

Indications

Coronary artery bypass surgery.

Contraindications

- IMA usage, particularly if bilateral, can be associated with increased risk of sternal wound problems in patients with diabetes, chronic obstructive pulmonary disease, and smokers.
- Patients with prior mediastinal radiotherapy or limited life expectancy are often revascularized with venous conduits.

Preoperative preparation

As for 'Median sternotomy' (p. 582).

Position and theatre set-up

Table raised and tilted away, often with the surgeon seated.

Procedure

- Place the mammary retractor and progressively open it, elevating the hemi-sternum to expose the IMA (Fig. 12.5).
- Mobilize the pleura off the anterior thoracic wall and identify the IMA by inspection and palpation.
- Make longitudinal incisions along either side of the IMA to produce the pedicle.
- Develop the plane between the chest wall and the IMA by pulling downwards on the pedicle and freeing up the IMA from the chest wall using a combination of blunt, diathermy, and scissor dissection, clipping branches as they appear.
- The dissection is continued inferiorly to the level of the xiphioid process and superiorly to the level of the 1st rib or subclavian vein.

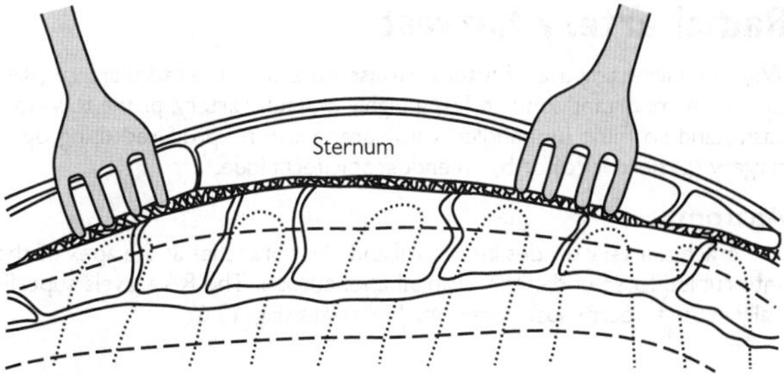
Sternum

Fig. 12.5 A 'surgeon's view' of the LIMA on the underside of the chest wall.

- After heparinization, ligate the distal end and divide the IMA from the chest wall, inspect to confirm good flow, clip any bleeding branches.
- Some surgeons employ topically or luminally applied papaverine to protect against arterial spasm.
- Ensure there is enough length of IMA to reach the target vessel (usually the LAD) and position in the pleural cavity away from the retractor.

Complications

- Subclavian artery or vein injury.
- Phrenic nerve injury.

Tips and tricks

- Be very careful at the cephalic end of the dissection, it is easy to injure the subclavian vessels and phrenic nerve.
- Develop the plane between the thoracic parietes and the IMA just behind a costal cartilage; there will be no anterior intercostal artery to injure.

Radial artery harvest

With the increasing use of arterial revascularization, the radial artery (RA) can be an important conduit. It is a highly muscular artery, prone to vasospasm, and so must be handled with care. It can be procured using open surgery (as described) or by an endoscopic technique.

Anatomy

The brachial artery divides into radial and ulnar branches at the apex of the ante-cubital fossa under the bicipital aponeurosis. The RA travels superficially in the forearm, just under brachioradialis (Fig. 12.6).

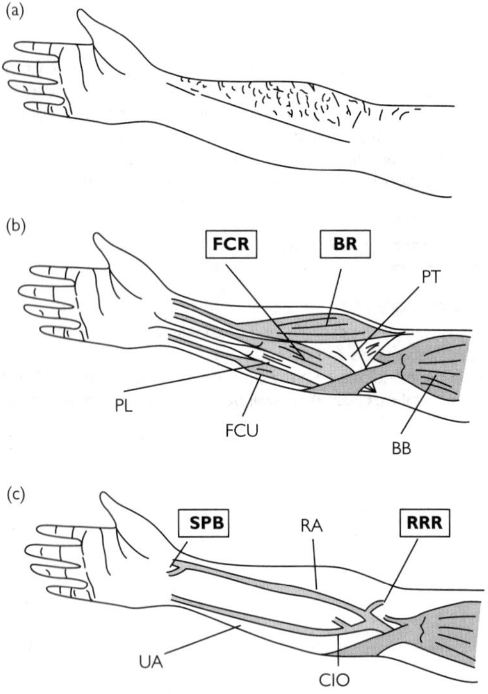
(a)
(b)
FCR
BR
PT
PL
FCU
BB
(c)
SPB
RA
RRR
UA
CIO

Fig. 12.6 (a) Incision; (b) muscular anatomy (arteries removed) with the two key muscles highlighted; (c) arterial anatomy with the two key arteries highlighted. FCR, flexor carpi radialis; BR, brachioradialis; PT, pronator teres; PL, palmaris longus; FCU, flexor carpi ulnaris; BB, biceps brachii; SPB, superficial palmar branch of radial artery; RA, radial artery; RRR, recurrent radial artery; UA, ulnar artery; CIO, common interosseus artery.

Indications

Coronary artery bypass surgery (CABG).

Contraindications

- Positive Allen's test.
- Atherosclerotic disease of RA.

Preoperative preparation

The palmar circulation can be assessed by the modified Allen's test, finger oximetry, or plethysmography, but all have limitations. Doppler ultrasonography can be a useful adjunct in patients with peripheral vascular disease or diabetes. Procure the artery from the non-dominant arm.

Position and theatre set-up

Arm on a sideboard at 70–80° to the torso.

Procedure

- Sterile field consisting of most of the upper limb, leaving the wrist visible.
- Make a curvilinear incision from just distal to the brachial pulse to the radial pulse along medial edge of brachioradialis.
- Divide the fat, incise the fascia, and develop the plane between the brachioradialis and the flexor carpi radialis.
- Carefully mobilize the RA and its venae commitantes with minimal handling, from below the brachial bifurcation (not proximal to recurrent radial artery) to before the superficial palmar branch of the RA.
- Clip and divide side branches.
- Apply artery clips to both ends of the RA and excise it.
- Flush with heparinized blood or saline with a vasodilator (e.g. papaverine) and ligate/repair any missed branches.
- Immerse the graft in heparinized blood or saline with a vasodilator.
- Transfix and ligate the stumps with a non-absorbable monofilament.

Closure

Absorbable suture to superficial fascia and skin.

Complications

- Nerve or arterial injury.
- Hand ischaemia.
- Compartment syndrome.

Tips and tricks

- Handle the RA with great care, it is vulnerable to spasm.
- An intraoperative Allen's test can be useful to confirm an adequate palmar anastomosis: needle the RA distal to a bull-dog clamp. If there is pulsatile flow, the collateral circulation is adequate.
- Avoid closing the deep fascia to prevent compartment syndrome.
- Consider prescribing a calcium channel-blocker postoperatively.

Cardiopulmonary bypass overview

- Cardiopulmonary bypass (CPB) assumes the function of the heart and lungs, allowing safe surgery on the heart. CPB with cardioplegic arrest provides a still and bloodless field in which to repair acquired or congenital defects. Once the repair has been effected, the cross-clamp can be released and the heart can then be weaned from bypass to reassume its role.

Indications

- Most cardiac surgery.
- Most surgery of the great vessels.
- Non-cardiac procedures such as complex cerebral aneurysms and renal tumours.
- Emergency scenarios (e.g. low cardiac output or arrest due to severe hypothermia).

Basic design

The CPB circuit is composed of (Fig. 12.7):

- Venous cannula and tubing connected to the reservoir to passively siphon systemic venous blood.
- A reservoir to collect the venous effluent.
- A heat exchanger to warm or cool the blood.
- A pump to drive oxygenated blood back to the body via the oxygenator and filter.
- A membrane oxygenator to add O_2 and remove CO_2.
- A filter to remove air bubbles and other emboli.
- Tubing and an arterial cannula to return pressurized blood to the systemic arterial circulation.

Adjuncts

Additional capabilities include:

- Facilities for monitoring temperature, pressure, flow, haemoglobin saturation, and blood gas content.
- Ports for sampling blood and administering drugs and fluids,
- Pump suckers for salvaging blood from the operative field and venting the heart.
- A system for delivering cardioplegia.
- Tubing delivering medical air, oxygen, and anaesthetic volatile agents.

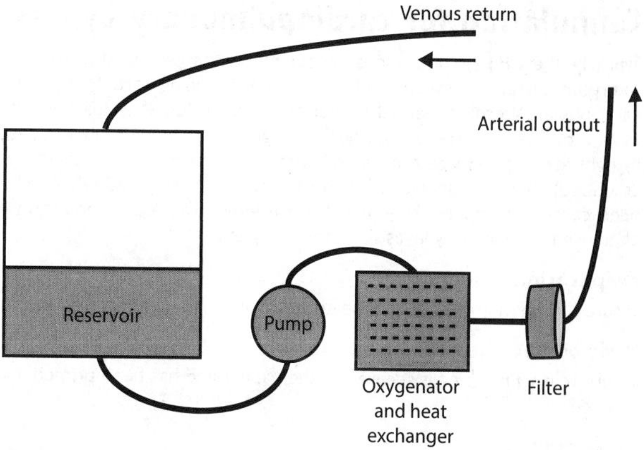
Venous return
Arterial output
Reservoir
Pump
Oxygenator
and heat
exchanger
Filter

Fig. 12.7 A simplified representation of the essential elements of the cardiopulmonary bypass circuit.

Cannulation for cardiopulmonary bypass

Typically, the CPB circuit siphons venous blood passively to the reservoir and returns filtered, oxygenated blood to the ascending aorta by the arterial cannula. Alternate arterial cannulation sites include the axillary, subclavian, or femoral arteries. Venous drainage is most commonly achieved by right atrial appendage cannulation with a two-stage venous cannula (as described). Bi-caval cannulation with caval snaring is required when right-sided cardiac chambers are entered, while femoral venous cannulation is often used for minimally invasive or redo surgery.

Preparation

Ensure that all members of the theatre team are ready for cannulation.

Position and theatre set-up

Ensure that CPB tubing is secured to the patient and has been primed and de-aired.

Procedure

- After administration of heparin, epiaortic ultrasound (or pre-operative imaging) can be used to select a cannulation site free from atheroma.
- Using a polypropylene suture, insert two partial thickness purse-strings on the aorta and a single purse-string suture at the right atrial appendage—large enough to accommodate the cannula (Fig. 12.8).
- Cut the needles off and feed the purse-string sutures through a tourniquet (also called a snugger) using a snare.
- Clamp and divide the bypass circuit lines to the appropriate lengths.
- With the systolic blood pressure <100mmHg, perform a controlled full thickness stab incision through the aortic wall, taking care to stay within the purse-string, and gently insert the aortic cannula. It is possible to control the arteriotomy by using the forceps to grasp the adventitia and maintain apposition of the two edges.
- Once inserted, orient the arterial cannula with the bevel pointing downstream and ask your assistant to hold it whilst you tighten the tourniquets–secure the tourniquets to the cannula with a heavy tie.
- Place a clamp on the cannula, remove the plastic cap, and de-air by gently loosening the clamp to allow blood to flow into a dish.
- Remove the clamp on the arterial line from the bypass circuit and ask the perfusionist to push a small amount of prime fluid so that you can connect the line to the cannula without leaving air bubbles.
- Once connected, remove the cannula clamp and ask the perfusionist to confirm correct positioning by inspecting the pressure waveform.
- Make an atriotomy within the purse-string and divide any muscular bands impeding insertion.
- Insert the two-stage cannula, passing it into the IVC until the atrial stage lies within the atrium.
- Tighten the purse-string, tie the tourniquet to the cannula with a heavy tie, and attach the cannula to the venous line (Fig. 12.9a).
- Remove the venous line clamp when you are ready to go on bypass.

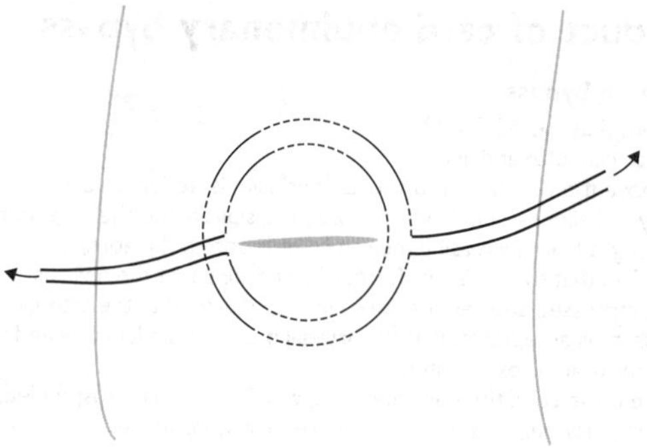

Fig. 12.8 Aortic purse-string. Dotted lines are suture within the media.

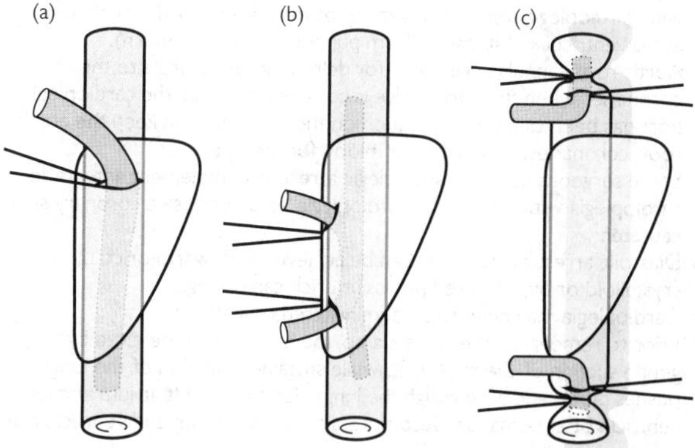
(a)
(b)
(c)

Fig. 12.9 The three principle methods of gaining access for venous return: (a) two-stage atrio-caval cannula with side holes in the atrial portion; (b) bi-caval un-snared cannulation with atrial puncture; (c) direct caval puncture with caval snaring.

Complications

- Particulate embolism (clot, cholesterol, air bubbles).
- Massive air embolism.
- Aortic dissection, atrial or caval injury.

Conduct of cardiopulmonary bypass

Going on bypass

- Ensure that the ACT >400s.
- Check cannulae and lines.
- Remove the venous clamp and ask perfusionist to 'go on bypass'.
- They will allow systemic venous blood to siphon into the reservoir whilst gradually increasing the return of blood to the aorta.
- Confirm that bypass is satisfactory by checking that the heart is decompressed and venous drainage is adequate, that the arterial line pressure is acceptable, that the arterial pressure is adequate, and that the perfusate is oxygenated.
- Once these conditions are met, lung ventilation can be suspended, cooling may begin, and the procedure may be continued.

On bypass

- Most cardiac operations will require an arrested heart, and so once bypass is established, the aorta is cross-clamped and the heart arrested with cardioplegia, often with venting of the left side of the heart to avoid ventricular distension (from pulmonary venous return).
- Aortic root cannulae are useful for delivering cardioplegia to the coronaries when the aortic valve is competent—once the cardioplegia port has been clamped, aspiration on the root vent can keep the aortic root, coronaries, and LV free of blood for the operation.
- Some surgeons achieve cardioplegic arrest or complement antegrade cardioplegia with retrograde cardioplegia via an occlusive coronary sinus catheter.
- Diastolic arrest of the heart can be achieved with warm or cold, crystalloid or blood-based potassium-rich cardioplegia.
- Cardioplegia may need to be administered repeatedly.
- Prior to removal of the cross-clamp, the heart can be de-aired by gentle suction of the root vent, while sustained inflation of the lungs pushes blood and air through the lungs clearing the left atrium and left ventricle of air—manual decompression of the atrium and ventricle can complement this process.
- After the clamp is released it is often worth continuing to vent the root as the patient comes off bypass, as some air may still be ejected from the left ventricle as the heart takes over the circulation.
- Alternative vent sites include the LV apex and the left atrium via the right superior pulmonary vein or trans-septally.

Coming off bypass

- Before the heart can be weaned from bypass, ensure the following conditions are met (a useful mnemonic is TRAVEL):
    - Temperature: is the patient re-warmed to at least 36°C?
    - Rate and Rhythm: is there a reasonable rate of sinus rhythm or is pacing required? Attach epicardial wires and pace if needed.
    - Air: has the heart been fully de-aired?

   - Ventilation: is the anaesthetist happy with the ventilation?
   - Electrolytes: has the potassium, calcium, acid base, and blood gas status been optimized?
   - Level: is the perfusionist happy with the level in the reservoir or do they need to add volume?
- When ready, ask the perfusionist to 'come off bypass'. They will slowly occlude the venous line and gradually reduce the arterial return, thus allowing the heart to fill and eject blood.
- Monitor haemodynamics and confirm the heart is contracting well and not over-filled.
- Inotropes are sometimes required to support ventricular function and overcome the effects of any ischaemia-reperfusion injury.
- Once the heart has stably resumed function, clamp and remove the venous cannula and tighten the purse-string using the tourniquet.
- Ask the anaesthetist to administer protamine at a dose of 1mg/mg of heparin (watch the heart and BP, as protamine may cause systemic hypotension and/or pulmonary vasoconstriction).
- Once heparin has been satisfactorily reversed, the venous cannulation site may be over-sewn, the aorta de-cannulated and the aortotomy over-sewn.

Coronary artery bypass grafting—overview

By revascularizing myocardium, CABG aims to achieve either improvement of symptoms or improvement of life-expectancy or both. CABG may be performed 'off-pump' (OPCAB), minimally invasively through a small anterior thoracotomy (MIDCAB), or totally endoscopically (TECAB). These variants all have advantages and disadvantages but, worldwide, CABG is still most commonly performed using cardiopulmonary bypass on the arrested heart: this procedure is described.

Anatomy

Typically two coronary arteries arise from two of the three sinuses of the aortic root (Fig. 12.10). The right coronary artery (RCA) is usually dominant, gives rise to the posterior descending artery (PDA), and supplies the majority of the right ventricle via acute marginal branches, as well as some of the inter-ventricular septum via the PDA (Fig. 12.11). The left main stem (LMS) travels behind the pulmonary trunk before emerging and branching into the left anterior descending artery (LAD) and circumflex artery. The LAD supplies most of the septum and a large amount of the anterior wall of the LV via its diagonal branches. The circumflex supplies the lateral and posterior walls of the LV via its obtuse marginal branches. When the left system is dominant, the inferior part of the septum is supplied by the PDA coming off the circumflex artery.

Indications

- Significant (>70%) left main stem stenosis.
- Left main stem equivalent (>70% proximal left anterior descending + proximal circumflex stenoses).
- Three-vessel disease.

Those at highest risk have the greatest potential benefit—left ventricular failure, diabetes, and prior myocardial infarction. The optimal therapeutic strategy of ischaemic heart disease will usually be decided at a multidisciplinary meeting or the 'Heart Team'.

For a comprehensive list of indications refer to the 2011 ACCF/AHA Guideline for Coronary Artery Bypass Graft Surgery.

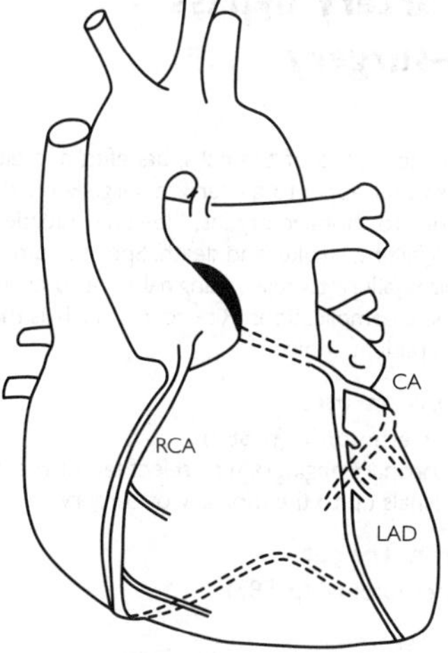
CA
RCA
LAD

Fig. 12.10 Coronary anatomy in context. Right dominant with three main branches labelled.

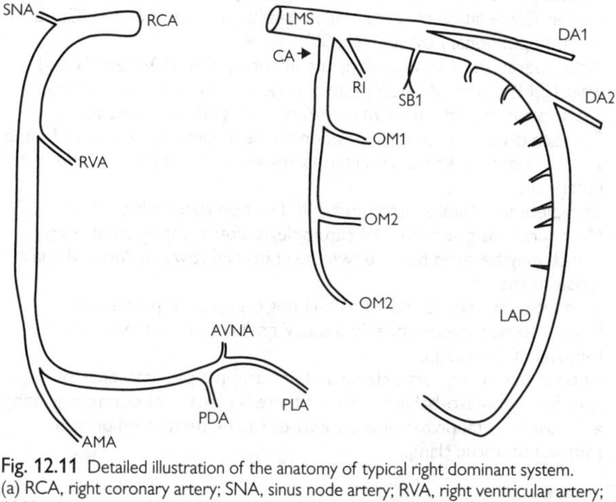
(a)
SNA
RCA
RVA
AVNA
PLA
PDA
AMA
(b)
LMS
DA1
CA
RI
SB1
DA2
OM1
OM2
OM2
LAD

Fig. 12.11 Detailed illustration of the anatomy of typical right dominant system. (a) RCA, right coronary artery; SNA, sinus node artery; RVA, right ventricular artery; AMA, acute marginal artery; AVNA, AV node artery; PDA, posterior descending artery; PLA, posterolateral ventricular artery; (b) LMS, left main stem coronary artery; CA, circumflex coronary artery; LAD, left anterior descending artery; RI, ramus intermedius; OM, obtuse marginal artery; SB Septal branch; DA, diagonal artery.

Coronary artery bypass grafting—surgery

Consent

Patients should be appraised of the risks, benefits, and alternatives to surgery. General risks that apply to all cardiac surgery need to be discussed, these include: injury to thoracic organs, bleeding, infection, wound failure, thrombosis, organ failure, stroke, and death. Specific complications of coronary bypass include: failure to relieve anginal symptoms, myocardial infarction, and conduit site complications. Risk scores, such as the Euroscore, may be used to inform patient choice.

Preoperative preparation

- As per 'Median sternotomy' (p. 582).
- Scrutinize the coronary angiogram to select target vessels.
- Give all anti-anginals up to the morning of surgery.

Position and theatre set-up

As per 'Median sternotomy' (p. 582).

Procedure

- As per 'Median sternotomy' (p. 582) and 'Conduct of cardiopulmonary bypass' (p. 598).
- Harvest and prepare conduits and give heparin.
- Open the pericardium, inspect the heart, and examine each target coronary artery for a suitable site for grafting.
- As per 'Cannulation for cardiopulmonary bypass' (p. 596) and 'Conduct of cardiopulmonary bypass' (p. 598).
- Most operations involve grafting the inferior (RCA/PDA) and lateral walls (OM) of the ventricle (requiring significant manipulation of the heart) prior to performing the LIMA to LAD graft anastomosis.
- For each distal anastomosis, position the heart optimally using packs and your assistant, make a small arteriotomy with a scalpel and extend with Potts' scissors.
- Complete the distal anastomosis with fine non-absorbable suture.
- Most surgeons give a dose of cardioplegia after completion of each graft (which may be given partly down the graft) and rewarm during the last anastomosis.
- Remove aortic clamp and LIMA bull-dog clamp to re-perfuse the heart—some surgeons needle the LSV grafts to de-air them prior to removal of the clamp.
- Apply a side-biting aortic clamp and perform the proximal anastomoses with fine non-absorbable suture—if there is concern about manipulating a diseased aorta, proximal anastomoses can be performed prior to removal of aortic clamp.

Closure

As for 'Median sternotomy' (p. 583).

Postoperative care

- Remove drains and pacing wires as per unit protocol.
- Reintroduce anti-platelet agents and (re-)start beta-blocker and ACE inhibitor therapy as haemodynamics permit.

Complications

- Early and late graft occlusion/stenosis.
- Arrhythmia.
- Ischaemic myocardial dysfunction.
- Conduit harvest site complications.

Tips and tricks

You should be able to complete an anastomosis (without needing any extra sutures) in less than 15min; practice is essential.

Aortic valve replacement—overview

Aortic valve replacement is the second commonest cardiac surgical procedure and is associated with large absolute risk reductions in death compared to medical management. Multiple pathologies can affect the valve and multiple options are available to replace or indeed repair it. A mechanical valve confers life-long durability at the cost of requiring anticoagulation, while a repaired valve or bio-prosthesis spares the need for anticoagulation but may deteriorate over time. The recent development of percutaneous trans-catheter aortic valve implantation (TAVI) has opened intervention up to those who may not have been previously deemed fit for open surgery. Aortic valve repair may also be contemplated in certain circumstances. Open aortic valve replacement will be described.

Anatomy

The aortic valve is a tricuspid semi-lunar valve found at the junction between left ventricle and aorta. It has a complex three-dimensional structure (Fig. 12.12). The cusps are attached just below the expanded portion of the aortic root—the three sinuses of Valsalva, two of which give rise to the coronary arteries. The zones on the aorta, where two adjacent cusps meet, are termed commissures. The commissure between non-coronary and right coronary cusps is particularly important as it is above the membranous septum where the bundle of His is located. The aortic valve, like the pulmonary valve, opens and closes passively, while the mitral and tricuspid valves have papillary muscles that hold the valves closed in an energy-dependent manner during ventricular systole.

Indications

- Symptomatic aortic stenosis.
- Asymptomatic severe aortic stenosis with impaired LVF, abnormal exercise test, or aortic valve area <0.75 cm^2.
- Symptomatic severe aortic regurgitation.
- Asymptomatic severe aortic regurgitation with LV failure.
- Aortic valve endocarditis, without root involvement.
- Moderate aortic stenosis or severe regurgitation in those undergoing cardiac surgery for another reason.

For a comprehensive list of the indications for aortic valve replacement, consult the 2012 ESC/EACTS Guidelines on the management of valvular heart disease.

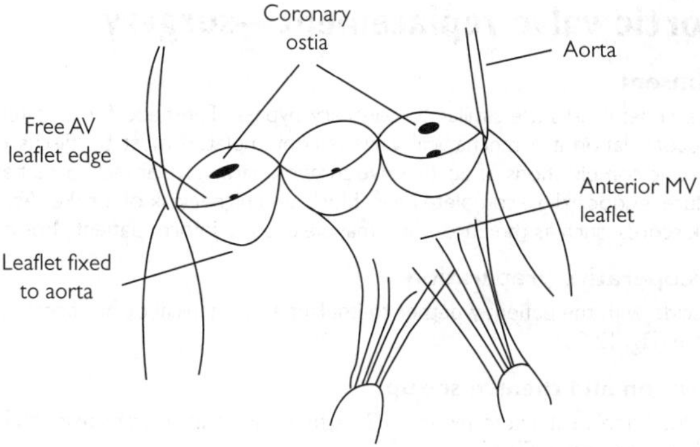
Coronary ostia
Aorta
Free AV leaflet edge
Anterior MV leaflet
Leaflet fixed to aorta

Fig. 12.12 Aortic valve and root anatomy.

Aortic valve replacement—surgery

Consent

The general risks are similar to coronary bypass. The need for long-term anticoagulation if a mechanical valve is contemplated must be discussed. Specific complications of aortic valve surgery: para-valvular leak, prosthesis failure, endocarditis, complete heart block, and higher risk of stroke. Again, risk scores, such as the Euroscore, may be used to inform patient choice.

Preoperative preparation

Decide with the patient whether to implant a mechanical or bio-prosthetic valve (Fig. 12.13).

Position and theatre set-up

As for 'Median sternotomy' (p. 582) with intraoperative transoesophageal echocardiography (TOE).

Procedure

- As for 'Median sternotomy' (p. 582), 'Cannulation for cardiopulmonary bypass' (p. 596), and 'Conduct of cardiopulmonary bypass' (p. 598).
- After cardioplegic arrest, make an transverse or hockey-stick aortotomy to expose the aortic valve.
- Excise the valve cusps and debride as much calcium as is safely possible (send valve cusps to laboratory for culture and sensitivities if operating for endocarditis).
- Size the aortic annulus and select an appropriate prosthesis.
- The valve sewing ring is sewn to the aortic annulus (Fig. 12.14) and secured with either continuous, interrupted, or plegeted interrupted non-absorbable sutures and normal leaflet motion is confirmed.
- Prior to release of the cross-clamp, the aortotomy is closed and the heart is de-aired.
- Separate from bypass as for 'Conduct of cardiopulmonary bypass' (p. 598) and assess heart function and new valve with TOE.

Closure

As for 'Median sternotomy' (p. 583).

Postoperative care

- Once the patient is stable, has been discharged from intensive care, and drains and pacing wires have been removed, begin oral anticoagulant therapy if a mechanical valve has been implanted. Some surgeons elect to prescribe a temporary course of anticoagulation following bioprosthesis insertion. Anticoagulation protocols will however vary by unit.
- If endocarditis—continue antibiotic therapy as per advice of microbiologist and rationalize therapy when sensitivity results available.

Complications

- Complete heart block.
- Cerebrovascular accident.
- Prosthetic valve endocarditis.
- Para-valvular leak.
- Structural deterioration.

Tips and tricks

In severe aortic regurgitation, antegrade cardioplegia via the root cannula is unlikely to work and so retrograde cardioplegia or direct cannulation of the coronary ostia after opening the aortic root may be necessary.

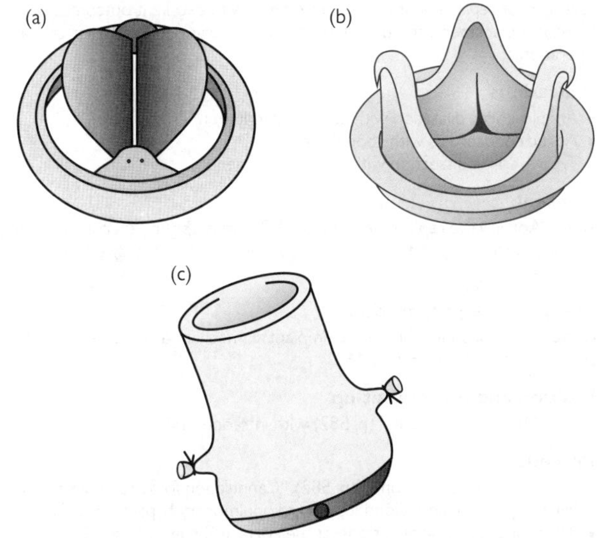
(a)
(b)
(c)

Fig. 12.13 Options available for AVR: (a) mechanical prosthesis; (b) bio-prosthesis; (c) stentless bioprosthesis or homografft.

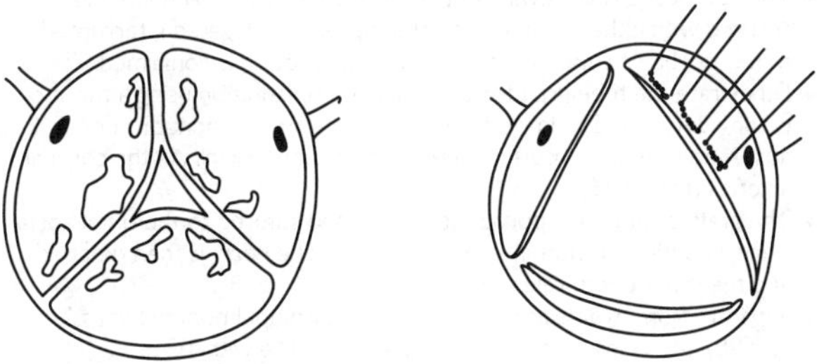

Fig. 12.14 Surgical views of stenosed aortic valve and beginning of placement of valve sutures in the annulus after excision of the valve leaflets.

Aortic root replacement

The aortic valve cusps form only a part of a functionally unitary aortic root that starts at the aortic annulus and ends at the sino-tubular junction (STJ; Fig. 12.15). The aortic wall of the root may dilate in isolation or in association with aortic incompetence or ascending aortic dilation. Although valve sparing root replacement can be performed with excellent outcomes, aortic root replacement, the Bentall procedure, remains an important cardiac operation.

Indications

- Annulo-aortic dilatation with aortic regurgitation.
- Aortic endocarditis with root abscess.
- Type A aortic dissection with root involvement.

Consent

As for 'Aortic valve replacement' (p. 606). There is a significant risk of major bleeding with this operation. During mobilization, the coronary arteries may be injured.

Preoperative preparation

Decide with patient whether to implant a mechanical or bio-prosthetic composite prosthesis (Fig. 12.16).

Position and theatre set-up

As for 'Median sternotomy' (p. 582) with intraoperative TOE.

Procedure

- As for 'Median sternotomy' (p. 582), 'Cannulation for cardiopulmonary bypass' (p. 596), and 'Conduct of cardiopulmonary bypass' (p. 598).
- After cardioplegic arrest, transect the aorta at the level of the STJ and open the aneurysm vertically.
- Carefully mobilize the coronary arteries and detach them from the aorta with a generous button of aortic tissue.
- Excise cusps and excess aneurysm tissue and size aortic annulus.
- The composite root sewing ring is sewn to the aortic annulus and secured with either continuous, interrupted, or plegeted interrupted non-absorbable sutures and normal leaflet motion is confirmed.
- Fenestrate the tube graft for coronary re-implantation using a thermo-cutting device and re-implant the coronaries with continuous non-absorbable suture, ensuring there is no tension or kinks in the coronary arteries (Fig. 12.16).
- The graft is cut to an appropriate length and sutured to the distal aorta using a continuous non-absorbable suture. The heart is then de-aired and the cross-clamp released.
- Separate from bypass as for 'Conduct of cardiopulmonary bypass' (p. 598) and assess heart function and new valve with TOE.

Closure

As for 'Median sternotomy' (p. 583).

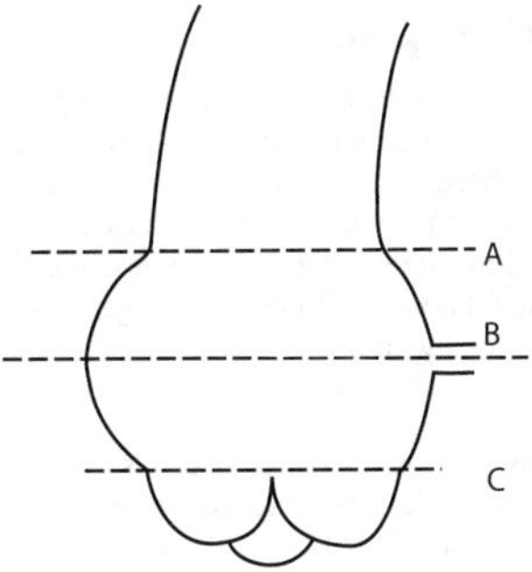
A
B
C

Fig. 12.15 Aortic root anatomy: A is the sinotubular junction, B is the width of the root at the sinuses of Valsalva, C is the diameter of the aortic 'annulus'.

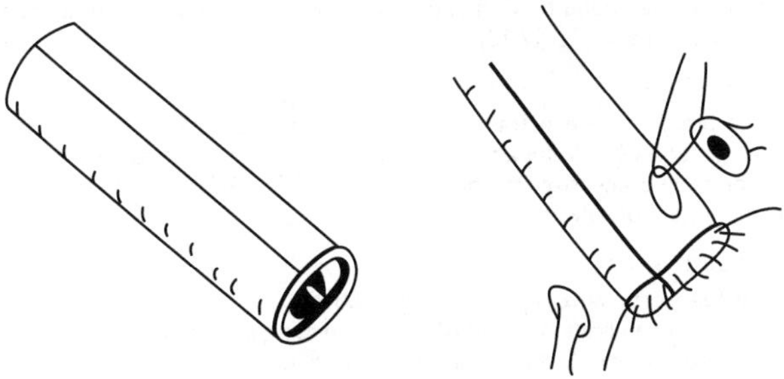

Fig. 12.16 Mechanical valved conduit and schematic of coronary re-implantation.

Postoperative care

As for 'Aortic valve replacement' (p. 606).

Complications

- As for 'Aortic valve replacement' (p. 606).
- Aortic pseudoaneurysm.

Tips and tricks

Bleeding is frequently problematic following this operation. Be very careful with haemostasis of the left coronary button, as this is inaccessible after release of the cross-clamp.

Mitral valve repair

Mitral regurgitation (MR) from myxomatous degeneration, ischaemic/functional MR, or endocarditis is the second most frequent valve disease requiring surgery. There is widespread agreement that in degenerative disease, mitral valve repair is superior to replacement. It carries a lower risk of mortality and morbidity than replacement and obviates the need for anticoagulation. Patients with MR unfit for surgery may be considered for percutaneous mitral intervention.

Anatomy

The mitral valve has a complex anatomy and is composed of two leaflets, anterior and posterior, that are attached circumferentially to the saddle-shaped mitral valve annulus (Fig. 12.17). The ventricular surfaces of the leaflets are anchored to two papillary muscles by tendinous cords. Adequate competence of the mitral valve is dependent on all aspects of the valve functioning properly—the leaflets, the cords, the papillary muscles, and the LV itself. Understanding the anatomy and the way in which regurgitation occurs, as described by Carpentier's classification, is essential to effect a good valve repair (Fig. 12.18).

Indications

Symptomatic severe mitral regurgitation or asymptomatic severe mitral regurgitation with LV impairment, AF, or pulmonary hypertension.

For a comprehensive list, consult the 2012 ESC/EACTS guidelines on the management of valvular heart disease.

Consent

- As for 'Aortic valve replacement' (p. 606).
- Specific complications: residual or recurrent regurgitation, systolic anterior motion (SAM) of the anterior leaflet.

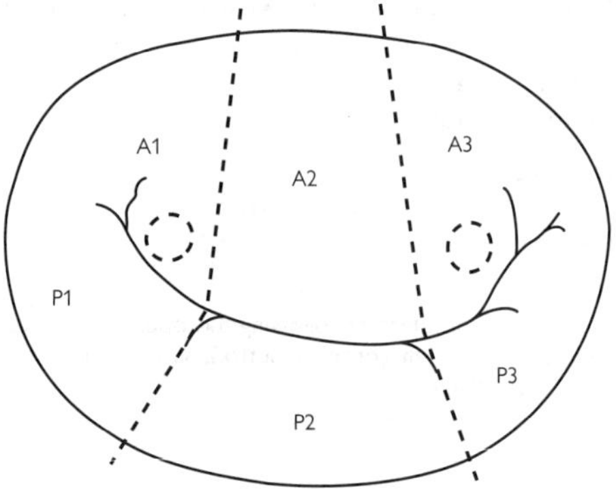
A1
A2
A3
P1
P2
P3

Fig. 12.17 A schematic of the normal mitral valve. The presence of two clefts within the posterior leaflet forms the three scallops of the posterior leaflet named P1–3. The corresponding areas in the anterior leaflet are likewise described as A1–3. The dotted circles represent the papillary muslces.

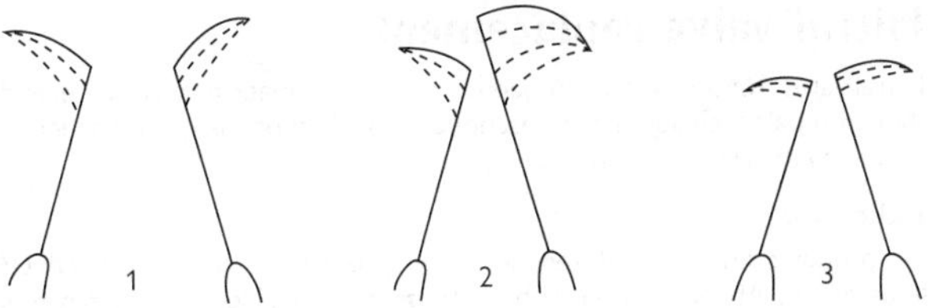
1
2
3

Fig. 12.18 Carpentier classification of lesions causing mitral regurgitation. Type 1 is characterized by normal leaflet motion but a dilated annulus. Type 2 is characterized by excessive leaflet motion. Type 3 is characterized by restricted leaflet motion.

Preoperative preparation

- As per 'Median sternotomy' (p. 582).
- Detailed preoperative assessment of valve morphology.

Position and theatre set-up

As for 'Median sternotomy' (p. 582) with intraoperative TOE.

Procedure

- As for 'Median sternotomy' (p. 582), 'Cannulation for cardiopulmonary bypass' (p. 596), and 'Conduct of cardiopulmonary bypass' (p. 598).
- Venous cannulation is by unsnared bi-caval cannulation if the valve is approached via the left atrium, though the cavae need to be snared if a trans-septal approach is utilized.
- A careful assessment of the valve is undertaken using nerve hooks and saline testing to determine the nature of the lesion.
- Repair is effected with a combination of leaflet resection/repair, chordal replacement/augmentation, and annuloplasty.
- Annuloplasty rings or bands are usually sized to the anterior leaflet and sewn in with interrupted non-absorbable sutures.
- After the repair is completed, valve competency is confirmed with saline testing.
- The atrium is closed prior to release of the cross-clamp, and the heart is de-aired.
- Separate from bypass as for 'Conduct of cardiopulmonary bypass' (p. 598) and assess heart function and new valve with TOE.

Closure

- As for 'Median sternotomy' (p. 583).

Complications

- Residual or recurrent regurgitation.
- Cerebrovascular accident or endocarditis.
- SAM of the anterior leaflet causing LVOT obstruction.

Tips and tricks

If your repair isn't right on TOE following cessation of bypass, recommence bypass and fix it or replace the valve.

Mitral valve replacement

Mitral valve stenosis is most frequently due to rheumatic heart disease, and though repair techniques are described, mitral stenosis is most frequently treated with valve replacement.

Indications

Symptomatic severe mitral stenosis or asymptomatic mitral stenosis with LV impairment, AF, or pulmonary hypertension, unsuitable for percutaneous commisurotomy.

For a comprehensive list of the indication for aortic valve replacement consult the 2012 ESC/EACTS guidelines on the management of valvular heart disease.

Consent

As for 'Mitral valve repair' (p. 610), except that residual regurgitation is not a concern.

Preoperative preparation

Decide with patient whether to implant a mechanical or bio-prosthetic valve but. It is worth noting that mitral bio-prostheses can have a shorter lifespan than those in the aortic position.

Position and theatre set-up

As for 'Median sternotomy' (p. 582) with intraoperative TOE.

Procedure

- As for 'Mitral valve repair' (p. 611).
- It is advisable to preserve as much of the subvalvar apparatus as possible, though in patients with fibrotic, calcified, and distorted valves, preservation may not be possible.
- Size the valve to the annulus.
- The valve sewing ring is sewn to the mitral annulus and secured with either continuous, interrupted, or plegeted interrupted non-absorbable sutures. Care is taken to avoid damaging the circumflex coronary artery, AV node, and the non-coronary aortic valve leaflet.
- The atrium is closed prior to release of the cross-clamp, and the heart is de-aired.
- Separate from bypass as for 'Conduct of cardiopulmonary bypass' (p. 598) and assess heart function and new valve with TOE.

Closure

As for 'Median sternotomy' (p. 583).

Complications

- Atrio-ventricular (AV) dehiscence.
- Complete heart block, circumflex coronary artery, or aortic valve injury.
- Cerebrovascular accident or endocarditis.
- Structural failure, paravalvular leak, or pannus formation leading to valve dysfunction.
- LV outflow tract obstruction.

Postoperative care

- Once patient is stable, has been discharged from intensive care, and drains and pacing wires have been removed, begin oral anticoagulant therapy if a mechanical valve has been implanted. Some surgeons elect to prescribe a temporary course of anticoagulation following bio-prosthesis insertion. Anticoagulation protocols will however vary by unit.
- If endocarditis—continue antibiotic therapy as per advice of microbiologist and rationalize therapy when sensitivity results available.

Tips and tricks

Once separated from bypass do not lift the heart as this can cause AV dehiscence.

Repair of atrial septal defect

Atrial septal defects (ASD) in adults are usually of the secundum type but can be sinus venosus or primum defects as well. Significant left-to-right shunting at atrial level causes right-sided volume overload with chamber dilatation, tricuspid regurgitation, and can lead to atrial fibrillation. Percutaneous trans-catheter ASD closure now plays a major role in the management ASD but is not suitable for all.

Indications

- ASD with pulmonary flow: systemic flow ratio >1.5.
- ASD with evidence of paradoxical embolism or atrial fibrillation.

Contraindications

Fixed, elevated pulmonary vascular resistance.

Consent

- As for 'Aortic valve replacement' (p. 606).
- Endocarditis of the patch and residual shunt are other specific risks.

Preoperative preparation

As for 'Median sternotomy' (p. 582).

Position and theatre set-up

As for 'Median sternotomy' (p. 582).

Procedure

- As for 'Mitral valve repair' (p. 611) with aortic and bicaval cannualtion.
- Harvest a pericardial patch if not planning a simple sutured closure.
- After cross-clamping and cardioplegic arrest, the cavae are snared and the ASD approached via right atrial incision.
- Inspect the ASD and confirm that all pulmonary veins are connected to the left atrium.
- If not simply suturing a small defect, trim the pericardial patch to an appropriate size and suture the patch to close the defect using continuous non-absorbable sutures, taking care to avoid the conducting tissue, and leaving the coronary sinus on the right side of the patch.
- The atrium is closed prior to release of the cross-clamp, temporary pacing wire are placed, and the heart is de-aired.
- Separate from bypass as for 'Conduct of cardiopulmonary bypass' (p. 598) and check the integrity and function of the repair using TOE.

Closure

As for 'Median sternotomy' (p. 583).

Complications

- Heart block.
- Embolism.
- Endocarditis.
- Residual or recurrent ASD.
- Cyanosis.
- Pulmonary hypertension.
- Congestive cardiac failure.
- Stroke.

Tips and tricks

It is important to clearly differentiate the inferior rim of the defect from the Eustachian valve as this can lead to baffling of the IVC blood to the left atrium and severe cyanosis.

Orthotopic cardiac transplantation

Heart transplantation remains a key therapeutic option in the management patients with end-stage heart disease. Recently, there has been increasing use of mechanical support devices as a bridge to transplant or recovery, or in patients unsuitable for transplant, as destination therapy.

Indications

The assessment of patients referred for consideration for cardiac transplantation is a multidisciplinary process. Though there are a number of disease processes that may benefit from transplantation, the indication for cardiac transplantation remains symptomatic end-stage heart failure, refractory to all other therapies.

Contraindications

- Advanced age or co-morbidities that curtail life-expectancy irrespective of cardiac transplantation.
- Irreversible pulmonary hypertension.

Consent

There has usually been extensive discussion of the merits, demerits, and alternatives to transplantation prior to admission and so consent usually involves discussion related to organ rejection and immunosuppressant medications.

Preoperative preparation

- As per 'Median sternotomy' (p. 582), though in many cases re-do sternotomy is necessary.
- Administer induction immunosuppression as per protocol.

Position and theatre set-up

- As per 'Median sternotomy' (p. 582) with intraoperative TOE.

Procedure

- Ensure that the heart is en route with an estimated time of arrival before starting. Aim to complete recipient cardiectomy as the allograft arrives.
- As for 'Repair of atrial septal defect' (p. 614), cross-clamp the aorta and snare the cavae.
- Excise the heart leaving enough right atrial, left atrial, pulmonary artery, and aortic tissue to accommodate the new heart (Fig. 12.19).
- Some surgeons perform bi-caval right atrial anastomoses, while some leave atrial cuffs and create atrio-atrostomies.
- Trim the atrial, pulmonary, and aortic tissue of the new heart to complement the native tissue.
- Most surgeons complete atrial anastomoses first, followed by the pulmonary artery and aortic anastomosis.
- Prior to release of the cross-clamp the heart is de-aired.
- Separate from bypass as for 'Conduct of cardiopulmonary bypass' (p. 598) often utilizing pulmonary vasodilators.

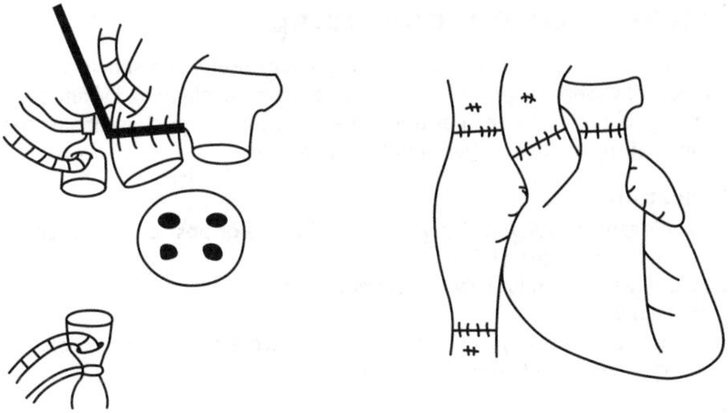

Fig. 12.19 Appearances post-recipient cardiectomy (with vessels and posterior left atrial wall ready for anastomosis) and post-transplant.

Closure

As for 'Median sternotomy' (p. 583).

Postoperative care

- This is complex and multidisciplinary.
- Wean inotropic support.
- Ensure that maintenance immunosuppression is prescribed and given.

Complications

- Severe sepsis.
- Renal failure requiring renal replacement therapy.
- Acute rejection.
- Chronic rejection usually characterized by allograft coronary disease.
- Complications of chronic immunosuppression.

Tips and tricks

Some surgeons complete the left sided anastomoses first, to facilitate early cross-clamp removal.

Intra-aortic balloon pump

The intra-aortic balloon pump (IABP) is a very useful and simple way of temporarily supporting the heart. It functions by diminishing LV afterload and augmenting coronary perfusion pressure, thus favourably tipping the balance of myocardial oxygen supply and demand.

Indications

- Cardiogenic shock due to myocardial ischaemia or post-cardiac surgery (as an aid to weaning CPB).
- Acute ischaemic mitral valve regurgitation or post-infarct ventricular septal defect.
- Preoperative 'prophylaxis' in those with severe left main stem coronary artery stenosis and poor LV function.

Contraindications

- Aortic valve regurgitation.
- Aortic dissection (or presence of stents).
- Severe peripheral vascular disease.

Consent

Written consent is not normally obtained as the patient will typically be either anaesthetized or critically ill. The principle risks are related to bleeding and thrombosis and are listed on p. 619.

Preoperative preparation

- Most cardiac units will have commercially available pre-prepared insertion packs and sterile drapes.
- Ensure clotting and platelet count acceptable.
- The patient should be lying supine, fully monitored, and with at least one good femoral pulse.

Procedure

- Create a sterile field with both groins exposed and the full length of legs covered. If the patient is awake make sure they are comfortable and infiltrate local anaesthetic at the puncture site.
- Flush the manometer line, remove the guard wire from the IABP, and aspirate the balloon fully.
- Cannulate the femoral artery over the femoral head, feed in the guide wire, remove the needle, and feed the IABP over the guide wire to the predetermined distance so that the tip of the IABP sits roughly level with the second intercostal space.
- Remove the guide wire, attach the manometry line, clear, flush, and zero the line.
- Confirm a good arterial trace and connect the balloon channel to the console and commence the balloon pump at the appropriate ratio and stimulus.
- Fix the IABP to the skin and dress the puncture site.
- Confirm correct positioning of IABP with CXR, prescribe anticoagulation as per unit policy.

Removal

- Once the patient has been weaned to 1 in 3 augmented beats, the IABP should be removed.
- Stop augmenting.
- Disconnect the helium inflow and aspirate on this port to ensure that the balloon is deflated.
- Pull the IABP out and apply direct pressure to the arterial puncture site (not the skin puncture site, which will be 1 or 2cm distal to the hole in the artery) for at least 30mins.

Postoperative care

- Regular assessment of the peripheral circulation is mandatory.
- Platelet count and clotting should be regularly checked at least daily.

Complications

- Peripheral ischemia due to thrombosis.
- Balloon rupture.
- Sepsis.
- Pseudoaneurysm of puncture site.

Tips and tricks

Although the IABP is usually inserted percutaneously and peripherally (as described), it can be inserted via open surgery either at the groin or directly antegrade into the ascending aorta. Surgically sited IABPs should be removed surgically.

Intercostal drain insertion

Anatomy

The safest area for insertion is the 4h or 5th intercostal space in the anterior axillary line, at the level of the nipple—this is often referred to as the 'triangle of safety' (Fig. 12.20).

Indications

Acute/emergency

- Pneumothorax in all patients on mechanical ventilation.
- Tension pneumothorax or spontaneous pneumothorax, if large or clinically significant.
- Haemo-pneumothorax after oesophageal rupture into pleural space.

Elective

- Malignant pleural effusion for cytology and pleurodesis.
- Para-pneumonic effusion or empyema.
- Chylothorax.

Contraindications

Relative contraindications include a risk of bleeding in patients taking anticoagulants or in patients with a predisposition to bleeding.

Consent

Obtain written consent if practical. Explain the benefits, risks and alternatives. The principle complications are listed on p. 621.

Preoperative preparation

- If time permits obtain written consent, this may not be possible when the need for chest-tube insertion is urgent.
- Most hospitals have packaged chest-tube insertion sets.

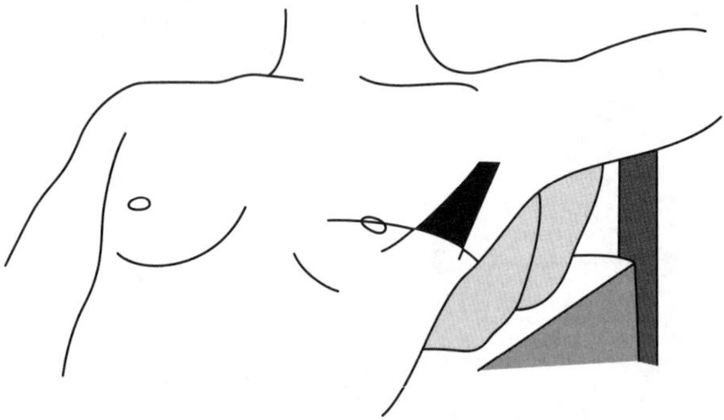

Fig. 12.20 The triangle of safety bordered by the pectoralis major and latismus dorsi.

Position and theatre set-up

- Position the patient in either a supine or a semi-recumbent position.
- Maximally abduct the arm or place it behind the patient's head.
- Use full barrier precautions to create a large, sterile field and select an appropriately sized chest-drain.
- Use local anaesthetic to infiltrate the skin, subcutaneous tissues, intercostal muscles, and periosteum of rib below the intercostal space for insertion.

Procedure

- Grasp proximal free end of the chest tube with artery forceps.
- Isolate triangle of safety by palpating the clavicle, then work downward along the ribcage, counting down the rib spaces to the 4th or 5th space.
- Make a 2cm incision in line with the rib, one intercostal space below the chest-tube insertion site.
- Use the artery forceps to bluntly dissect a path, diagonally upwards, to find the top of the rib of the anaesthetized intercostal space. Use of a trocar to aid insertion of the drain is discouraged.
- Gently push through the parietal pleura, enlarge tract with blunt dissection, and confirm entry into the pleura by finger palpation.
- Insert tube along tract using artery forceps, aiming the tube apically for evacuation of a pneumothorax or basally for evacuation of fluid.
- Seldinger drains are becoming increasingly popular as they substitute the blunt dissection of a standard tube for an over the wire, serial dilation technique.
- Make sure the last side hole of the drain is within the chest and secure tube to chest wall using non-absorbable sutures. Place an additional horizontal mattress suture for subsequent closure of incision.
- Cover with a dressing and connect the distal end of the chest tube to an underwater seal pleural drainage system and unclamp the drain.
- Many surgeons use low-pressure suction to aid cavity evacuation and lung inflation.

Postoperative care

Obtain a CXR to confirm placement.

Complications

- Bleeding and haemothorax due to intercostal artery injury.
- Perforation of major blood vessel, lung, heart, diaphragm, or intra-abdominal organs.
- Subcutaneous emphysema.
- Re-expansion pulmonary oedema.
- Infection of the drainage site or pleural cavity (empyema).

Tips and tricks

- Prior to removal of drain, any bubbling must have stopped, the lung must be fully expanded on CXR, and the drainage should usually be below 100ml/day.
- A forced Valsalva manoeuvre, after a full exhalation at the time of drain removal, will decrease the chance of residual pneumothorax.

Thoracotomy

The best surgical incision provides sufficient exposure to complete the proposed operation and requires consideration of both the goals of the operation and the individual patient characteristics. The thoracic cavity can be accessed in a variety of ways for a vast number of indications.

Anatomy

- Preoperative imaging studies are helpful in directing the location of the incision.
- In the case of lobar or segmental resection, the incision must provide exposure of the hilum.

Indications

- Anterior thoracotomy is an appropriate approach for right middle lobe resection and open-lung biopsy on critically ill patients.
- Bilateral anterior thoracotomy with transverse sternotomy, the clamshell incision, is popular for double-lung transplantation.
- Postero-lateral thoracotomy is suitable for more complicated pulmonary and oesophageal resections such as extra-pleural pneumonectomy, superior sulcus tumours, tracheal surgery, single lung transplantation, and resection of advanced malignancy after induction therapy.

Preoperative preparation

- The patient is placed in lateral position and the ipsilateral arm positioned anteriorly with the table slightly flexed under the torso to widen the rib interspaces; 'breaking the table'.
- The dependent leg is slightly flexed at the hip and knee, and a pillow is placed between the legs. The non-dependent leg is kept straight.

Procedure

- Make a curvilinear incision extending from as far anteriorly as the base of the axilla to as far posteriorly as the base of the neck midway between the scapular edge and the spine, depending on the operative approach (Fig. 12.21).
- After division of the subcutaneous fascia, the chest wall muscles are divided depending on the approach: pectoralis major anteriorly, serratus and latissimus laterally, and trapezius and rhomboids posteriorly.
- The rib space for entry is often decided by the nature of the surgery and diathermy is used to incise the intercostal muscles from the superior aspect of the rib below the interspace.
- The pleural cavity is entered bluntly to prevent injury to lung.
- Once the lung is collapsed or retracted, the rest of the interspace can be opened anteriorly and posteriorly to improve exposure.

Closure

- Site chest drains.
- Re-approximate ribs with pericostal absorbable sutures and re-approximate muscle layers carefully.
- Absorbable suture to facia and skin.

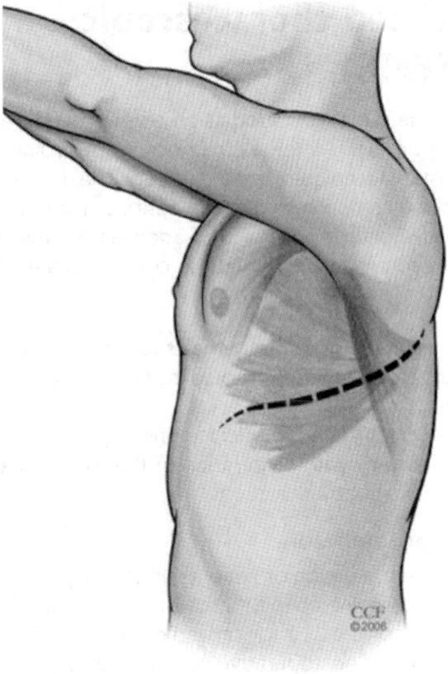
CCF
©2006

Fig. 12.21 Thoracotomy incision.

Postoperative care

- Some surgeons use low suction and perform a CXR after thoracotomy as a routine.
- Local anaesthesia delivered either by a wound, pleural or epidural catheter improves patient comfort and postoperative ventilation.
- It is essential to follow up on pathology results.

Complications

- Thoracotomy wound infection is rare and so when it occurs, an empyema draining spontaneously through the wound should be suspected.
- Wound seromas are common with muscle-sparing incisions, but obliterating dead space and using soft drains can be helpful.
- Avoid rib fractures as they create wound instability, increasing the amount of pain making effective coughing difficult.
- Post-thoracotomy neuralgia remains a troublesome problem.

Tips and tricks

- Muscle-sparing entry may be associated with improvements in postoperative respiratory function and decreased pain.
- For extended resections, it may be necessary to resect a rib to enhance exposure by incising the periosteum longitudinally and shelling the rib out using periosteal elevators before excising the bone.
- The intercostal muscles can be left attached to the vascular pedicle and used to cover a bronchial stump.

Video-assisted thoracoscopic surgery (VATS)

VATS should be the same operation as an open procedure except for the minimal access approach. All the basic principles regarding anatomy, tissue handling, and surgical techniques are unchanged. The need for safe, effective surgery must not be compromised by the desire to maintain minimal access and if any operative difficulty arises, or if adequacy of the resection seems doubtful, the surgeon must not hesitate to convert to a full thoracotomy.

Indications

- The indications for VATS are the same as for conventional approaches to thoracic surgery but consent should include conversion to an open thoracotomy.
- Tumour size >6cm, inability to tolerate single-lung ventilation, and previous thoracotomy with obliteration of the pleural space are considered relative contraindications.

Preoperative preparation

- The preoperative evaluation of patients undergoing VATS is similar to that of those undergoing open thoracotomy procedures.
- Diffusion capacity of the lung for carbon monoxide (DLCO) is a sensitive predictor of postoperative complications.
- The basic components of all VATS systems include one or two large monitors with recording capability and a light source. Most surgeons employ rigid 5–10mm wide 0° or 30° thoracoscopes.
- Endoscopic staplers enhance the surgeon's ability to perform minimally invasive pulmonary resections, particularly with tissue reinforcements that buttress the staple line.

Procedure

- The patient is positioned as for thoracotomy.
- VATS is usually performed under general anaesthesia with single-lung ventilation facilitated by double-lumen endotracheal intubation.
- There is great variability in port site position but the incisions should be placed such that a triangular configuration is achieved and the utility incision, if needed, is positioned over the hilum (Fig. 12.22).
- The camera port incision is usually in the 7th or 8th intercostal space between the mid and anterior axillary lines.
- The second incision is often used as the utility port for lung resection or biopsy and is often in the 4th intercostal space anterior to the latissimus dorsi.
- The third incision is a posterior instrument port and may be made in the 7th or 8th intercostal space in the posterior axillary line.

Postoperative care

- Patients who undergo resections via the VATS approach experience less immediate postoperative pain than those having the thoracotomy approach but adequate pain control is an essential part of recovery and can be aided by local anaesthetic application to intercostal spaces and incisions.

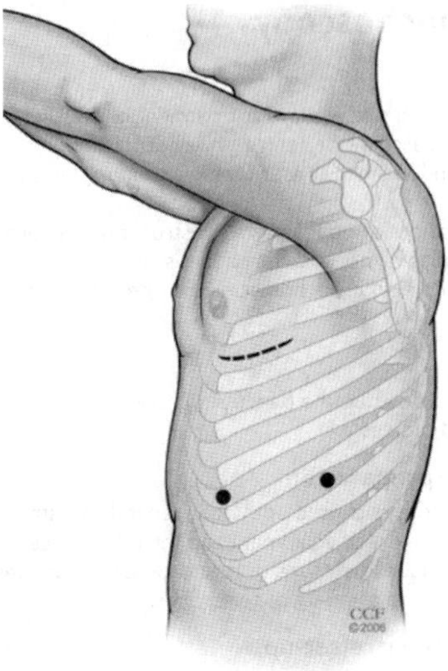
CCF
©2006

Fig. 12.22 Port sites for VATS showing an anterior camera port, a posterior instrument port, and an incision as a utility port and for retrieving resected tissue.

- After most procedures suction is applied to the drain and a CXR performed.
- As with thoracotomy, it is essential to follow up on pathology results.

Complications

Thoracoscopic procedures tend to be less physiologically stressful than open thoracotomy, with fewer cardiopulmonary complications such as atrial fibrillation or myocardial infarction.

Tips and tricks

In patients with loculated effusion, the port placement must sometimes be modified. The preoperative chest CT scan should help ensure that the ports are placed in areas where the lung is not adherent to the chest wall.

Rigid bronchoscopy

Indications

- Establishment of a safe airway for treatment of massive haemoptysis, foreign body, malignant or benign airway obstruction.
- To facilitate endobronchial laser therapy, stenting and tracheobronchial toilet.
- In certain instances of upper airway obstruction, rigid bronchoscopy may be the only way to save the patient's life.
- The flexible and rigid bronchoscopes are often complementary instruments.

Consent

It is important to describe the benefits and complications of any additional endobronchial therapies.

Preoperative preparation

- Rigid bronchosopy is carried out under general anaesthesia.
- Before induction, check equipment and the light source.
- Basic set-up includes two sizes of bronchoscopes, suctioning tubing, biopsy forceps, and a variety of telescopes.

Position and theatre set-up

- After induction, a muscle relaxant is administered.
- Placement of the patient's head on a pillow with neck extension facilitates introduction of the scope.
- The examiner's thumb should always protect the patient's upper teeth from injury from the scope.
- After intubation, the pillow is removed taking care to prevent injury to the cervical spine and teeth.

Procedure

- The most common form of ventilation used during rigid bronchoscopy is the Venturi technique via a side port of the scope, where a high-pressure jet of oxygen entrains surrounding ambient air, thus ventilating the patient through the lumen of the scope (Fig. 12.23).
- The scope is inserted through the mouth and advanced to the posterior median groove of the tongue under direct vision.
- The tip of the bronchoscope is used to gently elevate the tongue and is slowly advanced until the epiglottis is visible.
- The epiglottis is lifted anteriorly with the tip of the bronchoscope and the posterior part of the laryngeal inlet, arytenoids, and vocal cords identified.
- As the cords are approached, the scope is turned 90° and gently advanced through the larynx into the upper airway and rotated back to the original orientation so that the trachea and carina can be examined.
- To inspect the left or right main bronchus, the patient's head is turned away from the side to be examined.

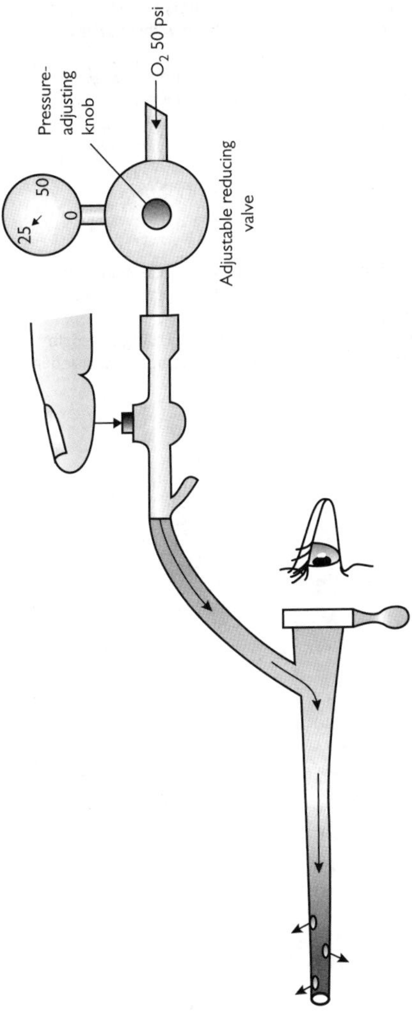
Pressure-adjusting knob
O_2 50 psi
Adjustable reducing valve
25
0
50

Fig. 12.23 Ventilation during rigid bronchoscopy.

- Endobronchial obstruction may be improved by the use of large-bore suction equipment to clear blood and clots, and debridement with biopsy forceps, laser, cryotherapy, or electrocautery.
- Focal stenosis of the bronchial tree can be dilated with bougies or balloons with or without stenting.
- Small amounts of bleeding can be controlled by adrenaline injection while major haemorrhage, particularly in cases of carcinoid, may necessitate thoracotomy.

Complications

- Injury to the lips, gums, teeth, pharynx, and upper airway.
- Bleeding.

Tips and tricks

- Removal of the rigid bronchoscope is performed as carefully as its insertion and the opportunity taken to examine the entire airway carefully on the way out.
- This is especially important for the proximal trachea and the subglottic, glottic, and supra-glottic areas, which may not have been visualized in detail on the way in.

Flexible bronchoscopy

Flexible bronchoscopy

- The flexible scope has become an invaluable tool in the diagnosis and management of tracheobronchial and pulmonary diseases but it does not replace the rigid scope.
- Flexible bronchoscopy has its greatest utility in diagnostic procedures because it is relatively easy to learn to use and because it can be performed without general anaesthesia.

Indications

- Diagnosis of a wide variety of airway entities, including laryngeal abnormalities, vocal cord paralysis, benign and malignant tumours, foreign bodies, inhalation injury, extrinsic compression, tracheal stricture, and tracheomalacia.
- Facilitation of biopsy, laser therapy, photodynamic therapy, and brachytherapy.

Consent

Although considered a low risk procedure, there are occasionally major complications (see p. 531). Remember the risks of sedation (if used) and also the risks of any delivered endobronchial therapy.

Preoperative preparation

- The basic set-up consists of a flexible fibre-optic bronchoscope, light source, biopsy forceps, and suction apparatus.
- Video-bronchoscopy provides excellent visualization and is ideal for teaching.
- The suctioning and clearing of secretions is best accomplished through larger scopes with wider working channels, but the ability to reach very distal airways to obtain direct biopsies is greater with smaller scopes.

Position and theatre set-up

- The theatre should be equipped with oxygen, cardiorespiratory monitoring, and supplies for cardiopulmonary resuscitation.
- The necessary drugs for sedation and topical anaesthesia.
- Appropriate solutions and containers for cytology, microbiology, and pathology specimens.

Procedure

- Specimens may be obtained by direct forceps' biopsy, washings, needle biopsies, or transbronchial biopsies.
- Flexible bronchoscopy can be performed with the patient in either the seated or the supine position.
- Patients may be pre-medicated and should have local anaesthetic applied topically to the nasal and oral mucosae.
- Insertion of the bronchoscope is through the nares or orally through a bite-block. In the intubated patient, the scope is inserted through a connector to the endotracheal tube.

- At bronchoscopy, systematically evaluate the entire tracheobronchial tree, including the vocal cords.
- Several additional procedures may be carried out after inspection of the airways, including washings, broncho-alveolar lavage, protected brushings, biopsies, and transbronchial biopsies.

Postoperative care

- Post-bronchoscopy respiratory failure may be anticipated in patients who are already verging on the need for intubation and mechanical ventilation
- The relative risks and benefits must always be carefully weighed in each patient who is being considered for a bronchoscopic procedure.

Complications

- Asthma and bronchial oedema can be triggered by bronchoscopy.
- Major complications such as respiratory arrest, pneumonia, pneumothorax, and airway obstruction are infrequent.
- Pneumothorax and bleeding are more likely in patients receiving transbronchial lung biopsies.

Tips and tricks

Epinephrine is useful for haemostasis via the working channel of the bronchoscope when mild to moderate bleeding occurs.

Lung biopsy

- Interstitial lung disease (ILD) is a heterogeneous group of lung conditions of both known and unknown aetiology broadly divided into infectious, occupational, iatrogenic, granulomatous, malignant, autoimmune/connective tissue disorder–related, and idiopathic categories.
- Two image-guided wedge biopsy samples should be obtained from separate lobes when investigating ILD in an ambulatory patient. Multiple biopsies are not necessary for the acutely ill, immunocompromised, or febrile patient, where the underlying process is more likely to be diffuse.
- Current CT imaging techniques and relatively non-invasive bronchoscopic biopsy strategies have reduced the need for surgical biopsy. Although surgical biopsy may not be necessary for some cases of idiopathic pulmonary fibrosis, it remains essential for more than one-third of patients.

Consent

Explain the need for biopsy clearly; usually other non- or less-invasive modalities will have been explored. The principle risk of the biopsy itself is continued air leak.

Preoperative preparation

As for 'VATS' (p. 624) or 'Thoracotomy' (p. 622).

Position and theatre set-up

As for 'Thoracotomy' (p. 622).

Procedure

- As for 'VATS' (p. 624) with single lung ventilation or as for 'Thoracotomy' (p. 622).
- The lung is inspected and the proposed site for biopsy, based on the CT scan, is identified.
- Lung staplers, particularly with pericardial buttresses, allow for ample biopsy size from multiple sites.
- Because the critically ill patient is unlikely to tolerate single-lung ventilation, a limited thoracotomy with brief periods of apnoea is often used to permit successful biopsy.
- A haemostatic survey, chest tube placement, and wound closure are standard, as for any thoracotomy or VATS.

Postoperative care

- As for 'VATS' (p. 623) or 'Thoracotomy' (p. 622).
- Specimens are often guided by the referring physician but can be sent for immunohistochemistry, fungal stains, flow cytometry, or electron microscopy.

Complications

- Procedure-related morbidity and mortality in the elective setting are uncommon for VATS lung biopsy but many patients referred for lung biopsy often have multiple co-morbidities and can represent a significant anaesthetic risk.
- Complications include bleeding, requiring re-exploration, and persistent leak, requiring prolonged chest tube drainage.
- Operative mortality in ICU patients may approach 50% and the benefit of histological diagnosis needs to be certain.

Tips and tricks

- Use of a more inferiorly placed port site or incision may facilitate the geometry of the biopsy.
- Brief episodes of apnoea during application of the stapler may help decrease pleural injury and subsequent air leak.

Pulmonary lobectomy

- Resectability refers to the amount of lung tissue and tumour that can be safely removed without developing respiratory insufficiency—it depends directly on the amount of pulmonary reserve of the patient.
- Operability refers to the ability of a patient to survive the proposed procedure and its perioperative complications—it depends on the patient's comorbid conditions.

Anatomy

- The right pulmonary artery passes anterior to the major bronchi, whereas the left pulmonary artery arches superior to the left main bronchus.
- The pulmonary veins are similar on the both sides with the superior pulmonary vein as the anterior structure in the hilum on both sides.

Indications

- In addition to carcinoma and carcinoid tumours, indications for lobectomy include congenital malformations and chronic infections such as fungal, mycobacterial, or bronchiectasis.
- Patients with early stage non-small cell lung cancer are clear candidates for primary surgical resection, while selected patients with more advanced disease may also benefit from surgery as part of multi-modality therapy.

Consent

Explain the benefits of resection, the alternatives (including non-operative management), and the risks. These relate to the wound (see 'Thoracotomy', p. 622 and/or 'VATS', p. 625) and the pulmonary resection, in particular the potential need for pneumonectomy (see p. 639).

Preoperative preparation

- The clinical stage is assessed using CT and positron emission tomography, though cervical mediastinoscopy still has an important role in preoperative staging.
- The patient's fitness to tolerate surgery is determined by history, physical examination, cardiac assessment, and full pulmonary function tests.

Position and theatre set-up

- Many surgeons perform routine bronchoscopic examination to evaluate the anatomy of the airway and verify the location of endobronchial tumour.
- The patient is ventilated intraoperatively with a double-lumen endotracheal tube and placed into the lateral decubitus position.
- Shoulder rolls will help ensure excellent access to the thoracic cavity

Procedure

- As per 'Thoracotomy' (p. 622) or 'VATS' (p. 624).
- The presence of the tumour in the lobe is confirmed.

- Hilar dissection begins with identification and dissection of the three primary vascular structures: the pulmonary artery, bronchus, and the pulmonary vein (Fig. 12.24).
- Anatomic resection requires division of the appropriate branches of the pulmonary artery, pulmonary vein, and lobar bronchus, as well as division of the lung parenchyma that forms any incomplete fissures.
- The sequence of exposure and vision of vessels and airway is not always uniform and tumour size or location sometimes mandate altering the sequence of the procedure.
- Lymphadenectomy is routinely performed by most surgeons.
- There are a number of nuances to video-assisted lobectomy but the anatomic features and principles should be identical to those of the open surgery.

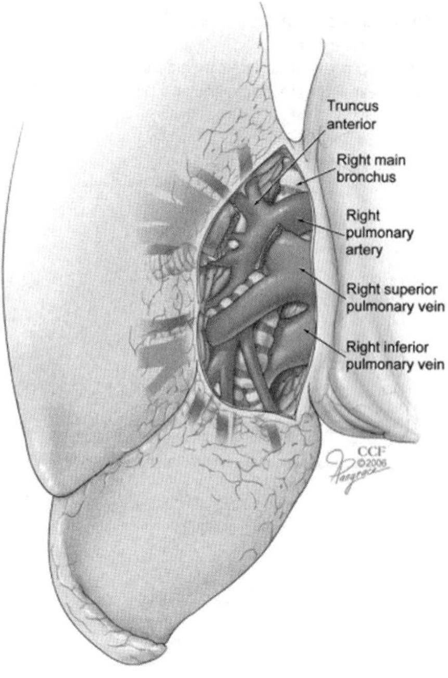
Truncus
anterior
Right main
bronchus
Right
pulmonary
artery
Right superior
pulmonary vein
Right inferior
pulmonary vein
CCF
©2006

Fig. 12.24 Right hilar anatomy.

Postoperative care

- It is important that the chest tubes are adequate to re-expand the lung and to evacuate air and fluid.
- Chest tube size, number, time for placement to water seal, and time of removal are all subject to debate.

Complications

- Major bleeding from the pulmonary artery during pulmonary resection can rapidly become life-threatening—direct gentle pressure with a finger can temporarily control most bleeding while proximal and distal control is obtained.
- Atrial fibrillation and venous thromboembolism are frequent occurrences after thoracotomy for malignancy and can cause significant morbidity, increase the risk of mortality, and prolong length of stay.

Tips and tricks

- Intra-pericardial dissection must be carried out if control cannot be obtained extra-pericardially.
- Techniques to help prevent air leaks include careful creation of the fissures with a clean, straight staple line and buttressing of this line with bovine pericardium.

Pneumonectomy

The decision to perform pneumonectomy may be made preoperatively based of the type or location of the pathology, the imaging, or endoscopic findings; however, often the decision may be made intraoperatively. In either situation the possibility of performing a lesser resection through the use of bronchoplastic or angioplastic sleeve resection should be considered because of the morbidity associated with pneumonectomy

Anatomy

The main stem bronchus is divided as proximally or as close to its origin as possible to avoid the problem of a long bronchial stump because the majority of the blood supply to the bronchial stump comes from the bronchial vessels

Indications

- Pulmonary malignancy that cannot be removed by lobectomy in patients who are fit enough to tolerate pneumonectomy.
- Pneumonectomy for inflammatory lung disease, bronchiectasis, tuberculosis, and other non-malignant conditions is uncommon in the modern era.

Consent

Explain the benefits of resection, the alternatives (including non-operative management), and the risks. These relate to the wound (see 'Thoracotomy', p. 622) and the pulmonary resection (p. 639).

Preoperative preparation

The patient's fitness to tolerate surgery is determined by history, physical examination, cardiac assessment, and full pulmonary function tests.

Position and theatre set-up

- The most common incision used for the removal of the lung is a postero-lateral thoracotomy with access to the pleural cavity via the 5th intercostal space, permitting access to all areas of the lung, both posterior and anterior.
- Median sternotomy carries the advantage of less postoperative compromise of pulmonary function and allows good access to the hilar structures for right pneumonectomy but it can be very difficult to perform left pneumonectomy through this approach.
- VATS has been employed in a limited manner to perform pneumonectomy.

Procedure

- As for 'Pulmonary lobectomy' (p. 634).
- The main PA and both pulmonary veins are divided as per 'Pulmonary lobectomy' (p. 634) (Fig. 12.25).
- After division and closure of the bronchus, the suture line is tested under water for air leaks.
- Any pericardial defect may need to be patched to avoid cardiac herniation and critical compromise of venous return.

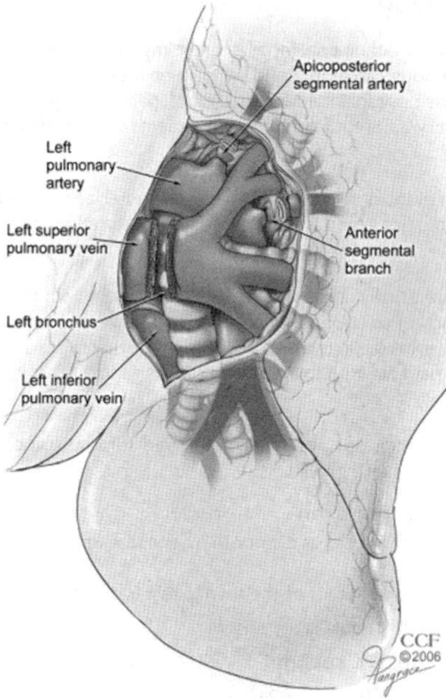
Apicoposterior
segmental artery
Left
pulmonary
artery
Left superior
pulmonary vein
Anterior
segmental
branch
Left bronchus
Left inferior
pulmonary vein
CCF
©2006

Fig. 12.25 Left hilar anatomy.

Postoperative care

Some surgeons elect to leave a chest tube in the empty hemi-thorax to achieve balancing of the mediastinum—it is absolutely essential that no suction be applied to the drain.

Complications

- Pneumonectomy carries a significantly higher operative morbidity and mortality than lesser resections mostly due to the cardiorespiratory compromise of removal of an entire lung.
- Broncho-pleural fistula.
- Cardiac herniation.

Tips and tricks

Intra-pericardial pneumonectomy is often much safer in patients with central lesions.

Thymectomy

Thymomas may be either benign, as seen in myasthenia gravis, or malignant, with squamous carcinoma and lympho-epithelial the most common tumours. The demographic characteristics of patients with thymic carcinoma are not very different from those of patients with myasthenia.

Anatomy

The thymus is a bi-lobar structure located in the anterior mediastinum that contains lymphoid tissue and is the site of T-cell maturation in early life.

Indications

- Thymomas are usually asymptomatic but can present with thoracic outlet obstruction or upper airway compromise.
- Thymectomy is the definitive treatment for myasthenia gravis, while the prognosis of patients with thymic carcinoma is generally poor.

Consent

The benefits may relate to potentially improved survival (cancer) and/or quality of life (myasthenia gravis).

Preoperative preparation

- Thymomas usually appear as a smooth mass in the upper half of the CXR.
- CT will delineate the extent of the thymic tissue, as well as any lymph node involvement.

Position and theatre set-up

As per 'Median sternotomy' (p. 582).

Procedure

- As per 'Median sternotomy' (p. 582).
- The entire thymic mass is resected en bloc to include any pericardial or cardiac involvement, taking care to avoid injury to the phrenic nerves.
- Achievement of a complete resection for thymoma is of paramount importance but is not possible in some cases of thymic carcinomas.

Post-op care

Remove any drains as per unit protocol.

Complications

- As per 'Median sternotomy' (p. 582), but increased risk of phrenic nerve injury.
- When there is intra-pericardial involvement injury to cardiac structures is also a risk.

Tips and tricks

- The use of a VATS approach for thymomas remains controversial.
- Careful follow up of pathology samples is essential.

VATS bullectomy and pleurectomy

VATS bullectomy and pleurectomy

- Blebs form when an alveolus ruptures and air subsequently leaks out from the lung tissue, but is contained by the fibrous tissues of the visceral pleura.
- A bulla is a coalescence of blebs and is the usual cause of a primary spontaneous pneumothorax.
- Rarely, bullae enlarge to such a degree that they occupy a significant proportion of the hemi-thorax.

Anatomy

Bullae tend to develop in the apical segment of the upper lobe and the superior segment of the lower lobe, with or without associated emphysematous changes in the remaining lung.

Indications

- Prolonged air leak—when bullae rupture the resultant air leak can settle with insertion of a chest tube; however, patients with an air leak lasting longer than 4–7 days merit surgery.
- Recurrent pneumothorax or first time pneumothorax in patients living in isolated areas or with certain occupations.

Consent

As for 'VATS' (p. 625), but additional risks of failure and recurrence should be mentioned in patients with prior pneumothorax.

Preoperative preparation

- As for 'VATS' (p. 624) or 'Thoracotomy' (p. 622).
- CXR or CT scanning is often helpful to confirm and localize the pneumothorax/bullae.

Position and theatre set-up

As for 'Thoracotomy' (p. 622).

Procedure

- Resection of the bullae and obliteration of the pleural space are the two major goals in the surgical treatment of spontaneous pneumothorax.
- Wedge resection of the apex, even if no bullae are seen, decreases the rate of recurrence.
- Pleurodesis can be achieved by using parietal pleurectomy, mechanical pleural abrasion, chemical pleurodesis, or a combination of these techniques.
- A full postero-lateral thoracotomy is seldom necessary for the surgical treatment of spontaneous pneumothorax and most centres perform VATS.
- Three ports are often necessary to introduce a rigid telescope and instruments to perform the bullectomy, pleurectomy, or pleural abrasion.

Postoperative care

- The chest drain management is guided by the presence of an air-leak or significant drain output. Once any leak has resolved and the drainage is minimal, the drain can safely be removed.
- It is essential to follow up on the any pathology results.

Complications

The principal complication is recurrence of pneumothorax and is higher in VATS compared with open procedures, possibly because pleurectomy stimulates the formation of denser and more complete and permanent adhesions.

Tips and tricks

- If a pneumothorax recurs after wedge resection and pleurodesis, it is more often caused by the inadequacy of the pleurodesis rather than the formation of new blebs.
- Anti-inflammatory analgesics should not be used postoperatively as they may lessen the effect of the pleurodesis.

Chapter 13

Neurosurgery

Lumbar puncture

Key points

- A common procedure for sterile and safe withdrawal of cerebrospinal fluid (CSF).
- Safer and less prone to infection than a ventricular drain, where there is a choice. This procedure is less invasive than the insertion of an external ventricular drain. It should only be done when obstructive hydrocephalus is ruled out.
- Requires complete sterility.

Indications

Diagnostic

Examination of CSF

- Subarachnoid haemorrhage.
- Meningitis—bacterial, viral, or neoplastic.
- Immune disorders—Guillain–Barre syndrome, transverse myelitis, multiple sclerosis.

Measurement of CSF pressure

- Communicating hydrocephalus.
- Idiopathic intracranial hypertension.

Therapeutic

Withdrawal of CSF

- Communicating hydrocephalus.
- Idiopathic intracranial hypertension.

Administration of therapeutic agents

- Spinal anaesthesia.
- Intrathecal chemotherapy.

Contraindications

- Intracranial space occupying lesion, e.g. tumour or abscess—associated risk of transtentorial or transforaminal herniation.
- Coagulopathy or therapeutic anticoagulants or antiplatelet agents.
- Infective lumbar skin lesion.
- Obstructive hydrocephalus.
- Deformity, e.g. scoliosis, kyphosis or advanced spondylosis.

Consent

Obtain written consent explaining the associated risks:

- Post-lumbar puncture headache (up to 40%). Usually transient and rarely requires a blood patch to treat.
- Epidural or intradural haemorrhage (rare).
- Nerve root injury (rare).
- Low back pain.

Equipment

- Sterile pack.
- Antiseptic.
- 22-gauge spinal needle with stylet.
- Disposable sterile manometer.
- Disposable three-way tap.
- Containers for laboratory investigations.
- Needle and syringe for contemporary blood sample.

Position

A comfortable right or left lateral position with the knees flexed to the chest, the neck flexed, and the patient assuming the foetal position (Fig. 13.1) at a height to suit the operator. This distracts the spinous processes optimizing access to the intervertebral space. The sitting position is a good alternative, especially for spinal anaesthesia, but is unsuitable for measurement of CSF pressure.

Procedure

- Reassure the patient and explain the procedure.
- Choose and mark the L3/4, L4/5, or L5/S1 intervertebral disc level, avoiding higher levels as the spinal cord ends at L1. A line between the superior iliac crests (the intercristal line) lies at the level of the body of the L4 vertebra in most subjects (Fig. 13.2).
- Employ sterile technique.
- Inject local anaesthetic (LA) at the chosen level in small aliquots, aspirating before each injection to avoid injecting into epidural veins or the intrathecal space.
- Wait for the LA to take effect.
- The spinal needle with its trocar is directed towards the umbilicus, bevel upwards, parallel to angle of the spinous processes. A 'give' is felt at the ligamentum flavum, and cerebrospinal fluid is obtained after withdrawal of the trocar.
- Connect the manometer via a three-way tap to measure the opening pressure if required. Allow the CSF to drain spontaneously. Collect

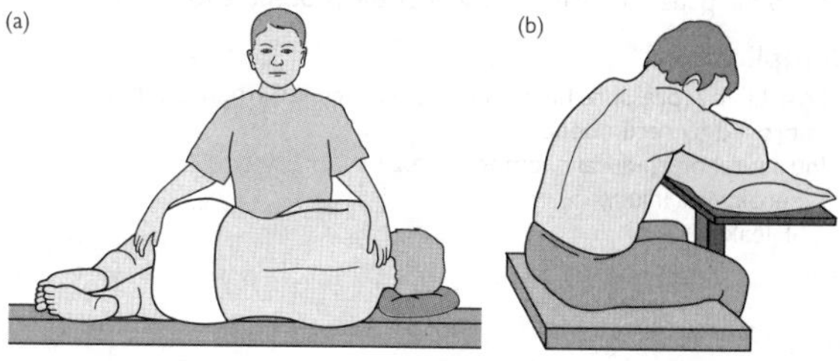
(a)
(b)

Fig. 13.1 Positioning for lumbar puncture: (a) lateral decubitus; (b) sitting position.

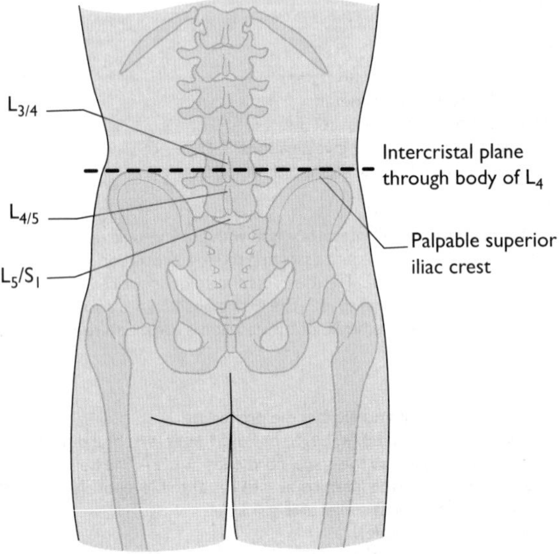
L3/4
Intercristal plane through body of L4
L4/5
Palpable superior iliac crest
L5/S1

Fig. 13.2 Surface landmarks for lumbar puncture.

CSF for microbiological and biochemical analysis. Three serial samples are obtained to distinguish a traumatic tap (diminishing red cell count) from bloodstained CSF (persistently raised red cell count with xanthochromia) in subarachnoid haemorrhage (Table 13.1).
- Measure the closing pressure if required.
- Replace the trocar and remove the needle. Apply firm pressure to the entry point.
- Keep the patient on flat bedrest after the procedure for 1h.

Complications

- Post-LP low pressure headache—usually worse when erect and improved by recumbency.
- Intradural or epidural haemorrhage.
- Neurological injury.
- CSF leak.

Table 13.1 CSF findings on lumbar puncture in common conditions

Diagnosis	Appearance	WBC	Glucose	Protein
Subarachnoid haemorrhage	Blood-stained. Positive for xanthochromia (confirmed with spectrophotometry)	Normal to mildly elevated (lymphocytes slightly predominate)	Decreased	Elevated or high normal
Bacterial meningitis	Turbid	Elevated (polymorphonuclear leukocytes predominate)	Decreased	Elevated
Viral meningitis	Clear	Elevated (lymphocytes predominate)	Normal	Elevated
Tuberculous meningitis	Turbid	Normal to elevated (lymphocytes predominate)	Decreased	Elevated
Fungal meningitis	Clear–Turbid	Normal to elevated (lymphocytes predominate)	Normal to decreased	Elevated

Tips and tricks

- Patients dislike this procedure so minimize the frequency of it. Use adequate local anaesthesia, or make use of a forthcoming general anaesthetic if available.
- Reassure the patient and clearly explain the procedure.
- Position with the lumbar spine well flexed.
- Locate the midline and do not deviate from it.
- Consider the use of the image intensifier in difficult cases.
- In the lateral decubitus position, the spine should be at the edge of the bed so that it is supported by the bed frame, preventing lateral curvature.

Lumbar drain insertion

Key points

- Useful for temporary, continuous CSF diversion where a ventricular drain is not required.
- A more comfortable choice for the patient than repeat lumbar punctures.

Indications

- Treatment of *communicating hydrocephalus*, especially of acute onset, e.g. subarachnoid haemorrhage; meningitis. Obstruction within the ventricular system should be excluded by radiological assessment.
- Treatment of a *CSF fistula*. Serves to decompress a CSF leak or the recent repair of a leak, promoting healing. Complies with the surgical principle that a fistula will heal best when the pressure gradient across it is reduced.
- Treatment of a pseudomeningocele.
- Preoperatively—to reduce intracranial pressure and *to allow brain relaxation*, e.g. for selected intrinsic tumours, skull base tumours, or for clipping of an aneurysm.
- To provide a *controlled increase in intracranial pressure* (ICP), e.g. when delivering the dome of a suprasellar tumour into the pituitary fossa. Small infusions of saline can be injected into the drain to achieve this.

Consent

As for 'Lumbar puncture' on p. 646. Additional rare risk of a foreign body within the spinal canal in the event of catheter fracture. Higher infection rate than a lumbar puncture alone.

Position of patient and equipment

As for 'Lumbar puncture' on p. 647 with the addition of:

- Tuohy needle and stylet. The needle has a 90° angle at the tip to direct the lumbar catheter in the required direction.
- Lumbar catheter and guide wire.

Procedure

- Preparation and access to the subarachnoid space is as for 'Lumbar puncture' on p. 647.
- The Tuohy needle is then introduced with the bevel angled in a cranial direction.
- Once CSF flow is obtained, the stylet is withdrawn and a fine lumbar catheter is inserted, fenestrated end first, with a luminal guide wire in place to provide rigidity.
- When an adequate length of the drain has been passed, the internal guide wire is removed from the drain and spontaneous distal flow of CSF from the drain is confirmed.
- *Important*: If distal flow is *not* confirmed, *do not* withdraw the catheter within the Tuohy needle, as the needle bevel can transect the catheter, leaving a foreign body within the canal. In this event, withdraw both the needle and the catheter together and start again.

- When distal flow is confirmed, the Tuohy needle is removed over the drain, leaving the latter in place.
- Firmly secure the catheter to the skin with a suture.
- Cover the catheter entry point with a clear occlusive dressing. Attach the distal end to a drainage bag via a three-way tap, for intermittent drainage, or to a manometric closed collection set for continuous drainage.
- For continuous drainage the collection set is positioned at a fixed height (typically 10cm) on free drainage when the patient is in bed. Alternatively, a fixed maximum hourly drainage (typically 10ml/h) is stipulated.
- The drain is turned off when the patient is upright or mobilizes to prevent over-drainage of CSF.
- Keep the drain in for the shortest time necessary, to minimize the risk of infection.

Removal

A purse-string monofilament skin suture is placed on removal of the drain to prevent a CSF leak.

Complications

- Low pressure headache. Common. Avoid over-drainage to minimize this.
- Blockage.
- Intrathecal or intracranial haematoma.
- Neurological injury (rare).
- Pneumocephalus.
- Infection.

Tips and tricks

- Ensure that the drain is firmly anchored in place with a skin suture.
- As with all external CSF drains, utilize the device for the shortest time necessary to minimize the infection risk.

Burrhole access to the cranial cavity

Key points

- A safe and rapid technique to provide access to the cranial cavity.
- The 'burr' in 'burrhole' refers to the spherical manual cutting bit traditionally used for this procedure to minimize the risk of a 'plunge' injury. A powered automatic-releasing cranial perforator provides this protection with modern equipment.
- In a drowsy or deteriorating patient, *this is an emergency procedure*. In this situation, liaise with the theatre and anaesthetic teams to get the procedure done as soon after diagnosis as possible. Take the patient directly to theatre from the CT scanner when required.

Anatomy

- The skull is composed of two layers of compact (cortical) bone: the outer table and inner table. These are separated by the cancellous bone of the diploe, which contains red marrow. The skull thickness varies considerably depending on the region of the skull, being thinnest at the temporal squama and thickest in the midline at the external occipital protuberance.
- The calvarium of the skull is covered with scalp in five layers (mnemonic = SCALP: Skin; Cutaneous tissue; Adipose tissue; Loose areolar tissue; and Pericranium). In the temporal region the scalp overlies the temporalis muscle and its covering layer of fascia.

Indications

- Insertion of external ventricular drain.
- Drainage of chronic subdural haematoma or partial evacuation of acute extradural or acute subdural haematoma.
- Needle biopsy of cerebral lesion.
- Insertion of intracranial pressure (ICP) bolt.
- Drainage of cerebral abscess or subdural empyema.
- Intracranial endoscopic procedures.
- Insertion of a deep brain stimulator (DBS) for movement disorders.
- It may be the first step in a craniotomy.

Consent

Obtain written consent explaining the following risks: haemorrhage or haematoma requiring reoperation; recollection of target collection requiring reoperation; infection; seizures. In emergency cases, a consent form for patients lacking capacity is often necessary.

Equipment

- Powered cranial perforator (pneumatic or electric). An automatic-releasing perforator bit may be used that cuts out when the burrhole is complete leaving a thin 'bone pad' on the dura, or a freehand high-speed cutting 'rose' burr. The latter enables small cosmetically favourable burr holes to be drilled (Fig. 13.3).
- Hudson hand brace and bit. This comprises a perforator bit to penetrate the inner table and a spherical burr to enlarge the hole. This combination minimizes the risk of a plunge injury. Slower than a power drill.

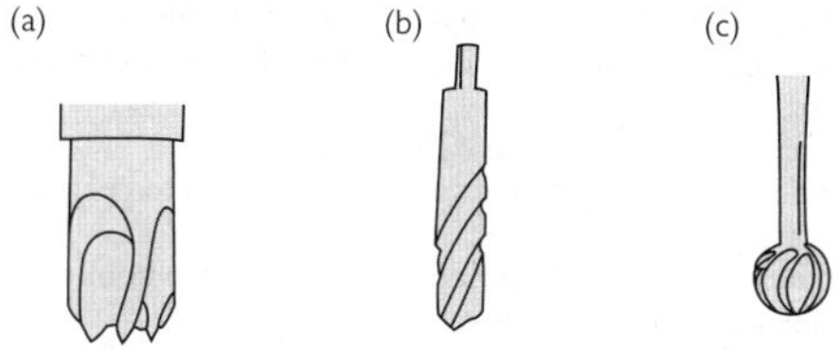
(a)
(b)
(c)

Fig. 13.3 Cranial perforators: (a) Powered drill: automatic releasing perforator; (b) Hudson brace—perforator; and burr (c).

Procedure

- Conduct the WHO checklist paying particular attention to the side of the procedure.
- Shave the hair, mark the chosen site, and prepare with antiseptic solution.
- Make a 2–3cm incision in the scalp straight down to the bone. Strip the pericranium with a periosteal elevator and control scalp bleeding with bipolar diathermy. Place a self-retaining retractor.
- Test the drill.
- The drill should be held firmly perpendicular to the skull and firm constant pressure is applied to the rotating drill bit. An assistant should steady the head.
- With the automatic perforator a change in noise intensity is heard when the drill goes through the outer table. The bit stops automatically after the inner table is breached leaving a thin bone pad on the dura.
- When using the manual drill, hold the Hudson brace firmly perpendicular to the bone surface and apply firm pressure whilst rotating the perforator bit (Fig. 13.4). Stop as soon as the dura is exposed in the middle of the hole. Change the bit to the burr, starting with the smallest available burr. Enlarge the hole until complete.

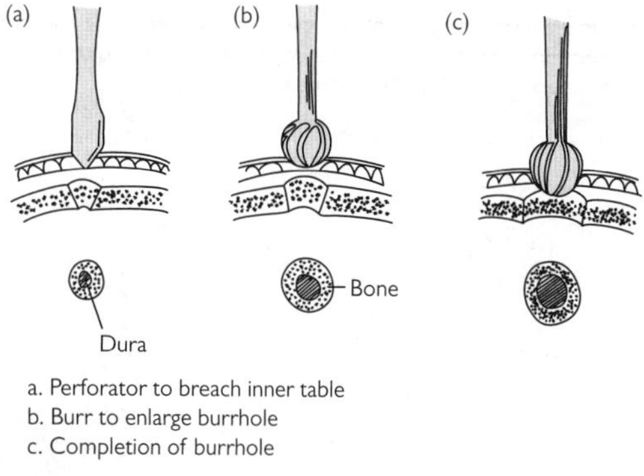
(a)
(b)
(c)
Bone
Dura
a. Perforator to breach inner table
b. Burr to enlarge burrhole
c. Completion of burrhole

Fig. 13.4 How to drill a burr hole with a Hudson brace.

A circular trajectory with the upper handle of the Hudson brace produces a parallel-sided burrhole. Caution should be exercised to avoid a plunge injury.

- Control any bleeding from the diploe with bone wax.
- Apply bipolar diathermy to the surface of the dura to coagulate the surface vessels.
- Elevate the centre of the exposed dura with a sharp hook to protect the brain then incise the dura with a small blade.
- Enlarge the durotomy to fully expose the arachnoid and pia beneath the hole. Apply diathermy to the edges of the durotomy, which will retract to complete the exposure.
- After the procedure, the dura is not closed but haemostatic material such as oxidized cellulose mesh may be placed to protect the brain. The cosmetic result may be optimized by replacing bone dust or by placing a titanium burrhole cover.
- Close the galea with 2/0 absorbable polyfilament and the skin with clips or 3/0 monofilament.

Postoperative care

- Dress the wound.
- As with all intracranial procedures, ensure regular postoperative neurological observations are done every 15min for the first 4h, then hourly for 24h, to detect clinical evidence of raised ICP.
- Act quickly to protect the airway and obtain an urgent scan in any patient with a postoperative decline in their Glasgow Coma Score (GCS).
- Remove staples or sutures at 5 days.

Complications

- Plunging of the drill—minimize this risk with an automatic perforator or with careful technique with the brace.
- Bleeding.
- Infection.
- Seizure.
- Cosmetic—a visible or palpable dimple often remains after the burrhole has healed. Bone dust or a burrhole cover may be placed to minimize this. Choose a site behind the hairline whenever possible.

Evacuation of chronic subdural haematoma

Key points

Indications

Procedure

Post-operative

Evacuation of chronic subdural haematoma

Key points

- Chronic subdural haematoma is a common condition in the elderly age group.
- The condition develops following an initial, commonly asymptomatic, acute subdural haemorrhage overlying the cerebral hemisphere, which matures to produce a symptomatic collection of chronic subdural fluid enclosed within a subdural membrane.
- Risk factors include increasing age, cerebral atrophy, antiplatelet therapy, anticoagulation therapy, and excess alcohol intake.

Indications

- Focal neurological symptoms and signs or evidence of raised ICP in association with a radiologically significant chronic subdural haematoma.
- Non-specific neurological dysfunction in the presence of a radiologically significant collection with failure to resolve over time.

Consent

As for a standard burrhole plus: risk of recurrent chronic subdural collection requiring redrainage (10%).

Equipment

- Irrigating syringe and saline irrigation.
- Soft catheter, e.g. Jacques' for intraoperative irrigation of the cavity and postoperative drainage.

Procedure

- A single burrhole will suffice for a unilateral non-loculated collection. Multiple burrholes are required for bilateral haematomas or for loculated fluid collections.
- The dura is opened as described under 'Burrhole access to the cranial cavity' (p. 652). A subdural membrane is identified beneath the dura and can be distinguished from the brain by the absence of sulci and cerebral vasculature—this is coagulated with bipolar diathermy and incised. The liquid subdural haematoma is evacuated, often under pressure.
- The cavity is thoroughly irrigated with normal saline at body temperature via the Jacques' catheter until the effluent runs clear.
- The irrigating catheter is secured and left in the subdural space.
- Closure is as described above (p. 654).

Postoperative care

- The subdural catheter is removed when drainage ceases, typically after 24h.
- A postoperative CT scan may be done to assess brain re-expansion or investigate ongoing neurological symptoms.

Complications

- Recollection requiring reoperation—the risk is reduced by use of an external drainage catheter.
- Infection including subdural empyema—should be suspected in cases of recurrent collection with features of infection.

Alternatives

Small asymptomatic collections may safely be observed whilst they resolve. Serial imaging may be done to monitor resolution.

Tips and tricks

- Consider local anaesthesia in patients with significant co-morbidities who cannot tolerate general anaesthesia.
- Seek haematological advice in patients on aspirin or with a coagulopathy before proceeding and consider appropriate blood products.

Insertion of external ventricular drain

Key points

- An external ventricular drain (EVD) provides rapid access to the largest intracranial CSF compartment.
- CSF infection is a common complication. Use meticulous aseptic technique and employ the drain for the shortest time necessary.
- Consider alternatives such as lumbar puncture or a lumbar drain when these simpler options are suitable.

Indications

Emergency

- Acute obstructive hydrocephalus. Common causes include:
  - Subarachnoid haemorrhage (SAH).
  - Tumour, e.g. posterior fossa tumour; pineal region tumour.
  - Cerebellar infarct.
  - Colloid cyst of the third ventricle. In this condition, obstruction is at both foraminae of Monro requiring bilateral EVDs.
- Head injury—continuous drainage of CSF helps reduce raised intracranial pressure. ICP monitoring may be done via the catheter.
- CSF infection—provides a temporary portal for administering intrathecal antibiotics directly into the ventricle, where indicated.

Elective

CSF diversion in elective tumour surgery where temporary impairment of CSF drainage is anticipated, e.g. large posterior fossa tumour.

Contraindications

A high blood load in the ventricles following haemorrhage may preclude drain placement.

Equipment

- Powered craniotome or Hudson brace and bit.
- Single-use ventricular catheter with stylet.
- Disposable closed CSF drainage system.
- An image-guidance system may be indicated with small ventricles or atypical anatomy.

Position

Supine in neutral with the head supported by a horseshoe or padded head ring.

Procedure

- Select the insertion site:
  - Kocher's point (Fig. 13.5) is the commonest site in the right frontal region. This is in the non-dominant side away from the speech cortex and is sited anterior to the motor strip, minimizing the risk of symptomatic injury. It also avoids major surface veins. The contralateral side is used if there is a contraindication for right sided placement (Table 13.2).
  - Frazier's point in the occipital region is an alternative (Fig. 13.5). This is readily accessible for a patient undergoing cranial surgery in the supine position.

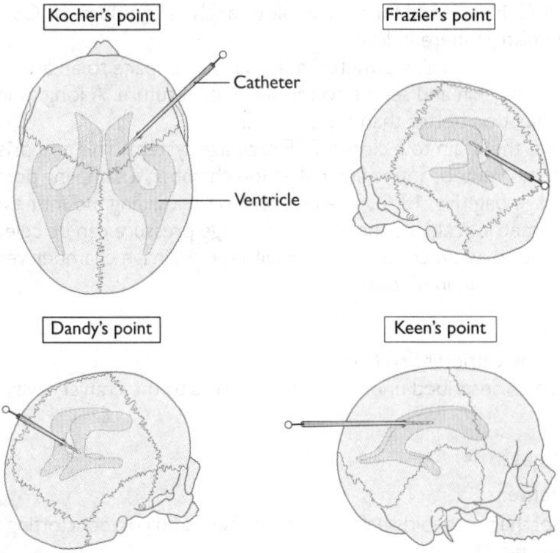
Kocher's point
Catheter
Ventricle
Frazier's point
Dandy's point
Keen's point

Fig. 13.5 Options for burrhole placement for ventricular cannulation.

Table 13.2 Surface landmarks for burr hole sites in drain and shunt placement

Site	Entry Point	Trajectory and Course
Frontal (Kocher's point)	2–3cm from the midline, midpupillary line, 1cm anterior to coronal suture—into the frontal horn	Perpendicular to the skull, medial canthus in the coronal plane, external auditory meatus (EAM) in the sagittal plane
Parietal (Keen's point)	3cm posterior and superior to the pinna—into the trigone	Perpendicular to the skull
Occipital (Frazier's point)	6–7cm above the inion, 3–4cm from the midline—into the occipital horn	Parallel to the skull base, aiming for the middle of the forehead
Dandy's point	3cm above the inion, 2cm lateral to the midline—into the occipital horn	Perpendicular to the skull

- Make a burrhole as described under 'Burrhole access to the cranial cavity', p. 652.
- Make a short pial incision to expose the cortex.
- Pass the ventricular catheter with stylet perpendicular to the tangent at the entry point. CSF should be encountered at around 3cm. A 'give' is felt when the catheter enters the ventricle. Advance the catheter so that about 6cm is within the brain. The catheter is marked at 5cm intervals to facilitate this.

- Collect CSF and send for microbiology analysis, cytology, or CSF biochemistry where indicated.
- Tunnel the ventricular catheter in the subgaleal space to an area of sterile scalp skin and secure to the skin with a suture. A long tunnel may resist infection better than a short one.
- Connect the drain to a closed CSF drainage system. This comprises a calibrated, vented, anti-reflux collection chamber, a sampling port, and a drainage bag (Fig. 13.6). The chamber is on a sliding mount next to a manometric scale, so the chosen drainage pressure can be selected. Take care to avoid contact of CSF with the drainage chamber vent which can result in blockage.

Closure

- Secure the catheter firmly to the skin.
- Closure as described under 'Burrhole access to the cranial cavity', p. 654.

Complications

Intraoperative

- Haemorrhage—avoid surface vessels; check and correct clotting before proceeding.
- Suboptimal siting—do not exceed the depth of the ventricle indicated by the imaging. Consider image guidance with small ventricles.

Postoperative

- Disconnection.
- Infection (ventriculitis)—ensure all CSF sampling from ports is done using a no-touch technique.
- Obstruction—consider CT scanning to confirm.

Tips and tricks

- Image guidance may be required in cases with small ventricles.
- 'Soft' passage of the catheter, by withdrawing the stilette as the catheter is advanced, is the safest mode of placement once CSF is obtained.
- Measure the required catheter length from the scan and take care not to exceed this to avoid damage to deep white matter structures.

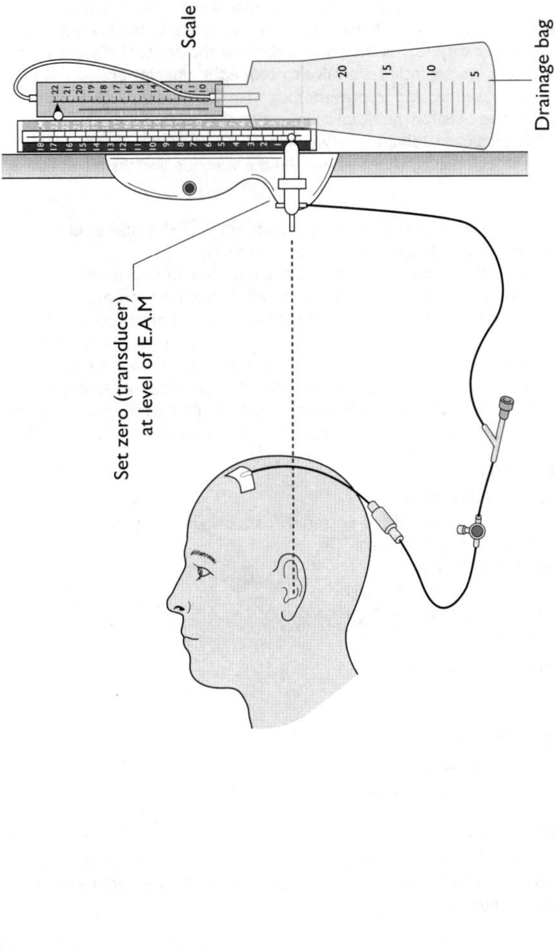
Scale
Drainage bag
Set zero (transducer)
at level of E.A.M

Fig. 13.6 Set-up for external ventricular drain (EVD).

Insertion of adult ventriculoperitoneal shunt

Key points

- Hydrocephalus is an increase in the volume of CSF within the ventricles. It is most commonly due to an obstruction in the CSF drainage pathway (obstructive hydrocephalus) or reduced CSF absorption in the presence of a patent anatomical CSF pathway (communicating hydrocephalus).
- A ventriculoperitoneal (VP) shunt is a permanent implanted drainage catheter that diverts CSF from the lateral ventricle of the brain to the peritoneal cavity. CSF is then reabsorbed via the peritoneal membrane. The shunt system includes a valve to define the opening pressure, to prevent backflow, and to prevent excessive CSF loss through siphoning.
- Alternative sites for the distal shunt catheter include:
  - Ventriculoatrial shunt—between the ventricle and the right atrium.
  - Ventriculopleural shunt—between the ventricle and the pleural cavity.

Anatomy

- CSF is actively secreted by the ependymal cells of the lateral ventricles at a rate of 0.5ml/kg/h (average of 500ml/day).
- The normal lateral ventricles contain about 25ml of CSF each.
- From the lateral ventricles, the CSF flows through the foramen of Monro into the 3rd ventricle, and then through the aqueduct of Sylvius into the 4th ventricle. CSF flows out of the 4th ventricle via the midline foramen of Magendie and the lateral foramina of Luschka. It then passes into the cisterna magna, before entering the subarachnoid space.
- CSF circulates over the cerebral hemispheres to be absorbed back into the cerebral venous system via the arachnoid villi which lie close to the midline.

Indications

Obstructive hydrocephalus

- Tumours, especially of the posterior fossa or pineal region.
- Colloid cyst of the 3rd ventricle.
- Aqueductal stenosis.
- Intraventricular haemorrhage.
- Posterior fossa haemorrhage.
- Chiari malformation.

Communicating hydrocephalus

- Subarachnoid haemorrhage.
- Meningitis.
- Traumatic brain injury.

Increased CSF secretion (rare)

- Choroid plexus papilloma.

Alternatives

Endoscopic 3rd ventriculostomy may be considered when appropriate to avoid the complications of blockage and infection associated with an implanted shunt system.

Contraindications

- CSF infection—an external ventricular drain is required in such cases until infection is completely clear.
- Coagulopathy—correct before proceeding.
- Peritoneal adhesions from previous surgery.

Consent

Written consent involves explaining the following risks:

- Shunt blockage requiring revision—most commonly due to proximal obstruction.
- Shunt infection requiring externalization and antibiotic therapy with shunt revision—these complications are significantly more common in children than adults.
- Slit ventricle syndrome.
- Shunt tract haemorrhage.
- Subdural haemorrhage.
- Bowel injury.

Equipment

- Shunt system comprising:
  - Ventricular catheter.
  - Valve.
  - Distal catheter.
- Disposable tunnelling device with trocar.

Position

- Supine with the head rotated so that the proximal entry point, usually on the right, is uppermost (Fig. 13.7).
- A sandbag is placed under the ipsilateral shoulder.

Procedure

- The cranial entry point is marked, in the parietal (commonest) or frontal location. A frontal site will usually require an additional intermediate scalp incision.
- A short, horizontal subcostal incision is marked on the ipsilateral side.
- Hair is clipped from the scalp and the whole tract from the scalp to the subcostal region is prepared and draped.
- The shunt system is preferably assembled and immersed in saline prior to commencing the procedure.
- A small inverted U-shaped incision is made behind the ear. The site is about 3cm posterior and superior to the pinna. A burrhole is fashioned as described under 'Burrhole access to the cranial cavity', p. 652.
- A short ipsilateral subcostal transverse incision is made and a muscle-splitting approach is made to the peritoneum.
- The peritoneum is elevated between artery clips, and incised.
- The proximal burrhole is elevated, as above. The tunneller is passed under the skin and guided from the abdominal incision to the cranial incision in the subcutaneous layer, over the ribs and clavicle so that it presents adjacent to the cranial burrhole.

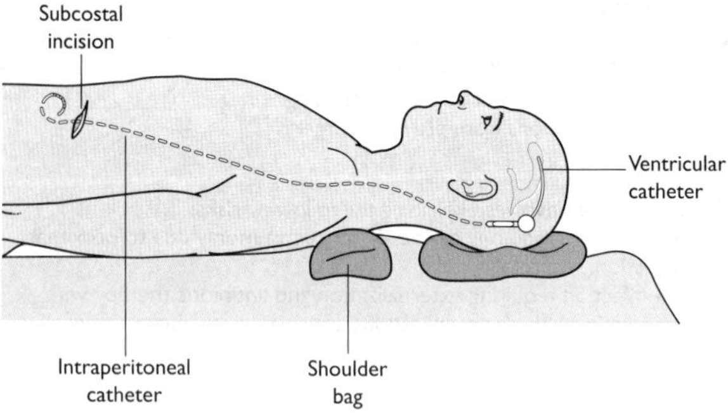
Subcostal
incision
Ventricular
catheter
Intraperitoneal
catheter
Shoulder
bag

Fig. 13.7 Positioning for insertion of ventriculoperitoneal (VP) shunt.

- The distal end of the catheter is passed though the tunneller, and the tunneller is then removed leaving the catheter in situ.
- A cruciate durotomy is made, and the ventricular catheter is passed into the ventricle. The distal end of the catheter is observed to confirm spontaneous CSF drainage.
- CSF sample is collected and sent for microscopy, glucose and protein measurements.
- The peritoneal end is internalized and closure is done in layers.

Closure

- The peritoneum is closed in a 'purse-string' fashion to retain the shunt tip. The abdomen is closed in layers with non-absorbable suture to the fascia.
- Scalp closure as described on p. 654.

Postoperative care

- Record the shunt type prominently in the patient's notes; programmable shunts require a valve check and reset following future MRI scans.
- A baseline postoperative CT head may be obtained to confirm catheter location and ventricular decompression.

Complications

Intraoperative

- Haemorrhage—intraparenchymal or subdural haematoma.
- Suboptimal placement of the ventricular catheter.
- Bowel perforation.
- Skin perforation from the tunnelling trocar.

Postoperative
- Infection.
- Shunt under-drainage or over-drainage.
- Seizures.
- Slit ventricle syndrome—a syndrome of over-drainage commonest in children. A programmable shunt valve may allow treatment of this without requiring valve revision.

Tips and tricks
- Position the patient so that the head, neck, chest, and trunk are in an approximate straight line to facilitate passage of the trocar.
- Ventricular CSF should be sent for microbiology, glucose, and protein analysis, plus tumour markers where indicated.
- Confirm spontaneous distal drainage before internalizing the distal catheter.

Insertion of intracranial pressure (ICP) bolt

Key points

- An ICP monitor is a device for the invasive measurement of ICP within the skull.
- The goal is to identify a rise in ICP early, to permit active treatment and therefore to optimize the outcome of the acute brain condition being treated.
- The cranial vault is a rigid box, and volume change of any of the three non-compressible components within it (brain, blood, and CSF) causes a compensatory reduction in the others (Monro–Kellie doctrine). When this compensation fails, the ICP rises. A rise in ICP impairs cerebral blood flow and is associated with increased neurological morbidity from ischaemia.
- The normal ICP is in the range of 0–20cm$H_2$0, but varies for physiological reasons.

Location and types of monitor

- Locations for placement include intraparenchymal, subdural, or intraventricular (Fig. 13.8).
- Various types of device are in use including:
  - Fibre-optic catheter tip transducer (e.g Camino).
  - Implanted microchip sensor (e.g. Codman).
  - External fluid-coupled transducer connected to a ventricular catheter.

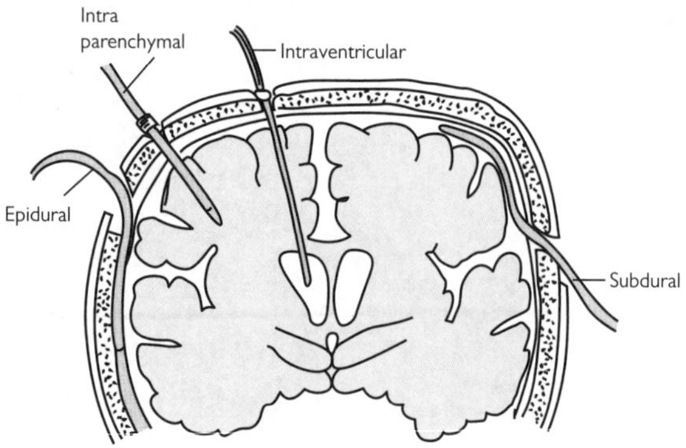
Intra
parenchymal
Intraventricular
Epidural
Subdural

Fig. 13.8 Options for ICP monitor placement.

Indications

- Severe head injury.
- SAH.
- Idiopathic intracranial hypertension (also known as 'benign intracranial hypertension' or 'pseudotumour cerebri').
- Cerebral infarct.

Equipment required

- Disposable ICP monitor.
- Twist drill and bit.
- Sterile dressing kit.

Contraindications

- Coagulopathy or anticoagulant therapy.
- Scalp infection.

Consent

If the patient is conscious, alert and oriented, explain why the procedure is being done and how long the monitoring would last (usually 48 hours). The surgeon should highlight the possible complications during discussion with the patient and/or family.

Procedure

- General or local anaesthetic.
- Select the insertion point—most commonly Kocher's point on the non-dominant side.
- Prepare the skin with betadine or chlorhexidine antiseptic. Infiltrate 1% lignocaine with adrenaline.
- Make a short incision and a twist drill hole.
- The ICP monitor bolt is screwed into the skull.
- The monitor is placed according to the manufacturer's instructions, depending on the device type. Some devices require zeroing prior to insertion.
- The ICP waveform is confirmed on the monitor.

Complications

Intraoperative

- Haemorrhage—intraparenchymal or subdural haematoma.
- Technical malfunction—a normal ICP trace should have a triphasic waveform and should show a variation in baseline with this respiratory cycle.

Postoperative

- Infection—usually Gram-positive cocci (*Staphylococcus* spp.).

Tips and tricks

- Confirm a clear 'triple' waveform is present on the monitor to confirm intracranial placement.
- A rise in ICP on the brief application of external jugular venous compression helps confirm satisfactory placement and function of the monitor.

Craniotomy—supratentorial

Key points

- A craniotomy is the creation of an opening in the skull in which the bone flap is elevated temporarily to gain access to the intracranial cavity, and then replaced. The flap may remain attached by a muscular pedicle (osteoplastic flap) to optimize the blood supply or may be completely free.
- An emergency craniotomy is most commonly fronto-temporal to expose the lateral convexity of the hemisphere. This is a common location for a traumatic extradural or subdural haematoma. There is good access to the branches of the middle meningeal artery and the cerebral bridging veins of the cerebral hemisphere.
- An elective craniotomy is a planned procedure to provide access to the intracranial cavity to approach a wide range of intracranial pathology. The location is tailored to the pathology.
- General anaesthesia is usually employed but local anaesthetic with sedation may be used ('awake craniotomy'), especially for elective surgery in eloquent locations, to aid in minimizing neurological deficits.

Indications

- Symptoms and signs of acutely raised intracranial pressure with a remediable intracranial mass lesion:
  - Deteriorating conscious level with decreasing Glasgow coma score.
  - Hypertension and bradycardia.
  - Altered pupil responses especially unilateral pupillary dilatation (a late sign).
  - Radiological evidence of raised ICP.
  - A natural history suggesting that an imminent rise in ICP is likely, e.g. recent contusion; intracranial pus.
- Common emergency pathologies (Fig. 13.9):
  - Haematoma—extradural, subdural or intracerebral.
  - Cerebral contusion.
  - Compound skull fracture including penetrating injury to the brain, e.g. knife or ballistic injury.
  - Cerebral abscess or subdural empyema.
  - Tumours or cysts with evidence of acutely raised intracranial pressure.
- Common elective pathologies:
  - Open biopsy, debulking, or resection of intrinsic or extrinsic brain tumours.
  - Clipping of cerebral aneurysms.
  - Resection of intracranial vascular malformations, e.g. arteriovenous malformation (AVM) or cavernoma.
  - Surgery of epilepsy.

Consent

Written patient consent must be obtained with an explanation of the following risks:

- Haemorrhage or haematoma.
- Infection.
- Seizure (commonest in the first 24h postoperation).
- CSF leak.

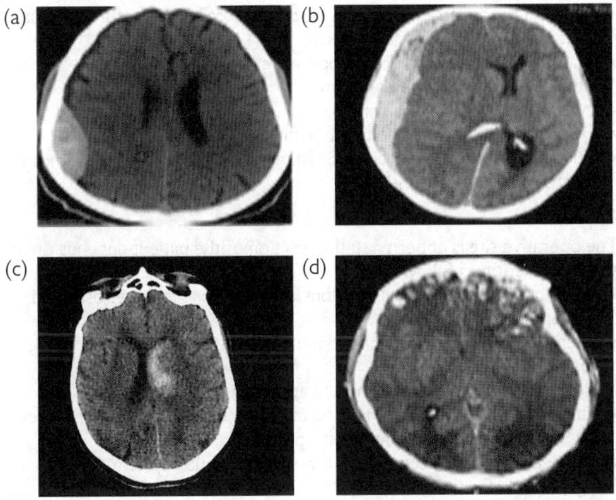
(a)
(b)
(c)
(d)

Fig. 13.9 Common indications for emergency craniotomy: (a) extradural haematoma; (b) acute subdural haematoma; (c) intracerebral haematoma; (d) cerebral contusions.

- New neurological deficit relating to site of surgery.
- Risk to life (around 2% depending on the procedure and the patient's co-morbidities).

Preoperative preparation

- Anticoagulant and antiplatelet therapy is discontinued for the perioperative period. Aspirin and clopidogrel are stopped 1 week before the procedure, while warfarin is either discontinued 36h prior to surgery in elective cases or reversed urgently in emergency cases.
- A preoperative course of oral dexamethasone (steroid medication) is given in tumour cases to reduce peritumoural oedema.
- Haematological, clotting, and biochemical parameters are checked and corrected. A group and save sample is sent to the haematology laboratory.
- Staging investigations appropriate to the suspected pathology. This may include CT of the chest, abdomen, and pelvis. There is a low threshold for this investigation, as primary and secondary brain tumours can have similar appearances.
- Depending on the patient's pathology and co-morbidities, other investigations are done, e.g. CXR, respiratory function tests, ECG, echocardiogram, sickle test, etc.

Equipment

- High-speed drill and craniotome attachment.
- Craniotomy set.
- Scalp clips (e.g. Raney) for haemostasis.
- Suction.
- Monopolar and bipolar diathermy.

- Haemostatic agents, e.g. bone wax, oxidized cellulose mesh, absorbable gelatin sponge, haemostatic sealant.
- Image-guidance system or intraoperative image-guidance with ultrasound or MRI, where indicated.
- A self-retaining retractor system.
- Operating microscope and micro-instruments.
- Dural substitute where indicated. Titanium miniplates or skull clamps to secure the replaced bone flap.

Position

The operative site is uppermost; the position of the patient depends on the site of the lesion as follows:

- *Supine position* for pterional, subfrontal, bifrontal or simple retrosigmoid approaches.
- *Lateral or 'Park-bench' position* for subtemporal or retrosigmoid approaches.
- *Prone position* for posterior midline approach.
- *Sitting position*—uncommonly used for supratentorial procedures—see ➔ 'Craniotomy—posterior fossa', p. 674.
- The head is immobilized using a three-point fixation system, e.g. Mayfield fixation clamp.
- The head is positioned above the heart to avoid venous hypertension ('reverse Trendelenburg' position).
- Potential pressure points are padded and protected.
- Intermittent calf compression boots are applied.

Principles of selection of scalp flap

There are three main considerations:

- Optimum exposure of the surgical lesion.
  - Consider using an image-guidance system to plan the best location and minimum size of the flap.
- Good neurovascular supply to the scalp and bone flap.
  - The scalp flap is curved with an inferior base; the length of the flap should not be greater than twice the width of the base.
  - Avoid intersecting incisions on the scalp during revision surgery to prevent areas of scalp ischaemia.
  - Use an osteoplastic (pedicled) bone flap where available to optimize blood supply to the bone.
- Optimum cosmetic result.
  - The incision should be made behind the hairline where possible.
  - Autologous bone dust is replaced in the burrholes or titanium burrhole covers may be utilized to optimize the postoperative cranial contour.

Procedure

- Conduct the WHO checklist with particular attention to the side of the craniotomy.
- Place a urinary catheter with antibiotic cover—this is essential for lengthy operations or when IV mannitol is to be given.

The following describes the procedure for a fronto-pterional trauma flap, the commonest emergency approach to the cranial cavity:

- Position the patient supine with the head rotated to bring the operative site uppermost.

- The head is placed above the heart to optimize venous drainage from the head (the 'reverse Trendelenburg' position).
- A three-point cranial immobilization system, such as a Mayfield clamp, is used to provide complete stability of the skull. This is important when cutting the flap and during intracranial microdissection.
- Carry out a minimal head shave along the incision line.
- Mark the pterional (fronto-temporo-parietal) flap. This is typically a large question-mark shaped incision with the posterior limit lying just above the root of the zygoma, 1cm in front of the tragus, coursing upwards and anteriorly to end behind the hairline, at or just across the midline.
- Prepare and drape the surgical field.
- On induction/prior to incision:
  - Give IV antibiotics according to local protocol.
  - Give 8mg IV dexamethasone with all brain tumours. A preoperative course of dexamethasone is given where indicated.
  - Give mannitol 20% IV in a dose of 0.5–1.0g/kg where required to control raised ICP.
  - Optimize pCO_2 in the range 4–4.5kPa.
- Make the incision straight down to the bone. Haemostasis of the scalp edges is achieved with bipolar diathermy and scalp clips (Fig. 13.10).
- Elevate the scalp flap by sharply dividing the loose areolar tissue layer beneath the galea. Temporalis muscle together with its fascia remains attached to the bone to form an osteoplastic flap. A pedicle is formed of the inferior fibres of temporalis which are separated from the underlying bone.
- Make the burrholes with a high-speed drill. Separate the dura from beneath the margins of each burrhole with a dissector.
- Connect the burrholes using the craniotome and divide the isthmus of bone beneath the temporalis pedicle.
- Raise the bone flap, carefully peeling the dura from beneath with a dissector to avoid dural injury.
- Extradural haemostasis is achieved with diathermy, bone wax to bleeding bone edges, haemostatic agents, and hitch sutures. A dry field is essential prior to durotomy.
- The bone and scalp flap are cleaned and retracted out of the operating field.

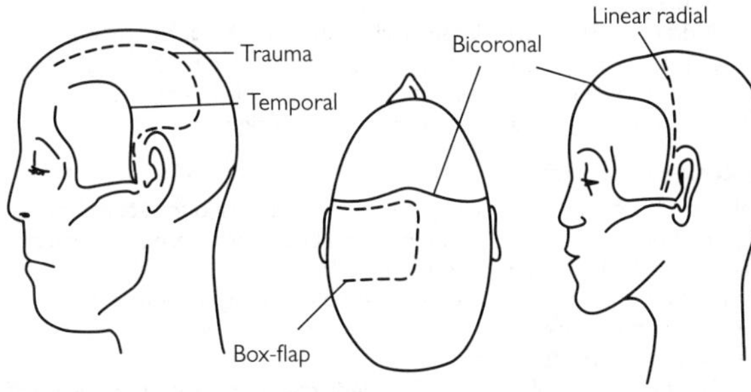
Trauma
Temporal
Box-flap
Bicoronal
Linear radial

Fig. 13.10 Common supratentorial craniotomy incisions.

- In an extradural haematoma, a thick blood clot will be seen overlying the dura, which is sucked and washed away. The arterial dural bleeding point, commonly a branch of the middle meningeal artery, is identified and coagulated with diathermy.
- For intradural lesions, a durotomy is done. A sharp hook is used to elevate the dura away from brain. A knife is then used to commence the durotomy. Toothed forceps and scissors are used to complete the dural opening, taking care to protect the underlying cortex and its vessels.
- Hitch sutures are placed to retract the dura.
- The intracranial pathology is treated as required.
- Key principles of surgical treatment of brain lesions:
  - Brain relaxation is achieved by consideration of the following either separately or in combination: preoperative steroids; CSF drainage via a lumbar drain or directly by opening the arachnoid of the basal cisterns; administration of IV mannitol on induction (0.5–1g/kg of 20% mannitol IV); optimum ventilation.
  - The operating microscope is preferred for all elective brain surgery, to promote optimum visualization and to minimize trauma to brain, cranial nerves, and vessels.
  - The subarachnoid plane, cerebral fissures, and sulci are employed wherever possible to approach cerebral lesions to minimize cerebral retraction and injury.
  - Where an intrinsic lesion must be approached directly through the cortex, the shortest trajectory available through non-eloquent brain is the preferred route.
  - Minimal retraction is applied to the brain to minimize cerebral ischaemia. 'Dynamic retraction' is preferred to fixed retraction.
  - Exposed cortex is protected with saline-moistened patties to prevent dehydration.
  - Bipolar diathermy is used throughout the intradural phase to minimize collateral thermal injury to neural tissue.
- Closure of the craniotomy is in layers:
  - Watertight dural closure is done with monofilament suture. This may be augmented with a dural graft, oxidized cellulose mesh or hydrogel sealant.
  - The bone flap is secured with titanium miniplates or clamps, or with sutures.
  - A drain may be placed beneath the galea, which is a common site of postoperative haematoma. The drain is tunnelled to the sterile scalp and sutured in place. Low pressure suction only is employed. The drain is removed early to minimize the infection risk.

Postoperative care

- Neuro-observations. The Glasgow coma scale is used to record best eye response, best speech response, and best motor response—every 15min for the first 4h, then hourly for 24h.
- In the event of neurological deterioration following craniotomy:
  - Secure the airway.
  - Obtain an urgent CT brain.
  - Treat any cause of raised ICP immediately, with a return to theatre if necessary.

- Postoperative neurological deterioration may be due to:
  - Intracranial haematoma requiring urgent return to theatre, e.g. intra-cavity haematoma; extradural haematoma; subdural haematoma.
  - Cerebral infarction.
  - Acute hydrocephalus.
  - Seizures.
  - Delayed ischaemic deficit in conjunction with subarachnoid haemorrhage.
  - If these are excluded, also consider non-CNS causes of a deteriorating conscious level such as hypoxia, metabolic derangement, or sepsis.
- Haemoglobin, clotting function, and electrolytes are measured and corrected; clotting derangements may occur following cerebral surgery and after significant blood loss.
- The subgaleal drain is removed at 24h.
- The urinary catheter is removed.
- Early mobilization is promoted, TED stockings are worn until discharge, and low molecular weight heparin is commenced 24h after surgery, to minimize the risk of venous thromboembolism. Heparin may be omitted in patients with unsecured vascular lesions.

Complications

Intraoperative

- Bleeding.
- Brain swelling.
- Nerve injury.
- Risks of anaesthesia.

Postoperative

- New neurological deficit.
- Seizure.
- Cerebral swelling.
- Hydrocephalus.
- Meningitis.
- Infection including wound infection, bone flap infection, subdural empyema, or cerebral abscess.
- CSF leak via the wound or CSF rhinorrhea via the frontal sinus or the mastoid air cells.
- General risks including:
  - DVT; PE.
  - Respiratory or urinary tract infection
  - Cardiac complications.

Tips and tricks

- A successful outcome from craniotomy depends as much on correct patient selection and meticulous patient workup as it does on the conduct of the procedure.
- Take care with placement of three-pin fixation, avoiding the thin skull at the temporal fossa floor, the suboccipital plate, and any previously placed shunt system.
- The scalp is highly vascular; minimize blood loss on opening with meticulous haemostasis and the use of scalp clips or haemostats.

Craniotomy—posterior fossa

Key points

- The posterior cranial fossa is the postero-inferior compartment of the skull bounded by the tentorium cerebelli superiorly and the foramen magnum inferiorly. It contains the cerebellar hemispheres, the medulla, and the pons together with the origin and part of the course of eight of the twelve cranial nerves from the trochlear nerve to the hypoglossal nerve.
- The posterior fossa is a key location for many pathologies that present with a highly variable combination of the following symptoms:
  - Symptoms of obstructive hydrocephalus from impairment of CSF circulation.
  - Cerebellar dysfunction such as clumsiness of upper or lower limbs or distinctive halting 'cerebellar' speech.
  - Cranial nerve dysfunction, e.g. trigeminal neuralgia, hemifacial spasm, diplopia, facial numbness, impaired gag and swallow, tongue wasting.
- It contains important elements of the CSF pathway, including the aqueduct of Sylvius, the 4th ventricle, and the foraminae of Luschka (lateral to midline) and Magendie (midline) through which CSF circulates onto the convexity of the cerebral cortex.
- Major intradural venous sinuses are located at the boundaries of the fossa, including the torcula, the transverse sinus, the sigmoid sinus, and the superior and inferior petrosal sinuses.

Indications

- Surgery of posterior fossa tumours.
  - Adult:
    - —Cerebellar metastasis.
    - —Cerebellar haemangioblastoma.
    - —Meningioma.
    - —Vestibular schwannoma.
    - —Choroid plexus papilloma.
    - —Epidermoid cyst.
    - —Dermoid tumour.
  - Paediatric:
    - —Pilocytic astrocytoma.
    - —Primary neuroectodermal tumours, including medulloblastoma.
    - —Ependymoma.
    - —Brainstem glioma.
- Microvascular decompression of cranial nerves, e.g. in:
  - Trigeminal neuralgia.
  - Hemifacial spasm.
- Posterior fossa haemorrhage.
- Congenital malformations. e.g:
  - Chiari malformation.
  - Arachnoid cyst.

Consent

As for 'Craniotomy—supratentorial' on p. 668, plus: risk of venous air embolism (entry of air into one of the major dural venous sinuses); increased risk of CSF wound leak because of the higher CSF pressure at the lower skull opening; risk of CSF rhinorrhoea following breach of mastoid air cells; risk of postoperative hydrocephalus following fourth ventricular obstruction; postoperative haematoma presents a higher risk than in the supratentorial compartment because of the proximity of the brainstem and respiratory centre.

Preoperative preparation

As for 'Craniotomy—supratentorial' on p. 669.

Equipment

As for 'Craniotomy—supratentorial' on p. 669, plus cranial nerve monitor. In posterior fossa surgery involving skull base tumours with cranial nerve involvement, e.g. vestibular schwannoma, intraoperative monitoring is mandatory to facilitate early identification of involved cranial nerves and provide electrical evidence of continuity of nerves during tumour resection.

Position

- *Prone position* for posterior midline approach.
- *Lateral or 'Park-bench' position* for retrosigmoid, posterolateral, or far lateral approach.
- *Supine position* for translabyrinthine approach or for the retrosigmoid approach.
- *Sitting position* for posterior midline approach—most commonly employed in paediatric patients whose risk of venous air embolism, an important complication of this approach, is less than in adults. Significantly reduces intraoperative blood loss by reducing intracranial venous pressure.

Procedure

The following describes the procedure for a midline suboccipital posterior fossa craniotomy:

- The patient is prone with the head stabilized with three-pin fixation.
- A midline incision is made in the avascular intermuscular plane and deepened down to the C2 spinous process and to the bone of the occipital plate (Fig. 13.11).
- Monopolar cutting diathermy is used and self-retaining retractors are placed and advanced for good visualization.
- A Cobb elevator is used to dissect the subperiosteal plane. The muscular and ligamentous attachments are stripped laterally off the occipital plate and the posterior elements of the C1 and C2 vertebrae. Tissue attachments are divided with monopolar diathermy.
- Laterally, at C1 and C2, caution is required to avoid injury to the vertebral artery and its encasing venous plexus, which emerge from the superior opening of the foramen transversarium on each side to course medially and upward around the lateral mass of C1, entering the cranial cavity by passing through the suboccipital membrane.

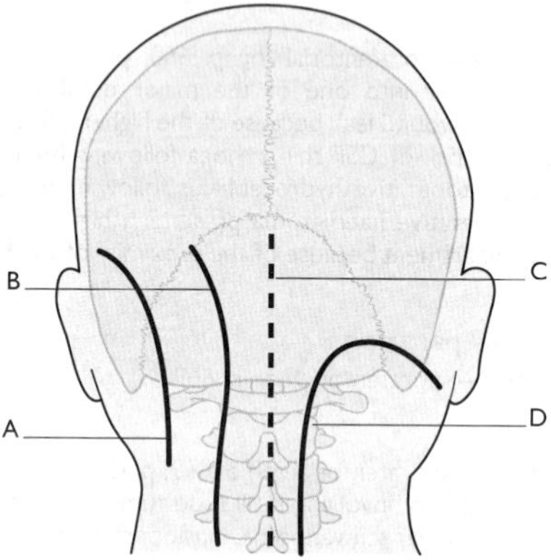
B
C
A
D

Fig. 13.11 Common infratentorial craniotomy incisions: (a) retrosigmoid craniotomy incision; (b) lateral suboccipital (paramedian craniotomy incision); (c) midline suboccipital craniotomy incision; (d), hockey-stick craniotomy incision.

- When the occiput and the first two laminae are adequately exposed, burrholes are drilled. These are connected to produce a free craniotomy flap. This is carefully separated from the underlying dura to avoid venous sinus injury.
- Kerrison rongeurs may be used to enlarge the bony opening and expose the venous sinuses where required.
- A high-speed drill may also be used for removing bone. (This is the preferred tool for approaching the dura in complex skull base approaches requiring temporal bone resection or skeletalization of the major venous sinuses.)
- Meticulous haemostasis is completed using bipolar diathermy, bone wax, and cellulose mesh before opening the dura.
- The dura is usually opened in a 'Y-shaped fashion. A midline venous sinus is commonly present, which requires control with ligating clips and diathermy prior to division.
- The dural flaps are elevated with hitch sutures to expose the posterior fossa contents.
- CSF is drained to relax the cerebellum. This is facilitated by incising the arachnoid of the cisterna magna at the inferior limit of the fossa, which promotes copious CSF drainage.
- The intradural phase of the operation is completed (see ➲ 'Key principles of surgical treatment of brain lesions', p. 672).
- Watertight dural closure is preferred; the thin native posterior fossa dura is usually inadequate for this. An autologous dural substitute, such as pericranium or fascia lata, may be used. Numerous proprietary dural substitutes, including bovine collagen matrix, bovine pericardium, and ePTFE, are also available. The closure may be reinforced with tissue glue.

- The bone flap is replaced in a craniotomy. In a decompression of the foramen magnum or when swelling of the cerebellum is anticipated, e.g. following infarction, a craniectomy is preferred.
- Multilayered muscle and fascial closure is with 1/0 and 2/0 absorbable polyfilament. Subcutaneous closure is with multilayered 2/0 absorbable polyfilament. Staples or sutures to skin.

Postoperative care

As for 'Craniotomy—supratentorial' (p. 669), plus carry out an urgent CT brain in the event of a decrease in conscious level because of the risk of postoperative hydrocephalus following posterior fossa surgery.

Complications

As for 'Craniotomy—supratentorial' (p. 673), plus:

- Intraoperative—venous air embolism. This rare complication occurs when air enters an opening in a dural venous sinus. It is suspected when a fall in end-tidal CO_2 is noted by the anaesthetist and a high-volume embolism may precipitate cardiac arrest. The treatment is to pack the posterior fossa immediately with a large, wet swab and place the patient head-down to raise the intracranial venous pressure, whilst initiating appropriate resuscitation.
- Postoperative—CSF fistula. CSF wound leaks are common, especially in children where the soft tissue layers available for closure are thinner than in adults. Meticulous dural and wound closure is the key to prevention. Replacement of the bone flap may reduce the incidence of leaks. CSF rhinorrhea may result from CSF entering the mastoid air cells at the lateral limit of the craniotomy opening. Thorough waxing of all exposed mastoid air cells and watertight dural closure help prevent this.

Tips and tricks

- Close the mastoid air cells, dura, and wound meticulously to minimize the risk of CSF leak. Wax the air cells and employ multilayered muscle and fascial closure is key.
- Optimize analgesia requirements in the postoperative period as pain is a common complication of the muscle-splitting approach to the posterior fossa.
- Be alert for signs of postoperative hydrocephalus (new headache, drowsiness, visual impairment, loss of upgaze paresis) and investigate with a CT scan where suspected.

Decompressive craniectomy

Key points

- A surgical means of controlling raised ICP when non-surgical management fails.
- A free calvarial bone flap is removed in a technique similar to a craniotomy (see ➲ 'Craniotomy—supratentorial', p. 668) but with non-replacement of the bone.
- The procedure reduces the magnitude of the rise in ICP that occurs in cerebral swelling. The perfusion pressure of the injured brain is thus improved, which may reduce neurological morbidity and prevent coning.

Indications

- Diffuse brain injury with raised intracranial pressure.
- Focal brain injury with lobar swelling, especially fronto-temporal swelling.
- May be indicated as a prophylactic measure in traumatic injury.
- Malignant cerebral infarction of a single arterial vessel territory following an occlusive stroke, e.g. middle cerebral artery infarction.
- Certain infections, e.g. subdural empyema; meningitis; acute encephalitis; toxoplasmosis, where associated with refractory brain swelling

Consent

This is often an emergency procedure in a sedated patient. Consent may be recorded on the appropriate form for patients lacking capacity, after discussion with relatives.

Equipment

As for 'Craniotomy—supratentorial' (p. 669).

Position

- Bifrontal craniectomy: supine in neutral.
- Fronto-temporo-pterional craniectomy: supine with neck rotated to bring the operation site uppermost. Avoid over-rotation which may impede cerebral venous drainage.
- 'Reverse Trendelenburg' (head up) position to promote venous drainage.
- See Fig. 13.10 for bicoronal and pterional (trauma flap) craniotomy incisions.

Procedure

The following describes a bicoronal decompressive craniectomy:

- Following a minimal shave of the incision line, a bicoronal incision is made from one zygomatic arch to the other, commencing 1cm in front of the tragus on each side.
- The scalp flap is raised by sharp dissection in the subgaleal plane.
- The pericranium around the margins of the free flap is incised with monopolar diathermy and peeled from the bone with an inferiorly based pedicle.

- A generously sized bone opening is essential to prevent cortical injury from cerebral herniation through an inadequate defect. The ideal diameter of the flap should be at least 12cm.
- Burrholes are placed at the margins of the flap, and connected with the craniotome. Two of the burrholes are sited either side of the superior sagittal sinus posteriorly; the sinus may then be carefully separated from the inner table without injury, prior to dividing the bone.
- A midline bridge of bone may be left in situ over the superior sagittal sinus, in which case two separate craniectomies are fashioned. The dura is opened widely, with two large dural flaps based on the superior sagittal sinus.
- Superior sagittal sinus should be cut low on the anterior fossa floor to adequately release pressure.
- Measures to prevent excessive brain swelling on dural opening include positioning the patient head-up, administering intravenous mannitol, and optimizing ventilation to control PCO_2.
- In cases of uncontrolled brain herniation, a limited lobectomy may be necessary to facilitate closure.
- Haemostasis is secured.
- The dural flaps are re-approximated but not closed. The dural defects are reinforced with absorbable cellulose mesh.
- The scalp is closed in layers in a watertight fashion.
- A subgaleal drain may be left in. A subdural ICP monitor may be left in situ for postoperative monitoring.
- If an autologous cranioplasty is planned, the bone may either be removed, sterilized, and stored or may be placed in a subcutaneous abdominal pocket for subsequent retrieval.

Postoperative care

- Patients are usually electively ventilated following the procedure on the neuro-intensive care unit.
- Intracranial pressure monitoring is used to direct medical therapy.
- The wound dressing is non-constrictive and is marked 'no bone flap'; direct pressure on the site is avoided.

Complications

Intraoperative

- Bleeding.
- Herniation of the brain with secondary cortical injury. This can occur through an inadequate defect and can result in local ischaemia and necrosis of brain tissue.

Postoperative

- Infection.
- Subdural hygromas—the cause of this is not clear but different postulations have been made, e.g. altered CSF circulation dynamics after the decompression, injury to the arachnoid-dura interphase, and increased cerebral perfusion pressure.

- Contralateral haematomas (subdural or extradural)—these occur due to the shift of brain parenchyma from the change in pressure.
- Wound dehiscence.
- Post-traumatic hydrocephalus.
- Seizures.
- 'Syndrome of the trephined'—cognitive, neurological, or psychological deficits. This can develop as a late feature and may be improved by subsequent cranioplasty.

Tips and tricks

- Do not delay the craniectomy in urgent cases. Complete resuscitation and arrange immediate transfer to theatre for surgery.
- Ensure an adequate craniectomy. An inadequate opening can cause local brain injury from herniation.

Elevation of depressed skull fracture

Elevation of depressed skull fracture

Key points

- The aim of the procedure is to clean and debride the injured area of scalp and skull to minimize the risk of infection, to achieve watertight dural closure, and to reconstruct the calvarium to achieve the best cosmetic result.
- A full trauma assessment according to ATLS guidelines is required to include CT cranial imaging with brain and bone windows prior to surgery.
- The scalp is highly vascular and scalp haemorrhage may be life-threatening if not controlled early. Therefore, significant scalp bleeding requires suturing of the wound in the emergency department prior to transfer to theatre.

Indications

- Any compound depressed fracture where a breach of cranial dura is suspected, e.g. in-driven fragments, visible CSF leak, haemorrhage, seizure, neurological deficit, penetrating foreign body, pneumocephalus evident on CT.
- Any non-compound depressed fracture with significant cosmetic deformity. More than 5mm of skull depression in a cosmetically prominent area may warrant elevation.
- In addition—gross wound contamination or any compound skull fracture requires exploration and debridement, even if elevation of the depressed skull fragment is not indicated.

Consent

Written consent is obtained, including risks of infection, haemorrhage, seizure, postoperative CSF leak.

Procedure

- Tetanus and antimicrobial prophylaxis are given prior to surgery.
- The patient is positioned with the injury uppermost and the head elevated. Avoid over-rotation of the cervical spine, to optimize venous drainage from the head (Fig. 13.12).
- Non-alcoholic antiseptic preparation is used when a dural breach is suspected.
- Anticonvulsants are either given prophylactically or may be reserved for patients with seizures, depending on local practice.
- The existing scalp laceration, if present, is extended to expose the fracture. For non-compound injuries a scalp flap is turned.
- Debridement of the compound wound is done with excision of non-viable or detached scalp. As much healthy scalp as possible is preserved.
- Bone fragments are removed and cleaned.
- Bone fragments are frequently impacted and require elevation. Access is gained by placement of an adjacent burrhole or burrholes.
- In some cases, a partial lobectomy might be required for brain swelling.

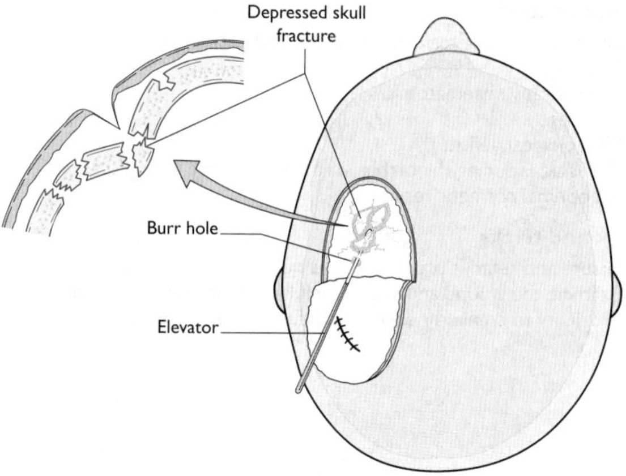
Depressed skull fracture
Burr hole
Elevator

Fig. 13.12 Elevation of depressed skull fracture (burrhole to aid elevation).

- Any herniated non-viable brain is resected.
- Lacerated dura is repaired primarily or patched with pericranium or dural substitute.
- The bone fragments are re-assembled using titanium miniplates.
- There are two special cases:
  - *Involvement of a dural venous sinus*. Copious bleeding is likely on elevating the depressed bone fragments. The patient is placed head-up and immediate control of haemorrhage is achieved with haemostatic sponge and surface pressure. Large defects in the venous sinus may require formal repair with monofilament suture or a tissue graft. The lumen of the superior sagittal sinus must be preserved in its middle and posterior thirds.
  - *Involvement of a cranial air sinus*. The affected sinus is stripped of mucosa and sealed before replacement of the calvarial bone. This may be done with a layer of pericranium or fascia lata, reinforced with hydrogel tissue glue. The advice of the maxillofacial team is sought for significant sinus or maxillofacial involvement.
- In cases of major scalp loss a rotation flap or free flap may be required for closure.
- Wound closure is in layers as for craniotomy. Monofilament skin sutures are removed at 5 days.

Postoperative care

- As for 'Craniotomy—supratentorial' on p. 672.
- Be alert for signs of wound or intradural infection.

Complications

- Infection including scalp infection, osteomyelitis or meningitis.
- Bleeding.
- Postoperative haematoma.
- Seizures.
- Neurological deficit.
- CSF leak, including rhinorrhea via a breach of the frontal sinus
- Suboptimal cosmetic result.

Tips and tricks

- Ensure anti-tetanus prophylaxis has been given.
- Examine the wound and scans carefully—for foreign body and for proximity to cranial air sinuses and dural venous sinuses.

Anterior cervical discectomy

Key points

- The removal of a cervical disc is most safely done from an anterior approach to avoid retraction of the cervical spinal cord.
- A posterolateral disc protrusion may also be safely accessed via a posterior foraminotomy with nerve root retraction.

Indications

- Relief of neural compression in:
  - *Cervical myelopathy* from compression of the cervical spinal cord.
  - *Cervical radiculopathy* from compression of a cervical nerve root.
- Disc removal as part of more complex surgery with internal fixation, e.g. cervical corpectomy, treatment of cervical fracture, or for cervical instability from facet joint disease.
- The procedure is most commonly elective but may be required as an emergency when the history is rapidly progressive.

Consent

Explain the procedure to the patient explaining the following risks:

- Oesophageal or vascular injury on approach.
- Risk of neurological complication such as weakness or numbness of the index nerve root.
- Small risk of cord dysfunction, including risk of paralysis below the operated level (rare).
- Bleeding, infection, hoarseness of voice due to recurrent laryngeal nerve injury.
- Displacement or infection of any implant used requiring revisional surgery.

Equipment

- High-speed drill and cutting 'rose' burr.
- Interbody pin retractor system, e.g. 'Caspar'.
- Soft tissue cervical retractor system, e.g. 'Black Belt'.
- Pituitary and upcut-type ronguers.
- Bone curettes.
- Operating microscope.
- Disc space implant—see p. 688.

Procedure

- Position with the neck slightly extended and the nape of the neck supported.
- An incision is made parallel to an anterior cervical skin crease to the right of the midline as follows:
  - C3/4: level with the hyoid bone.
  - C4/5: level with the thyroid cartilage.
  - C5/6: level with the cricoid cartilage.
- The correct skin level is confirmed with a radio-opaque marker and a lateral X-ray using the image intensifier.

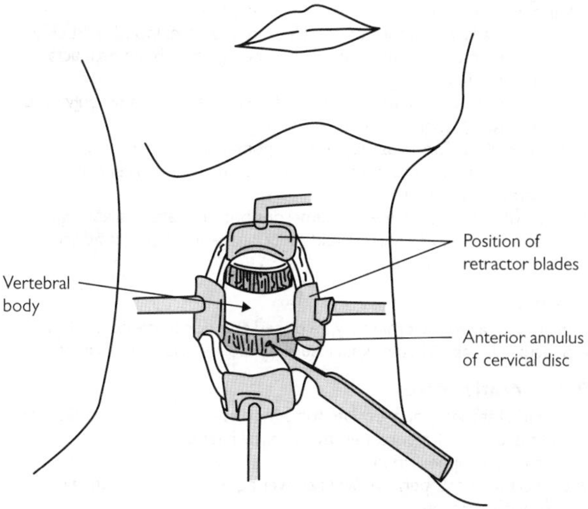
Position of retractor blades
Vertebral body
Anterior annulus of cervical disc

Fig. 13.13 Anterior cervical discectomy.

- Skin incision is made and a self-retaining retractor is placed. Platysma is exposed and incised perpendicular to its fibres. Sternocleidomastoid is retracted laterally (Fig. 13.13).
- The cervical strap muscles are mobilized parallel to their fibres. The carotid sheath is identified by inspection and palpation of the carotid pulse. The approach to the spine is between the carotid sheath laterally and the trache-oesophageal bundle medially.
- The anterior cervical spine is exposed. A needle with a double 90° bend is placed in the annulus of the most prominent disc and a further lateral X-ray is taken to confirm the correct level.
- Screw pin cervical distractors are placed in the adjacent vertebral bodies and soft tissue cervical retractors are placed beneath the elevated medial edges of longus colli.
- The operating microscope is introduced.
- The disc is incised and cleared with rongeurs and curettes. The superior and inferior end-plates are curetted until cleared of all cartilage.
- Anterior and posterior osteophytes are removed with a high-speed rose burr.
- The longitudinal fibres of the posterior longitudinal ligament are incised horizontally and the underlying dura is exposed and cleared of any remaining disc material.
- The lateral recesses are explored and cleared to fully decompress the nerve roots. The root foramen should easily accommodate a probe anterior to the root on each side.

- Various options are available for the interspace:
  - *Cage*—a large number of products are available, including PEEK and metallic implants, augmented with bone graft or bone products to promote fusion.
  - *Autograft*—bone harvested from the iliac crest. Uncommonly used because of donor site complications.
  - *No implant*. Fusion usually occurs spontaneously.
  - Any implant may be augmented with *an anterior cervical plate* to increase fusion rate.
  - *Cervical disc replacement*—numerous products are available with the aim of preserving motion and reducing the incidence of adjacent segment degeneration.

Closure
- In layers—a wound drain may be placed anterior to the cervical spine.
- Subcuticular absorbable skin closure or subcuticular monofilament.

Postoperative care
- An HDU setting is appropriate for 24h to promote early identification and treatment of a postoperative cervical haematoma which can obstruct the upper airway.
- Be alert for postoperative wound swelling or stridor suggesting upper airway obstruction.
- A wound haematoma in this location can result in life-threatening upper airway compromise and requires immediate treatment.
- Secure the airway and carry out urgent wound drainage if a significant haematoma is suspected
- Wound drain removed at 24h.
- Cervical spine X-ray is obtained on day 1 to confirm satisfactory implant placement.

Complications
- Wrong level surgery.
- Dural tear.
- Oesophageal perforation.
- Hoarseness of voice from recurrent laryngeal nerve impairment.
- New neurological deficit of cord or nerve root.
- Upper airway obstruction from cervical haematoma.

Tips and tricks
- The neck should be slightly extended, and the shoulders depressed (tape may be used for traction) to facilitate intraoperative lateral radiographs.
- Important structures, e.g. oesophagus, carotid artery, internal jugular vein, lie within the operative field; keep to the avascular loose areolar tissue planes between fasical bundles during the approach.
- Ensure meticulous haemostasis before closure to minimize the risk of a prevertebral cervical haematoma. This is a dangerous event because of the risk of airway compromise and always warrants immediate treatment.

Lumbar microdiscectomy

Key points

- The commonest neurosurgical spinal procedure. Surgical treatment of sciatica caused by a herniated lumbar disc is considered after an initial period of conservative management has proved ineffective.
- The aim is to relieve lower limb pain associated with radicular symptoms, such as myotomal weakness or dermatomal sensory impairment, and to restore normal lower limb function.

Indications

- Elective: sciatica without resolution, in the presence of physical signs of a lumbar radiculopathy and a correlating posterolateral disc protrusion demonstrated on lumbar MRI. A posterolateral protrusion impinges upon the nerve root crossing the disc space. A far lateral or foraminal disc protrusion may impinge on the exiting nerve root.
- Emergency: established or incipient cauda equina syndrome—this is a neurosurgical emergency. Features include: bilateral sciatica; bladder impairment, including painless urinary retention or incontinence; bilateral altered sacral sensation. Note that finding normal ankle power and sensation does not exclude cauda equina syndrome as a central disc can spare the S1 nerve roots, and impinge only on roots S2-4.

Consent

Obtain written consent including the risks of:

- New weakness or numbness of the index nerve root—usually temporary but may be permanent.
- Major neurological injury including permanent loss of bladder, bowel, or sexual function (rare).
- CSF leak requiring bedrest or repair.
- Haemorrhage or haematoma.
- Infection, including discitis requiring prolonged antibiotic therapy.
- Risk of visceral or vascular injury (rare).
- Non-resolution of symptoms despite technically satisfactory surgery.
- Risk of recurrent disc herniation.

Equipment

- Image intensifier.
- Monopolar and bipolar diathermy.
- Cobb periosteal elevator.
- Self-retaining lumbar retractor, e.g. McCulloch.
- Pituitary and upcut-type bone rongeurs.
- High-speed drill with rose cutting burr.
- Operating microscope.

Position

Prone on a Wilson frame to promote lumbar flexion.

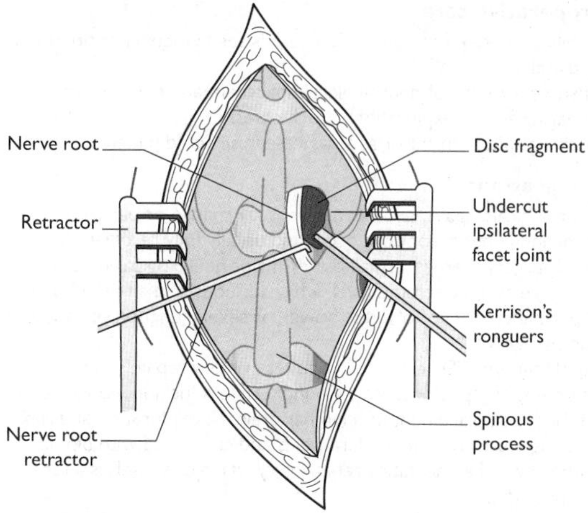
Nerve root
Retractor
Nerve root retractor
Disc fragment
Undercut ipsilateral facet joint
Kerrison's ronguers
Spinous process

Fig. 13.14 Lumbar microdiscectomy (approach to a protruded disc).

Procedure

- A radio-opaque marker is placed on the skin and a lateral radiograph is taken with the image intensifier to confirm the level of the incision.
- The short vertical incision is made through skin and subcutaneous tissue and deepened to the spinous processes.
- A unilateral muscle strip is done as follows: The monopolar diathermy is used to detach the midline fascial attachment and the Cobb elevator is used to carry out a subperiosteal strip of the paraspinal muscles from the posterior elements on the side of the disc (Fig. 13.14).
- A radio-opaque marker is placed at the level of the bone and a second lateral radiograph is obtained to confirm the correct level.
- The self-retaining unilateral lumbar retractor is placed and the operating microscope is introduced.
- The inferior edge of the superior lamina is debulked with a high-speed cutting burr to create a window (laminotomy) to access the ligamentum flavum. Bony haemostasis is with bone wax.
- The ligamentum flavum is carefully incised and removed taking care to avoid injury to the underlying dura. The epidural plane is defined using a Watson–Cheyne dissector.
- The epidural space is explored to identify the nerve root laterally and the disc protrusion beneath. The nerve root is the most lateral dural structure within the canal. It is located in contact with the pedicle.
- The annulus of the disc is incised and the prolapsed disc is removed with rongeurs. Sometimes a single large sequestrated fragment of disc is encountered and removed en bloc.
- Any dural CSF leak is repaired.
- Closure is in layers with polyfilament absorbable suture; clips or sutures to skin.

Postoperative care

- Mobilize early except when a CSF leak is seen when a period of bed rest is advisable.
- Observe for signs of neurological impairment and consider early reimaging and re-exploration in such cases.
- Discharge after 1 night or as a day case in selected patients.

Complications

- Neurological impairment—minor sensory change or partial weakness of the index nerve root can occur and usually fully resolves. As with all spinal surgery there is a small risk of major neurological impairment of any nerve at the operated level, which includes a small risk (1% or less) of permanent loss of bladder, bowel, or sexual function or of lower limb paralysis.
- Dural tear and CSF leak—this requires primary repair. Options for treatment of a postoperative wound CSF leak include wound resuture and bed rest; placement of a lumbar drain; re-exploration and repair.
- Bleeding—usually from epidural veins and controlled with bipolar diathermy or haemostatic agents. Injury to major vessels is a rare complication.
- Infection—consider discitis in cases of severe postoperative axial pain in the presence of raised inflammatory markers or systemic signs of infection. MRI imaging may assist diagnosis. A prolonged course of IV antibiotics is required until resolution.

Tips and tricks

- Carry out two lateral radiographs prior to removing disc material—one radiograph is for placement of the skin incision and a second radiograph is done at the level of the bone after opening. Obtain further X-rays if in any doubt about the level at any stage—wrong level surgery is a cause of avoidable morbidity and litigation in lumbar disc surgery.
- Ensure an adequate bony decompression and a mobile nerve root before removing disc material to minimize nerve root trauma. This especially applies in large central disc protrusions.
- Take care to preserve the pars interarticularis of the superior facet to minimize the risk of future instability.

Laminectomy

Key points

- A procedure for obtaining access to the spinal canal to relieve neurological compression or to access epidural or intradural pathology.
- The procedure is tailored to the level of the spinal canal involved—the local anatomy varies according to spinal level, but the principles that follow are common to all spinal levels.
- The aim is to remove part or all of the lamina at one or more levels. The midline spinous processes are removed in a full laminectomy but may be spared in a unilateral 'hemilaminectomy' approach. Partial medial debulking ('undercutting') of the facet joints may also be done to decompress the lateral recess of the spinal canal, especially in the lumbar region. Preservation of the majority of the facet joints including the pars interarticularis helps prevent instability following surgery.
- The procedure may be augmented with placement of spinal instrumentation or bone graft when a stabilization procedure is required.

Indications

- Cervical or thoracic myelopathy secondary to disc protrusion or congenital or degenerative spinal canal stenosis.
- Intradural or intraspinal extradural spinal tumours.
- Decompression of the cervico-thoracic cord or evacuation of a haematoma following trauma.
- Evacuation of spontaneous epidural haematoma.
- Evacuation of infective collections—especially bacterial or mycobacterial.
- Open surgical treatment of spinal vascular abnormalities, e.g. excision of dural arteriovenous fistula; removal of intramedullary cavernous angioma.
- Decompression of congenital or degenerative lumbar canal stenosis to treat neurogenic spinal claudication.

Consent

Obtain written consent including the following risks:

- CSF leak requiring bedrest or repair.
- Neurological deterioration, including permanent worsening of neurological function—the nature of the risk depends on the level of the laminectomy.
- Epidural haematoma requiring evacuation.
- Infection.
- Late instability or kyphosis.

Equipment

- Image intensifier.
- Mono-polar and bi-polar diathermy.
- Cobb periosteal elevator.
- Self-retaining spinal retractors.
- High-speed drill with rose cutting burr.
- Upcut-type bone ronguers.
- Operating microscope.

Position

- Prone on a Montreal mattress or Wilson frame.
- For cervical surgery the head and neck are supported in three-pin skull fixation.

Procedure

(See Fig. 13.15)

- A radio-opaque marker is placed on the skin and a lateral radiograph is taken with the image intensifier to confirm the level of the incision.
- A vertical incision tailored to the length of the decompression is made through skin and subcutaneous tissue, and deepened to the spinous processes. Self-retaining retractors are advanced to aid the approach. Haemostasis is with bipolar diathermy.
- Monopolar diathermy and a Cobb elevator in the subperiosteal plane are used to strip the paraspinal muscles on both sides of the laminae.
- The image intensifier is used for a repeat radiograph with a radio-opaque marker at the level of the bone.
- The laminae are exposed laterally as far as the medial part of the facet joint. Swabs are placed ahead of the elevator to aid haemostasis and muscle retraction. These are removed.
- The high-speed cutting burr or bone rongeurs are used to remove the spinous processes at the required levels. The leading edge of the required lamina is then undercut with Kerrison type rongeurs or with the drill.

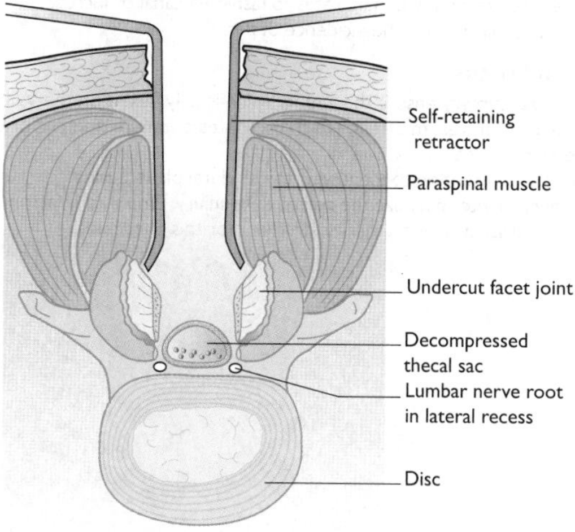
Self-retaining retractor
Paraspinal muscle
Undercut facet joint
Decompressed thecal sac
Lumbar nerve root in lateral recess
Disc

Fig. 13.15 Intraoperative axial view following decompressive lumbar laminectomy.

- The ligamentum flavum is segmental at each level and is removed to expose the dura.
- The epidural plane is regularly defined with a dissector as bone removal proceeds.
- The laminectomy is completed with piecemeal removal of bone to expose the ligamentum flavum.
- Haemostasis of epidural veins is done with bipolar diathermy.
- An epidural vacuum drain at low pressure is optional. Closure is in layers as described above.

Postoperative care

- Mobilize early with TED stockings in place and subcutaneous low molecular weight heparin from day 1.
- Observe for signs of neurological impairment and consider early reimaging and re-exploration in such cases.

Complications

Early

- Neurological impairment—see ➲ 'Lumbar microdiscectomy', p. 692.
- Dural tear and CSF leak—see ➲ 'Lumbar microdiscectomy', p. 692.

Late

- Postoperative spondylolisthesis—may occur if the facet joints are compromised. Medial facetectomy avoids this complication and in the lumbar region the pars interarticularis is spared whenever possible.
- Postoperative kyphosis—seen especially in the cervical spine in young patients as a late complication. Cervical laminoplasty, where the laminar bone is reattached with miniplates to fashion a canal of increased diameter, may reduce the incidence of this.

Tips and tricks

- In lumbar surgery ensure the lumbar spine is fully flexed on the Wilson frame or Montreal mattress, which promotes optimum opening of the interspinous space.
- Pay careful attention to identifying the epidural plane during laminectomy to minimize the risk of dural injury. Employ a Watson-Cheyne dissector or a similar instrument for this purpose.

Carpal tunnel decompression

Key points

- Carpal tunnel syndrome is the most common cause of median neuropathy.
- The distribution of altered sensation in a median neuropathy will be over the thumb, index, and radial half of the long finger, and involving the palm of the hand but not the dorsal surface.

Anatomy

(See Fig. 13.16)

- The carpal tunnel is a fibro-osseous tunnel deep to the palmaris longus tendon (if present), and is bordered on three sides by the carpal bones, and on the palmar surface by the transverse carpal ligament.
- The carpal tunnel contains the median nerve, the flex-or pollicis longus (FPL) tendon, four flexor digitorum profundus (FDP) tendons, and four flexor digitorum superficialis (FDS) tendons.
- The transverse carpal ligament (also known as the flexor retinaculum) is attached to the pisiform and the hamate on the medial side, and to the tubercle of the scaphoid and the crest of the trapezium on the lateral side.

Clinical features

Risk factors

- Manual workers, especially those using vibration tools.
- Endocrinopathies, e.g. diabetes mellitus/thyroid deficiency.
- Previous wrist injury.
- Soft tissue masses occupying the carpal tunnel.
- Acromegaly.

Physical signs

- Episodic pain and 'pins and needles' sensations in the radial two-and-a-half digits of the hand—classically wakes the patient at night and is relieved by mobilizing the affected hand.
- Positive Tinel's sign—paraesthesia in the median nerve distribution is elicited after tapping on the wrist.
- Positive Phalen's sign—wrist flexion for about a minute elicits paraesthesia in the median nerve distribution.
- Late signs that usually do not reverse after treatment are wasting of the thenar eminence and the dorsal interossei.

Consent

Obtain written consent including the risks of: wound infection; weakness of the thenar eminence; non-resolution of symptoms due to atypical nerve anatomy; reflex sympathetic dystrophy of the upper limb (rare).

Equipment

- Bipolar diathermy.
- Nerve stimulator.

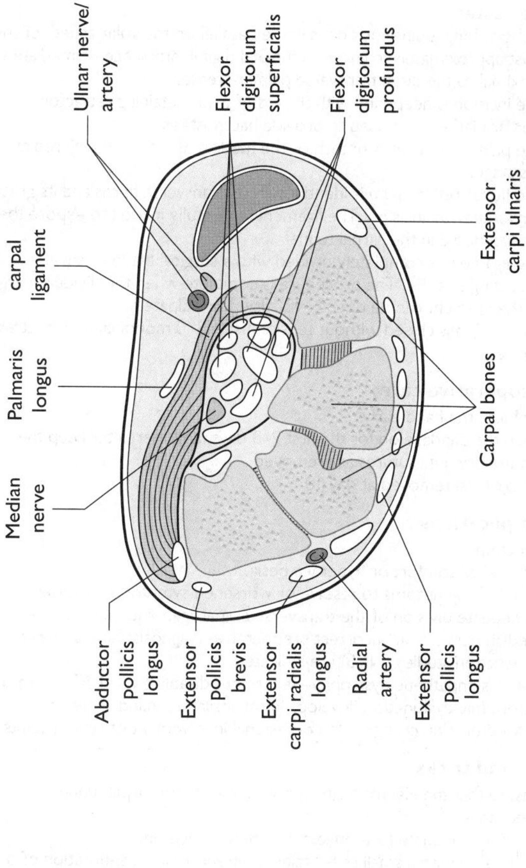
Transverse carpal ligament
Palmaris longus
Median nerve
Ulnar nerve/ artery
Flexor digitorum superficialis
Flexor digitorum profundus
Extensor carpi ulnaris
Carpal bones
Abductor pollicis longus
Extensor pollicis brevis
Extensor carpi radialis longus
Radial artery
Extensor pollicis longus

Fig. 13.16 Schematic cross-section through the carpal tunnel at the wrist.

Preoperative preparation

Antiplatelet agents and anticoagulants are discontinued prior to surgery.

Position

Patient is in supine position and the hand is held outstretched.

Procedure

- Day case with local anaesthetic. Regional or general anaesthesia are alternatives.
- A short, longitudinal incision is made parallel on the volar aspect of the wrist approximately in line with the 3rd digital interspace, immediately proximal to the distal transverse palmar crease.
- The incision is deepened with the aid of a self-retaining retractor. Bipolar diathermy is used to provide haemostasis.
- The palmar cutaneous branch of the median nerve can be injured at this stage.
- The flexor retinaculum is identified by its transverse fibres and its gritty consistency on incision. The ligament is carefully incised to expose the median nerve in the carpal tunnel.
- The ligament is completely divided with a surgical blade or small dissecting scissors. The procedure is complete when the divided margins of the ligament can be directly visualized or palpated.
- The wound is closed without tension using 3/0 monofilament mattress sutures.

Postoperative care

- Mobilize the hand early.
- Keep the bandage on for the first 2–3 days, and thereafter keep the wound dry until sutures are removed.
- Sutures are removed at day 10.

Complications

- Infection.
- Wound discomfort or hyperaesthesia.
- Failure of symptoms to resolve or worsened symptoms—implies inadequate division of the transverse carpal ligament, injury to the median nerve or an incorrect preoperative diagnosis. Repeat nerve conduction studies (NCS) are indicated.
- Reflex sympathetic dystrophy—a rare but disabling condition in which autonomic dysfunction develops in the ipsilateral hand. There are autonomic skin changes with occasional involvement of several joints.

Tips and tricks

- Ensure that the electrodiagnostic studies confirm carpal tunnel syndrome.
- Confirm adequate local anaesthesia before incision.
- Retraction with a small self-retaining retractor aids identification of the transverse carpal ligament.
- Mobilize the hand early following surgery.

Ulnar nerve decompression

Key points

- The commonest site of ulnar nerve compression is in the cubital tunnel where the nerve passes behind the medial epicondyle of the elbow.
- Ulnar nerve decompression is performed when there is correlation between the clinical symptoms and signs and nerve conduction studies which indicate a conduction block at the elbow.

Anatomy

The cubital tunnel is bordered by the medial epicondyle of the humerus, the olecranon process of the ulna, and the tendinous arch joining the humeral and ulnar heads of the flexor carpi ulnaris (FCU).

Consent

Obtain written consent including the risks of: bleeding; recurrence, wound infection; atrophy of the hypothenar eminence; non-resolution of symptoms due to atypical nerve anatomy; reflex sympathetic dystrophy of the upper limb (rare).

Clinical features

- Motor weakness. Physical signs include:
  - Wasting of the hypothenar eminence.
  - Guttering (wasting of the interossei of the hand).
  - Froment's sign.
  - Wartenberg's sign.
  - An ulnar 'claw hand' with extension at the 4th and 5th MCP joints and flexion at the corresponding DIP and PIP joints.

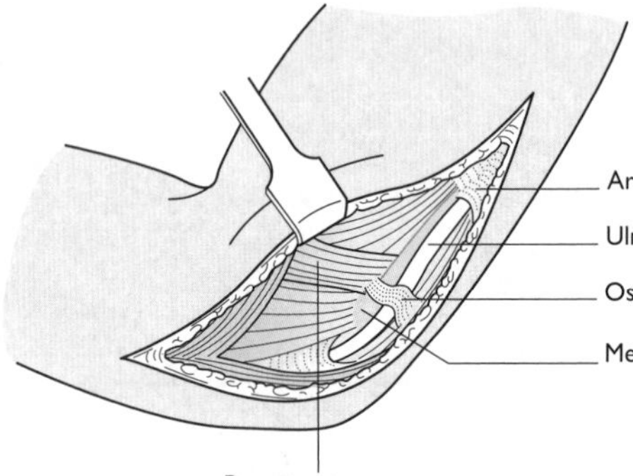
Arcade of struthers
Ulnar nerve
Osborne's fascia
Medial epicondyle
Pronator teres

Fig. 13.17 Operative exposure of the cubital tunnel.

- Diminished sensation or active sensory symptoms 'pins and needles' in the lateral two-and-a-half fingers of the hand.
- Positive Tinel's sign at the elbow—paraesthesia is elicited in the C8/T1 dermatomal distribution when percussing the ulnar nerve in the cubital tunnel in the elbow.
- Risk factors include a history of trauma to the elbow.

Equipment

- Bipolar diathermy.
- Silicone nerve sling.
- Upper limb support.
- Nerve stimulator.

Pre-operative preparation

- Day-case.
- Off anticoagulants/antiplatelet agents.
- Nerve conduction study available indicating slowing of ulnar nerve conduction across the elbow.

Procedure

(See Fig. 13.17)
The following describes a simple decompression of the cubital tunnel:

- The patient is supine.
- General anaesthesia or a regional nerve block such as a Bier's block.
- Position:
  - The upper limb is placed with the forearm supinated on an arm table or
  - The upper limb is supported above the patient's chest on a 90° arm support. The elbow is flexed to expose the posteromedial aspect.
- A curvilinear 7–8cm incision is made over the posteromedial aspect of the elbow.
- The incision is advanced through the subcutaneous tissue with the aid of a self-retaining retractor.
- The nerve is identified distal to the ulnar tunnel in the proximal forearm. The nerve stimulator can be used to confirm the location of the nerve.
- The ulnar nerve in the cubital tunnel is identified and the ligament forming the roof of the tunnel is exposed.
- The fascial roof of the cubital tunnel is opened.
- Haemostasis with bipolar diathermy.
- The skin flap can be closed with subcuticular absorbable sutures, or with mattress non-absorbable sutures. Dress with wool and crepe bandage. A high arm sling and early mobilization minimize postoperative swelling.

Alternatives

Anterior subcutaneous transposition of the ulnar nerve, endoscopic surgery, or medial epicondylectomy..

Postoperative care

- The bandage may be removed at 2 days. Thereafter keep the wound covered until the sutures are removed.
- Sutures can be removed after 10–14 days.
- Promote early mobilization.

Complications

- Infection.
- Wound discomfort or hyperaesthesia.
- Failure of symptoms to resolve or worsened symptoms—implies inadequate decompression of the nerve, injury to the ulnar nerve, or impairment of the ulnar nerve elsewhere in its course. Repeat NCS may be indicated.
- Reflex sympathetic dystrophy—a rare but disabling condition in which autonomic dysfunction develops in the ipsilateral hand. Skin joint changes could also occur.

Tips and tricks

- Ensure that the electrodiagnostic studies confirm cubital tunnel syndrome.
- Identify the medial epicondyle and olecranon before making the incision; the ulnar nerve lies between these two important landmarks.
- Confirm adequate local anaesthesia before incision.
- Mobilize the limb early following surgery.

Chapter 14

ENT

Aural microsuction

Overview

Aural microsuction is commonly performed both in the outpatient setting to treat impacted wax or otitis externa and also in the operative setting as the first step in a larger operation on the ear.

Anatomy

The ear canal is approximately 2.5cm long. It is divided into a cartilaginous external part and a bony internal part. It is slightly curved with a prominent anterior bulge associated with the temporo-mandibular joint. It is bordered medially by the tympanic membrane (Fig. 14.1).

Indications

Removing wax, debris, infection, and foreign bodies from the ear canal.

Equipment

- Binocular microscope.
- Toumarkin speculum (various sizes).
- Suction unit with Zoellner sucker and fine end inserts.
- Ear swab for microbiology if in the context of infection.
- Bart's wax hook, Jobson–Horne probe, crocodile forceps may be required.
- Antibiotic drops and ointment can be considered.
- Pope wicks may be used in infection with severe oedema of the ear canal.

Consent

Implied consent is usually satisfactory. Patients should be warned of the noise, and advised that in the context of infection, the procedure can be uncomfortable.

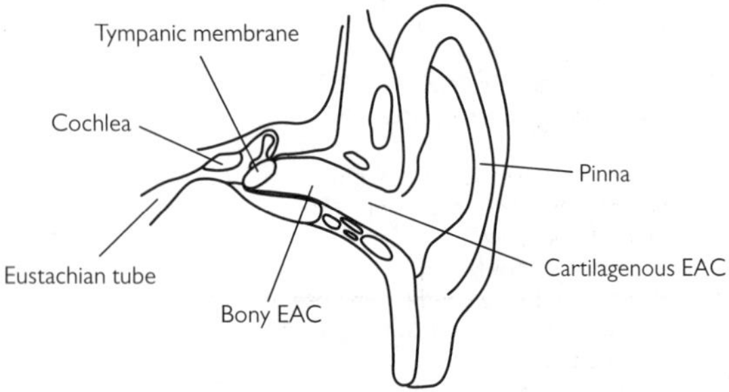
Tympanic membrane
Cochlea
Pinna
Cartilagenous EAC
Eustachian tube
Bony EAC

Fig. 14.1 Coronal view of ear canal and middle ear.

Preoperative preparation

Equipment is prepared and brought close to hand. It may be beneficial to have an assistant to clear blocked suction and pass pieces of equipment.

Position and theatre set-up

Position the patient supine on the examination couch in a comfortable position with their head turned slightly away from you.

Procedure

- Visually inspect the pinna and the ear canal skin looking for signs of eczema and infection.
- Holding the pinna posteriorly and superiorly, gently introduce an appropriately sized Tumarkin speculum.
- Assess the canal for the presence of wax or infected debris. If infected debris or discharge is present, swab this for microbiology culture.
- Debris and wax can then be gently suctioned out, being careful not to traumatize the ear canal wall or tympanic membrane.
- Otitis externa should be treated with topical antibiotic drops (some contain anti-fungals and also steroids) but in cases with significant inflammation it is best to instil an antibiotic, steroid, or combination ointment into the ear canal.
- A Jobson–Horne probe or Bart's wax hook may be required if the wax is relatively firm.
- Foreign bodies can be removed with the crocodile forceps, wax hook, or suction. The wax hook is best for round objects such as beads (a common ear foreign body in children).
- If the ear canal skin is swollen and consequently limiting access to the ear canal, a Pope wick may be required. Insert this slowly with a pair of crocodile forceps until it lies within the narrowed area. This can then be soaked in an antibiotic solution to open up the wick and treat any underlying infection.

Postoperative care

- Patients may often feel dizzy during and immediately after microsuction due to a temperature-related caloric effect. Patients should be sat up slowly and be advised to wait until feeling steady before standing up.
- Patients with otitis externa will need a course of topical antibiotic drops and follow-up to chase the swab results and perform further microsuction as required.

Complications

Care should be taken to avoid traumatizing the ear canal skin or the tympanic membrane. If there is a perforation care should be taken around microsuctioning close to the perforation.

Tips and tricks

When clearing debris from close to the drum switch to a fine-end suction tip to have better control of the tip and to reduce the sound of the suction. In severe infection or inflammation, steroid ointment can be instilled. This ointment fills the canal and the patient returns a few days later to have the ointment removed.

Dix Hallpike testing and the Epley manoeuvre

Overview

Both this diagnostic test and therapeutic manoeuvre are based on manipulating otoliths within the semicircular canals to bring on the symptoms of benign paroxysmal positional vertigo (BPPV) and then to relocate the otoliths to prevent them causing symptoms again.

Indications

The Dix Hallpike test should be carried out in all patients undergoing assessment for vertigo. If the Dix Hallpike is positive, then a therapeutic Epley manoeuvre can be performed.

Consent

It is important to explain to the patient that the process may bring on their symptoms and they might feel extremely dizzy. Patients should always be asked how they got to hospital as they may feel too dizzy to drive home themselves.

Preparation

A couch is placed in the centre of the room with enough space for the tester to examine the patient during the steps of the manoeuvre.

Position

The patient sits on the couch initially.

Procedure

- Ask the patient to sit on the examination couch upright with their legs flat on the couch.
- The patient is then asked to rotate their head 45° in the sagittal plane to the tested side.
- Ask the patient to find an object on which to fix their gaze and then quickly lower the patient down so that their head is hanging supported just beyond horizontal over the edge of the couch.
- Observe their eye movements for 60s looking for rotatory nystagmus with latency and fatiguability.
- If no nystagmus is observed, the test is considered to be negative and the patient is returned to the sitting position. The test may now be performed with the patient facing the other direction to test the contralateral ear.
- If rotatory nystagmus is observed, or the vertiginous feeling is elicited, a therapeutic Epley manoeuvre may be conducted.
- The patient then rotates their head 45° from the sagittal plane to the alternate side (a rotation of 90°). The patient is again brought into a position where their head hangs over the edge of the table.

- This position is held for 60s.
- The patient then rolls on to their shoulder, with the head at 45° to the body, such that the patient is almost looking at the ground.
- This position is held for 60s.
- From this position the patient is slowly brought up to a sitting position.

The patient may feel unstable for some minutes after the procedure and should be given time to recover. Patients are advised to avoid bending down/leaning rapidly for 1 or 2 days after the procedure.

Tips and tricks

- Frenzel glasses may be worn, which make it easier to view any nystagmus that may be elicited.
- Care should be taken in patients with limited mobility of the cervical spine.
- The Dix Hallpike test can also elicit nystagmus in rare cases of anterior canal BPPV (downbeat) and lateral canal BPPV (horizontal).

Myringoplasty

Overview

Myringoplasty operations are performed to close perforations of the tympanic membrane. The aetiology of a tympanic membrane perforation should be considered, as, if it is indicative of poor Eustachian tube function, then failure of the reconstruction is more likely and a more robust method of closure can be considered.

Anatomy

The tympanic membrane has three layers: an inner mucosal layer, middle fibrous layer, and external epithelial layer. The ossicles are deep to the tympanic membrane in the postero-superior quadrant. The chorda tympani is intimately related to the tympanic membrane in the postero-superior quadrant. The anterior part of the tympanic membrane is more medial than the posterior part. The border of the tympanic membrane is robust, and referred to as the fibrous annulus. It lies within a groove of bone referred to as the bony annulus.

Indications

Tympanic membrane perforations can be closed if they predispose the patient to recurrent infections. Such infections often manifest as foul otorrhoea. Perforations may also be closed to attempt to improve hearing, but this is a weaker indication, as hearing may not improve subsequent to surgery (Fig. 14.2).

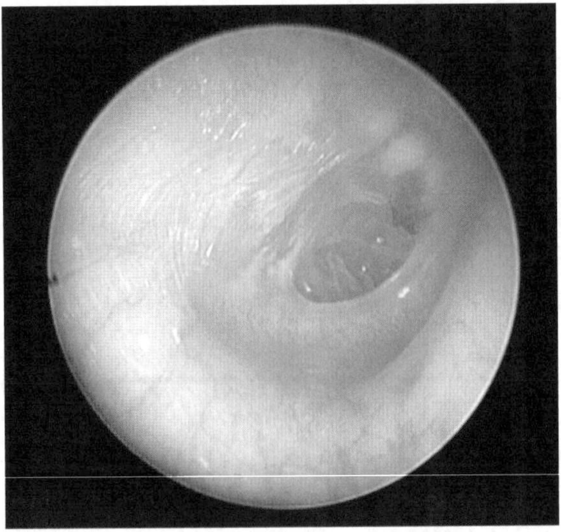

Fig. 14.2 Tympanic membrane perforation.

Equipment

- Drapes.
- Operating microscope.
- 10 blade and 15 blade scalpels.
- Forceps, scissors, needle holder, bipolar diathermy.
- 1st incision knife/'spud' knife.
- Freer's elevator.
- Biel's and Hughes' elevator.
- Rosen's drum elevator.
- Plester 'D' knife may be used.
- Middle ear scissors.
- Middle ear needles.
- Sickle knife.
- BIPP (bismuth iodoform paraffin paste) packing.
- Cotton wool balls (small), with topical adrenaline.
- Zoellner suction with a range of fine ends.
- Block for the preparation of grafts.
- Other middle-ear instruments may be useful.
- Exogenous grafting materials may be used.

Consent

The indication and success of the operation should be discussed. Success rates in closure of perforations are variable, and depend on the size and location of the perforation, and also the age of the patient. A figure of 80–90% may be reasonable. A proportion of patients who have a residual perforation may also have a smaller perforation that becomes asymptomatic. Hearing may improve and declines only infrequently.

Infection and bleeding are infrequently problematic. A scar may result from the operation, depending on the approach taken and the source of an endogenous graft. Injury to the chorda tympani may occur, but may be subclinical, although patients can complain of a metallic taste some months postoperatively. The procedure is usually performed under general anaesthesia.

Loss of hearing through ossicular or inner ear damage, or damage to the facial nerve, is exceptionally rare, and is not always discussed.

Preoperative preparation

The audiogram is checked, and the patient examined. There is controversy as to whether intercurrent infection is a contraindication to surgery. Success rates are likely to be unchanged, but the operation may be more technically challenging.

The approach to the surgery, nature of reconstruction, and choice of graft should be considered. The operation may be conducted via a permeatal, endaural, or post-auricular approach. Endogenous grafts may include tragal or conchal cartilage, temporalis fascia, perichondrium, or a variety of exogenous materials. Reconstruction methods include underlay, overlay, and inlay techniques. Broadly, the graft can be placed under the tympanic membrane, usually anchored by a proportion of the graft lying under the fibrous annulus, the graft can be placed on top of the perforation, although this has a higher failure rate, or the graft can be fashioned to sit within the perforation.

For the purposes of this chapter, a permeatal tragal cartilage underlay with perichondrium will be discussed.

Position and theatre set-up

The patient is supine with the head turned away to present the ear canal to the surgeon. The ear is prepared with cleaning solution such as betadine. The head and ear are then draped to provide a sterile field.

Procedure

- The perforation is examined, and the edges freshened using a needle.
- The tragus is infiltrated with local anaesthetic with adrenaline.
- An incision is made over the tragus, and a graft of cartilage and perichondrium is harvested.
- The graft can then be checked and prepared.
- The ear canal is injected with local anaesthetic with adrenaline.
- A sagittal incision is made around the postero-inferior 6–11 o'clock of the ear canal, around 6–8mm from the tympanic membrane.
- Adrenaline covered cotton wool is used to control bleeding.
- The Biel's is then used to gently elevate the skin from the bone of the ear canal.
- The skin flap that is raised is very fragile, and should not be directly suctioned, but blood can be cleared through using a fine-end tip on a Zoellner sucker, and administering suction behind an elevator or cotton wool ball.
- The skin flap is elevated to the point of the fibrous annulus.
- The fibrous annulus is identified, and elevated. Middle ear mucosa is seen deep to this.
- The middle ear mucosa is perforated with a needle and the middle ear space is entered. The elevated flap is now referred to as a tympanomeatal flap.
- The Rosen's drum elevator may then elevate the fibrous annulus from the bony annulus.
- In the postero-superior part of the tympanic membrane, the chorda tympani may be encountered, and should be freed from the tympanomeatal flap, and preserved.
- Once the tympanomeatal flap has been raised sufficiently, it is replaced, and the location of the perforation is confirmed.
- The cartilage graft is placed in position deep to the perforation.
- Gelfoam may be placed in the middle ear to support the graft and hold it in position.
- The perichondrium is placed over or under the perforation to cover any areas of the perforation not in direct contact with the cartilage graft.
- The integrity of the reconstruction is checked by replacing the tympanomeatal flap.

Closure

Pieces of BIPP ribbon gauze packing are placed in the ear canal to hold the reconstruction in place. The tragal incision is closed with a Prolene® or Monocryl® stitch.

Postoperative care

The procedure is usually undertaken as a day-case. Dizziness is not uncommon. The BIPP packing is removed after 2 weeks. The hearing is checked after 2 months.

Complications

Failure of the graft may require revision surgery. It is likely that cartilage is more robust than fascial or exogenous grafting materials.

Tips and tricks

Small perforations may be managed using a cartilage inlay graft. In this case, the cartilage is cut slightly larger than the size and shape of the perforation. A groove is then cut in the side of the graft, and the graft is placed in the perforation, with the margins of the perforation sitting within the groove. This is known as a 'butterfly' graft.

Exploratory tympanotomy

Overview

The steps of exploratory tympanotomy are similar to those of myringoplasty and form a central part of otologic practice. Exploratory tympanotomy usually leads on to other operations, discussed on p. 730, such as ossiculoplasty and stapedectomy.

Anatomy

In addition to the anatomy of the ear canal and tympanic membrane, the anatomy of the ossicles and the medial wall of the tympanic cavity should be considered (Fig. 14.3).

Indications

This procedure is most commonly performed to assess and subsequently treat conductive hearing loss of an unknown aetiology. The procedure may also be undertaken to remove lesions of the tympanic cavity, or implanted foreign bodies.

Equipment

- As for 'Myringoplasty' (p. 711).
- Currettes.
- Additional middle ear instruments may be beneficial.

Consent

The indication of the operation, and likelihood of achieving success, should be discussed. Infection and bleeding are rarely problematic. The chorda tympani is potentially vulnerable. Depending on any intervention in the tympanic cavity, the facial nerve, ossicles, and vestibulocochlear system are potentially at risk. Rarely, a tympanic membrane perforation may result.

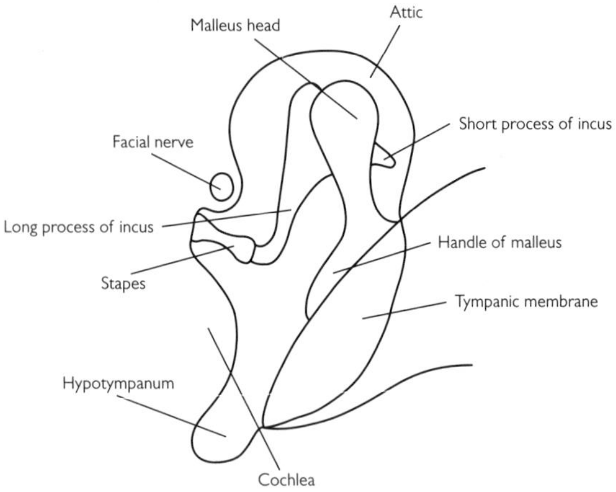
Attic
Malleus head
Short process of incus
Facial nerve
Long process of incus
Handle of malleus
Stapes
Tympanic membrane
Hypotympanum
Cochlea

Fig. 14.3 Middle ear ossicles.

Preoperative preparation

- The audiogram should be checked. A clear plan should be formulated based on the predicted findings. Preoperative imaging is important in the assessment of middle ear tumours.
- A permeatal approach is used most frequently for this operation.

Position and theatre set-up

- The patient is supine with the head turned away to present the ear canal to the surgeon.
- The ear is prepared with cleaning solution such as betadine.
- The head and ear are then draped to provide a sterile field.

Procedure

- The canal is injected (LA) and a tympanomeatal flap is raised (see ➲ 'Myringoplasty', p. 712).
- The flap is raised superiorly, to allow visualization of the postero-superior part of the tympanic cavity.
- The mobility of the ossicles, and their continuity, is checked. This is performed using the needle to move the handle of the malleus and stapes. It should be remembered that the handle of malleus may move in otosclerosis due to some laxity in the malleoincudal and incostapedial joints.
- In order to improve visualization of the ossicles, currettes may be used to remove the margins of the lateral ear canal. Great care should be taken to avoid trauma to the ossicles or the chorda tympani.
- Lesions arising from the promontory, such as small glomus tumours, may be removed, but the risk of bleeding should be considered, and appropriate measures prepared should such a step be undertaken.

Closure

After the operation is completed, the tympanomeatal flap is replaced, and the ear is packed with pieces of BIPP ribbon gauze.

Postoperative care

The BIPP is removed at 2 weeks, and the hearing is checked at 2 months.

Complications

The likelihood of complications depends on the extent of intervention within the middle ear.

Tips and tricks

The nature of the pathology will determine the location and size of a tympanomeatal flap. Large first incisions or spiral incisions may allow greater access to the tympanic cavity.

When assessing for movement of the stapes, it may be possible to detect movement in the region of the round window, indicating transfer of pressure through the stapes and cochlea.

Tympanoplasty

Overview

Tympanoplasty and myringoplasty operations are often considered synonymously. Indeed, by Wullstein's original classification, a myringoplasty could be termed a 'type 1 tympanoplasty'. The distinction can be thought of in terms of intervention within the middle ear. A tympanoplasty indicates that the surgeon intends to address pathology within the middle ear, in addition to any perforation that may or may not be present within the tympanic membrane.

Anatomy

- The anatomy of the external ear canal, tympanic membrane, medial wall of the tympanic cavity, and also the hypotympanum and epitympanum should be considered.
- When planning on harvesting conchal cartilage, the anatomy of the pinna is important.

Indications

The indications for tympanoplasty are broad. The procedure may be undertaken for discharging perforations or hearing loss, in a similar fashion to myringoplasty. The distinction is that tympanoplasty is done in those patients where middle ear mucosal or squamous disease is suspected. The procedure may also be performed to clear adhesions or sclerotic areas that are impeding the ossicles and leading to hearing loss (although recurrence is common). Retraction pockets that are thought to be symptomatic, problematic, or potentially prone to leading to cholesteatoma, may also be addressed using this method.

Equipment

- As per 'Exploratory tympanotomy' (p. 714).
- Periosteal elevators.
- Self-retaining clamps.

Consent

The risks of the procedure depend on the degree and nature of intervention in the middle ear cavity. The chorda tympani is at risk. The facial nerve may be injured rarely. If the stapes is manipulated, then there is rarely a small risk of 'dead ear', leading to permanent profound deafness, and medium-term vertigo. In this context, whether the ossicular chain is intact or not is an important consideration when manipulating the incus or malleus.

The procedure is often, but not always, performed using a post-auricular approach, and this will leave a post-auricular scar. Bleeding and infection should be mentioned, and when they occur, they are usually related to this incision.

Implantation cholesteatoma may occur as a result of surgery to remove atelectatic retraction pockets. This may be mentioned, however, the role of surgery in these cases may be to prevent cholesteatoma, and this should also be considered.

Preoperative preparation

The audiogram should be checked. Preoperative imaging is sometimes employed, and should be reviewed if it has been performed. A plan should be made to determine interventions for adhesions or ossicular erosion. A plan for reconstruction can be considered preoperatively or at the time of surgery, depending on the findings.

Position and theatre set-up

The patient is supine with the head turned away to present the ear canal to the surgeon. The ear is prepared with cleaning solution such as betadine. The head and ear are then draped to provide a sterile field.

Procedure

- The post-auricular area is infiltrated with local anaesthetic with adrenaline.
- The microscope is used to assess the ear canal and tympanic membrane.
- The edges of any perforations are freshened.
- The location and depths of a retraction pocket, if present, is determined.
- A post-auricular incision is made.
- The subcutaneous fat and post-auricular muscles are noted and divided.
- A plane is raised overlying the temporalis muscle and fascia overlying the mastoid perichondrium. The root of the zygoma is identified.
- Cymba concha cartilage may be harvested by placing a finger in the concha, and dissecting through the elevated pinna to the cartilagenous layer. Care is taken not to cut through the skin of the lateral aspect of the pinna.
- A piece of fascia overlying temporalis may be harvested by making an incision into temporalis, using a Freer's elevator to develop a plane between temporalis and its overlying fascia, and then removing a piece of the fascia.
- An incision is made posterior to the root of the zygoma, parallel to the inferior border of temporalis. A parallel incision below the ear canal is made, staying within the limits of the palpable mastoid. A perpendicular incision is made posteriorly to join these incisions.
- A periosteal elevator then elevates this periosteal and fascial flap, referred to as a Pulva flap (anteriorly based in this case).
- This flap is raised until the ear canal is reached, and then the flap is raised in continuity with the ear canal.
- This flap is secured in place using a self-retaining clamp.
- A 're-entrant' incision is made using a 15 blade, or middle ear scissors. The tympanic membrane may now be visualized.
- A tympanomeatal flap is raised (see ➲ 'Myringoplasty', p. 712).
- Care should be taken to determine the location of perforations and retractions whilst the flap is raised.
- The middle ear cavity is exposed (see ➲ 'Exploratory tympanotomy', p. 715).
- The ossicles are assessed (see ➲ 'Exploratory tympanotomy', p. 715).

- Retraction pockets are extracted from the ossicles and medial wall of the tympanic cavity. This may be done using a Hughes' elevator with a slightly curved needle, or a Biel's. If a retraction pocket enters the attic, then the pocket may be controlled by removing the 'scutum'—the superomedial lip of the ear canal.
- The chorda tympani should be identified, and where possible, preserved.
- Adhesions may be cleared from the middle ear to allow visualization of the ossicles, mobilization of retraction pockets, and access to any perforations.
- Retraction pockets, once elevated, may be excised or reinforced using cartilage grafts. Perforations can be closed (see ➲ 'Myringoplasty', p. 712).
- If there has been ossicular erosion, then the reinforced tympanic membrane may not be positioned on the handle of the malleus. Rather, the tympanic membrane may lie on the incus, stapes, footplate, or oval window.

Closure

After the operation is completed, the tympanomeatal flap is replaced, and the ear is packed with pieces of BIPP ribbon gauze. The post-auricular wound is closed in layers, with absorbable polyfilament such as Vicryl® used to close periosteum, fascia, and the post-auricular muscles. Monofilament is used to close the skin.

Postoperative care

The BIPP is removed at 2 weeks, and the hearing is checked at 2 months.

Complications

Implantation cholesteatoma may occur as a result of surgery to remove atelectatic retraction pockets. If this is thought likely, or if the hearing outcome is poor, further surgery may be planned at an interval. This may be in the form of exploratory tympanotomy (discussed on p. 714), or ossiculoplasty (discussed on p. 730).

Tips and tricks

- Temporalis fascia is harvested early so it may be laid out and left to dry. Dry fascia is more rigid, and thus more amenable to use as a grafting material to ensure perforations are closed.
- Pieces of cartilage may be laid upon one another, in what is known as a 'palisade'. This may be used to position pieces of cartilage, and may be more effective at closure of difficult perforations.

Excision of external canal osteoma/exostosis

Overview

External ear canal osteomas and exostoses can be differentiated by the morphology, number, and position. Exostoses are multiple, at characteristic positions in the ear canal, and broad based. Osteomas, by contrast, are almost invariably solitary, and often arise from a narrow base.

Anatomy

The external auditory canal runs within the temporal bone. It includes areas of the tympanic, squamous, and petrous temporal bone. The ear canal is comprised laterally of its cartilaginous part, and medially of the bony part. The bony part is overlaid by very thin skin. The medial border of the ear canal is the tympanic membrane.

Indications

It is recommended that osteomas are removed. Histological diagnosis is important. They have a tendency to grow, which may be problematic. Exostoses may be removed if they are leading to recurrent otitis externa, or impeding clearance of wax and keratin from the ear canal.

Equipment

- Operating microscope.
- Aural speculum.
- Currettes.
- First incision 'spud' knife.
- Biel's elevator.
- Small cotton wool balls soaked in adrenaline.
- A high-speed operating drill may be required.

Consent

The risk of recurrence should be mentioned. The ear may have to be kept dry whilst it heals, which may take some weeks. Bleeding is rarely problematic. Rarely, a post-auricular or endaural approach may be needed, with consequent scarring and bleeding and infection risk.

Preoperative preparation

Preoperative imaging is not necessary, but should be reviewed if it has been performed.

Position and theatre set-up

- The patient is supine with the head turned away to present the ear canal to the surgeon.
- The ear is prepared with cleaning solution such as betadine.
- The head and ear are then draped to provide a sterile field.
- The procedure is often performed under GA, but may be safely performed under LA with a compliant patient.

Procedure

- The ear should be examined and any debris cleared with microsuction.
- Osteomas with a very narrow base may be excised using a curette at their base.
- Exostoses require a flap of ear canal skin to be raised.
- A sagittal incision in the ear canal is made, and skin is raised over the bony exostoses. Care is taken to preserve the skin.
- The high-speed drill, often with a 2mm burr, is used to remove the exostoses, and recreate the diameter of the external ear canal.
- The skin flap is then replaced.
- Specimens are sent for histology. This is not necessary for exostoses.

Closure

After the operation is completed, the tympanomeatal flap is replaced, and the ear is packed with pieces of BIPP ribbon gauze.

Postoperative care

The BIPP may be removed after 2–4 weeks. Histological results should be checked when they are available. The demineralization process may, however, take some weeks.

Complications

Complications are uncommon, but damage to the skin flap can potentially delay healing, and potentially lead to soft tissue stenosis of the ear canal.

Tips and tricks

Pieces of card can be used to hold the skin flap away from the bony ear canal and protect them from the burr. The use of a diamond burr may also reduce the trauma to the flap. The location of the initial incisions should be planned carefully to allow full access to exostoses.

Cortical mastoidectomy

Overview

Cortical mastoidectomy refers to the removal of the external/cortical part of the mastoid bone. In practice, it is taken as the removal of sufficient mastoid bone to allow opening of the mastoid antrum.

Anatomy

The petromastoid is one of the four parts of the temporal bone. It is bordered posteriorly by the sigmoid sinus and posterior fossa dura, and superiorly by middle fossa dura. The anatomy of the facial nerve, and its relation to the short process of the incus and the lateral semicircular canal, is crucial to perform the procedure safely (Fig. 14.4).

Indications

Cortical mastoidectomy is classically described as the treatment for acute mastoiditis. In this setting, removal of infected bone may alleviate infection, and prevent complications, including intracranial sepsis. However, there is an increasing understanding that intravenous antibiotics are sufficient to treat the majority of cases of uncomplicated acute mastoiditis.

Cortical mastoidectomy is otherwise performed as part of a formal mastoid exploration, commonly for cholesteatoma, or as part of an operation to access medial structures of the temporal bone. A common setting in which it is used is in cochlear implantation, as it allows a posterior tympanotomy to be performed, and thus the cochlea and round window to be accessed. It may also allow access to the bony labyrinth or facial nerve.

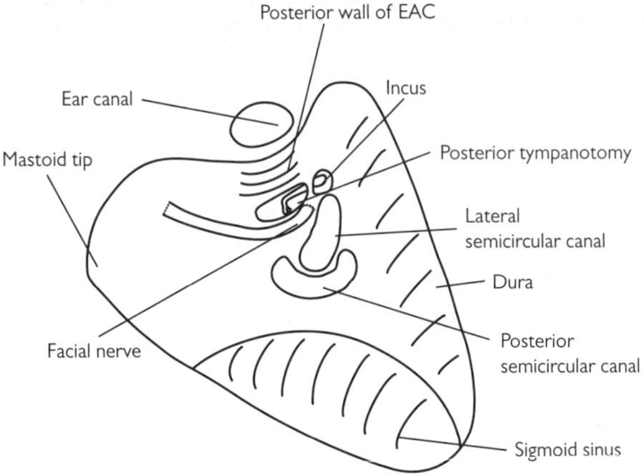
Posterior wall of EAC
Ear canal
Incus
Mastoid tip
Posterior tympanotomy
Lateral
semicircular canal
Dura
Facial nerve
Posterior
semicircular canal
Sigmoid sinus

Fig. 14.4 Cortical mastoidectomy (operative schematic view of left ear) performed with structures exposed.

Equipment

- Scalpel with 10 blade and 15 blade.
- Scissors, bipolar forceps, forceps, self-retaining clamps.
- Periosteal elevators.
- High-speed drill with irrigation.
- Drill bits depending on size/age of patient.
- Zoellner suction.
- Middle ear instruments may be helpful.

Consent

The indication of the procedure is discussed. There is a risk of damaging the structures that surround and run through the mastoid. These risks may be higher in the context of acute mastoiditis and therefore in this setting, it is common for a limited cortical mastoidectomy to be performed.

The structures that may be injured include facial nerve, chorda tympani, lateral semicircular canal, sigmoid sinus, posterior wall of the ear canal, and dura. It should be noted that all of these complications are exceptionally rare when a cortical mastoidectomy is performed.

Infection and bleeding may occur. There will be a post-auricular scar. The procedure is almost invariably conducted with GA, although may be conducted under LA if the patient is very compliant.

Preoperative preparation

Preoperative imaging may be necessary and should be reviewed if it has been performed. If it is possible, an audiogram should be performed.

Position and theatre set-up

- The patient is supine with the head turned away to present the ear canal to the surgeon.
- The ear is prepared with cleaning solution such as betadine.
- The head and ear are then draped to provide a sterile field

Procedure

- The post-auricular region is infiltrated with LA with adrenaline.
- A post-auricular incision is made and a plane elevated overlying temporalis fascia and fascia overlying periosteum.
- An anteriorly based Pulva flap is raised and the periosteal elevator is used to expose the bony cortex of the mastoid.
- The ear canal should be identified.
- Initial bone cuts with the high-speed drill are made in most patients with a 5mm cutting burr.
- Irrigation is essential, and suction is required to remove the irrigation fluid and bone dust.
- Bone cuts follow the temporal line, posterior wall of the ear canal, and a tangential line between the two.
- Drilling should occur in parallel with the underlying structures to facilitate early identification and avoidance.
- In clinical practice it is not necessary to expose the dura or sigmoid sinus unless that is required to gain adequate access to the antrum.

- After the superficial air cells have been removed, Korner's septum, the petrosquamosal lamina may be encountered. This is a plate of bone that may occur as an embryological remnant, and may give the incorrect impression that the antrum has been reached. If present (which it is not always), it should be removed.
- The mastoid is removed until the antrum is opened, and the lateral semicircular canal can be seen. The short process of the incus lies anterosuperior to the lateral semicircular canal.

Closure

The post-auricular wound is closed in layers with absorbable polyfilament such as Vicryl® used to close periosteum, fascia, and the post-auricular muscles. Monofilament is used to close the skin.

Postoperative care

In acute mastoiditis, the patient will need to continue antibiotic treatment for at least one week subsequent to the surgery.

Complications

The concerning complications in cortical mastoidectomy are damage to the sigmoid sinus, external ear canal, or dura. Should they occur, this damage needs to be repaired. Dural injury can lead to CSF leak and consequent meningitis. Cartilage and fascia may be used in combination with fibrin glue to repair these injuries. Perforation into the ear canal should also be repaired with cartilage to prevent ear canal epithelium retracting into the mastoid. Sigmoid sinus injuries may be challenging to manage, and require formal control of the sigmoid. Limited injuries can be managed with bone wax.

Tips and tricks

Larger burr sizes may be less prone to cause injury, as they tend to remove a shallower area of bone, allowing for earlier visualization of colour and pitch changes that may indicate an underlying structure. The sigmoid sinus is characteristically blue. Proximity to the dura may be indicated by a raise in drill pitch, an increase in bleeding, and a slightly pink colouration of the bone.

Mastoid exploration

Overview

There is a significant amount of variation in the terms used to describe surgery in the tympanic cavity and mastoid cavity to remove cholesteatoma. These include 'combined approach tympanoplasty', 'modified radical mastoidectomy', and 'mastoid exploration'. Many of the principles and measures are similar to those described under 'Tympanoplasty' (p. 716) and 'Cortical mastoidectomy' (p. 722).

Anatomy

It is important to be familiar with the anatomy of the tympanic and mastoid cavities when undertaking surgery for cholesteatoma. These are discussed in previous sections. The most important structure to consider in this operation is the course of the facial nerve in the temporal bone, which may be encountered at many stages throughout this operation. The facial nerve passes from the cerebellopontine angle through the internal acoustic meatus. It enters its intralabyrinthine portion and passes anterior to the cochlear, where it has its geniculate ganglion. Here it makes its first genu (turn), and heads posteriorly, immediately superiorly to the stapes footplate, until it lies inferior to the lateral semicircular canal. At this stage, it turns again, the second genu, and heads inferiorly, through the mastoid to the stylomastoid foramen (Fig. 14.5).

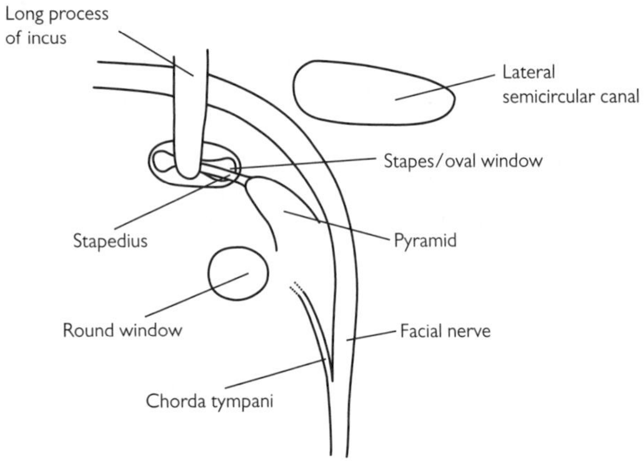
Long process of incus
Lateral semicircular canal
Stapes/oval window
Stapedius
Pyramid
Round window
Facial nerve
Chorda tympani

Fig. 14.5 Schematic of the path of the facial nerve around the second genu.

Indications

Mastoid exploration is most commonly performed for the removal of cholesteatoma.

Equipment

- As per 'Tympanoplasty' (p. 716).
- As per 'Cortical mastoidectomy' (p. 723).
- A facial nerve monitor is commonly used.

Consent

The nature of the proposed surgery should be discussed. This often includes the intention to preserve, remove, or reconstruct the posterior canal wall. This has implications for long-term ear care and hearing outcomes. Removal of the posterior canal wall may, however, reduce the incidence of residual and recurrent cholesteatoma.

The chorda tympani is frequently relatively inactive due to persistent infection of the tissues through which it runs. Risks of injury to the facial nerve, CSF leak, damage to the semicircular canals or cochlea, and 'dead ear' are all very uncommon risks. Bleeding and infection may occur. Hearing may be improved, deteriorate, or be broadly similar to the preoperative level.

Preoperative preparation

Imaging is commonly, but not always, performed prior to mastoid exploration. This is almost invariably in the form of high resolution CT scanning of the temporal bone. Diffusion weighted MRI may have some role to play in the assessment of cholesteatoma.

Position and theatre set-up

The patient is supine, with the head elevated, and turned away from the surgeon.

Procedure

The steps of surgery depend on the extent of the disease, and the decision on whether to preserve or remove the posterior canal wall. A combined approach tympanoplasty may involve many of the same steps as a cortical mastoidectomy and a tympanoplasty. Cholesteatoma is identified in both of these approaches, and is removed, with the tympanic membrane being reconstructed.

Closure

As per 'Tympanoplasty' (p. 718).

Postoperative care

As per 'Tympanoplasty' (p. 718). When the canal wall is preserved, or the middle ear is hidden through the use of opaque reconstruction materials such as cartilage, it is not uncommon to recommend '2nd look' surgery to detect and remove any residual disease. This is often undertaken ~1 year subsequent to the original surgery.

Patients who have undergone canal wall down surgery may need intensive care in the postoperative period, with frequent clinic appointments and dressing changes.

Complications

Facial nerve injury may require grafting in extreme cases, or when it occurs postoperatively, may mean packing has to be removed from the ear and possibly re-exploration of the cavity.

CSF leaks should be repaired at the time with fascia used as an underlay graft in the middle cranial fossa. Fibrin glues can be useful in increasing the success of such repairs.

Tips and tricks

There are many approaches to cholesteatoma surgery, and familiarity with all approaches may allow the surgeon to offer his patient the most appropriate approach for their pathology. The approach described is the post-auricular approach; however, an alternative is the endaural approach, where an incision is made between the tragus and root of the helix. This allows wide access into the bony ear canal. The bone of the posterior ear canal can then be removed to expose and remove cholesteatoma, leaving a cavity that is dependent on the extent of disease.

Stapedectomy and ossiculoplasty

Overview

Operations directed at the correction or replacement of the ossicles are designed to improve hearing.

Anatomy

The handle of the malleus is adherent to the tympanic membrane. Movement of the tympanic membrane causes movement of the body of the malleus and articulation with the body of the incus. This in turn, causes movement of the long process of the incus and movement of the stapes' footplate on the oval window. This process amplifies sounds as they pass through the middle ear.

Indications

- Stapedectomy is undertaken in patients with hearing loss caused by otosclerosis. Specifically, it is undertaken in those patients who have had insufficient benefit from hearing aids, or who have other reasons for declining hearing aids in favour of surgical management.
- Ossiculoplasty is undertaken to improve hearing in patients who have ossicular injury, commonly due to the sequelae of chronic otitis media.

Equipment

- As per 'Tympanoplasty' (p. 716).
- A 'skeeter' drill may be necessary.
- Lasers may be used in stapedectomy.
- Ossicular replacement prostheses may be needed.
- Stapes' piston prostheses may be needed.

Consent

The indication is the restoration of hearing. Stapedectomy can usually restore hearing to near normal levels for that individual. It should be noted that this will not address any concomitant age- or noise-related hearing loss. Ossiculoplasty is likely to improve hearing but usually not to the extent of stapedectomy.

Stapedectomy carries a risk of dead ear associated predominantly with perforating the bony footplate of the stapes. This risk is often quoted as 1%, although in practice it is likely to be significantly less than this. The chorda tympani may be damaged, but injury to the facial nerve is exceptionally uncommon. The operation is usually undertaken by a permeatal approach.

Ossiculoplasty is often conducted as part of another operation for chronic otitis media, such as tympanoplasty or mastoidectomy and the consent will be discussed in combination with these other operations.

Preoperative preparation

Preoperative audiometry is mandatory. Stapedial reflexes may be undertaken. High-resolution CT of the temporal bone may give valuable information about the integrity of the ossicular chain and sites of discontinuity. It may also help to confirm a clinical diagnosis of otosclerosis.

Position and theatre set-up

Supine with the head elevated and turned away from the surgeon.

Procedure

- As per 'Exploratory tympanotomy' (p. 715).
- Fixation of the stapes is confirmed by palpation.
- The incudo-stapedial joint is dislocated.
- Stapedius tendon is divided using the KTP laser or microscissors.
- The laser may be used to weaken the posterior crus of the stapes.
- This is then fractured.
- The anterior crus is fractured—the laser may be used to facilitate this.
- The laser is used to weaken the footplate.
- A perforator is used to make a small, round hole in the stapes' footplate.
- A stapes' prosthesis is inserted into the stapedotomy, and the hook is secured to the long process of the incus.
- Movement of the ossicular chain is confirmed.
- The tympanic membrane is replaced and the ear canal packed.

Closure

The ear canal may be packed with BIPP ribbon gauze.

Postoperative care

The packing is removed after 2 weeks, and an audiogram is conducted at 2 months.

Complications

Perilymph leaks are rare, but may require re-exploration and the use of fascial grafts to cover the oval window. Failure of the procedure may necessitate revision surgery.

Tips and tricks

There are many different prostheses that may be used in stapes' surgery. Familiarity with the prosthesis is essential.

Cochlear implantation

Overview

Cochlear implantation is a highly effective procedure at providing the sensation of hearing to those patients with profound sensorineural hearing loss. The procedure involves inserting an electrode into the scala vestibuli, and securing the unit of the cochlear implant on the surface of the temporal bone. This involves a cortical mastoidectomy, posterior tympanotomy, and either entry into the middle ear through the round window, or otherwise a cochleostomy.

Pinnaplasty

Overview
Prominent ears usually become evident during the first few months of life, and are noticed by parents. They may be splinted at this stage, but should they persist, then they may cause embarrassment for the child around the age of six.

Anatomy
The anatomy of the concha should be considered (Fig. 14.6).

The cause of prominent ears is usually an absence of the antihelix.

Indications
Cosmetic correction of prominent ears causing embarrassment or distress.

Equipment
- Needle and ink.
- 15 blade scalpel.
- Toothed forceps, needle holders, iris scissors.
- Freer's elevator.
- Sutures.

Consent
The indication should be confirmed and the wishes of the child and parents should be discussed. The procedure involves a scar behind the ear. There are risks of infection and bleeding, including pinna haematoma. There is a risk of over-correction.

Preoperative preparation
The ear should be manipulated to the desired position. The degree of excision of skin and scoring of cartilage should be assessed and discussed.

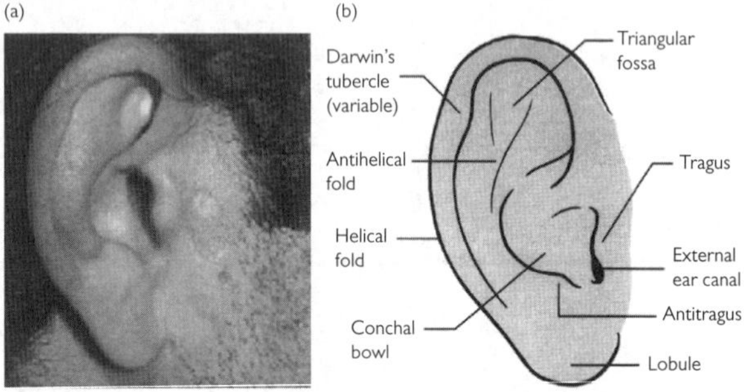
(a)
(b)
Darwin's tubercle (variable)
Triangular fossa
Antihelical fold
Tragus
Helical fold
External ear canal
Antitragus
Conchal bowl
Lobule

Fig. 14.6 Diagram of the pinna. Reproduced from Corbridge, Rogan, and Steventon, Nicholas, Oxford Handbook of ENT and Head and Neck Surgery 2e, 2010, with permission from Oxford University Press.

Position and theatre set-up

- The patient is supine with the head turned away.
- A head up position may diminish venous bleeding.
- The site of the anti-helix is marked with ink and then tattooed through the ear with a needle. The posterior skin excision is marked also.
- As the procedure is most frequently performed on children, GA is advised. In adults, LA may be used.

Procedure

- An incision is made in the sulcus of the ear, and an ellipse of skin from over the posteromedial surface of the pinna is excised. This has been premarked.
- The posteromedial skin overlying the pinna is elevated until the tattooed markings for the antihelix are identified.
- An arcuate incision within the cartilage is made about 0.5–1cm posterolateral to the marks, extending inferiorly and superiorly.
- The incision through the cartilage is completed with a Freer elevator to avoid damage to the skin overlying the anterolateral aspect of the pinna.
- The anterolateral pinna skin is elevated from the cartilage.
- The cartilage forming the central part of the pinna is now free, and is manipulated posteriorly into its desired position.
- The cartilage is scored using multiple parallel marks in the plane of the antihelix.
- The upper helical margin is partially transected at the point of the superior crus.
- The position of the ear is checked. Occasionally it may be necessary to cross score the helical fold.

Closure

An absorbable or non-absorbable monofilament may be used to close the incision site. The ear is protected with dressings, and a head bandage is placed.

Postoperative care

Non-absorbable sutures are removed at 10 days along with the head bandage. A headband may be worn for some weeks after this.

Complications

Pinna haematomas require drainage. Skin necrosis can be avoided by ensuring that the newly prominent antihelix is protected by dressings when the head bandage is placed.

Tips and tricks

More limited operations may be performed in some cases. A needle may be used to score the cartilage percutaneously—although this requires significant experience of this technique. Equally, skin excision and the placement of non-absorbable sutures may pre-empt the need for a cartilage flap, although this procedure can have its own complications.

Adult rigid nasal endoscopy

Indications

- Diagnostic: viewing nasal cavity, middle meatus for sinus drainage pathways, post-nasal space.
- Therapeutic: in functional endoscopic sinus surgery, biopsies, dacrocystorhinostomy (DCR), foreign body removal, etc.

Equipment

- Rigid Hopkins' rod endoscope (2.7mm in children, 4mm in adults)—0°, 30°.
- Light source and cable.
- Anti-fog.
- LA spray with decongestant, e.g. 5% lidocaine with phenylepherine 0.5% (Co-phenylcaine®).

Procedure

- Spray the Co-phenylcaine® spray into both nostrils and allow at least 2min for this to work.
- With the endoscope connected to the light source, dip the end in the anti-fog.
- Three-pass technique:
  - First pass: gently introduce the endoscope along the floor of nasal cavity, view of inferior turbinate, view of inferior surface of middle turbinate, view of post-nasal space, including Eustachian tube opening and adenoids.
  - Second pass: withdraw the endoscope and then pass medial to the middle turbinate inspecting the septum, the medial part of the middle turbinate, and sphenoid ostium.
  - Third pass: the endoscope is passed to look at the middle turbinate and the middle meatus. Angled scopes can be rotated to better view the lateral wall of the nasal cavity looking at the uncinate and inspecting for any discharge, polyps, or masses.

Postoperative care

After using LA sprays in the nose, the patient should be advised not to eat or drink for at least 30min as the anaesthetic may have affected the throat impairing the gag reflex.

Complications

Potential trauma to the nasal mucosa may cause bleeding.

Nasal cautery

Overview

Nasal cautery is commonly used for the management of active, or recurrent, epistaxis.

Anatomy

Little's area describes an area in the anterior septum that has a particular tendency for bleeding. This is due to the anastamosis of the nose's numerous arterial supplies in this area. The anterior nasal valve is also found at this area, meaning that airflow is significant, and this may encourage bleeding.

Indications

Recurrent epistaxis. Acute management of epistaxis that is persistent despite conservative measures.

Equipment

- Headlight.
- Thudicum's nasal speculum.
- Silver nitrate cautery.
- Co-phenylcaine® spray.
- Cotton wool.
- Gauze with saline.

Consent

Verbal consent is usually sufficient for the procedure. The risk of ongoing bleeding should be mentioned. There is a very small risk of bleaching the skin on the upper lip, and a remote possibility of septal perforation.

Preoperative preparation

Adequate consent should be taken. Co-phenylcaine® should be applied to the nose, both for anaesthetic and vasoconstrictive properties.

Position

The patient is seated in a stable chair, facing the surgeon.

Procedure

- The bleeding point is identified.
- A silver nitrate cautery stick is passed in a 'halo' around the bleeding point.
- Multiple cautery sticks may be required.
- A cautery stick is then applied to the bleeding point.

Postoperative care

If dark fluid leaks from the nose on to the skin of the upper lip, this should be immediately wiped with gauze with saline. This inactivates the silver nitrate and prevents bleaching of the skin in this area.

Complications

Nasal cautery to both sides of the septum should be avoided where possible due to the possibility of this causing septal perforation.

Tips and tricks

In active bleeding, a small piece of cotton wool with Co-phenylcaine® can be applied to the bleeding point to cause vasoconstriction, reduce bleeding, and make cautery more likely to be successful.

Reduction of simple nasal fractures

Overview

Nasal fracture reduction allows a potentially severe cosmetic injury to be repaired simply and rapidly.

Anatomy

The nasal bones lie at the upper third of the nose. They are commonly fractured. Their relationship to the midfacial skeleton should be considered (Fig. 14.7).

Le Fort fractures of the midfacial need more formal intervention, and these patients should be appropriately referred on. Equally, patients with a history of head or cervical spine injury should be assessed initially with a view to, clinically or radiologically, excluding intracranial haemorrhage.

Indications

Nasal fracture causing clear visible cosmetic deformity. The timing of the injury is important. Manipulation can be performed at the time of injury (within 30min), or secondarily within 21 days after injury. Subsequent to this, healing will make manipulation of the nasal bones extremely challenging, and manipulation is likely to fail.

Equipment

- Steristips, thermoplastic splints, plaster of Paris, or whatever the surgeon's chosen nasal dressing may be.
- It may be necessary to use Walsham's forceps to elevate a depressed nasal bone.
- It can also be useful to have nasal packing materials available.

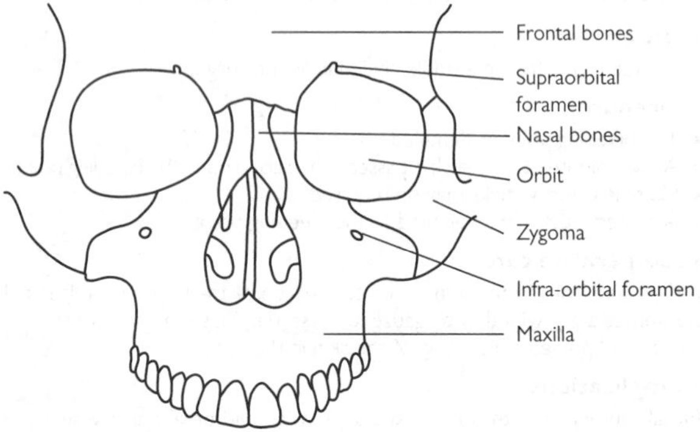
Frontal bones
Supraorbital foramen
Nasal bones
Orbit
Zygoma
Infra-orbital foramen
Maxilla

Fig. 14.7 Bony anatomy of facial skeleton.

Consent

The likelihood of successful manipulation should be discussed. Further bruising and swelling is possible. Epistaxis is uncommon, but may be problematic.

Preoperative preparation

Clinical photographs are not required but may be considered. The patient should confirm their previous nasal shape and the nature of the deviation should've discussed.

Position and theatre set-up

The procedure may be performed in the anaesthetic room, with either a brief GA or, less commonly, LA. Local anaesthetic involves lignacaine within the fracture, and infiltrated towards to supra- and infraorbital nerves.

Procedure

- The nose is examined.
- The fracture may be mobilized by pushing the nose and worsening the apparent deviation.
- The nose is then pushed into the midline firmly.

Closure

A dressing, or external splint, is placed over the nose for 1 week. The nature of dressing depends on the surgeon's choice and the mobility of the nose.

Postoperative care

The patient should abstain from contact sports for 2–3 months.

Complications

Epistaxis may be problematic and can require nasal packing. Very rarely, a surgical procedure may be indicated to treat epistaxis, and in severe facial trauma it may be that the anterior ethmoid artery needs to be ligated.

Tips and tricks

When performing a secondary manipulation, some days after the injury, the earlier the procedure can be performed, the more likely that the procedure will be successful. A period of about 5 days is considered to allow settling of swelling associated with the injury, and thus allow the deformity assessment and manipulation to be more precise. Whilst there is a limit of 21 days, it is preferable to perform manipulation at 5–10 days. Patients with tender fractures are also more likely to be successfully manipulated.

Manipulation can be performed under LA with injection around the infra and supra orbital nerves, and the fracture site.

Septoplasty

Overview

Septoplasty procedures have largely superseded submucosal resection (SMR) for the treatment of symptomatic nasal septal deflection.

Anatomy

The nasal septum is comprised of membranous, cartilaginous, and bony parts. Their relation to each other is shown here (Fig. 14.8).

Indications

- Symptomatic nasal septal deflections, often resulting in unilateral nasal obstruction. This may also be refractory to treatment with topical nasal steroid.
- Septoplasty may also be performed to facilitate access to a nasal cavity for other surgical procedures, such as sinus surgery.
- Septoplasty is rarely performed to reduce the incidence of recurrent epistaxis.

Equipment

- Dental syringe with needle.
- Local anaesthetic.
- Killian's or Cottle's nasal speculum.
- 15 blade scalpel.
- Freer's elevator.

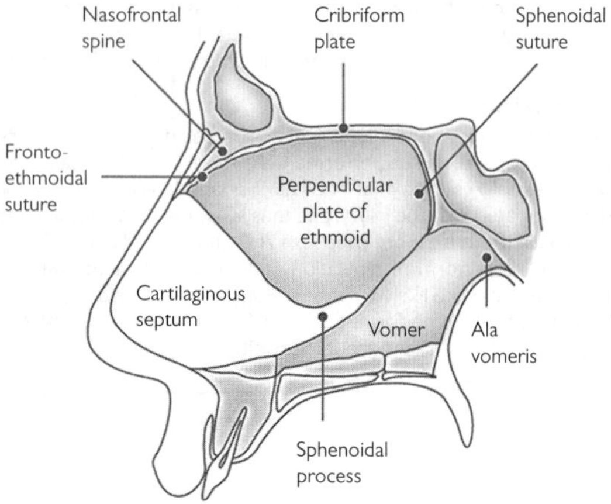
Nasofrontal spine
Cribriform plate
Sphenoidal suture
Fronto-ethmoidal suture
Perpendicular plate of ethmoid
Cartilaginous septum
Vomer
Ala vomeris
Sphenoidal process

Fig. 14.8 Sagittal schematic of nasal septum. Reproduced from Warner, G., et al., Otolaryngology and Head and Neck Surgery, 2009, with permission from Oxford University Press.

- Hockey stick elevator.
- Tilley–Henckel forceps.
- Turbinectomy scissors.
- Fishtail gauge and mallet.
- Jansen–Middleton forceps.
- Needle holder and 4-0 Vicryl Rapide™.

Consent

The success rates should be discussed. They are generally high by subjective measures, but mixed by objective measures of nasal patency and airflow. Nasal adhesions are relatively common and may limit the effectiveness of the operation. They can, however, be easily removed. Sometimes, silastic splints are left in the nose to prevent adhesions. The patient should be forewarned of this possibility, and the possibility of nasal packing. The nose is usually much more blocked for some weeks after the operation due to postoperative swelling.

Risks include bleeding, which may lead to septal haematoma, and infection, including septal abscess. These complications, in addition to poor healing that may be related to surgical factors, may lead to septal perforation. This may be asymptomatic, but can lead to whistling, crusting, a tendency to epistaxis, or when large, saddling of the nose. The external appearance of the nose may also change if the medialization of the septum moves the nasal dorsum to the midline. This change, however, is uncommon and rarely problematic.

A small proportion of patients will have postoperative anosmia, due to manipulation of the ethmoid bone causing bony injury around the olfactory niche. Equally, bony injury of the maxillary crest, performed to correct anterior deflections, may lead to paraesthesia or numbness of the anterior upper incisors.

The procedure generally requires a GA, with its consequent risks.

If a concomitant turbinate reduction or outfracture of the inferior turbinates is planned, this should be discussed.

Preoperative preparation

The patient's consent is obtained, and the nose examined.

Position and theatre set-up

- The patient is supine with the face turned slightly towards the surgeon.
- A head ring supports the head in position.
- A 25° head-up tilt minimizes intraoperative venous bleeding.

Procedure

- Infiltration of the subperichondrial layer of the nose.
- Outfracture of the inferior turbinates may be performed at this stage.
- An incision is made. This is commonly on the left, as this is technically easier for a right-handed surgeon. The incision can be made on the dorsum of the cartilaginous septum, slightly to one side (a hemitransfixion), or further posteriorly (a Killian's incision).

- The subperichondrial plane is found, and dissected posteriorly and inferiorly, over the anterior vomer and maxillary crest. This flap may be raised on one side, or both. Complicated deflections may require bilateral flaps. Otherwise, the flap is usually raised on the left, or otherwise the side of the convexity of the deflection.
- Individual spurs may be excised, making sure to preserve the integrity of the flap on each side.
- To straighten the septum it is frequently important to free the septum posteriorly and inferiorly. The bony-cartilaginous junction may be dislocated posteriorly, and the anterior vomer excised to free the cartilagenous septum. Inferiorly, the septum can be freed from the maxillary crest.
- Excess cartilage may be excised, sutures, and (rarely) scoring may be used to bend the cartilage into a midline position.
- If the septum is removed anteriorly from the maxillary crest, it should be reattached using a dissolvable suture.
- Excised cartilage may be replaced into the nose if there are large areas without cartilage present. This allows the structural integrity of the nose to be preserved.

Closure

The incision should be closed with 4-0 Vicryl Rapide™ suture, and then in continuity, the suture is used to quilt the mucosa to the straightened septum. This is performed by passing the suture back and forth between each side to hold the mucosa onto the cartilage.

Postoperative care

If silastic splints are inserted to prevent adhesions, these are removed after 1 week.

Complications

- A proportion of septoplasty will need to be revised to achieve the desired result. This is a much more challenging procedure, and should be performed by an experienced surgeon. The postoperative scarring makes elevation of the flap more difficult, and the incidence of perforation is likely to be higher.
- Symptomatic perforation is the most common significant complication of septoplasty. The incidence may be around, or slightly below, 1%. They tend to be symptomatic due to either a loss of the support of the nose, or otherwise through causing turbulent airflow at the margins of the perforation. Very small perforations may whistle, and can be managed by enlarging them so they do not whistle. Perforations may also be managed by inserting silastic buttons to close the hole. Operations to close the peroration may include mobilizing septal or turbinate mucosa to place over the perforation. If there is saddling of the nose as a consequence of the perforation, however, then an external augmentation septorhinoplasty may be necessary.

Tips and tricks

Septoplasty is a challenging operation.

The cartilage at the dorsum of the nose, and the structural integrity of the connection between the tip of the nose and the maxillary crest, are crucial. Loss of cartilage in these areas may lead to saddling, or collapse of the nasal dorsum. In particular, loss of cartilage at the keystone area at the junction of the nasal bones and dorsal cartilaginous septum may be exceptionally difficult to correct.

Elevation of the subperichondrial flap over the maxillary crest is more difficult, as the mucosa is quite adherent at the junction of the cartilage and bone. There is a limited role for sharp dissection at this point.

Endoscopic sinus surgery and polypectomy

Overview

Enodoscopic sinus surgery (ESS), often termed as functional ESS (FESS), is a term used to describe procedures to open or remove the bony paranasal sinuses. The principles and anatomy of such surgery may also be used to address structures around the nose, including the skull base and orbit.

Anatomy

It is essential to be familiar with sinonasal anatomy when undertaking ESS. Figures 14.9–14.13 present endoscopic images demonstrating key landmarks.

Indications

- The most common indication for ESS is the management of chronic rhinosinusitis, with or without nasal polyposis.
- It is also used to manage fungal sinusitis, and its extended applications include the removal of sinonasal tumours, accessing the skull base and the orbit, and treating complications of acute sinusitis, including endoscopic orbital abscess management.

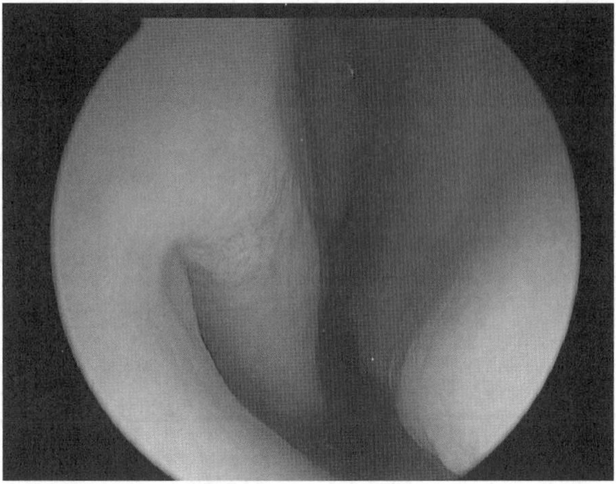

Fig. 14.9 View of right nostril. The inferior turbinate is clearly seen, and the middle turbinate is also visible postero-superiorly.

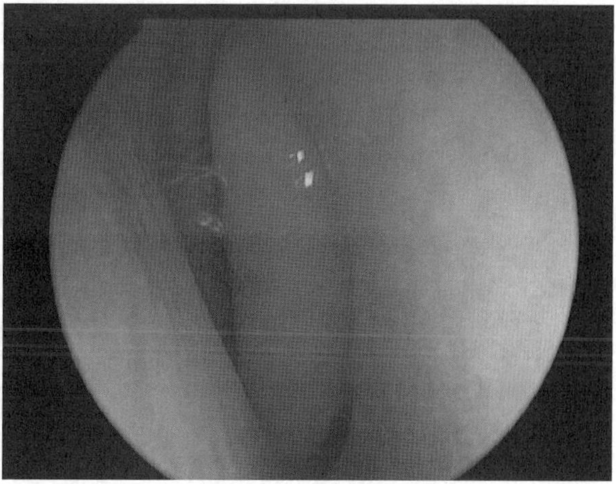

Fig. 14.10 View of right nostril. A close view of the anterior aspect of the right middle turbinate. The middle meatus is can be entered immediately lateral to the middle turbinate.

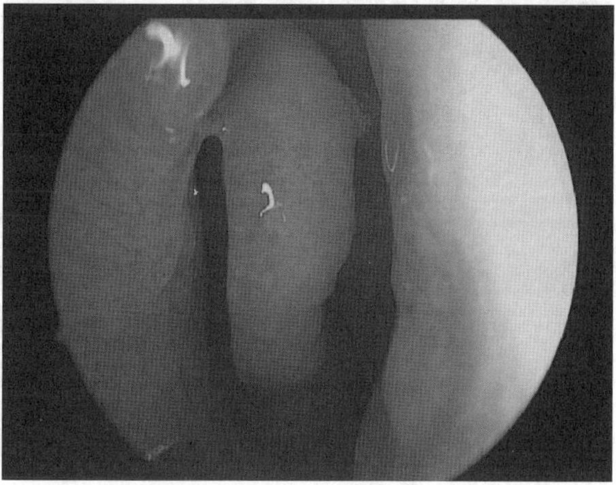

Fig. 14.11 View of left nostril. There is erythema around the middle meatus in keeping with chronic rhinosinusitis.

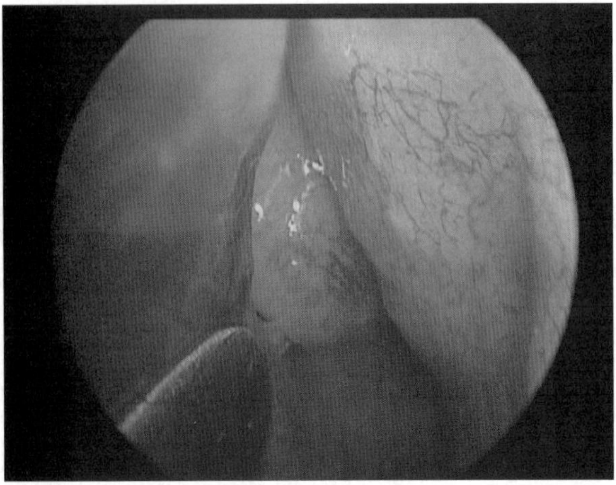

Fig. 14.12 View of left nostril. As the middle turbinate is moved medially, the uncinate on the lateral wall is seen, and the bulla ethmoidalis is seen posteriorly.

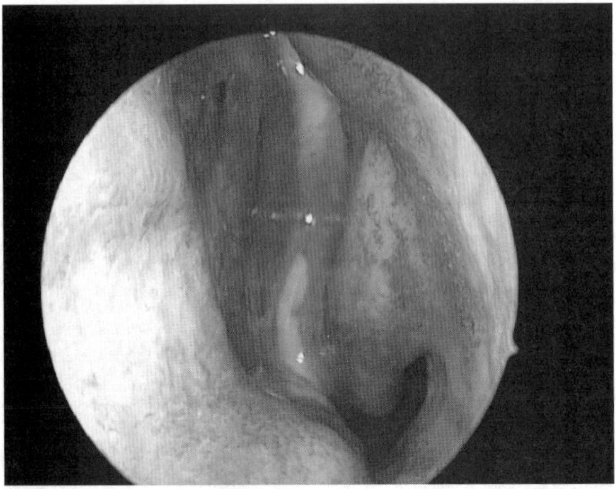

Fig. 14.13 Pus emanating from the middle meatus is a sign of acute infection and also chronic rhinosinusitis.

Equipment

- Blakesley forceps (straight and upturned).
- McKay through-cutting forceps.
- Sinus seeking probe.
- Freer elevator.
- Zoellner suction.
- Fraser suction.
- Downbiting forceps.
- Backbiting forceps.
- Tilley dressing forceps.
- Sickle knife.
- Adrenaline-soaked patties.
- Microdebrider.
- Endoscopic bipolar forceps.

Consent

Consent should include discussion of the indication for the operation. Medical alternatives for surgery should be discussed to ensure that the patient has decided to have surgery in the full knowledge of the alternatives.

Potential complications include infection and bleeding. Orbital injury and CSF leak are the most feared complications. Orbital injury, or injury of the anterior ethmoidal artery may lead to retro-orbital haematoma (discussed on p. 750), diplopia due to injury of the medial rectus, or most concerning, visual loss associated with damage to the optic nerve. CSF leak is rare, and can be repaired endoscopically at the time of surgery, but may predispose to intracranial sepsis, such as meningitis.

More common complications include nasal adhesions, epiphora, or (uncommonly) septal perforation.

Preoperative preparation

Cross-sectional imaging of the sinuses is mandatory. CT scans give the best resolution of the bony structures of the nose, and may allow important structures to be identified and, if necessary, avoided. Furthermore, the CT will identify which sinuses are affected by disease processes, and allow the surgery to be planned.

Topical nasal decongestant can be inserted prior to surgery, usually after the induction of anaesthetic. Options include Co-phenylcaine® and cocaine, including solutions such as Moffat's solution—typically 100mg of cocaine (1ml of 10%), 1mg adrenaline (1ml of 1:1,000), and normal saline and/or sodium bicarbonate.

Position and theatre set-up

- The patient is supine with the head supported by a head ring, and turned towards the patient.
- A head-up tilt minimizes intraoperative venous bleeding.

Procedure

This describes an operation to remove polyps and open maxillary and anterior ethmoid sinuses. Sinuses should only be opened if it is thought they are contributing to the disease process. Further sinuses, the posterior ethmoid, sphenoid, and frontal sinuses may also need to be opened.

- The nose is examined.
- Topical decongestant or Moffett's solution inserted.
- Nasal polyps are removed from the nasal cavity using the microdebrider, or otherwise Tilley or Blakesley forceps.
- The endoscope is inserted into the middle meatus. It may be necessary to medialize the middle meatus to insert the endoscope, but this should be avoided if possible.
- The uncinate process is identified. It may be removed 'anterograde' using a freer to excise it at its root, 'retrograde' using a backbiter to free it inferiorly and superiorly, and then anteroflexing the uncinate and removing it with the Blakesley forceps.
- A sinus-seeking probe is used to identify the natural maxillary ostium at the level of the inferior border of the middle turbinate. The natural ostium is enlarged using through-cutting forceps or downbiters. If an accessory ostium is present, then the natural and accessory ostia are joined.
- The bulla ethmoidalis is identified and opened at the inferiomedial portion of the anterior face.
- Anterior ethmoidal cells are then opened, with care taken at the lamina papyracea near the orbit. The maxillary sinus is used to identify the lamina.
- The anterior ethmoidal artery may lie within the anterior ethmoidal cells on a bony mesentry. This should be avoided.
- The posterior limit of the anterior ethmoids is the basal lamella (sometimes termed the ground lamella), which is a part of the middle turbinate, as it rotates from its vertical part to its horizontal part. Identification of the basal lamella therefore relies on assessment of the middle turbinate.
- The posterior ethmoids are opened through the basal lamella. Care should be taken due to their proximity to the skull base, and the possibility of sphenoethmoidal cells that may contain the optic nerve.
- The sphenoid may be identified through the posterior ethmoids, or more commonly through the nasal cavity, superior to the choana. The frontal sinus drains through the frontal recess, which lies anterior to the ethmoid bulla.

Closure

Haemostasis should be ensured, usually with topical adrenaline patties. Nasal packing may be used. Absorbable packing, such as nasopore, is often used.

Postoperative care

- Regular nasal saline douching is important.
- Regular review in clinic with cleaning of the cavity may reduce adhesions, but has a limited evidence base to support the practice.
- Topical nasal steroids may commence shortly after the operation to reduce the recurrence of symptoms.
- Occasionally, systemic steroids are given in the postoperative period.

Complications

The most feared complications are breach of the anterior skull base resulting in CSF leak, or orbital injury. These are rare, but may require urgent treatment.

CSF leaks should be identified, and may be repaired using local tissue flaps, underlay grafts with fat plugs or cartilage, and tissue glues. The patient will need systemic antibiotics, and may need to be nursed at 45° head-up for some days after surgery to maximize the chance of healing. Laxatives and a catheter are often used in this period.

Orbital injury may be indirect due to division of the anterior ethmoidal artery. This causes the artery to retract to within the orbit, and causes retrobulbar haematoma and an orbital compartment syndrome. Lateral canthotomy and inferior cantholysis may relieve tension in the orbit. Mannitol and steroids may play a role in relieving consequent pressure on the optic nerve. Removal of the lamina papyracea and release of the orbital periosteum will allow the haematoma to drain into the nose. Haematoma may, however, be caused by direct injury, and this should also be considered. Direct injury may also injure the medial rectus leading to diplopia. The optic nerve may be injured within the sphenoid, or if it runs through sphenoethmoidal cells.

Tips and tricks

FESS is usually undertaken as a bilateral operation. When bleeding obscures a view of one side, packing with adrenaline-soaked patties, and moving to the other side to progress the operation is advisable to save time. Passing back and forth between the sides can allow an optimized field, and also give some insights into a patient's anatomy (although this is uncommonly asymmetrical).

Drainage of orbital abscess

Overview

Orbital abscesses are a complication of periorbital cellulitis. This is most commonly sinugenic in origin, although it may occur as a result of skin infection (and in this case is less likely to lead to orbital abscess).

Anatomy

- Orbital cellulitis is characterized by its position in relation to the orbital septum, a fibrous band of tissue running from the orbital rim to the eyelid.
- Orbital abscesses are most commonly subperiosteal—below the periosteum overlying the lamina papyracea. This reflects the common origin of sepsis from the adjacent sinuses. They may extend into the orbit, breaching the peristeum, but they almost invariably have a connection with this space.
- An uncommon variant is lacrimal gland abscesses, which are uncommon, rarely require surgical intervention, and are on the superolateral aspect of the orbit.

Indications

Conventional advice holds that all orbital and subperiosteal abscesses should be drained. Abscesses are identified on CT, which is requested on clinical grounds. Nasal endoscopic drainage may be performed but if not amenable then open drainage is appropriate.

Equipment

- Scalpel with 15 blade.
- Iris scissors, toothed forceps, needle holder.
- Freer's elevator and small periosteum elevator.
- Sort malleable retractors for retracting the globe.
- Bipolar diathermy.
- Drain.
- Drain suture.
- Endoscope and FESS equipment (see p. 747) may be used alternately.

Consent

- There are risks of orbital haematoma, diplopia, and visual loss. An external approach involves a small scar.
- These risks are significantly outweighed by the removal of pus, and consequent improvement of infection.

Preoperative preparation

- The imaging should be checked.
- The side and site of the abscess should be confirmed, and a surgical plan made.
- Experienced endoscopic surgeons can perform this operation through the nose. This is described on p. 747.

Position and theatre set-up

- Supine with the head turned towards the surgeon.
- A head ring is used.

Procedure

- Infiltration of LA.
- An Lynch–Howarth incision is made between the medial canthus and the nose, extending towards the orbital rim.
- Care is taken to avoid the medial canthal ligament and the trochlea of the superior oblique, which is repaired if cut.
- Dissection down to the lacrimal bone, and then a subperiosteal flap is raised.
- This is developed into the abscess cavity.
- The abscess is aspirated, contents sent for culture, and the cavity washed out.
- A drain is usually placed.

Closure

Closure is with 5-0 Prolene®, although if a drain is placed, this will leave a small open area. This, if necessary, can be closed after removal of the drain.

Postoperative care

It is important to monitor the eye to ensure that swelling settles, and vision does not deteriorate.

Complications

Complications are uncommon, and are usually more likely in untreated disease. Orbital abscesses may cause intracranial sepsis, notably cavernous sinus thrombosis.

Tips and tricks

This approach may be used for access to other medial orbital pathologies.

Sphenopalatine artery ligation

Overview

Sphenopalatine artery (SPA) ligation is one of the most commonly performed surgical procedures for the management of persistent or recurrent epistaxis.

Anatomy

- The SPA is the largest of the terminal branches of the maxillary artery, which itself is one of the terminal branches of the external carotid artery.
- The SPA enters the nasal cavity posterior to the maxillary sinus, having run in the pterygomaxillary fissure. There is a bony prominence immediately anterior to its entrance called the crista ethmoidalis.

Indications

- Persistent epistaxis that is uncontrollable with nasal cautery and packing (this is an emergency indication).
- Persistent epistaxis that is controllable with packing, but which persistently recurs on removal of packing, despite nasal cautery.
- Recurrent epistaxis over a long period, which is resistant to topical treatment and nasal cautery.

Equipment

- As per FESS (p. 747).
- Endoscopic clip applicators.
- Endoscopic bipolar cautery.

Consent

- The procedure is effective in the management of epistaxis. However, there will be cases of persistent bleeding after surgery.
- The risks of the procedure are similar to those of FESS surgery, although the risk of CSF leak will be much lower, and risk of orbital injury is likely to be slightly diminished.

Preoperative preparation

- Active bleeding should be controlled where possible, as operating in the context of active bleeding is challenging.
- Replacement blood products should be available.
- A CT scan of the sinuses may be beneficial to outline any atypical anatomy.

Position and theatre set-up

- The patient is supine, with the head and upper body elevated to about 20°.
- The head is turned towards the surgeon.

Procedure

- Nasal preparation is instilled if possible.
- Packs are removed.
- The nose is examined (see p. 736). The middle meatus is entered with the endoscope. It may be packed with adrenaline soaked ribbon gauze.
- A middle meatal antrostomy may be made.
- An incision to bone is made in the mucosa immediately posterior to the maxillary sinus. This is extended along the height of the maxillary sinus.
- This flap is elevated, over the crista ethmoidalis. It is often helpful to pack adrenaline ribbon gauze into this flap.
- The crista ethmoidalis may be removed with a curette to improve access to the vessel.
- The SPA is identified and the flap is progressed inferiorly and superiorly.
- The artery may now be clipped, or diathermy may be used to cauterise the vessel.
- The vessel may, or may not, now be divided, depending on the surgeons preference. The flap is replaced.

Closure

An absorbable pack, such as nasopore, may be placed to hold the flap in place over the sphenopalatine artery.

Postoperative care

The patient is monitored for bleeding.

Complications

As per FESS (p. 749).

Tips and tricks

It is not uncommon for the SPA to have a number of branches that may arise prior, or subsequent, to its entry into the nasal cavity; the surgeon should therefore examine this area closely to identify all branches.

Closed septorhinoplasty

Overview

Septorhinoplasty (SRP) is a procedure performed to address cosmetic and functional issues of the nasal bones and nasal septum. It may be performed primarily as a cosmetic procedure, or primarily to address nasal obstruction.

Anatomy

The nose lies in the centre of the face, and is therefore highly significant for cosmesis. The position of the nasal bones in relation to the maxilla and frontal bones should be considered.

Indications

SRP can be undertaken for a combination of functional and cosmetic indications. These may be associated with deviation of the nose to one side, or prominence of certain parts of the nose—either within the airway or on the external nose, which may have cosmetic implications. There may be combinations of all of these issues.

Equipment

- A for 'Septoplasty' (p. 740).
- Headlight.
- Dental syringe and needle.
- LA with adrenaline.
- Scalpel with 15 blade.
- Curved scissors.
- Foman's scissors.
- Aufricht's retractor.
- Alar retractor.
- Osteotome (various sizes).
- Mallet.
- Rasp.

Consent

Consent in SRP is crucial in achieving a satisfactory result. The patient's wishes, particularly surrounding cosmetic issues, should be closely addressed. The surgeon should, as much as possible, avoid preconceptions of what the position and shape of the nose 'should' be. The consent is usually taken over a period to allow time for the patient to consider their requests.

The risks of the procedure are similar to those as 'Septoplasty' (see p. 741), these should be discussed. Also, the risk of poor cosmetic results should be discussed. Skin necrosis, peri-orbital bruising, CSF leak, or collapse of the nose is possible and should be mentioned.

Revision procedures are possible, but are much more challenging, and the patient's desired result may not be achieved.

Preoperative preparation

Preoperative photos are almost invariably taken. They allow a record of the preoperative nose and may also guide the surgeon when intraoperative swelling obscures the assessment of the nose.

The role of psychological review of the SRP patient is controversial. A very small proportion of patients seeking predominantly cosmetic nasal operations will have concomitant psychiatric illness, such as body dysmorphic disorder. These patients will not benefit from surgery, and indeed may worsen a preoccupation with a perceived disorder of the nose. These patients should be highlighted and managed appropriately.

Position and theatre set-up

As per 'Septoplasty' (p. 741).

Procedure

- Removal of the hairs lining the nasal vestibule.
- The nasal septum, columella, and dorsum of the nose is infiltrated with LA with adrenaline. Infiltration is also placed laterally, percutaneously, at the midpoint of the pyriform aperture and the medial canthus.
- Septoplasty is now performed (see p. 741).
- Intercartilagenous incisions are made within the nose at the scroll area where the upper lateral and lower lateral cartilages meet.
- The dorsum of the nose is degloved using either a scalpel or scissors.
- The Aufricht's retractor is placed into the degloved nasal dorsum to allow access to the nose.
- Any dorsal hump, which may or may not be addressed, is now reduced with an osteotome or a rasp.
- The procerus muscle is palpated on the nasal bones and elevated. If this is not performed, this may lead to this muscle pulling the nasal bones superiorly after they have been mobilized.
- Medial osteotomies are made between the septum and nasal bones. The upper lateral cartilages may also be divided from the nasal septum (Fig. 14.14).
- Lateral osteotomies are made percutaneously in the frontal process of the maxilla as it joins the nasal bones. The nasal bones are relatively small, and osteotomies placed too medially may lead to a step when the nasal bones are manipulated. A stab incision is made in the skin, and the osteotome is inserted onto the bone, then used to scour the periosteum. The bone is 'postage-stamped' to weaken it.
- Superior osteotomies are made between the canthus and the nasion in the same way.

The nose is then held firmly and fractured into the midline. This process also 'closes' an open book deformity if removal of a dorsal hump has left a flattened area on the dorsum, which enters into the nasal cavity.

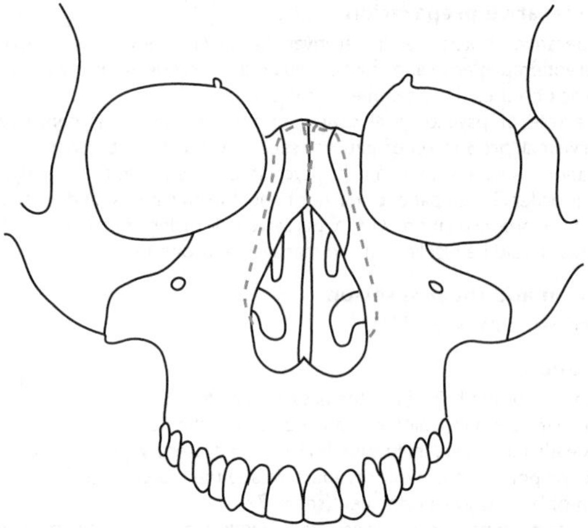

Fig. 14.14 Location on facial skeleton of osteotomies.

Closure

- Closure and quilting of the septum is undertaken, and the intercartilagenous incisions are also closed.
- Plaster of Paris or a thermoplastic splint is placed over the nose to hold it into position. If plaster of Paris is used, then steristrips are used under the splint to protect the nose. The splint is then secured over the nose with tape.

Postoperative care

The patient is reviewed at 1 week to remove the splint.

Complications

Poor functional and cosmetic results may be challenging to address. Commonly an open approach where the skin is elevated off the nose from the columella may be used for these cases.

Tips and tricks

Replacing the skin over the nose and assessing the likely postoperative appearance several times during surgery may inform if further resection may be needed.

Dacrocystorhinostomy

Overview

Dacrocystorhinostomy (DCR) is a surgical procedure performed for the relief of epiphora.

Anatomy

The lacrimal gland lies on the upper lateral aspect of the orbit. The lacrimal sac lies on the inferomedial aspect of the eye (Fig. 14.15).

Indications

- Nasolacrimal duct obstruction.
- Recurrent dacrocystitis.

Equipment

- As per FESS (p. 747).
- Endoscopic drill.
- Lacrimal light probes/fibre-optic endoilluminator.

Consent

Consent should mention the risks of infection, bleeding, nasal adhesions, and failure of the procedure. Orbital injury is exceptionally rare.

Preoperative preparation

- Topical nasal decongestant is used, as per FESS (p. 747).
- Imaging should be reviewed, including investigations to confirm the cause of epiphora.

Position and theatre set-up

Supine on a head ring.

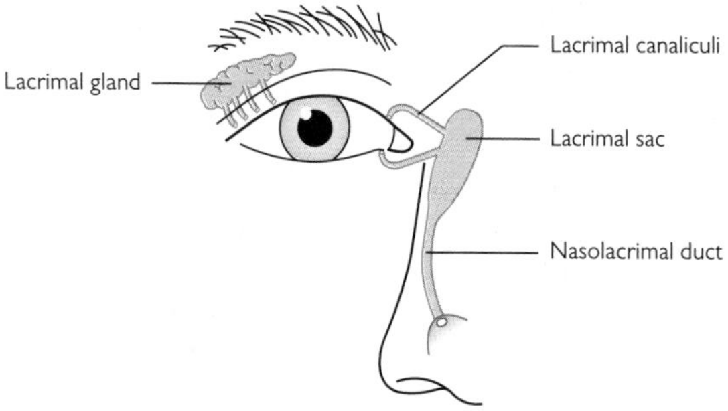
Lacrimal gland
Lacrimal canaliculi
Lacrimal sac
Nasolacrimal duct

Fig. 14.15 Lacrimal apparatus.

Procedure

- The fibre-optic endoilluminator is inserted though the lacrimal canaliculi and into the lacrimal sac. This movement is initially perpendicular to the lid, and then turns sharply to face medially and enter the sac. Care should be taken to avoid trauma, which may cause persisting epiphora. This process allows endonasal visualization of the location of the sac.
- The nose is examined, and the nasal mucosa adjacent to the lacrimal sac is incised, and a posteriorly based flap is raised. This flap is positioned lateral to the middle turbinate for protection.
- The drill is used to remove the lacrimal bone in the lateral aspect of the nasal cavity.
- The mucosa of the exposed lacrimal sac is removed.
- The canaliculi may be used to irrigate the lacrimal system to ensure that sufficient patency has been achieved.
- Silicone stents are placed through the canaliculi and tied in the nose. These may be removed 4 weeks after surgery—usually as an outpatient procedure.

Closure

Nasal packing is rarely required.

Postoperative care

- Stent removal may be undertaken in outpatients.
- The silicone stent is secured at the medial canthus and divided.
- The stent is held within the nose and extracted through the nose.

Complications

- Restenosis or persistent epiphora may occur in around 10% of patients.
- This may, or may not, be amenable to revision surgery.

Tips and tricks

The procedure may be performed alone, but is not infrequently performed with an assistant/second surgeon. In these cases, one surgeon undertakes the endonasal steps, and the other cannulates the canaliculi as required.

Caldwell–Luc procedure

Overview

The Caldwell–Luc procedure allows entrance into the maxillary sinus. As endoscopic equipment, particularly angled scopes and curved instruments, improve and become more available, this procedure is used less frequently.

Anatomy

The anatomy of the midface has been discussed on p. 738. The position of the infra-orbital nerve is important to remember, as it should be avoided.

Indications

Access to the maxillary sinus for removal of lesions such as inverted papilloma.

Equipment

- Cheek retractors.
- Dental syringe and needle.
- LA with adrenaline.
- Scalpel with 15 blade.
- Periosteal elevators.
- Drill with cutting burr.
- Oscilating saw.
- Langenbeck retractors.

Consent

- The consent depends upon the reason for access to the maxillary sinus.
- Oro-antral fistula is not uncommon, as is parasthesia of the midface.
- The patient may take some days to return to tolerating a full diet, as mastication may be uncomfortable for some days and weeks after the operation.

Preoperative preparation

- Preoperative imaging is reviewed.
- A CT will allow preoperative planning and will be performed in all cases.

Position and theatre set-up

The patient is supine, with the head and upper body elevated to dismiss venous congestion and bleeding.

Procedure

- Infiltration of LA.
- An incision is made in the bucco-gingival sulcus between the contralateral incisor, and the ipsilateral second premolar.
- Dissection proceeds down to the bone, and a periosteum elevator is used to expose the anterior part of the maxillary sinus.
- The maxillary sinus is opened with the drill, and a window into the sinus is fashioned.

Closure
Closure is with a 4-0 absorbable polyfilament, such as Vicryl®.

Postoperative care
Nutritional support may be required until a full diet is tolerated.

Complications
Oro-antral fistula is uncommon, but can be managed relatively easily with a procedure to close the fistula. It may present with foul or watery nasal discharge, often linked to mastication.

Tips and tricks
The incision can be extended to the contralateral side, and combined with a rhinoplasty transfixion incision. This 'midface degloving' approach allows the elevation of the skin from the midface, and allows excellent access to the post-nasal space, pterygomaxillary fossa, and inferior sinonasal space. This approach may be used for the removal of tumours such as juvenile nasal angiofibromas.

Flexible nasolaryngoscopy

Overview

Flexible nasolaryngoscopy is one of the most commonly performed procedures by ENT surgeons. It is performed in outpatient and inpatient settings, and rarely in the operating theatre. It is an invaluable technique for the assessment of the pharynx, larynx, and the airway.

Anatomy

The flexible endoscope is passed through the nasal cavity into the nasopharynx. It is subsequently passed inferiorly into the oropharynx, and at this stage achieves a view of the larynx and hypopharynx.

It is important to recognize the nasal turbinates, Eustachian tube cushions, fossa of Rosenmuller, soft palate, base of tongue, tonsils, epiglottis, laryngeal cartilages, false and true vocal cords, subglottis, pyriform fossae, and the posterior pharyngeal wall (Fig. 14.16).

Indications

The indications for flexible nasolaryngoscopy are diverse, but include the assessment and diagnosis of patients with laryngeal and pharyngeal symptoms.

Equipment

- A flexible endoscope.
- A light source.
- Topical anaesthetic may be used.
- Lubricating gel may be used.
- Video or image capture may be used.

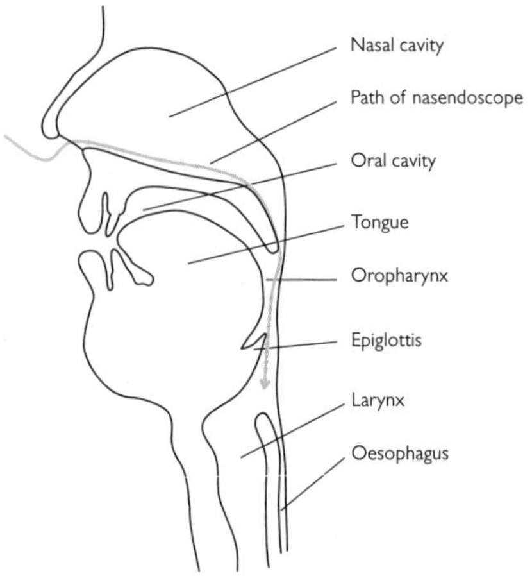
Nasal cavity
Path of nasendoscope
Oral cavity
Tongue
Oropharynx
Epiglottis
Larynx
Oesophagus

Fig. 14.16 Diagram of flexible endoscope passing through upper aerodigestive tract.

Consent

Verbal consent is usually sufficient for this procedure. The patient should be warned that the procedure may be uncomfortable, but should not last long. Gagging, coughing, and tearing are common.

Preoperative preparation

The patient is advised about the procedure. The indication of the procedure is confirmed, and any expected anatomical abnormalities are reviewed.

Position and theatre set-up

The patient is seated facing the surgeon. The head is in a neutral position, and may be supported from behind to prevent a tendency for the patient to back away from the surgeon.

Procedure

- Topical anaesthesia may be instilled.
- Lubricating gel may also be used.
- The scope is inserted into the nose. If there is a septal deviation, then the side with the more open airway is chosen.
- The scope is passed either medial to the middle meatus, or in the floor of the nose.
- When the post-nasal space is reached, the patient is asked to breathe in through the nose.
- The scope is angled downwards into the oropharynx.
- A view of the larynx and pharynx is now obtained.
- The scope may be extended down closer around the larynx or even between the cords to achieve the view desired.
- Manoeuvres such as turning the head, puffing out the cheeks, making sounds, and sniffing may move the larynx and pharynx to check cord mobility and examine the pharynx.

Postoperative care

NA.

Complications

Epistaxis is very rare after this procedure.

Tips and tricks

Tilting the head forward whilst puffing out the cheeks and turning the head away from the examined side may facilitate the best view of the piriform fossa.

Drainage of a peritonsillar abscess (Quinsy)

Overview

Quinsies are common complications of acute tonsillitis. They present with a painful swelling of the soft palate, most commonly superior and lateral to the tonsil. In addition to the symptoms of tonsillitis, patients may have otalgia and voice change.

Anatomy

The tonsil lies within a fascia-lined fossa. This leads to a potential space that may lead to abscess formation.

Indications

Transoral quinsy drainage is indicated for all patients with suspected or confirmed peritonsillar abscess. The contraindication for drainage is a suspicion of the peritonsillar swelling being caused by an aberrantly placed or aneurysmal carotid artery. This can be determined by palpation of the oropharynx.

Equipment

- Head light.
- Tongue depressor.
- Syringe with wide-bore needle.
- Scalpel.
- Kidney dish.
- Topical xylocaine spray.
- Lidocaine with needle and narrow bore syringe can be used.

Consent

Verbal consent is usually sufficient for this procedure. The rationale should be explained. The patient should be warned that the procedure may be uncomfortable, and they should expect some bleeding into the mouth. The possibility of not finding pus should be mentioned.

Preoperative preparation

- The patient is advised about the procedure.
- Xylocaine spray should be applied to the throat.
- A decision should be made whether to proceed with needle aspiration, incision and drainage, or a combination procedure.

Position and theatre set-up

- The patient is seated facing the surgeon.
- The head is in a neutral position, and may be supported from behind to prevent a tendency for the patient to back away from the surgeon.
- A kidney dish is present.

Procedure

- A tongue depressor is used, and the quinsy is visualized.
- The surgeon satisfies themselves as to the adequacy of the visualization and the lighting (a headlight is used).
- A needle is placed into the bulge of the soft palate next to the tonsil, and pus is aspirated.
- Three passes of repeated aspirations may be undertaken. Alternatively, an incision may be made to open the quinsy.

Postoperative care

The patient is examined after 5min to ensure any bleeding has settled.

Complications

Reaccumulation of quinsies may occur, and is more likely after aspiration than incision and drainage.

Tips and tricks

A combination procedure involves confirmation of the presence and location of a quinsy using a needle, and then subsequently using a scalpel to incise the collection.

Biopsy of small oral or skin lesion

Overview

Oral cavity biopsies are commonly performed in outpatient clinics when a diagnosis of malignancy is considered. Excisional biopsy of facial lesions is more frequently performed in an operating theatre, as in these cases it is important to consider postoperative cosmesis.

Anatomy

When assessing a facial skin lesion for excisional biopsy one should consider the relaxed skin tension lines of the face. These are lines that lie perpendicular to the long axis of the muscles of the face. Incisions that run parallel to these lines will give the best cosmetic results. Facial wrinkle lines are often the same as the relaxed skin tension lines. One must also be aware that in some areas branches of the facial nerve run quite superficially (e.g. over the zygoma or mandible, and medial to the parotid gland).

In the oral cavity you should consider the underlying structures where an incision is made. Most areas for small biopsy in the oral cavity are relatively safe but you must consider the underlying salivary ducts or, for deep biopsies, nerves and vessels.

Indications

Biopsies of skin or oral skin lesions will be used to determine histology and guide further management. Be aware that the ongoing management may include a more extensive excision and hence it is important to accurately document the location and orientation of the specimen to guide any subsequent operation. For some benign tumours, excision biopsy can also be considered curative.

Equipment

- A basic set of surgical instruments, including, at a minimum, a scalpel and 15 blade, toothed forceps, and needle holder.
- Skin preparation.
- Sutures for closure.
- Bioplar diathermy may be required for haemostasis.
- LA, which may be delivered by a dental syringe and needle.
- For very small lesions, a biopsy punch, or grasping forceps (Blakesley–Wilde in the oral cavity), may be selected.

Consent

Consent should mention the indication for surgery. Risks include scarring, which can affect cosmesis. Keloid and hypertrophic scars are a possibility. Infection and bleeding is rarely problematic. Occasionally, biopsy specimens are inadequate or not representative of the underlying tumour, and the procedure may need to be repeated. If there are any important nearby structures at risk of injury (e.g. submandibular duct) this should be mentioned.

Preoperative preparation

Mark out the lesion and incision lines prior to injecting LA as this can distort the area and make incision selection more difficult.

Position and theatre set-up

- Oral cavity biopsies in outpatients are commonly done with the patient seated, a surgical headlight, and instruments to hand.
- For excision biopsy of facial lesions, the patient is usually supine on an operating table.

Procedure

- Slowly infiltrate LA around the area to be excised. Give this time to work and check that the sensation to sharp stimuli is absent.
- Excise the area of skin bearing the tumour, or oral lesion. This is often performed in ellipse to facilitate closure.
- Orientate and the specimen for histological analysis.
- Use haemostasis as required.

Closure

For superficial biopsies a simple interrupted suturing technique for closure is used (absorbable sutures for the oral cavity and non-absorbable monofilament sutures for the facial skin).

Postoperative care

- For facial lesions, clean the area and cover the suture with brown tape.
- Ensure that if it is a non-absorbable suture that arrangements are made for it being removed either at the patient's GP practice or back in outpatients.
- The patient is then followed up with the results of histology.

Complications

- Poor cosmetic results are the most significant complication of facial skin lesion excisions. Local skin flaps may ameliorate some of these cases but, where possible, poor cosmesis should be avoided.
- Inadvertant ligation of salivary ducts may lead to sialadenitis. This can be managed conservatively, but may have a long-term impact on salivary production, which may be relevant if the patient receives radiotherapy to the oropharynx or neck.

Tips and tricks

Longer scars that are appropriately orientated may have a lesser effect on cosmesis than shorter, awkwardly placed scars

Tracheostomy tube change

Overview

Tracheostomy tube changes are performed on a routine, expedited, and emergency basis. The majority of tracheostomy tubes in current use have a license for use for ~1 month, and have to be regularly replaced in those patients with a long-term tracheostomy requirement. If patients develop tracheostomy-associated complications, or require a different size or type of tube, these changes may be expedited. In cases of unresolved blockage or dislodgement, it may be necessary to change a tracheostomy tube as a life-saving intervention.

Anatomy

When preparing to change a tracheostomy tube it is important to consider the depth of the trachea from the skin. This will vary from patient to patient, depending on their neck size. With patients with broader necks, the trachea may lie more deeply and it may be easier to create a false passage in front of the trachea. This is likely to have been considered by the surgeon who placed the tracheostomy tube and hence if an extra-long or adjustable flange tube has been used these should be used again. Furthermore, the degree of flexion and extension of the neck is variable, and those patients with cervical spinal pathology may be unable to extend their neck. Neck extension moves the trachea more anteriorly within the neck, making it more accessible.

So called 'stay sutures' are commonly used for paediatric patients when a tracheostomy is first placed. They are rarely used in adult patients. These are non-dissolvable sutures placed though the trachea wall and then stuck to the outside of the skin. These can be utilized to draw the trachea up to the skin and to open the tracheal slit or window to aid tracheostomy replacement (Fig. 14.17).

Indications

- Tracheostomy tubes are usually changed after at least 1 week after insertion. A week is left for an adequate tract to form and the tracheostomy is often sutured in position during this period.
- After the first change, the tracheostomy tube is replaced once a month to prevent excessive crusting or gross contamination of the tube.
- If a different size or type of tube is required, a tube change may be performed.
- A fenestrated tube may allow vocalization, for example.

Equipment

- Replacement tube of the correct size and type.
- Additional tube that is one size smaller.
- Water-soluble lubrication gel or sterile saline.
- Syringe for inflating/deflating the cuff of the tube (if cuffed tube present).
- Tracheal dilators.
- Suction (with endobronchial suction catheters and Yankauer).

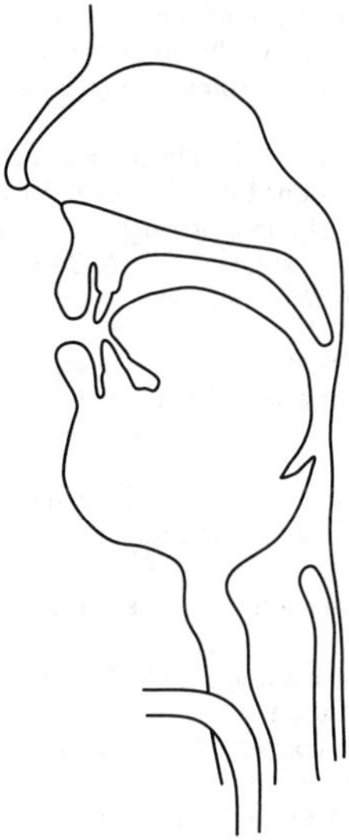

Fig. 14.17 Sagittal diagram of tracheostomy tube in situ.

- Personal protection equipment (gloves, gowns, eye protection may be considered).
- Gum elastic bougie or guide wire if the change is thought to be difficult.
- Flexible fibre-optic endoscope (optional but useful in confirming the location of the new tube or in placement if the tract is lost).

Consent

- Verbal consent is usually sufficient for this procedure or in emergency cases, where the procedure is undertaken as an immediate, life-saving measure.
- Complications are highly infrequent but potentially include tracheal trauma, airway bleeding, placing a tube into a false tract, and causing airway obstruction.

Preoperative preparation

- The indication for a tube change is confirmed, any factors that may make the change difficult are considered.
- The correct tube is determined.
- Equipment is gathered and prepared.
- The procedure requires at least two people to perform safely and should be performed in a controlled environment.

- If there is concern about the difficulty of the change or the patient is unstable, then the procedure should be performed in the operating theatre with the relevant equipment and personnel to open the wound if the tract is lost.
- If an NG tube is present this should be used to aspirate the stomach.
- The patient may be kept nil-by-mouth for some hours before the procedure to avoid aspiration, although this is not necessary in all cases.
- The patient may be pre-oxygenated on 100% O_2 before the procedure and oxygen levels can be monitored.

Position and theatre set-up

The patient is supine with the neck extended.

Procedure

- One hand is used to secure the current tracheostomy tube.
- The ties, sutures, or tapes that are currently securing the tube are removed.
- The tracheostomy is suctioned and the cuff (if present) is concomitantly deflated.
- The replacement tube has a small volume of lubricating gel placed on the tip and outer curvature.
- If the tracheostomy is connected to a ventilator, this is detached.
- The current tube is removed.
- The replacement tube is inserted into the stoma in a gentle curving motion, mimicking the curvature of the tube. If it is difficult to visualize the tract, a tracheal dilator may be inserted prior or subsequent to removing the tube, in order to hold the tract and the trachea open whilst the new tube is placed.
- With one hand securing the tube, if the tracheostomy was connected to a ventilator, this is now reattached.
- A suction catheter or flexible nasendoscope is passed to confirm position of the tube within the trachea. Patients may be asked if they feel that they can breathe easily and comfortably.
- With the tube still held in place by one practitioner, the tracheostomy tapes should be attached and firmly secured.

Postoperative care

- Once the position of the tube is confirmed, sedated patients should be returned to their previous nursing position. The patient should be closely observed for any respiratory changes due to potential complications, including aspiration and pneumothorax.
- When a cuff is used the pressure of this should be checked with a manometer to ensure it is in the correct range.
- Full documentation of the change should be written in the notes, including the sticker from the new tracheostomy pack with details of the size and whether any cuff or fenestrations are present on the tube. Plans for the next tracheostomy change should also be documented.
- Appropriate contact details should be clearly documented.

Complications

Complications are rare, but can be devastating. It is therefore important to be appropriately trained in this procedure. Potential complications include loss of airway with consequent hypoxia, haemorrhage into the airway, creation of false tract, cardiovascular instability, bronchospasm, aspiration, and tracheal trauma.

Tips and tricks

- In cases where a difficult change is expected or a false tract has previously been caused, the tracheostomy tube may be changed over a guide wire using a Seldinger technique.
- When changing tubes of differing manufacturers, pay particular attention to the tube outer diameter as tubes of defined inner diameter vary in outer diameter between brands.

Surgical tracheostomy

Overview

The development of percutaneous techniques for tracheostomy means that surgical approaches are less commonly utilized. They are considered a more controlled technique and although there is some evidence to suggest their short-term complications may be higher, this may be because they are commonly used in the more difficult cases. These may involve bleeding diasthesis, poor neck extension, cervical tumours, or adipose necks.

Anatomy

The trachea lies in the midline from the larynx superiorly, into the thorax. The layers of the neck are important to consider (Fig. 14.18).

Indications

The most common indication for tracheostomy in adults is a persistent requirement for ventilation in an ITU setting. In these patients it may also assist in weaning from ventilation. It is also indicated in cases of airway obstruction and as an adjunct to major head and neck resections, where it is thought that there will be, in the short term, significant aspiration of secretions and consequent respiratory compromise.

Equipment

- Scalpel with 10 and 11 blade.
- Dental syringe and needle.
- LA with adrenaline.
- McIndoe scissors, needle holders, toothed forceps.
- Head light.
- Langenback retractors.
- Self-retaining retractors.
- Suction with a Yankauer.
- Bipolar diathermy.
- 2-0 Vicryl® suture.

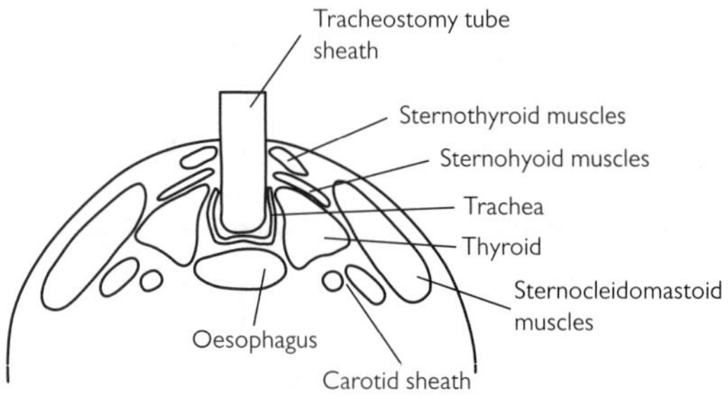
Tracheostomy tube sheath
Sternothyroid muscles
Sternohyoid muscles
Trachea
Thyroid
Sternocleidomastoid muscles
Oesophagus
Carotid sheath

Fig. 14.18 Transverse diagram of neck with tracheostomy tube in situ.

- 2-0 silk suture.
- Tracheostomy tubes.
- Sterile ventilation connector.
- Monopolar diathermy may be used.

Consent

Consent should consider the indication, and the risks and consequences of surgery. The procedure may be life-saving and is usually designed to replace an endotracheal tube, which has its own complications when in situ for a lengthy period.

Standard consent is often not always possible, as the procedure may be undertaken in best interests, if the patient lacks the capacity to make a decision on treatment. It is good practice, however, to consult with the family.

When the patient has capacity, the effect of a tracheostomy on airway, tracheal secretions, voice, and swallow should be considered. The care a tracheostomy requires should be mentioned. The potential for blockage and infection also mentioned, as well as the potential for fistula formation. In the short term, risks of bleeding, infection, unexpected decannulation, and pneumothorax should be mentioned.

Preoperative preparation

The indication is confirmed and an appropriate tube should be selected. This may be fenestrated or not, cuffed or not, have an inner tube, and be a variety of makes, shapes, and sizes.

Position and theatre set-up

- The patient is supine with a shoulder roll and head ring used to extend the neck.
- The head may be elevated to reduce bleeding.

Procedure

This describes an elective procedure for an intubated patient:

- Infiltration of LA with adrenaline.
- Skin crease incision at the midpoint of the cricoid and suprasternal notch (Fig. 14.19).
- Division of platysma.
- Identification of strap muscles and a plane is elevated superiorly and inferiorly.
- Anterior jugular veins are ligated and divided, if encountered.
- Straps are divided in the midline and the thyroid isthmus is exposed within the pretracheal fascia. The trachea is identified inferiorly and superiorly to the thyroid isthmus.
- A curved clip is placed deep to the isthmus to elevate a plane between thyroid and trachea.
- Two parallel clips are placed over the isthmus, which is then divided.
- The two free edges of the isthmus are transfixed with Vicryl®.
- Haemostasis is ensured.
- The cricoid and tracheal rings are identified.
- The endotracheal tube cuff is deflated.

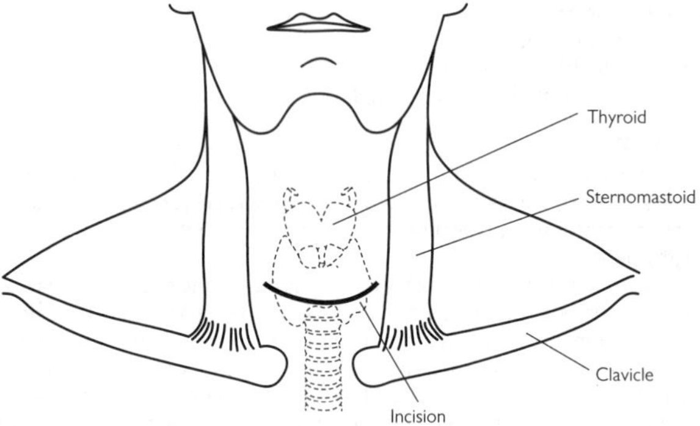
Thyroid
Sternomastoid
Clavicle
Incision

Fig. 14.19 Tracheostomy incision. Reproduced from McLatchie, G. and Leaper, D., Operative Surgery 2nd edition, 2006, with permission from Oxford University Press.

- A window of anterior tracheal wall, involving the 3rd and 4th tracheal rings, is excised. The height of this window may be variable. Care is taken to avoid the first tracheal ring (Fig. 14.20).
- The endotracheal tube is seen, and is slowly withdrawn to reveal the trachea. The tracheostomy tube is sited in the trachea. The ventilation circuit connector is attached and ventilation is confirmed with end tidal CO_2.

Closure

- Haemostasis is checked, whilst one hand continually secures the tracheostomy tube.
- Approximation of the skin at the edges of the tracheostomy is performed with silk.
- The tube is sutured to the skin of the neck with silk.
- Tracheostomy ties are placed.
- The hand can then be removed from the tracheostomy.

Postoperative care

- Humidification and regular saline nebulizers can help manage secretions in the tube along with regular suctioning and tube care.
- Appropriate replacement and smaller tubes should be available for cases of dislodgement or blockage.

Complications

Tracheo-cutaneous fistulae may be closed in layers excising a rim of epithelium from the tract. Rare but feared complications of tracheostomy include fistulae into great vessels, which may be very challenging to manage. Airway stenosis may occur as a long-term consequence of tracheostomy and this may be managed endoscopically or (rarely) with open surgery.

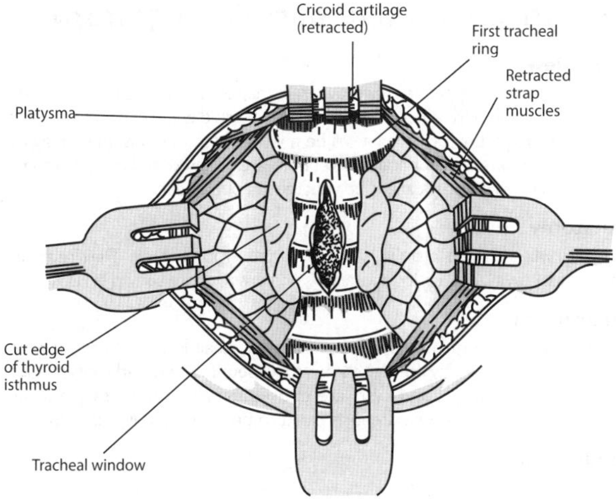
Cricoid cartilage
(retracted)
First tracheal
ring
Retracted
strap
muscles
Platysma
Cut edge
of thyroid
isthmus
Tracheal window

Fig. 14.20 Window created into the trachea for a tracheostomy tube. Reproduced from McLatchie, G. and Leaper, D., Operative Surgery 2nd edition, 2006, with permission from Oxford University Press.

Tips and tricks

The positioning of the patient is essential to achieve adequate surgical access. Neck extension is essential and, if it is not possible (e.g. in cervical fixation), the case will be more difficult, and a larger incision is advised.

Pharyngoscopy and microlaryngoscopy

Overview

Examination of the upper aerodigestive tract may be performed most easily on awake patients in clinic, often with the aid of a flexible endoscope. However, a very small proportion of patients will be unable to tolerate this, there may be cases where biopsies or surgical interventions are required, and there are some areas of the pharynx that cannot be visualized in outpatients.

Anatomy

The pharynx is divided into the naso-, oro-, and hypo-pharynx. Their relations to the nasal cavity, oral cavity, and larynx, and divisions are shown in Fig. 14.21.

Indications

Diagnostic or therapeutic for the excision of small lesions. In the larynx, microlaryngoscopy may frequently be therapeutic when pathologies such as granulomas, polyps, and cysts are excised. Small tumours may also be removed with laser. Airway stenosis can also be addressed in this manner.

Equipment

- Dedo pilling laryngoscope.
- Lindholm supraglottic laryngoscope.
- Pharyngoscopes may also be helpful.
- Light source.
- Light carrier.
- Suction.
- Gel and dental guard.
- Biopsy forceps.
- Bouchier microlaryngoscopy instruments and laser may be helpful if microlaryngoscopy proceeds to intervention.

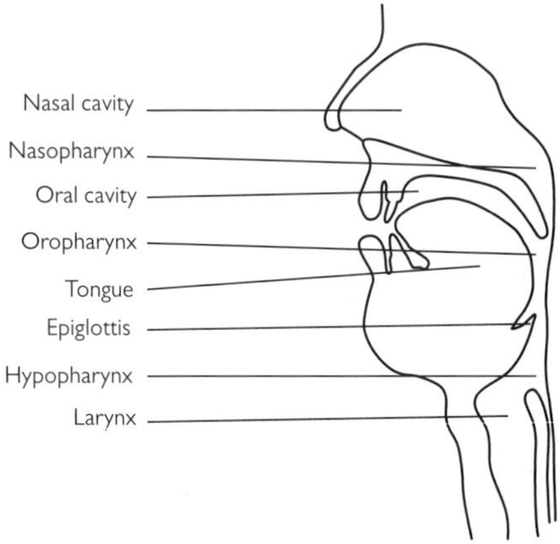
Nasal cavity
Nasopharynx
Oral cavity
Oropharynx
Tongue
Epiglottis
Hypopharynx
Larynx

Fig. 14.21 Upper aerodigestive tract.

Consent

The procedure itself carries a risk associated with anaesthesia, a risk of chipping or otherwise damaging the teeth, or dislocating the TMJ, and a chance that the desired view of the pharynx or larynx is not achieved.

Further intervention, such as biopsy or phonosurgery, carries additional risks, including infection and bleeding, vocal cord scarring leading to dysphonia, and (rarely) even swallow symptoms or swelling compromising the airway. The nature of these risks depends upon the expected intervention.

Preoperative preparation

The indications for the operation are checked. Records from clinic, including a record of flexible nasendoscopic examination, are important. In some ways these are better forms of examining the pharynx and larynx, and their findings can help target the examination.

Position and theatre set-up

The laryngoscopy position is supine on the operating table with the head on a head ring, thus extending the neck superiorly and adopting the 'sniffing the morning air' position.

Procedure

- Teeth are protected with a mouth guard or wet swab.
- Palpating of the base of tongue and tonsils is conducted.
- The laryngoscope is lubricated and inserted into the mouth.
- With care not to lever on the teeth, the tip if the laryngoscope is elevated and the epiglottis is identified.
- The oropharynx may now be examined, including the vallecula.
- The epiglottis is passed and both pyriform fossae are entered and examined.
- The intervening post-cricoid area is also examined.
- The larynx is then entered and examined.
- If microlaryngoscopy is performed, this area can be entered initially.
- If laryngeal surgery is going to take place, a suspension arm may be attached to support the laryngoscope in place whilst two hands are used to operate.

Closure

Not required.

Postoperative care

If phonosurgery is undertaken, voice rest for 2–3 days is usually advised.

Complications

Damage to the teeth can require dental input. Anterior glottic scarring after laryngeal surgery is difficult to manage, and can require a piece of silastic to be sutured into the anterior commisure for 1–2 weeks.

Tips and tricks

If a view of the larynx cannot be obtained, elevation of the head may facilitate access.

Branchial cyst excision and excision of a cervical lymph node for diagnosis

Overview

The excision of branchial cleft cysts is a relatively commonly performed procedure. Branchial cleft cysts commonly arise in the 2nd or 3rd decade and may be liable to recurrent infections. There is controversy surrounding their likely aetiology. They arise in level 2 almost invariably. In older patients, a differential diagnosis may be a cystic metastasis of an upper aerodigestive tract squamous cell carcinoma.

Cervical lymph nodes vary hugely in their location. Excision for diagnosis is most commonly performed in cases of suspected lymphoma as a diagnosis of SCC can usually be made on FNA. The nature of a procedure to excise such a lump will vary depending on their location.

Anatomy

The anatomy of the hypoglossal and spinal accessory nerves are important to consider (Fig. 14.22).

Indications

- Branchial cleft cysts are excised on the basis of confirming diagnosis, preventing their possible enlargement, and preventing recurrent infection.
- Lymph nodes may be excised when they are persistent and a diagnosis of a condition such as lymphoma or other lymphoproloferative or oncological diagnoses are considered.

Equipment

- Scalpel with 10 blade.
- McIndoe scissors.
- Toothed forceps.
- Needle holder.
- Bipolar forceps.

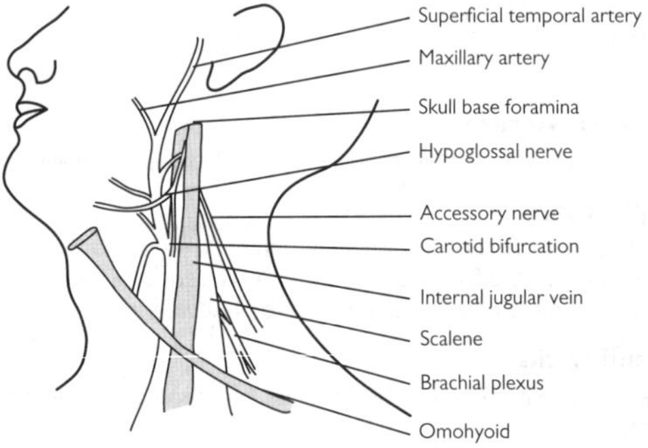
Superficial temporal artery
Maxillary artery
Skull base foramina
Hypoglossal nerve
Accessory nerve
Carotid bifurcation
Internal jugular vein
Scalene
Brachial plexus
Omohyoid

Fig. 14.22 Lateral neck anatomy.

- Self-retaining forceps.
- Langenbach retractors.
- Vicryl®.
- Monocryl®.

Consent

The small risk of nerve injury should be mentioned. Dependent on the location of the lymph node, other cranial nerves than the accessory may be at risk. If operating in level 4 on the left the thoracic duct is potentially at risk. These potential complications will depend on the site and depth of the node.

Bleeding and infection can be potentially problematic. An incision is required, usually in a neck crease in the region. Incomplete excision of the node or cyst can also be problematic, but is uncommon.

Preoperative preparation

The site is marked, and investigations are checked.

Position and theatre set-up

- GA.
- Patient supine, with the head turned away to improve access to the cervical tissues on that side.

Procedure

- Infiltration with LA and adrenaline is optional.
- The incision is marked.
- Division of skin.
- Division of platysma.
- Identification of lesion within fibro-fatty tissue of the neck.
- Extracapsular dissection around the lesion taking care not to rupture.
- Haemostasis.
- A drain may be placed.

Closure

Closure of platysma with Vicryl® and skin with Monocryl®.

Postoperative care

- A drain may be removed the next morning if there has been a sufficiently low output.
- Patients may have a day-care operation, or be kept for one night.
- Patients are seen in clinic for discussion of histology.

Complications

Accessory nerve injury is the feared complication. Should this occur, physiotherapy should be commenced at an early stage. Seroma may be managed conservatively.

Tips and tricks

An incisional biopsy of a lymph node may be necessary for very large conglomerate masses, as excision will often carry greater risks, and an incisional biopsy may well be sufficient for diagnosis.

Excision of thyroglossal cyst

Overview

Thyroglossal cysts are remnants of the embryological development of the thyroid.

Anatomy

Thyroglossal cysts occupy a tract between the thyroid and the foramen caecum in the tongue base. This is the course of descent of the thyroid in development. They may be classified by their relation to the hyoid.

Indications

Recurrent infection, confirmation of diagnosis.

Equipment

- Scalpel with 10 blade.
- Alice forceps.
- McIndoe scissors.
- Toothed forceps.
- Needle holder.
- Bipolar forceps.
- Bone-cutting forceps.
- Self-retaining forceps.
- Langenbach retractors.
- Vicryl®.
- Monocryl®.

Consent

- The risk of infection, bleeding, and the requirement for a scar should be mentioned.
- There is a risk of recurrence of these lesions, although surgical steps can be undertaken to minimize this risk.

Preoperative preparation

It is essential to confirm that there is functional thyroid tissue that does not lie within the thyroglossal cyst. In a minority of these patients, the deficit in descent of the thyroid leaves all functioning thyroid tissue within the cyst. Excision of the cyst would thus leave the patient hypothyroid. An ultrasound of the neck is usually considered sufficient to confirm the presence of a normal thyroid, although some units routinely perform other tests.

Position and theatre set-up

The patient is supine with a shoulder roll and head ring to allow neck extension.

Procedure

- Infiltration of LA is optional.
- A skin crease incision is made near the upper margin of the palpable cyst.
- Platysma is divided and the cyst is identified between the straps or, if necessary, the straps are divided.
- The inferior border of the cyst is dissected.
- A wide area of the central compartment of the neck is excised heading superiorly towards the hyoid.
- The middle-third of the hyoid is grasped with Allis forceps, skeletonized, and excised.
- The tract of the cyst is excised widely into the tongue base and diathermy is used to divide the tract near its root.
- Haemostasis is ensured. A drain is usually sited.

Closure

Closure in layers with Vicryl® and Monocryl®.

Postoperative care

The drain is removed the following morning if the output has been sufficiently low—usually <30ml by the next morning is considered acceptable.

Complications

Recurrent thyroglossal cysts are problematic as revision surgery is challenging and a greater volume of tissue may need to be excised.

Tips and tricks

Wide, local excision is essential to prevent recurrence. In some cases, this may even involve resection of a very small amount of the medial border of the strap muscles.

Uvulopalatopharyngoplasty

Overview

Uvulopalatopharyngoplasty, commonly termed UPPP, is a procedure designed to induce scarring in the soft palate and restrict its movement. Consequently post-procedure pain requires skilful management.

Anatomy

The operation occurs within the oropharynx (Fig. 14.23).

Indications

- Snoring resistant to treatment with conservative measures such as mandibular advancement splints.
- It may also be indicated in selected cases of obstructive sleep apnoea, most commonly if treatment with CPAP has failed.

Equipment

- As for 'Tonsillectomy' (p. 808).
- Monopolar diathermy.
- Otherwise CO_2 laser.

Consent

The postoperative recovery is painful, and this should be made clear to the patient. It is not always successful at stopping snoring, which is very common, and there is some evidence to suggest that its efficacy diminishes over time as the elasticity of the tissue recovers. Infection and bleeding can occur but are rarely problematic, unless concomitant tonsillectomy is also performed, in which case bleeding is a significant risk. Nasal regurgitation is uncommon, but may occur.

Preoperative preparation

Preoperative investigations should be confirmed.

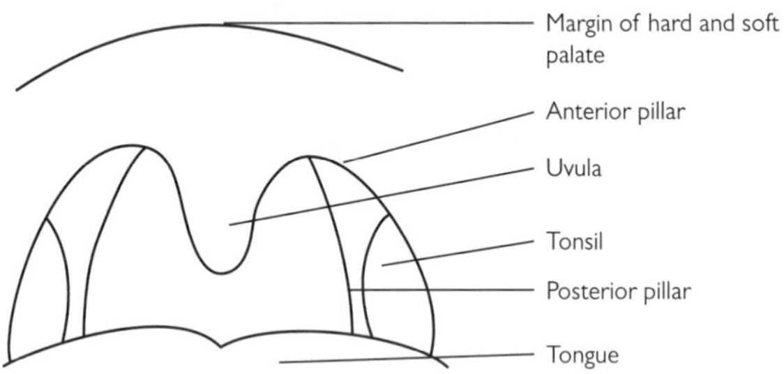
Margin of hard and soft palate
Anterior pillar
Uvula
Tonsil
Posterior pillar
Tongue

Fig. 14.23 Anatomy of the oropharynx.

Position and theatre set-up

Tonsillectomy position (p. 809).

Procedure

- Boyle Davis gag is inserted and secured with Draffin rods.
- If tonsillectomy is going to be performed, it is performed at this stage.
- Measurement and marking of the soft palate, so that two triangles of soft tissue are planned for excision. Vertical incisions extend superiorly no further than 25% of the whole soft palate length.
- The inferior half of the uvula is excised with mucosa between the incision and the tonsillectomy site preserved. The plane of excision is bevelled slightly, with the posterior part of the uvula preserved.

Closure

Not necessary.

Postoperative care

Postoperative analgesia is important. Some patients may benefit from one or two doses of dexamethasone.

Complications

Nasal regurgitation is usually managed conservatively, and almost invariably settles. Palatal surgery to correct such a problem is challenging, and may not be possible.

Tips and tricks

Measurement of the soft palate and uvula can allow precision, and potentially reduce the chance of persistent symptoms, or nasopharyngeal regurgitation.

Parotidectomy

Overview

Parotidectomy is an operation for the removal of tumours of the salivary gland. The parotid is divided into superficial and deep parts, divided by a fascial plane in which the facial nerve and its branches lie. Total parotidectomy, therefore, carries a high risk of facial nerve injury. More limited operations are commonly performed for the removal of these tumours, which are most frequently found in the superficial part of the gland. Unlike operations on the submandibular gland, parotidectomy is not performed for the management of siallorhoea.

Anatomy

The parotid gland lies in the posterior aspect of the cheek and drapes over the ramus of the mandible. Its position is shown. It's relation to the facial nerve is crucial (Figs 14.24 and 14.5).

When performing parotidectomy, landmarks for the detection of the facial nerve are important. It is at the same depth as the posterior belly of digastric. The tympanomeatal suture line may be palpated to give its point of origin, and the tracheal cartilage can indicate its direction (although this can be a slightly unreliable marker).

Indications

Removal of benign or malignant tumours from the parotid gland.

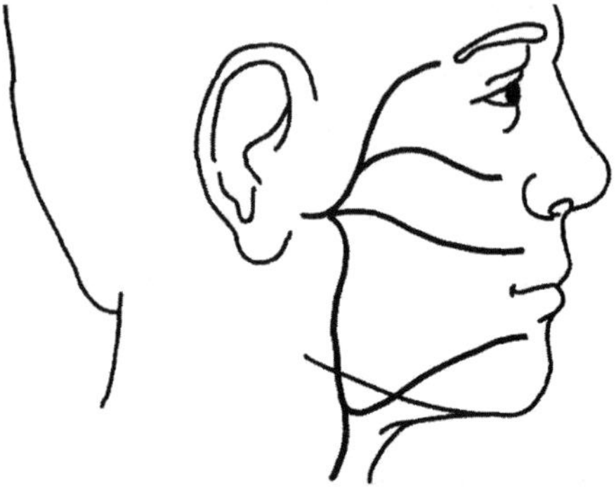

Fig. 14.24 Anatomy of the right facial nerve—typical pattern. Reproduced from McLatchie, G. and Leaper, D., Operative Surgery 2nd edition, 2006, with permission from Oxford University Press.

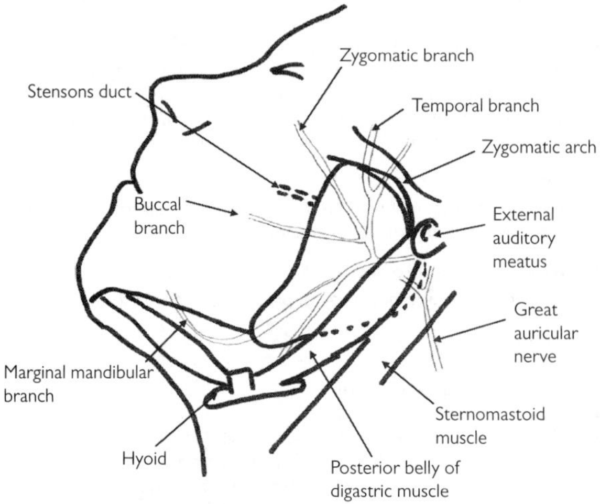
Zygomatic branch
Stensons duct
Temporal branch
Zygomatic arch
Buccal branch
External auditory meatus
Great auricular nerve
Marginal mandibular branch
Sternomastoid muscle
Hyoid
Posterior belly of digastric muscle

Fig. 14.25 Anatomy of the left parotid gland. Reproduced from McLatchie, G. and Leaper, D., Operative Surgery 2nd edition, 2006, with permission from Oxford University Press.

Equipment

- Scalpel with 10 blade.
- Mayo scissors.
- Alice forceps.
- McIndoe scissors.
- Toothed forceps.
- Needle holder.
- Bipolar forceps.
- Self-retaining forceps.
- Langenbach retractors.
- Vicryl®.
- Monocryl®.
- Prolene®.

Consent

The rationale for the operation is discussed. The most common indication is removal of a suspected pleomorphic adenoma. The rationale for the excision of these tumours is confirmation of diagnosis (and consequently ruling out malignancy), prevention of enlargement, and cosmetic removal of a cheek lump. Furthermore, a small proportion of pleomorphic adenoma will undergo malignant transformation over a lengthy period. These malignancies are characteristically very aggressive and challenging to manage.

The risks most notably relate to the facial nerve. Temporary paresis is seen in up to 15–20% of patients with permanent weakness in one or more branch of the facial being seen in around 2% (although individual surgeon's figures will vary significantly). Other risks include Frey's syndrome, salivary fistula, incomplete tumour excision/rupture of tumour capsule/recurrence of tumour, bleeding and haematoma formation, wound infection, and numbness of the earlobe (which may be permanent).

Preoperative preparation

- Preoperative imaging should be checked, and the diagnosis confirmed.
- A facial nerve monitor is recommended.

Position and theatre set-up

Supine with the head turned away to present the parotid to the surgeon.

Procedure

- Skin preparation.
- LA with adrenaline is optional.
- Draping of the operative field.
- Incision—modified Blair or otherwise facelift (Fig. 14.26).
- Raising of a plane over the capsule of the parotid.
- Dissecting the anterior border of sternocleidomastoid.
- Identification of the posterior belly of digastric.
- Exploration of pre-tragal plane towards the facial nerve.
- Identification of the facial nerve using the above stated landmarks.
- A plane superficial to the facial nerve is developed.
- The lump is manipulated and the parotid divided superficial to the identified facial nerve.
- Depending on the location of the lump, one, two, or more of the facial nerve branches may need to be followed.
- The parotid tissue, elevated off the facial nerve over one or more branches, is excised and sent for histology.
- Haemostasis is ensured. A drain is sited.

Closure

- Subcutaneous with Vicryl®, skin of the face anterior to the ear with 5-0 Prolene®, skin of the neck with Monocryl®.
- A head bandage is often used to provide pressure on the operative site.

Postoperative care

- The drain may be removed the next morning, depending on the output.
- The histology may be reviewed at two weeks.

Complications

- Facial nerve palsy may require eye care in the short term if the grade of the facial nerve palsy is sufficient to prevent complete eye closure. It will often recover over time, but may not, particularly if it is recognized that a branch has been cut. In these cases, there may be some facial and oculoplastic procedures to ameliorate the effect of the palsy.

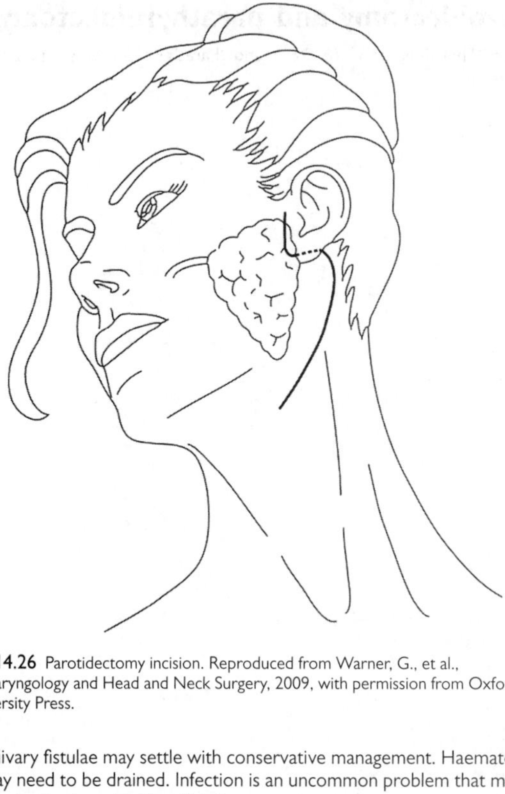

Fig. 14.26 Parotidectomy incision. Reproduced from Warner, G., et al., Otolaryngology and Head and Neck Surgery, 2009, with permission from Oxford University Press.

- Salivary fistulae may settle with conservative management. Haematomas may need to be drained. Infection is an uncommon problem that may require treatment with antibiotics.
- Frey's syndrome is a very common complication, but is rarely symptomatic or troublesome. It may be managed with botulinum toxin, or further surgery.

Tips and tricks

Closure of the parotid capsule, or use of local flaps such as fascial flaps or sternocledиomastoid flaps, may replace tissue defects and potentially limit Frey's syndrome.

Thyroidectomy and parathyroidectomy

➲ See 'Thyroidectomy' (p. 282) and 'Parathyroidectomy' (p. 290) in Chapter 6.

Submandibular gland excision

[illegible]

Anatomy

[illegible]

Lingual nerve

[illegible]

Submandibular gland excision

This topic is reproduced from McLatchie, G, and Leaper, D. Operative Surgery 2nd edition, Oxford University Press: 2006.

Anatomy

The deep part of the submandibular gland lies under cover of the medial border of the mandible, below the oral mucosa and above the mylohyoid muscle. The superficial part is covered by deep fascia, platysma, and skin. The larger superficial and smaller deep lobes are joined around the posterior edge of the mylohyoid muscle. The submandibular duct originates from the deep surface of the deep lobe and passes forwards into the floor of the mouth, where it opens as a papilla lateral to the lingual fraenum behind the lower incisor teeth. The facial artery and vein lie initially deep to the posterior pole and then run over the upper surface of the gland.

The lingual nerve lies above the gland but anteriorly loops around the infero-lateral aspect of the duct (Fig. 14.27) and can therefore be damaged during surgery causing tongue anaesthesia. The mandibular (or marginal) division of the facial (VII) nerve can be damaged during surgery causing ipsilateral weakness of the lower lip. Patients should be warned about possible damage to these two nerves.

Anatomically, the mandibular nerve crosses the facial artery at the lower border of the mandible. In 81% of cases the nerve lies at the level of the lower border posterior to the artery, while the remaining 19% lies anywhere up to 12mm below the mandible. For this reason the incision should be placed in a skin crease at least 2cm below the angle of the mandible. The nerve lies deep to platysma, enveloped in the deep fascia overlying the gland. Anteriorly it becomes more superficial at the angle of the mouth.

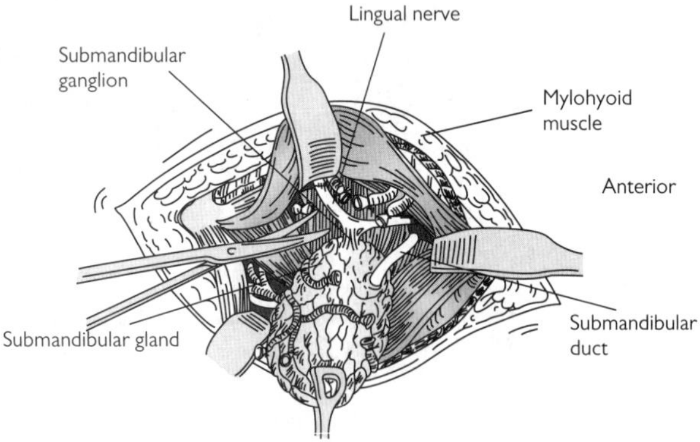
Lingual nerve
Submandibular ganglion
Mylohyoid muscle
Anterior
Submandibular gland
Submandibular duct

Fig. 14.27 Removal of the submandibular gland. Reproduced from McLatchie, G. and Leaper, D., Operative Surgery 2nd edition, 2006, with permission from Oxford University Press.

Indications

- Chronic sialadenitis.
- Stone in submandibular gland or posterior duct causing obstruction.
- Benign tumour arising from gland.
- Surgical management of intractable drooling in handicapped patients.
- Removal as part of radical or selective neck dissection.

Equipment

- Number 15 blade.
- Bipolar diathermy.
- Vacuum drain.
- Vicryl® ties and suture, 4-0 Prolene® suture.

Position

- Supine with head rotated to the opposite side supported by a head ring.
- Tilt the operating table into a head-up position.

Procedure

- Prepare the skin with betadine or chlorhexidine antiseptic. Infiltrate lignocaine subcutaneously with adrenaline to help haemostasis.
- Make a transverse incision placed in a skin crease at least 20mm below the angle of the mandible. Its posterior end should not extend beyond the posterior border of the mandible (Fig. 14.28).
- Divide skin, subcutaneous fat, and the platysma muscle. Continue dissection obliquely upwards through the deep fascia to the inferior aspect of the gland. Thereafter, dissection is continued on the capsule of the gland (except for tumours where the surrounding fascia should also be removed). This avoids damage to the mandibular branch of the facial nerve. Mobilize the gland from the anterior, posterior and inferior aspect.

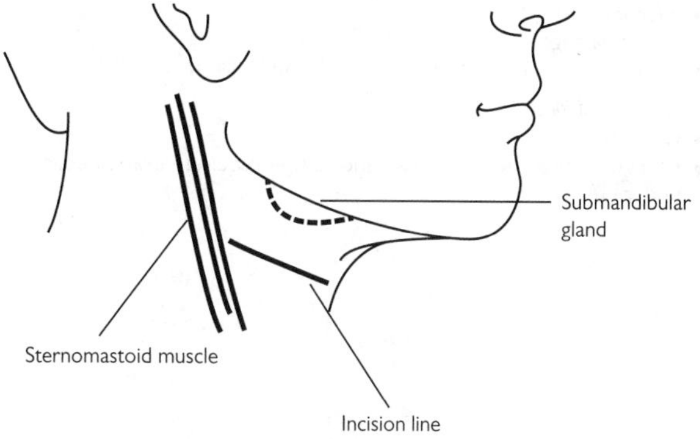
Submandibular gland
Sternomastoid muscle
Incision line

Fig. 14.28 Submandibular gland incision. Reproduced from McLatchie, G. and Leaper, D., Operative Surgery 2nd edition, 2006, with permission from Oxford University Press.

- Identify the facial vessels deep to the posterior part of the gland and divide them.
- Mobilize the superficial lobe of the gland anteriorly off the mylohyoid muscle and retract the muscle forwards. At this point the lingual nerve and submandibular duct can be identified on the deep surface of the mylohyoid muscle. The nerve is looped due to its attachment to the submandibular ganglion.
- Cauterize the attachments of the ganglion to the nerve and divide them. Continued dissection of the gland from the hyoglossus and mylohyoid muscle leaves the gland mobilized on its own duct. Divide the duct and ligate it as far forward into the mouth as possible.
- Carry out careful haemostasis; suture a vacuum drain in place. Close the platysma muscle with Vicryl® sutures and the skin with 4-0 Prolene®. Apply an Opsite dressing.

Postoperative care

Monitor blood loss in the drain. This can usually be removed the following morning and the patient should be discharged 3–4h later after checking that a haematoma has not developed.

Complications

Intraoperative

- Arterial haemorrhage if proximal end of facial artery not properly ligated.
- Damage to mandibular branch of facial nerve, which is usually temporary, due to retraction injury or accidental diathermy.
- Damage to lingual nerve if difficult to see, because of fibrosis following infection.

Postoperative complications

- Haematoma—this sometimes occurs after removal of drain.
- Infection.
- Nerve damage.
- Retained calculi in residual anterior submandibular duct.

Late complications

- Unsightly scar.
- Infection caused by calculi in anterior duct—requires intraoral excision under GA.

Neck dissection

Overview

[illegible]

Anatomy

[illegible]

Indications

[illegible]

Equipment

[illegible]

[illegible]

Neck dissection

Overview

Neck dissection is a term used to describe the bulk removal of cervical lymph nodes within fibro-fatty soft tissue in the neck. Terminology often revolves around which nodal levels are removed, and which structures are preserved. Traditionally, in a radical neck dissection, the spinal accessory nerve, sternocleidomastoid, and internal jugular vein were sacrificed. When these structures are preserved the procedure is termed a modified radical neck dissection or when specific lymph node levels are removed, a selective neck dissection.

Anatomy

Familiarity of the structures of the neck is essential for safely performing neck dissection. There are numerous important structures that usually need to be preserved. These include the carotid artery, vagus nerve, phrenic nerve, sympathetic chain, hypoglossal nerve, accessory nerve, internal jugular vein, thoracic duct, marginal mandibular nerve, and superior thyroid artery (Fig. 14.29).

Indications

Removal of confirmed or suspected metastatic lymph node deposits of tumour. The likelihood for the presence of undetected SCC required to perform prophylactic neck dissection is >20%. Neck dissection type operations may also be performed to facilitate access to the great vessels of the neck in the event of penetrating trauma, or to allow access for free-flap reconstruction.

Equipment

- Scalpel with 10 blade.
- Mayo scissors.
- Alice forceps.
- McIndoe scissors.
- Toothed forceps.
- Needle holder.
- Bipolar forceps.
- Artery clips.
- Self-retaining forceps.
- Langenbach retractors.
- Vicryl®.
- Monocryl®.

Consent

The indication for the operation should be confirmed, and the risks discussed. These are highly variable, depending on the extent of disease, experience of the surgeon, lymph node levels planned, and patient factors such as prior chemo radiotherapy.

In addition to bleeding and infection, cranial nerve injury and damage to the great vessels, the small chance of thoracic duct injury should be considered in level four on the left.

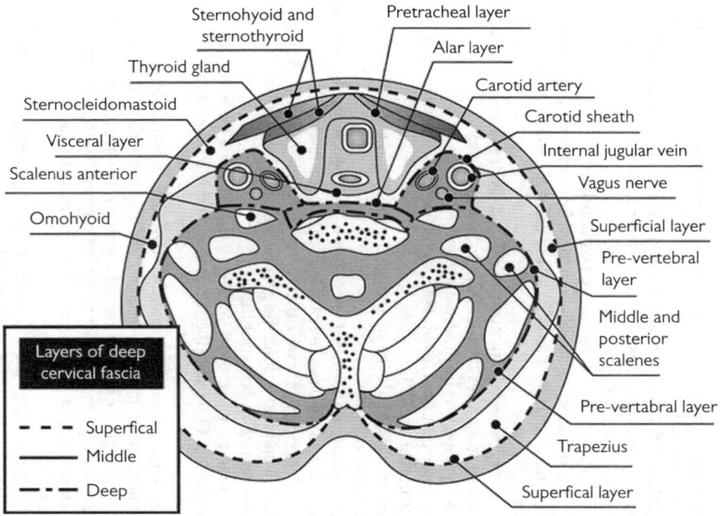
Sternohyoid and sternothyroid
Pretracheal layer
Alar layer
Thyroid gland
Carotid artery
Sternocleidomastoid
Carotid sheath
Visceral layer
Internal jugular vein
Scalenus anterior
Vagus nerve
Omohyoid
Superficial layer
Pre-vertebral layer
Middle and posterior scalenes
Layers of deep cervical fascia
Superfical
Middle
Deep
Pre-vertabral layer
Trapezius
Superfical layer

Fig. 14.29 Layers of the neck. Reproduced from Warner, G., et al., Otolaryngology and Head and Neck Surgery, 2009, with permission from Oxford University Press.

Preoperative preparation

- Review of indication and imaging.
- A headlight may be useful.
- An assistant is mandatory.

Position and theatre set-up

- Supine with the head turned away.
- The head may be elevated to diminish venous bleeding.

Procedure

- A neck crease incision is made at the midpoint of the zonal levels that are to be dissected.
- A subplatysmal flap is elevated over the zonal areas to be dissected. Care should be taken in level 1 to avoid the marginal mandibular nerve, which may run just deep to the platysma.
- Usually the dissection is commenced posteriorly.
- Level 5 may be accessed laterally, and freed from trapezius. The floor of the posterior triangle is found, and the tissue is elevated forwards towards SCM.
- The accessory nerve runs through level 5 and divides level 2, and may be identified as it passes through SCM to prevent injury.
- The level 5 tissue may be divided and sent separately.
- The posterior border of levels 2–4 may be found by dissecting over the anterior border of SCM.
- The tendon of SCM may be used to give an idea of the location of the accessory nerve.
- When the posterior border of levels 2–4 is identified, it may be elevated anteriorly and tissue dissected of the deep cervical fascia.
- The superior border of level 2 should be dissected—the digastric will mark level 1 and also protect the great vessels and hypoglossal nerve as they pass deep to its posterior belly.
- Omohyoid is identified, and if level 4 is included in the dissection, it may be divided. Otherwise this forms the inferior border of level 3 dissection.
- Levels 2–4 may be dissected anteriorly over the carotid sheath. Dissection is easier in a plane directly over the adventitia of the IJV.
- As the dissection specimen is peeled anteriorly, the hypoglossal nerve may be found high and anterior to the IJV running over the carotids.
- Once levels 2–5 have been removed, level 1 may also be removed in continuity.
- Level 1a is bounded by the anterior bellies of digastric on each side and hyoid inferiorly and can be removed safely.
- Level 1b can be moblized postero-inferiorly by dissection of the facial artery off the submandibular gland.
- The submandibular gland is mobilized and the duct is identified, ligated, and divided
- Deep and superior to the SMG lies the lingual nerve, which should be preserved.
- The SMG may be divided into two parts, and both superficial and deep parts should be removed.

Closure

Haemostasis should be ensured, and closure in layers with Vicryl® and Monocryl®.

Postoperative care

A drain may need to be removed. The patient is kept overnight.

Complications

- Sacrifice of the IJV may increase the ICP by a factor of 3. Bilateral sacrifice of the IJV will have a multiplicative effect, and increase ICP by a factor of 10.
- Carotid injury is exceptionally rare, but may occur in extensive disease if the procedure is being performed as part of a palliative plan. Furthermore prior chemo-radiotherapy may increase the risk of this happening. Carotid injury carries a significant injury of stroke.

Tips and tricks

Preservation of arterial pedicles, notably the facial artery, may be useful if a free-flap reconstruction is planned.

Total laryngectomy

Overview

Laryngectomy is removal of the larynx with the formation of a permanent tracheostomy and repair of the pharynx.

Anatomy

The larynx's main function is the prevention of aspiration. It has a secondary role in the production of voice. The larynx lies in the midline in the neck, with little in the way of important structures in the soft tissue overlying the larynx. Deep to the larynx, however, lie the hypopharynx and the upper oesophagus. Closure of this area is essential to laryngectomy, and an understanding of the musculature involved is essential to improving voice and swallow rehabilitation (Fig. 14.30).

Indications

Malignancy of the larynx, not amenable to organ preservation. It may also be performed for a non-functioning larynx, due to prior treatment of malignancy, or occasionally for neuromuscular disease.

Equipment

- Scalpel with 10 blade.
- Mayo scissors.
- Alice forceps.
- McIndoe scissors.
- Toothed forceps.
- Alice forceps.
- Needle holder.
- Artery clips.
- Bipolar forceps.
- Self-retaining forceps.
- Langenbach retractors.
- Vicryl®.
- Monocryl®.

Consent

Laryngectomy has a profound effect on life, and should be extensively discussed prior to proceeding with surgery. This is often done in a multidisciplinary fashion, and it is considered ideal if the patient has the opportunity to meet another patient who has undergone a laryngectomy.

In addition to the cosmetic implications of having an end stoma in the neck, there are implications for normal daily life. The loss of sense of smell and taste will result from lack of nasal airflow. The inability to swim again. The care the stoma requires. These will all need to be discussed.

In the short term the patient will have no voice, but over time the use of a speaking valve, or the development of oesophageal voice, may allow this to be rehabilitated to some extent.

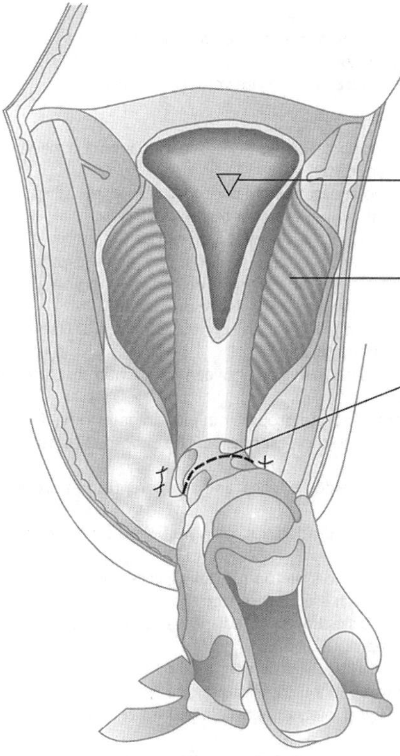
Pharyngeal lumen
Constrictor muscles
Line showing level of division of the trachea

Fig. 14.30 For total laryngectomy. Reproduced from Warner, G., et al., Otolaryngology and Head and Neck Surgery, 2009, with permission from Oxford University Press.

Whilst in patients with benign disease this procedure is designed to improve swallow function, it may take some time to regain swallow after the operation. A proportion of patients will develop stenosis at the site of the pharyngotomy, and this may be persistent.

Further possible risks include pharyngocutaneous fistula, bleeding, and infection. It is a significant operation and there is a very small mortality rate associated with it.

Preoperative preparation

- The indication for the operation is confirmed.
- A dose of antibiotics is usually given at induction.

Position and theatre set-up

- The patient is supine with a shoulder roll to extend the neck, and a head ring to support the head.
- The head may be elevated to alleviate venous bleeding.

Procedure

- A Gluck–Sorensen or apron incision with separate stoma is made.
- Subplatysmal flaps are raised.
- Anterior jugular veins are ligated and divided, as are all the strap muscles, including the omohyoid, to mobilize the larynx.
- If a concomitant hemithyroidectomy is undertaken (as it most commonly is in the case of laryngeal malignancy), then the ipsilateral hemithyroid is resected with the larynx. The recurrent laryngeal nerves may be sacrificed, but the parathyroids are preserved.
- The thyroid isthmus is divided and the contralateral thyroid lobe is mobilized away from the trachea.
- A 'gutter' is fashioned on each side between the carotid sheath and the larynx on each side.
- The trachea is transected and brought out into an end stoma. Care is taken to avoid injury to the oesophagus. The endotracheal tube is removed.
- A stitch supports the divided trachea, and a new ventilation circuit is attached.
- The superior part of the divided trachea is mobilized superiorly away from the oesophagus.
- The hyoid is identified and skeletonized, taking care not to injure the hypoglossal nerve, which is closely related to its greater cornu.
- From the hyoid, the dissection proceeds posteriorly to the anterior part of the root of the epiglottis.
- The epiglottis is held with an Alice forceps, and pulled downwards.
- Scissors are used to open the contralateral pharynx resect along the margins of the laryngeal inlet, and pass around the tumour (if it is close to the pharynx).
- As much pharyngeal mucosa as possible is preserved.
- The laryngeal framework may be grasped and moved to one side in order to dissect free the mucosa of the pyriform fossae from the posterior part of the thyroid cartilage.
- The larynx is dissected anteriorly from the pharynx.
- A finger is placed into the upper oesophagus and a fresh blade is used to cut down onto the finger and divide the cricopharyngeus.
- At this stage a tracheo-oesophageal puncture can be fashioned, and either a speaking valve or a nasogastric feeding tube is inserted into the puncture to maintain its patency and allow feeding.
- The pharyngotomy may be closed horizontally, vertically, or in a 'T-shape'. It is typically closed with an inverting mucosal suture and at least one more layer to reduce the chance of a fistula.

Closure

- Haemostasis is ensured and drains may be placed.
- Closure in layers, with care around the stoma to avoid wound necrosis.
- Non-dissolvable stitches are used in the stoma to hold its position.

Postoperative care

- A laryngectomy tube is placed in patients where swelling around the margins of the stoma may impair the airway.
- Swallow tests are conducted between 1 and 2 weeks after the procedure with water-soluble contrast to determine patency of the neopharynx and rule out a fistula. If this is adequate, feeding may then be commenced.
- It is usual to give the patient 1–5 days of antibiotics postoperatively.
- Venous thromboembolism prophylaxis is often required as the patient will be an inpatient for at least a week after the procedure.
- Drains may be removed the morning after theatre, depending on output.
- Stomal sutures are removed at 2 weeks.

Complications

Fistula formation is the most common significant complication. In addition to delaying discharge, and being unpleasant for the patient, it may be potentially lethal. It may predispose, notably in patients with prior radiotherapy, to carotid blowout. Treatment is by keeping the patient nil-by-mouth, possibly by using anti-muscarinics, such as hyoscine, and the use of antibiotics if there is an infective element. Maintaining nutrition will allow healing and the majority will settle spontaneously. Surgical management is rarely needed and when conducted is most commonly in the form of pedicled flap interposition.

Tips and tricks

- Vertical closure may be undertaken if horizontal closure is not possible. This increases the chance of stenosis at this point.
- If a significant volume of pharyngeal tissue is removed, a pectoralis major flap may be used to provide tissue to the area, and prevent stenosis. These flaps are also useful in preventing fistula formation and aiding healing in patients who have had prior chemo-radiation, or who have concomitant neck dissections. When a large amount of pharyngeal tissue is removed, a pectoralis major flap may be insufficient, and a free jejenum or tubed anterolateral thigh flap can be considered.

Removal of foreign body from nose of a child

Overview

Children between the age of 18 months and 4 years may present having put foreign bodies in the nose. Removal may be undertaken in primary care, A&E, ENT clinics, or in theatre. This may depend on the compliance of the child, the assistance of the mother and staff members, and the location and nature of the foreign body.

Anatomy

- Foreign bodies, depending on their shape, may become lodged in the anterior nasal valve. They are commonly found in the main part of the nasal cavity.
- Infrequently, they may be pushed into the inferior meatus or middle meatus. This is more common with malleable foreign bodies such as polythene or organic matter.

Indications

- All foreign bodies within the nose should be removed. If they are not removed, they act as a focus for infection. When presenting late, children may have a unilateral mucopurulent discharge.
- Batteries may lead to a chemical burn within the nose, and cause lasting damage to the nasal cartilages, and should be removed within a few hours at most.
- It is important to consider the possibility of nasal foreign bodies being aspirated into the trachea. This is uncommon, but can potentially lead to a more serious situation, and necessitate bronchoscopy.

Equipment

- Bart's wax hook.
- Zoellner suction.
- Crocodile forceps.
- Thudicum nasal speculum.
- In some cases, rigid nasal endoscope.
- In some cases, further nasal instruments such as Blakesley forceps.

Consent

There is a small risk of causing epistaxis. There is also a risk of leaving a retained foreign body. Depending on the setting, it is important to consider the risks of anaesthetic or the measures required to ensure the child's cooperation or restraint. This should be discussed prior to the procedure.

Preoperative preparation

- When undertaken using GA, the patient is supine.
- The procedure may be undertaken in the anaesthetic room.
- Outside of this setting, a compliant patient may be seated facing the surgeon. A patient who is not compliant may be restrained, most commonly by wrapping in a blanket. Assistance is required for this procedure.

Position and theatre set-up

- Supine or facing the surgeon.
- Equipment should be immediately available.

Procedure

- Visualize the foreign body.
- If using a hook, the hook should be passed beyond the foreign body, then engaged, and used to pull the foreign body out of the nose.
- The object may be grasped with forceps.
- The nose should be examined to ensure there is no evidence of a retained foreign body.

Closure

Not necessary.

Postoperative care

Patients can be discharged that day.

Complications

- Retained foreign bodies may require examination of the nose under GA.
- If the foreign body is dislodged into the pharynx or trachea, then these sites may need to be examined to prevent the possibility of leaving an inhaled foreign body.
- Epistaxis is uncommon and can usually be managed conservatively.

Tips and tricks

The tool used to remove the foreign body depends primarily on the nature and shape of the foreign body. Slim or flexible foreign bodies may be more amenable to forceps. Solid, round foreign bodies such as beads are more amenable to removal with a hook.

Myringotomy and insertion of grommet

Overview

Grommet insertion is one of the most frequently performed operations in ENT. Their principle is to allow ventilation of the middle ear cavity. Sometimes referred to as 'tubes', they hold open a perforation or myringotomy in the tympanic membrane. There are a number or types of ventilation tubes, the most commonly used in the UK is the Shah grommet. Less commonly used tubes include Permavent™, Paparella grommets or t-tubes. Shah grommets tend to be extruded after about 9 months in children (longer in adults). Other tubes are frequently designed to be more long-lasting.

Anatomy

Grommets are commonly inserted in the antero-inferior part of the tympanic membrane. This is to avoid proximity to the ossicles. They lie with an inner flange within the middle ear (Fig. 14.31).

Indications

- Grommets are most commonly inserted for management of hearing loss in the context of persistent glue ear (otitis media with effusion).
- Other indications include recurrent acute otitis media, management of severe retraction of the tympanic membrane, instillation of intra-tympanic medications or (rarely) in the context of complicated acute otitis media.

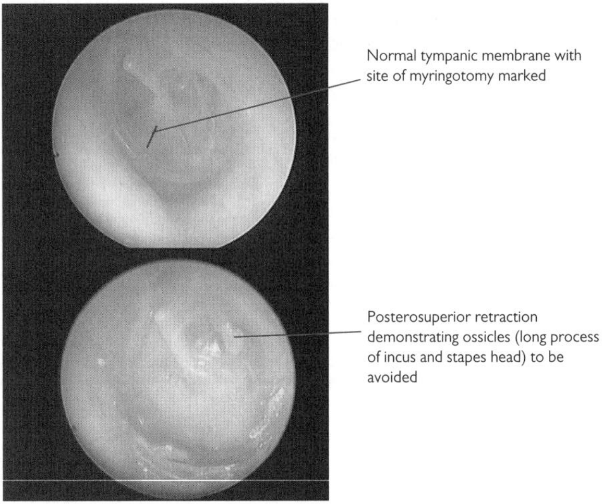
Normal tympanic membrane with site of myringotomy marked
Posterosuperior retraction demonstrating ossicles (long process of incus and stapes head) to be avoided

Fig. 14.31 Normal tympanic membrane demonstrating site of myringotomy and retracted tympanic membrane demonstrating osscíles to be avoided.

Equipment

- Aural speculum, appropriately sized.
- Myringotome.
- Slightly curved needle.
- Grommet.
- Crocodile forceps.
- Zoellner suction with fine end available.
- Jobson Horne probe to assist removal of wax.
- If performed under LA, equipment for this—LA creams or injection.
- Operating microscope.

Consent

- Bleeding is an uncommon risk associated with grommet insertion. A perforated tympanic membrane runs a higher risk of infection leading to otorrhoea. 'Water precautions' to ameliorate this risk are controversial due to their efficacy.
- Grommets may extrude before or after their usual or intended length of action. About 2% of patients will be left with a persistent perforation, which may or may not become problematic and require myringoplasty.
- A proportion of patients will not achieve the intended result of surgery, and a very, very small proportion may suffer damage to the auditory ossicles, with consequent hearing loss.

Preoperative preparation

The indication and audiograms should be checked, and the ear examined. If a unilateral grommet is inserted (this is uncommon), then the surgical side should be marked.

Position and theatre set-up

The patient is supine with the head turned away from the operated site, to provide a comfortable angle for the surgeon to access the tympanic membrane via the ear canal.

Procedure

- Microsuction clearance of the external auditory meatus.
- Incision of the tympanic membrane using a radial cut in the inferior or antero-inferior tympanic membrane.
- Suction, using a fine end, of the contents of the middle ear.
- The longer flange of the grommet is inserted into the myringotomy.
- The needle is used to push the grommet into position within the tympanic membrane.
- Ear drops, commonly ciprofloxacin, are inserted into the ear to prevent clot formation within the grommet with consequent blockage.

Closure

Not necessary.

Postoperative care

- The procedure is usually performed as a day case. It is important to perform an audiogram at the postoperative outpatient visit to ensure that the hearing has improved.
- Dry ear precautions may be recommended. These involve water proof ear plugs when using the bath or swimming.

Complications

Postoperative otorrhoea should be managed with topical antibiotics, usually ciprofloxacin.

Tips and tricks

The flange of the grommet may be manipulated to allow easy passage into the myringotomy. There are a variety of ways in which the grommet can be held when it is inserted into the tympanic membrane, by holding the grommet at its base, top or waist, and in a variety of orientations. Avoid injury to the canal wall and subsequent bleeding as the view can become more difficult.

Tonsillectomy

Overview

Tonsillectomy is one of the most commonly performed operations in ENT. It is commonly performed in both paediatrics and adult settings, but proportionally is more commonly performed in children.

Anatomy

The palatine tonsils lie within the oropharyngx on either side of the throat. They lie superior to the tongue base and lingual tonsils, inferiorly to the soft palate, posterior to palatoglossus (the anterior pillar), and anterior to palatopharyngeus (the posterior pillar). The tonsil is comprised of lymphoid tissue, and comprises part of the Waldemeyer's ring of lymphoid tissue around the upper aerodigestive tract. The tonsil has a fibrous capsule that is partially adherent to the underlying constrictor muscle. Lateral to this lies the carotid artery.

Indications

Tonsillectomy is most frequently indicated for the prevention of recurrent tonsillitis. In a paediatric population, it is also commonly used for the management of obstructive sleep apnoea (OSA). Multiple peritonsillar abcesses may also be managed with tonsillectomy, even in the acute setting. Less common indications include removal for suspected malignancy, to allow access to deeper structures, including the styloid ligament, or for PFAPA (periodic fever, adenitis, phayngitis, apthous ulcer) syndrome.

Equipment

- Boyle–Davis gag.
- Draffin rods.
- Gwynne–Evans tonsil dissector.
- McIndoe scissors.
- Curved Negus clip.
- Negus knot pusher.
- Straight Burkitt clip.
- 2-0 silk ties (60cm long).
- Dennis–Browne tonsil forceps.
- Toothed and non-toothed forceps (long).
- Mollison's pillar retractor.
- Bipolar forceps.
- Suction.
- Mastoid/tonsil swabs.
- Endobronchial suction catheter.

Consent

- Tonsillectomy is a painful procedure, and the pain usually lasts for 2 weeks after the procedure.
- It is important to eat and drink regularly in the postoperative period.
- Bleeding in the postoperative period is a significant complication associated with tonsillectomy, and occurs in about 5% of patients.
- About 1% require a further operation to stop the bleeding.
- Infection, injury to the teeth, tongue or lips, and GA risks should be mentioned.

Preoperative preparation

The indication of the operation is confirmed. It is important to ensure that the child does not have intercurrent infection that may elevate the risk of the operation.

Position and theatre set-up

The patient is supine on the operating table, with a shoulder roll under the shoulders, and the head resting on the operating table.

Procedure

- The Boyle Davis gag is inserted over the endotracheal tube or laryngeal mask airway, heading posteroinferiorly.
- The gag is placed over the teeth.
- With the tube, tongue, and gag in the midline, the gag is opened to allow a view of the oropharynx.
- The gag is held in position by Draffin rods, with the loops of the rods holding the tip of the gag.
- The first tonsil to be dissected is held with the Dennis–Browne forceps and pulled medially. This allows the lateral extent of the tonsil to become clear.
- An incision with scissors or bipolar is used to divide the mucosa between the medialized tonsil and it's lateral margin. The mucosa parallel and running inferior to the tonsil is divided (Fig. 14.32).
- The plane between tonsil and underlying constrictor is found, and the tonsil is dissected around.

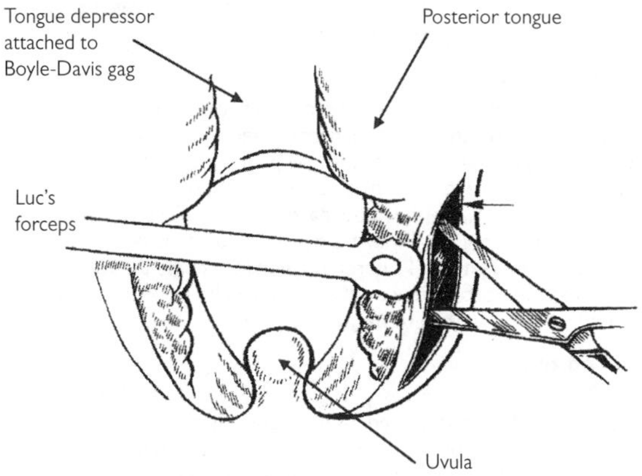
Tongue depressor
attached to
Boyle-Davis gag
Posterior tongue
Luc's
forceps
Uvula

Fig. 14.32 Initial incision. Reproduced from McLatchie, G. and Leaper, D., Operative Surgery 2nd edition, 2006, with permission from Oxford University Press.

- This may be done using a Gwynne–Evans tonsil dissector, or using bipolar forceps. It is important to remain close to the capsule of the tonsil to avoid excessive bleeding and unnecessary trauma to the lateral pharyngeal wall. When the superior pole of the tonsil is free, the tonsil is mobilized inferiorly to clarify its margins; continue dissection.
- The inferior pole may be dissected or clipped with a curved Negus clip. If clipped, the isolated tonsil may be removed with scissors, and a tie placed over the clip and tightened as the clip is removed. This is done using a Negus knot pusher.
- A tonsil or mastoid swab is placed in the tonsil fossa to control bleeding.
- The contralateral tonsil is now removed.
- The fossa is examined for signs of bleeding. The Mollison's pillar retractor can be used to expose the fossa.
- Bleeding is controlled with bipolar and ties, which require the straight Burkitt clip, and subsequently the curved Negus clip.
- Haemostasis is confirmed.
- The teeth and TMJ are checked.
- The post-nasal space is checked and suctioned for blood or clot that may have accumulated.

Closure

Not necessary.

Postoperative care

Patients are usually kept in hospital for a minimum of 4–6h postoperatively. If the procedure was indicated for OSA, then the residual anaesthetic agents may worsen pharyngeal tone and respiratory drive, and patients are therefore often kept overnight for monitoring of oxygen saturations. A clear and effective analgesic regimen is necessary.

Complications

Bleeding is the most common significant complication associated with tonsillectomy. Approximately 5% of patients suffer postoperative bleeding and most can be managed conservatively. All patients are admitted as about 1 in 5 of those who bleed will require emergency surgical management. This management is similar to the latter parts of a tonsillectomy, although the friable, inflamed tonsil fossa may be more difficult to handle. The anterior and posterior pillars may be sutured together to isolate the tonsil bed, and rarely, in extreme circumstances, the throat can be packed, the patient left intubated for 24h and then re-examined.

Tips and tricks

When it is not possible to easily hold the tonsil with the Dennis–Browne forceps, toothed forceps may be used. These may grasp a smaller, less flexible piece of tissue, but are more prone to causing trauma to the tonsil. Better access for haemostasis may be achieved by repositioning the tongue to the contralateral side.

Alternative dissection techniques are also used. These include coblation, which may incur less postoperative pain in the short term. The predominant indication for laser is in cases of tonsillar malignancy.

Adenoidectomy

Adenoidectomy

Overview

Adenoidectomy may be performed on its own, but is more commonly performed as an adjunct to tonsillectomy or grommet insertion.

Anatomy

The adenoids lie in the post-nasal space, as a line of about four prominent pieces of lymphoid tissue falling from near the choana onto the posterior pharyngeal wall.

Indications

- Adenoidectomy is indicated for the management of chronic otitis media with effusion, often being performed if a second set of grommets are required. It may also be undertaken for recurrent acute otitis media. It is thought its effect on the ears is more related to nasopharyngeal biofilms than obstruction of the Eustachian tube orifice.
- Adenoidectomy may also be undertaken in patients with nasal obstruction, and as part of an adenotonsillectomy for OSA.
- Adenoidectomy is almost invariably performed in a paediatric population due to the tendency for adenoid tissue to naturally regress in adolescence.

Equipment

- Boyle–Davis gag.
- Draffin rods.
- Adenoid curette and mirror.
- Monopolar adjustable suction diathermy.
- Endobronchial suction catheter.
- Tonsil/mastoid swabs.

Consent

Adenoidectomy is a relatively safe procedure. Risks of bleeding are low, particularly when suction diathermy adenoidectomy is performed. Infection is rarely problematic, although children usually have very smelly breath in the week after the operation. There are small risks to damaging the teeth, tongue or palate. There is a theoretical risk that injury to the Eustachian tube cushion will worsen middle ear ventilation.

Nasopharyngeal incompetence, or regurgitation, or hyponasal speech is rarely seen after adenoidectomy. This may be an indication of a pre-existing palatal weakness such as a submucus cleft palate.

Preoperative preparation

The patient is supine on the operating table, with no pillow or head ring. A shoulder roll may or may not be used at the discretion of the surgeon.

Position and theatre set-up

The indication of the operation is confirmed.

Procedure

- The Boyle–Davis gag is inserted and secured (see 'Tonsillectomy' on p. 809).
- The uvula and soft palate are inspected, and the soft palate and junction of soft and hard palate are palpated carefully to look for evidence of a submucous cleft palate (i.e. bifid uvula, zona pellucida, central hard palate notch). These may be challenging to recognize.
- An endobronchial suction catheter is inserted through the nose, until it passes into the oropharynx.
- The catheter is the retrieved through the mouth to move the soft palate anteriorly and allow access to the adenoids.
- A mirror is inserted into the oropharynx to allow a view of the adenoids.
- If a currette is used, then this is placed antero-superiorly to the adenoids, and removes the adenoid cushion with a single sweep.
- If suction diathermy is used then the device is bent to allow it to pass through the mouth to the adenoids. It is then placed within the adenoid tissue and activated.
- The adenoids are observed as they reduce in size, and are ablated by the monopolar.
- Care is taken to avoid the Eustachian tube cushion.
- Haemostasis is checked. Bleeding points can be addressed with diathermy, or by packing the post-nasal space.

Closure

- Cold water may be instilled into the nasopharynx to cool tissue that has been heated by monopolar diathermy.
- The teeth and TMJ are checked.

Postoperative care

Patients may have very smelly breath for a week after the procedure. This can be prevented with antibiotic treatment, but the balance of risk and benefit in this setting is very dubious, and antibiotics are therefore not used routinely.

Complications

Nasophayngeal regurgitation usually passes spontaneously. Hyper-nasal speech associated with an unrecognized submucus cleft palate may be addressed with palatoplasty under the care of a cleft team.

Tips and tricks

- The currette may remove adenoid tissue rapidly, but it has a high rate of bleeding, and it may prolong the procedure significantly.
- Coblation may also be used, and the use of microdebriders has been described in the literature.

Microlaryngoscopy + bronchoscopy (MLB)

Overview

MLB is a procedure used to visualize the airway between the pharynx and the first or second bronchial division. It is a dynamic procedure and findings may be best recorded using clinical imaging and video. A number of endoscopic interventions may be undertaken to improve the airway during an MLB, but these will be mentioned only in passing.

Anatomy

The anatomy of the airway in children is important to consider, notably, the parts of the airway that may be liable to compression or stenosis associated with airway pathologies.

Indications

- MLB is most frequently performed as a diagnostic procedure to investigate a chronically stridulous child. It may also be performed to assess children who are not stridulous, but are thought likely to have airway pathology.
- It may detect inhaled foreign bodies.
- It may also be undertaken prior to therapeutic endoscopic or open airway interventions.

Equipment

The gauge and length of the required equipment will depend on the age and size of the child, or adult, being examined.

- Rigid 0 degree Hopkins' endoscope.
- Long suction.
- Anaesthetic laryngoscope—straight and curved.
- Laryngeal probe.
- Age appropriate supraglottic laryngoscope (e.g. Baby Benjamin, Lindholm).
- Suspension arm.
- Rigid ventilating bronchoscope set with age-appropriate sizes should be available (This should include a light prism, suction caps, lenses and bridges).
- Optical grabbing forceps.
- Appropriately sized endotracheal tubes.
- The anaesthetist will require an endotracheal tube, which is placed through the nose into the oropharynx.

Consent

When a purely diagnostic procedure is planned, the risks are small. There is a small risk associated with the GA. There are small risks of dislocating the TMJ, or damaging teeth. Minor trauma can lead to bleeding or swelling in the larynx, which may affect the voice, or uncommonly, the airway.

When intervention, such as removal of papillomas, division and dilatation of stenotic areas, or laser of granulation tissue, the risks are higher. Swelling affecting the airway is more common, and the swallow is also rarely affected.

Preoperative preparation

- Anti-muscarinc medication may be given prior to the induction of anaesthesia. This reduces oropharyngeal secretions.
- A close working relationship between anaesthesia and the surgical team is important. A discussion of the anaesthetic technique, and measures to be taken in the event of desaturation can be discussed.

Position and theatre set-up

- The patient is supine with both a shoulder bolster and a head ring in position. This straightens the axis between the mouth and the carina.
- A suspension arm or table may be used when laryngeal intervention is planned, to support the laryngoscope.

Procedure

- Anaesthesia is induced.
- An endotracheal tube is inserted through the nose such that it lies in the oropharynx and may deliver oxygen if there is spontaneous ventilation with TIVA (total intravenous anaesthesia).
- If inhalational anaesthesia is used, then oxygen and sevoflurane may be administered to maintain oxygenation and anaesthesia in a patient that is self-ventilating.
- The mouth may be closed to allow the accumulation of oxygen and anaesthetic gases.
- When the anaesthetic team is comfortable, the mouth is opened, and an anaesthetic laryngoscope is used to obtain a view of the larynx.
- The rigid endoscope examines the supraglottis and the glottis, and then is advanced to examine the subglottis, trachea, and main bronchi.
- Images are taken at these steps to record the findings. Video may also be helpful (Figs 14.33–14.37).

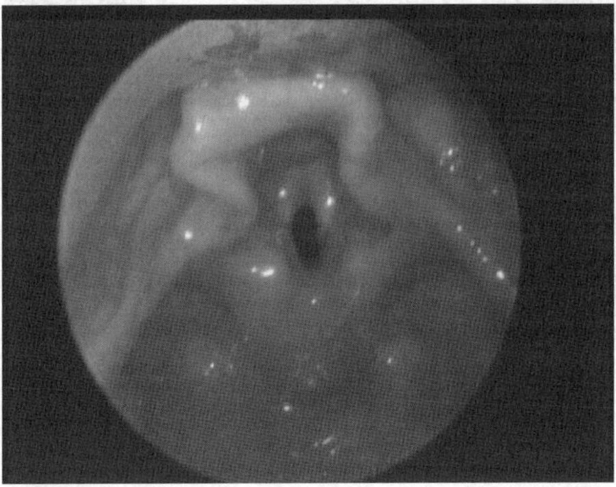

Fig. 14.33 View of supraglottis.

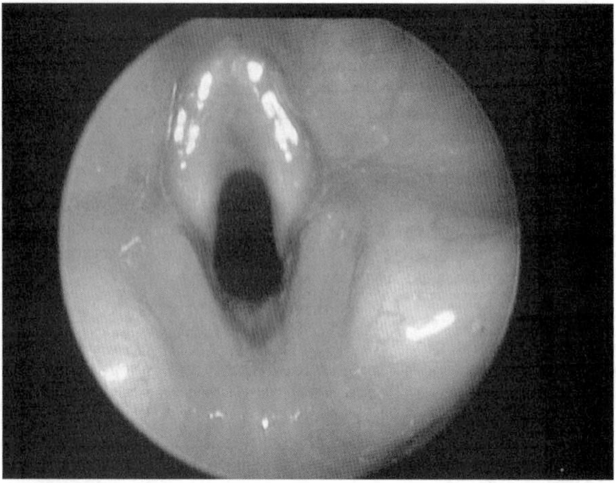

Fig. 14.34 View of glottis.

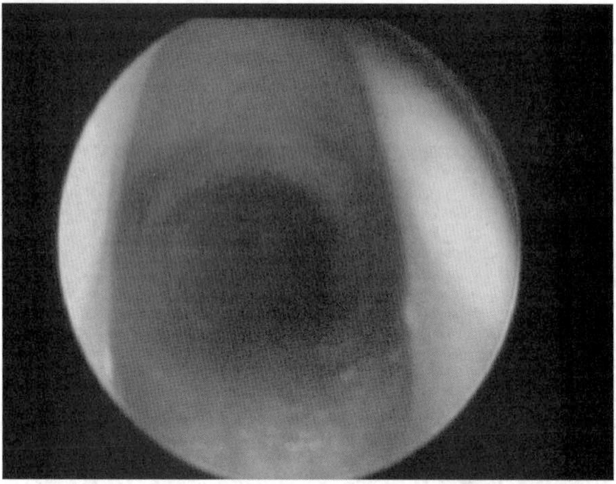

Fig. 14.35 View of subglottis.

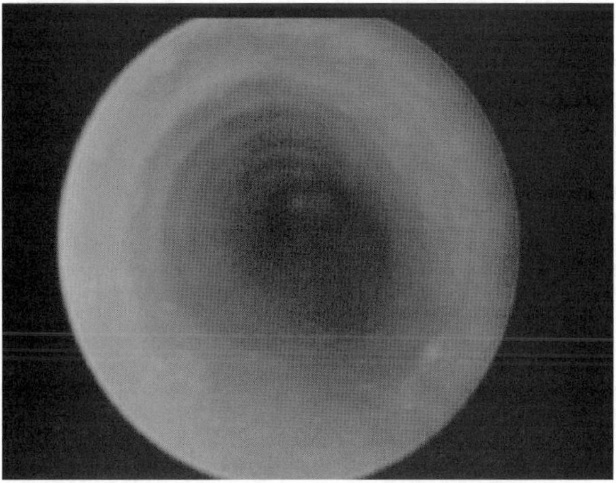

Fig. 14.36 View of trachea.

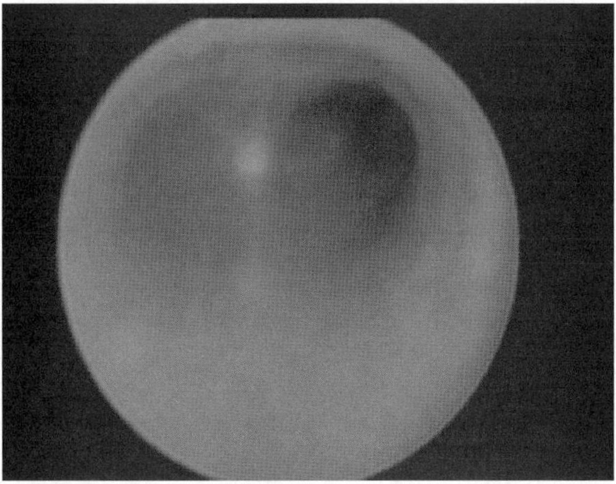

Fig. 14.37 View of carina.

- The laryngeal probe is used to palpate for crico-arytenoid joint mobility and laryngeal clefts.
- Bilateral vocal cord spontaneous movement should be observed.

Postoperative care

Patients are usually observed overnight, such that any potential airway compromise can be managed.

Complications

Minor trauma may lead to oedema and consequent airway obstruction. This can be managed with inhaled adrenaline and intravenous steroid. It is rare for the patient to require intubation, unless there is a pre-existing severe stenosis. This will usually be evident preoperatively, and in these cases it is not unusual for tracheostomy to be performed.

Tips and tricks

Close collaboration with the anaesthetic team is essential to conduct this procedure smoothly and safely.

Paediatric tracheostomy

Overview

Tracheostomies may be difficult to manage in an adult population, but they are much more challenging in paediatrics. Where possible, they are avoided, but there will invariably be children who require a tracheostomy on a short- or long-term basis.

Anatomy

Children tend to have a shorter, more adipose neck than adults. The trachea is smaller, and may be softer. The thyroid is also smaller, and less vascular than the adult organ.

Indications

Tracheostomies are usually inserted in patients with significant airway compromise that is not amenable to endoscopic or open management. This may be due to the size and age of the patient, or the nature of the pathology. Tracheostomy may also be recommended for the management of very severe OSA, most commonly in children with craniofacial syndromes. Tracheostomy can also be indicated as an adjunct to procedures that may affect the airway, such as mandibular advancement.

Equipment

- Age/size-appropriate tracheostomy tube, with the suction length checked.
- One size smaller tracheostomy tube.
- Sterile anaesthetic circuit connector.
- Scalpel with 10 and 15 blade.
- Forceps, McIndoe scissors, needle holder.
- Swabs.
- Paediatric self-retainer.
- Vicryl® and Prolene® sutures.
- Bipolar diathermy forceps.

Consent

- Having a tracheostomy is a major undertaking, but it may be necessary to preserve life, or to allow the child's development.
- When the tracheostomy is in, the child's cry will be very quiet, and many parents find this distressing. The impairment to laryngeal elevation may make swallowing more difficult. Tracheostomy tubes can become dislodged, or blocked, and this may precipitate life-threatening airway obstruction.
- There are small risks associated with bleeding and infection. There are very rare reports of pneumothorax and tracheal trauma leading to tracheo-oesophageal or tracheo-innominate fistula.
- A high proportion of patients with tracheostomies left for a significant period will have a persistent tracheo-cutaneous fistula.

Preoperative preparation

Appropriate consent is important. Paediatric tracheostomy requires a significant care requirement and this should be planned preoperatively. Prior to proceeding with this operation, the indication should be confirmed, and microlaryngoscopy and bronchoscopy should be considered to assess the current status of the airway.

A clear discussion should be had with the anaesthetist to discuss management of the airway during the procedure. If there is no airway compromise and the operation is being performed on an elective basis, the patient may be intubated or may already be intubated. Laryngeal mask airways may play a role, but subglottis stenosis may make ventilation difficult. Unlike adult patients, there is no role for attempted LA tracheostomy in a paediatric setting.

Position and theatre set-up

- The patient is supine, with a shoulder roll and head ring.
- It is important to ensure that there is sufficient neck extension to bring the trachea anteriorly in the neck and facilitate access.
- A tape is used to retract the adipose tissue of the neck superiorly and further facilitate access. This is necessary in younger children as they have a tendency to fatter necks.

Procedure

These steps are assuming a planned operation. Rarely, in life-threatening airway obstruction, an emergency procedure may need to be performed that does not include all of the below steps. A balance is made between the time taken to complete the procedure and the control of the airway and bleeding that a slower procedure will allow.

- Infiltration of LA with adrenaline.
- A vertical or transverse incision at midpoint between cricoid cartilage (more prominent than thyroid cartilage in children) and sternal notch.
- Removal of subcutaneous fat pad in area tracheostomy tube will sit.
- Transverse division of platysma.
- Dissection superiorly and inferiorly of the fascial plane overlying strap muscle.
- Lateral retraction of the strap muscles.
- Identification and division with bipolar cautery of the thyroid isthmus.
- Exposure of anterior trachea.
- Discussion with anaesthetics about subsequent airway steps. If present, the cuff of the endotracheal tube may be deflated.
- Placement of 2-0 Prolene® stay sutures in a paramedian position in the trachea. Sutures are clipped long, and the clips are placed on either side of the neck to bring the trachea anteriorly.
- Vertical slit in midline of trachea between the 3rd and 4th tracheal rings.
- Maturation sutures: 4-0 Vicryl® are placed between the margin of the incision and the margin of the skin to bring the trachea and skin edge together.
- Endotracheal tube is withdrawn until the tip lies just superior to the incision.

- The endotracheal tube is placed.
- A clean connector is placed between the tracheostomy tube and anaesthetic circuit.
- End tidal CO_2 is checked to confirm the position of the tube.

Closure

Cotton tracheostomy ties are placed around the neck to secure the tube. This should be done with the neck in a neutral position, after removal of the head ring and shoulder roll. They should be tied sufficiently tight that one finger can be placed between the neck and ties, but no more than one finger. A tracheostomy dressing is placed.

Postoperative care

- The patient is accompanied back to the ward and a clear handover is given, including the length of endobronchial suction catheter required for suction.
- A CXR is arranged.
- The inspired air or oxygen is humidified. Nebulizers are helpful. The tube should be suctioned regularly.
- The first change is performed no earlier than 1 week after the tracheostomy is sited by a trained person with assistance.

Complications

- Pneumothorax is an uncommon complication but should be checked with a CXR.
- Tracheal granulation may be a consequence of excessive suctioning, or an inappropriately sized tube.
- Tracheo-cutaneous fistulae may be closed in layers if they persist for some months after removal of the tube.

Tips and tricks

Close collaboration with anaesthetics is necessary to ensure that the airway is safely maintained whilst the operation is performed.

Laryngotracheal reconstruction and cricotracheal resection

Overview

Laryngotracheal reconstruction (LTR) and cricotracheal resection (CTR), or tracheal resection (TR) are considered the definitive open surgical procedures for subglottic stenosis.

Broadly speaking, LTR involves the dissection of the larynx and upper trachea, a vertical incision being made in the trachea, and cartilage grafts, usually taken from the costal margin, being placed in the margins of the cut trachea to hold the airway open. Concomitant stenting or intubation is performed to ensure the patency of the airway whilst healing occurs.

Tracheal resection involves resection of the stenotic segment and mobilization of the trachea to allow a tension free end to end anastomosis.

Chapter 15

Oral and maxillofacial surgery

Intra-oral nerve blocks

Nasopalatine and greater palatine nerve block

(See Fig. 15.1)

Anatomy

- The incisive canal, located under the incisive papilla, transmits the nasopalatine nerve, which supplies the anterior palate.
- The greater palatine nerve leaves its foramen 1–2cm medial to the 2nd/3rd maxillary molar and courses anteriorly supplying the ipsilateral side of the palate up to the canines

Procedure

- Insert the needle just lateral to the incisive papilla, a few mm in depth, aspirate and deposit 0.2ml LA.
- Repeat this just in front of the posterior border of the hard palate, approximately a finger's breadth medial to the teeth on each side.
- Full palatal anaesthesia can be achieved with these three injections.

Inferior dental nerve (IDB) and lingual nerve block

(See Fig. 15.2)

Anatomy

- The posterior division of the mandibular nerve gives rise to the inferior alveolar nerve (IAN) and lingual nerve.
- The IAN enters the mandibular foramen and supplies the teeth and labial gingiva of the ipsilateral half of the mandible.

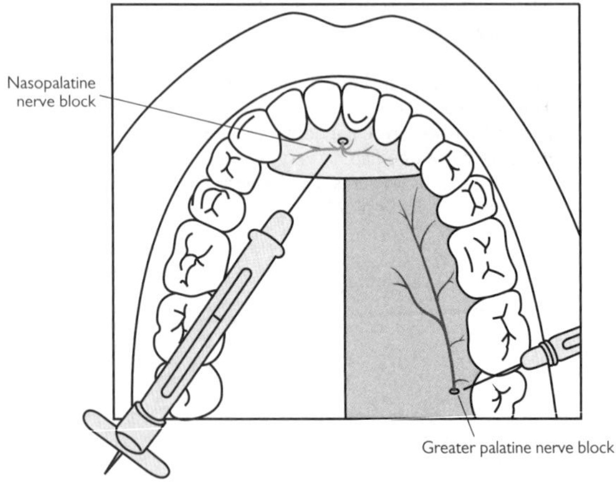
Nasopalatine nerve block
Greater palatine nerve block

Fig. 15.1 Anatomy and injection position for palatal anaesthesisa.

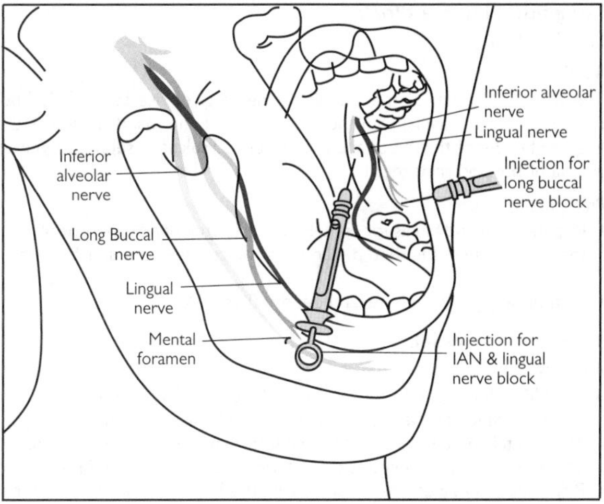
Inferior alveolar nerve
Lingual nerve
Injection for long buccal nerve block
Inferior alveolar nerve
Long Buccal nerve
Lingual nerve
Mental foramen
Injection for IAN & lingual nerve block

Fig. 15.2 Anatomy and injection position for IAN, lingual, and long buccal nerve blocks.

- The lingual nerve descends with the inferior alveolar nerve towards the mandibular foramen, but does not enter it, instead travelling anteriorly along the lingual surface of the mandible above mylohyoid to supply the lingual gingiva, floor of mouth and anterior two-thirds of the tongue.

Procedure

- Hold the mandible in the non-dominant hand, placing the thumb on the anterior border of the ramus above the 3rd molar intra-orally, and index finger extra-orally along the posterior border of the mandible.
- The mandibular foramen usually lies just posterior and superior to the thumb nail in this position.
- Approaching from the angle of the contralateral premolars, insert the needle just above and behind the thumb nail until bone is reached—this should be at a depth of 15–25mm.
  - Failure to hit bone requires altering the angle and position of the needle; reinsert approaching from the contralateral molars.
  - If bone is reached too soon then the needle is likely to be in front of the mandibular foramen, so re-approach from the angle of the contralateral canine.
- Withdraw slightly, aspirate, and deposit 1.5ml LA.
- For lingual nerve blockade, withdraw the needle halfway, aspirate again, and deposit a further 0.5ml LA.

Long buccal nerve block

(See Fig. 15.3)

Anatomy

The anterior division of the mandibular nerve gives rise to the long buccal nerve, which travels from the medial side of the mandible across the anterior border of the ramus and into the buccal sulcus to supply the buccal gingiva of the posterior teeth.

Procedure

- Palpate the mandible as for an IDB, but insert the needle in front of the ramus behind the third molar and advance a few mm until bone is reached.
- Withdraw slightly, aspirate, and deposit 0.5ml LA.

Mental nerve block

Anatomy

- The IAN bifurcates into the incisive and mental nerve at the mental foramen, which sits between the 1st and 2nd lower premolars.
- The mental nerve is sensory to the internal and external lip and chin.
- The incisive nerve innervates the anterior teeth and labial gingivae.
- Pulpal anaesthesia can be obtained with this block as anaesthetic enters the foramen to block the incisive nerve.

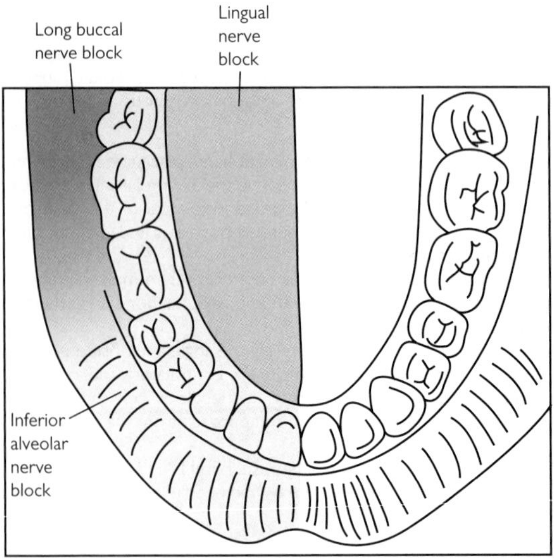
Long buccal nerve block
Lingual nerve block
Inferior alveolar nerve block

Fig. 15.3 Area of anaesthesia for IAN, lingual and long buccal nerve blocks.

Procedure

Palpate the mental foramen and insert the needle in the buccal sulcus just below before aspirating and depositing 0.5ml LA.

Buccal/labial and palatal/lingual infiltration

Used for isolating smaller segments (e.g. single tooth extractions).

Procedure

- For buccal/labial infiltration, retract the cheek and insert the needle into the buccal sulcus along the axis of the tooth, depositing 0.5ml LA next to where the apex is expected.
- Lingual infiltration uses the same technique on the lingual surface of the mandible but should be reserved for the anterior teeth to avoid damage to the lingual nerve.
- Palatal infiltration is similar to greater palatine nerve blockade, but just distal to the tooth required.

Nerve blocks of the face

Overview

Local anaesthetics are used frequently to close wounds and excise small lesions, and are often prepared with a vasoconstrictor to assist haemostasis (see Table 15.1). An awareness of the regional blocks described in this section (p. 830, p. 831) is extremely useful depending on location of the lesion.

Supraorbital/supratrochlear nerve block

(See Fig. 15.4)

Anatomy

- The supraorbital and supratrochlear nerves emerge from the supraorbital notch/foramen at the supraorbital ridge vertically above the medial border of the iris.
- Blocking these nerves will anaesthetize the forehead from the midline, extending laterally to the superior temporal line and superiorly to the middle of the scalp.

Procedure

- Palpate the supraorbital notch, holding some gauze between the eyelid and the supraorbital ridge (this will prevent swelling of the eyelid and LA contacting the eye).
- Insert the needle laterally and advance medially along the supraorbital ridge towards the foramen.
- Just prior to reaching the foramen aspirate and deposit 1ml of LA, before continuing to advance, and deposit a further 1ml just after the foramen.

Table 15.1 Common preparations and doses

	Onset (min)	Duration (min)	Max dose (mg/kg)	Max adult dose (mg)	Max adult dose (ml)
Lidocaine plain 1% or 2%	1–4	15–60	3	200	20 (1%) 10 (2%)
Lidocaine with 1:200,000 adrenaline	1–4	120–360	7	150	15
Lidocaine 2% with 1:80,000 adrenaline	1–4	120–360	4.4	308	15.4 i.e. 7 cartridges
Levobupivicaine 0.25% or 0.5%	10–15	120–240	2.5	150	60 (0.25%) 30 (1%)

Infraorbital nerve block

(See Fig. 15.4)

Anatomy

- The infraorbital nerve emerges from the infraorbital foramen, which can be palpated 4–7mm below the infraorbital rim in line with the medial border of the iris.
- Blocking the infraorbital nerve anaesthetizes the lower eyelid to the upper lip, extending medially to the lateral wall of the nose, and laterally about 15mm past the lateral commissure of the eye

Procedure

- Palpate the infraorbital notch.
- Insert the needle between the alar groove and nasolabial fold, and advance superiorly towards the infraorbital foramen.
- Alternatively, the infraorbital foramen can be approached intra-orally by inserting the needle into the part of the upper buccal sulcus closest to it and advancing superiorly towards the foramen.
- Just below the foramen, aspirate and deposit 1–2ml LA.

Complications

- Failed anaesthesia (wrong place, not enough or unusual anatomy).
- Intravascular injection (transient adrenergic effects, haematoma).
- Intra-neural injection (persistent anaesthesia/paraesthesia).
- Toxicity (headache, visual symptoms, twitching/tremor).
- Needle breakage (weakest at the hub).

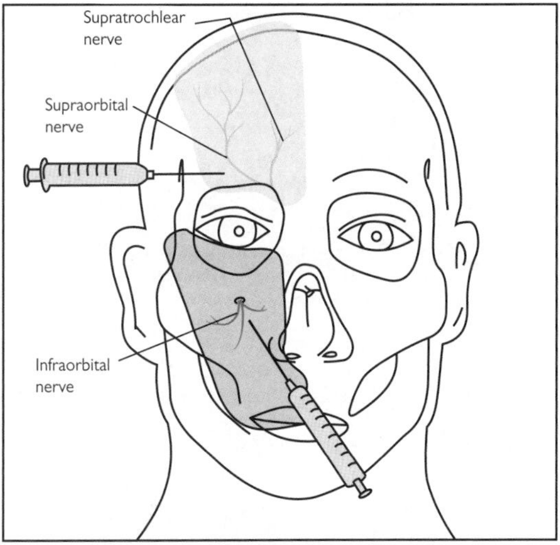
Supratrochlear nerve
Supraorbital nerve
Infraorbital nerve

Fig. 15.4 Position of needles for supraorbital/supratrochlear and infraorbital nerve blocks with anaesthetized areas highlighted.

Tips and tricks

- If possible use a dental syringe; it has a fine 30G needle and allows excellent control of speed for delivery, reducing patient discomfort.
- Aspiration of a dental syringe is achieved by applying pressure without injecting solution, then releasing pressure—blood enters the cartridge if the needle is intra-vascular.
- Cold anaesthetics delivered quickly are more painful, so warm the cartridge in your hand first and inject slowly.
- Give regional blocks first, then top up with local infiltration if needed as infiltrating an area with reduced sensation is less painful.
- If there is an open wound, inject from inside the wound through the dermis as this is less painful.
- Allow approximately 5min for vasoconstrictors to take effect.
- Use the smallest amount of the lowest concentration possible.
- Tend to use 1% lidocaine in children.
- Maximum dose of adrenaline is 500µg.
- A 1% concentration is equal to 10mg/ml.

Biopsies and excision of small lesions

Overview

Provisional clinical diagnosis is critical in determining correct biopsy technique (see Table 15.2), whilst careful tissue handling and good communication with the pathologist will greatly improve diagnostic value. In general, small, benign lesions undergo excisional biopsy, whilst most large or suspected malignant conditions undergo incisional biopsy to confirm diagnosis and allow appropriate treatment.

Indications (typical)

- Diagnosis ± treatment of skin or mucosal abnormalities, including:
  - Suspected malignancy.
  - Mucocutaneous lesions.
  - Precancerous lesions.

Consent

- Infection.
- Bleeding.
- Numbness around surgical site.

Table 15.2 Determining biopsy type and site

Suspected clinical diagnosis	Biopsy type	Site
Suspected SCC	Incisional, excisional if very small	Margin
Leukoplakia/ erythroleukoplakia	Incisional/punch	Worst affected area; consider multiple biopsies
Oral lichen planus	Incisional	Representative sample
Vesiculobullous lesions	Incisional, fresh for immunofluorescence	Unaffected peri-lesional tissue
Granulomatous disease	Deep incisional, fresh for microbiology	
Mucocele	Excisional	
Fibroepithelial polyp, pyogenic granuloma, epulis	Excisional	
Minor salivary gland tumour	Palate: deep incisional Lip: excisional	
Vascular lesions	Excisional	

NB Biopsies are often used to diagnose cancers. The principles of cancer excisions in the head and neck are the same as for anywhere else in the body, i.e. remove the lesion with the necessary margins taking into account all of the local anatomy. The specifics of tumour ablation are not described here as the range of surgical treatments is beyond the scope of this book. However, there are two excellent books that cover the subject (1, 2).

Preoperative preparation

- The lesion and skin margins should be marked and WHO surgical safety checklist completed.
- If direct immunofluorescence or a frozen section is required, the laboratory must be informed prior to the procedure

Margins

- BCC should be removed with a 3–5mm margin.
- Low-risk SCC should be removed with a 4mm margin. Risk may be determined as low by:
  - Position: sun-exposed skin, not including lip/ear.
  - Dimensions: <2cm wide and <4mm deep.
  - Differentiation: well differentiated.
  - Patient factors: immunocompetent patient.
- High-risk SCC should be removed with a 6mm margin.
- Malignant melanoma should undergo excisional biopsy with a 2–5mm margin and cuff of fat to allow accurate staging.
  - In large facial lesions a 5mm punch biopsy of the thickest part is sometimes acceptable.

Position and theatre set-up

- Generally supine or semi-supine depending on lesion position.
- Aqueous chlorhexidine skin preparation for extra-oral lesions.

Procedure

Soft tissue biopsy

- Inject LA either as a ring block around the lesion or a regional block.
  - Do not infiltrate the lesion itself as this distorts the tissues.
- If there is a possibility of the lesion being vascular, aspirate before beginning and consider further imaging (bleeding can be profuse).
- Place a loosely tied suture through the lesion to control the tissues.
  - Forceps are best avoided as they distort architecture.
- For incisional biopsies sample the lesion at its margin incorporating surrounding normal tissue.
- For excisional biopsies create an elliptical incision around the lesion with a no. 15 scalpel, ensuring the length is three times the width.
  - Intra-orally the long axis of the ellipse should be anteroposterior.
  - Extra-orally it should be in the axis of relaxed skin tension lines.
- Depth is to the necessary margin size with no bevelling.
- Leave any sutures in place to avoid artefacts, and consider adding loose positional sutures to orientate the pathologist.
- Place in an appropriate transport medium to reduce tissue autolysis.
  - Usually this is 10% neutral buffered formalin.
  - Use at least ×10 the volume of the specimen.
- The request form must include all information regarding appearance, position, orientation, and suspected diagnosis.
  - Drug, medical, and alcohol history can also help the pathologist and should be included.
- Close in layers with absorbable sutures (non-absorbable for skin).

Punch biopsy

- Anaesthetize as described for 'Soft tissue biopsy' (p. 835).
- Use a 4 or 5mm punch.
- At 90° to the surface gently insert with a rotating movement cutting a 3mm deep circular core; the bevel on the punch is 1mm.
- Thicker lesions may require a deeper core to include a few mm of lamina propria.
- Carefully grasp the core and use a scalpel or scissors to excise at the base.
- One or two 5-0 nylon sutures may be needed for closure of skin.

Postoperative care

Skin sutures should be removed in 5–7 days.

Complications

- Haematoma.
- Infection.
- Paraesthesia.
- Damage to submandibular duct for floor of mouth biopsies.

Further reading

1. Langdon, J., Patel, M., Ord, R., and Brennan P. (2010) *Operative Oral and Maxillofacial Surgery*, 2nd edn. London: Hodder Arnold.
2. Ward Booth, P., Schendel, S.A., and Hausamen, J. (2007) *Maxillofacial Surgery*, 2nd edn. St. Louis: Churchill Livingstone/Elsevier.

Simple tooth extraction

Indications (typical)

- Unrestorable tooth.
- Orthodontic purposes.
- Traumatic fracture compromising viability of tooth.
- Tooth compromising repair of fractured mandible/maxilla.

Consent

- Infection and dry socket.
- Bleeding.
- Damage to adjacent teeth.
- Communication with maxillary sinus.
- Tooth fracture requiring surgical removal of root.

Preoperative preparation

- Radiographs demonstrating root morphology and position of adjacent structures (e.g. maxillary sinus, IAN, mental foramen).
- Complete WHO checklist and consider VTE prophylaxis if necessary.
- LA ± IV sedation if anxious.
- Position patient supine with head stabilization ring.
- Rinse with chlorhexidine 0.2% mouthwash.

Position and theatre set-up

- For upper teeth position the patient with the maxillary arch at 60° to the floor.
- For lower teeth the patient should be positioned lower, with the mandibular arch parallel to the floor.
- Approach lower teeth that are on the side of your dominant hand from above; all other teeth are approached from the side of the patient.

Procedure

- Support the jaw around the tooth with the non-dominant thumb and index finger throughout the procedure to counter extraction forces and aid visualization.
- Place a luxator into the gingival margin, slightly angled towards the root surface and stabilize with a finger rest on a tooth.
- Use a rocking action with steady axial pressure to cut the periodontium and dilate the socket to two-thirds of its depth.
- Evenly dilate the socket by continuing luxation around the circumference of the tooth; avoid luxating the lingual surfaces to reduce risk of damage to the lingual nerve.
- Elevators are used perpendicular to the tooth root with the blade engaging cementum and rotating 90°; use the adjacent alveolar bone as a fulcrum and *not* an adjacent tooth (see Fig. 15.5).
- Forceps are specifically designed for each tooth to conform to its anatomy and aid positioning for the surgeon.
- Seat forcep beaks as far down the axis of the tooth as possible to expand crestal alveolar bone by a wedging effect.

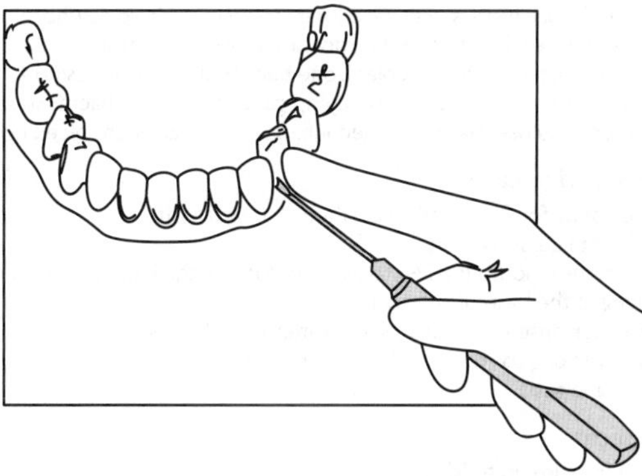

Fig. 15.5 Position of elevators.

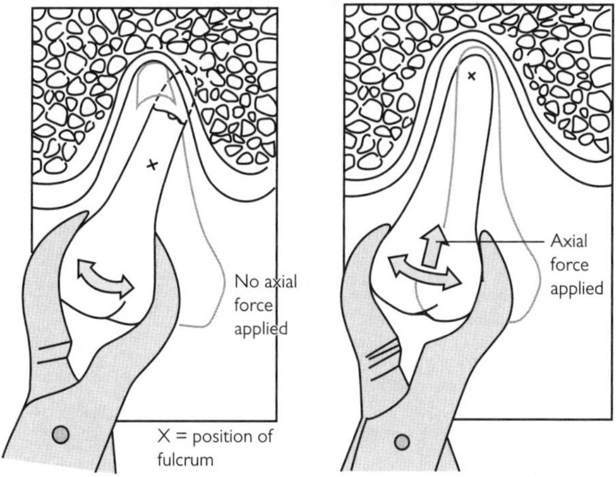
No axial
force
applied
X = position of
fulcrum
Axial
force
applied

Fig. 15.6 Application of forceps and direction of movement.

- Apply axial force through the long axis of the tooth to displace the centre of rotation as apically as possible; this reduces excess apical movement and subsequent apical fracture (see Fig. 15.6).
- Maintain this axial force and apply slow, purposeful outward pressure (buccally) then inward (lingually) to widen the socket.
- Rotation can also be used for conical-shaped, single-rooted teeth.
- Deliver tooth with a light tractional force in an outward occlusal direction.

- For mandibular molars with extensive crown loss, sharp cowhorn forceps that reach between the roots may facilitate extraction.
- Press the dilated crestal alveolar bone back to its original position.
- Ask the patient to bite down on damp gauze to achieve haemostasis.
- Oxidized cellulose may be packed into socket if persistent bleeding.

Postoperative care

- Avoid eating for 3–4h until anaesthetic has worn off.
- Avoid hot liquids for 24h.
- Do not rinse mouth for 24h to avoid dislodging the haemostatic plug forming at the base of the socket.
- Thereafter rinse with warm, salty water for 4–5 days.
- Avoid smoking to reduce risk of dry socket.
- Simple analgesia.

Complications

- Tooth fracture up to 20%.
- Alveolar osteitis ('dry socket') 10%.
- Postoperative bleeding 1%.
- Displacement of tooth into adjacent tissue space 0.1%.

Surgical tooth extraction

Anatomy

- Flap design should take into account adequate access, aesthetics, and avoidance of damage to adjacent structures,
- The mental nerve is inferior to the second mandibular premolar.
- The lingual nerve often lies close to the distal aspect of 3rd molars.
- The long buccal nerve crosses halfway up the anterior border of the mandibular ramus, although injury is rarely reported.
- Posterior roots may overlie the maxillary sinus or mandibular canal.

Indications (typical)

- Teeth or roots that cannot be extracted routinely with forceps.
- Unerupted or impacted third molars.

Consent

As for 'Simple tooth extraction' (p. 838), but also include:

- Dissolving stitches.
- Numbness to lip and tongue (<1%).

Preoperative preparation

As for 'Simple tooth extraction' (p. 838).

Position and theatre set-up

As for 'Simple tooth extraction' (p. 838).

Envelope flap

(See Fig. 15.7a)

- Used for superficial roots and almost all palatal procedures.
- An incision is made in the gingival sulcus starting distally and extending mesially beyond the surgical site with a no.15 blade.
  - Keep the blade vertical and slightly angled towards the tooth to reduce damage to the gingiva.
  - Preserve the papillae to aid repositioning and aesthetics.
- For unerupted teeth perform a crestal incision (see Fig. 15.7c).

Triangular (two-sided flap)

(See Fig. 15.7b)

- Used for almost all other minor oral surgical procedures.
- Create an envelope flap as above.
- Then make a full-thickness, oblique, relieving incision that includes the papilla in the flap.
  - The relieving incision is usually mesial as this gives better vision and access but can be distal depending on adjacent structures.
  - Do not extend further than 15mm posterior to mandibular 2nd molars as this risks damaging the long buccal nerve.

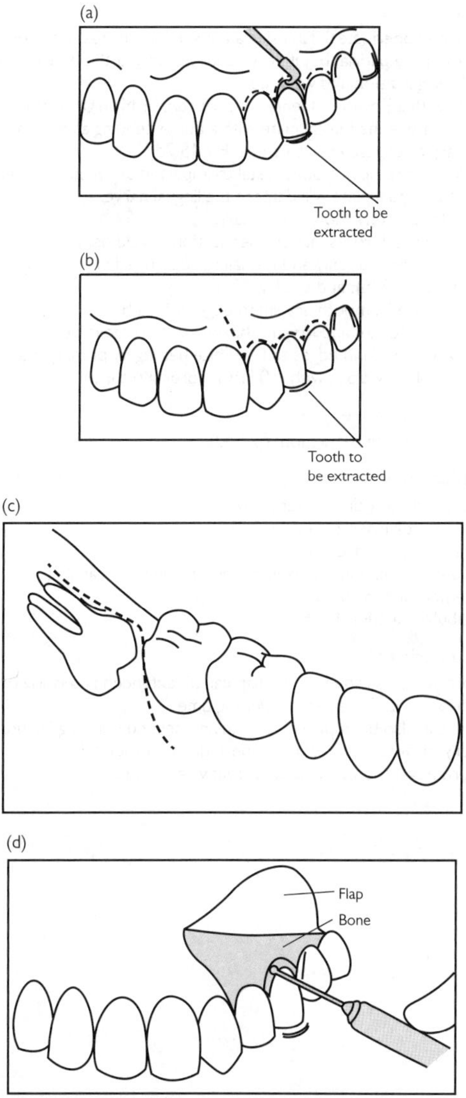
(a)
Tooth to be extracted
(b)
Tooth to be extracted
(c)
(d)
Flap
Bone

Fig. 15.7 (a) Gingival sulcus incision for envelope flap. (b) Triangular flap. (c) Flap design for unerupted teeth. (d) Bone removal.

Procedure

- Raise a mucoperiosteal flap using a Howarth periosteal elevator.
  - Start at the papilla, but if very adherent start at the base of the relieving incision and work up.
- Retract with a Bowdler–Henry rake, Austin, or Michigan retractor.
- Gently remove the buccal plate with a bur, extending as deep as necessary to engage elevators (see Fig. 15.7d).
  - Take care removing bone distal to impacted 3rd molars as perforating the lingual plate will damage the lingual nerve.
  - Use lingual retraction if necessary.
- Divide the tooth roots into smaller sections to aid delivery.
- Apply elevators buccally and mesially as described under 'Simple tooth extraction' (p. 838), and see Fig. 15.5.
- Once removed, smooth any sharp edges with a bur.
- Debride the socket and irrigate thoroughly to remove debris.
- Approximate wound edges to maximize healing by primary intention and meticulously close with 4-0 fast-resorbing sutures.

Postoperative care

As for 'Simple tooth extraction' (p. 840).

Complications

- Alveolar osteitis ('dry socket') 10%.
- Inferior alveolar nerve damage 0.3%.
- Lingual nerve damage <0.4%.
- Root displacement into maxillary sinus, mandibular canal or infratemporal fossa 0.1%.
- Mandibular fracture 0.005%.

Tips and tricks

- If more access is required, the flap can be extended anteriorly or posteriorly with no extended healing time
- Access can also be improved by adding a second relieving incision mesially or distally, creating a trapezoidal three-sided flap.
- Bone removal should be as conservative as possible.

Apicectomy

Overview

Apicectomy is a form of surgical endodontics combining root-end resection, apical curettage, and root-end filling to disinfect the pulp space and periradicular tissues where non-surgical root canal treatment is not appropriate (see Indications). RCS guidelines published in 2012 state that success rates vary from 44% to 95%.[3]

Indications (typical)

- Periradicular disease where non-surgical root canal treatment cannot be undertaken due to patient or technical factors.
- Visualization of tissues required when perforation or root fracture suspected.
- Biopsy of periradicular tissue required (e.g. odontogenic cyst).

Consent

- Infection.
- Bleeding.
- Loosening of tooth requiring early extraction.
- Late failure requiring tooth extraction.
- Localized gum recession.
- Communication with maxillary sinus.

Preoperative preparation

- Long-cone periapical (LCPA) radiographs demonstrating at least 3mm past apex.
- Complete WHO checklist and consider VTE prophylaxis if necessary.
- Chlorhexidine 0.2% mouth rinse.
- LA—regional block and local infiltration with vasoconstrictor.

Position and theatre set-up

- Supine.
- Surgical magnification should be used if available.

Procedure

- Raise a mucoperiosteal flap over sound bone as described for surgical tooth extractions (see ➲ 'Surgical tooth extraction', p. 842).
- Estimate the position of the apical third of the tooth and create a superficial osteotomy in the buccal cortical plate with curettes or a small round bur in a water-cooled handpiece.
- Remove sufficient bone to allow visualization and instrumentation of the apex and periradicular lesion.
- Remove periradicular soft tissue with curettes and transect ≥3mm of the root end with a fissure bur.
- Prepare a 3mm deep root-end cavity with ultrasonic scaler or drill.
- Place retrograde root filling (RRF) material in prepared cavity; mineral trioxide aggregate (MTA), glass ionomer, reinforced zinc oxide eugenol, or super-EBA cement (ethoxybenzoic acid) can be used.
- Close with 4-0 nylon sutures.

Postoperative care

- Removal of sutures 2–4 days.
- Chlorhexidine 0.2% mouthwash until toothbrushing comfortable.

Complications

- Infection.
- Success rate of 44–95%.
- Maxillary sinus perforation 10% (maxillary molars and premolars).

Tips and tricks

- Ensure root end transected at 90° to the root to reduce the number of dentinal tubules exposed.
- Place Surgicel into cyst cavity whilst condensing RRF for haemostasis and to catch debris.

Further reading

3. Evans, G.E., Bishop, K. and Renton, T. (2012) *Guidelines for Surgical Endodontics*. Royal College of Surgeons of England.

Odontogenic cyst enucleation and marsupialization

Overview

The jaws contain teeth and epithelial remnants of tooth formation, accounting for the much higher incidence of cysts than any other bone. The treatment of choice is enucleation with removal of the entire cyst lining. Marsupialization can be a sole procedure to decompress a cyst, promoting its shrinkage and infilling with bone, but is more usually followed by enucleation of a now smaller area.

Indications (typical)

Facilitation of histopathological diagnosis for persistent or enlarging radiolucencies.

Preoperative preparation

- Plain radiographs in two planes or cone-beam CT (CBCT); CBCT is excellent for visualization of position of the inferior alveolar canal and for diagnosis.
- Complete WHO checklist and provide VTE prophylaxis as necessary.
- GA may be required for extensive lesions.

Position and theatre set-up

Supine with head stabilization ring.

Consent

As for 'Apicectomy' (p. 846).

Procedure

- Aspirate the cyst with a 21G 40mm needle on a 10ml syringe and submit fluid for microbiology and histopathological examination.
    - If aspiration fails, or contains blood, reconsider diagnosis.

Enucleation ± peripheral ostectomy

- Raise a mucoperiosteal flap over sound bone as previously described (see ➲ 'Surgical tooth extraction', p. 842).
- Where a cyst has perforated the cortical plate, the cyst lining must be carefully separated from the flap with a Mitchell's trimmer.
- Use a water-cooled size 8 tungsten carbide round bur to remove a window of bone, taking care not to tear the underlying cyst lining.
- Non-vital teeth or those with a poor prognosis due to bone loss are extracted.
- Use a large curette to completely release the cyst lining from the bone.
    - Dissection is facilitated by keeping the cyst intact.
    - Damp gauze to push the cyst lining from bone can assist dissection.
- Deliver the cyst and irrigate the cavity with saline.
- Dry with gauze and visually inspect the specimen and cavity to ensure no residual lining remains.

- If a keratocystic odondogenic tumor (KCOT) is suspected, perform a peripheral ostectomy by instrumenting the cavity by hand or utilizing a round bur with the aim to remove 1–2mm of bone; applying Carnoy's solution further reduces the risk of recurrence.
- Place the cyst in 10% neutral buffered formalin and submit for histological examination.
- Smooth bony edges to transition smoothly with the bone surface.
- Blood clot will fill the cavity and eventually organize into bone, but brisk bleeding can be managed with diathermy, oxidized cellulose (Surgicel®), or bone wax.
- Close with absorbable sutures to complete a watertight seal.

Marsupialization

- If the cyst has perforated the cortical plate by more than a third of the cyst's dimensions, and no anatomical structures are at risk, use scissors or a no.15 blade to remove a soft tissue window of mucoperiosteum and cyst lining at the margins of the perforation.
- Otherwise expose the area as for enucleation, then excise a window of lining, evacuate cyst contents, place in fixative, and submit for histological examination.
- Irrigate with saline and dry with gauze.
    - Areas of ulceration or thickening may require additional biopsy.
- Suture the margins of the cyst lining to the mucosa (see Fig. 15.8).
- Gently pack the cavity to maintain the opening with 1/2in ribbon gauze impregnated with BIPP or Whitehead's varnish (compound iodoform paint).
- Oversew a pack to prevent displacement with a 4-0 silk suture.

Postoperative care

- Chlorhexidine 0.2% mouthwash QDS for 2 weeks.
- Re-pack marsupialized cysts every 2–3 weeks until the cavity is self-cleansing and easily irrigated by the patient.

Complications (specific to the procedure)

- Recurrence >8% for KCOT.
- Wound infection and dehiscence <5%.
- Fracture is unusual but can occur if the cyst is very large.

Tips and tricks

- The bone and mucosal window must be at least a third the size of the cyst for marsupialization to prevent closure and recurrence.
- A removable periodontal dressing material (Coe-Pak™) or acrylic bung can be used to maintain the window after the first pack change; as the cavity shrinks the patient is instructed to remove the dressing and rinse with chlorhexidine 0.2% after meals.
- Existing dentures can be modified with soft denture reline material (Coe-Soft™) to make an obturator.

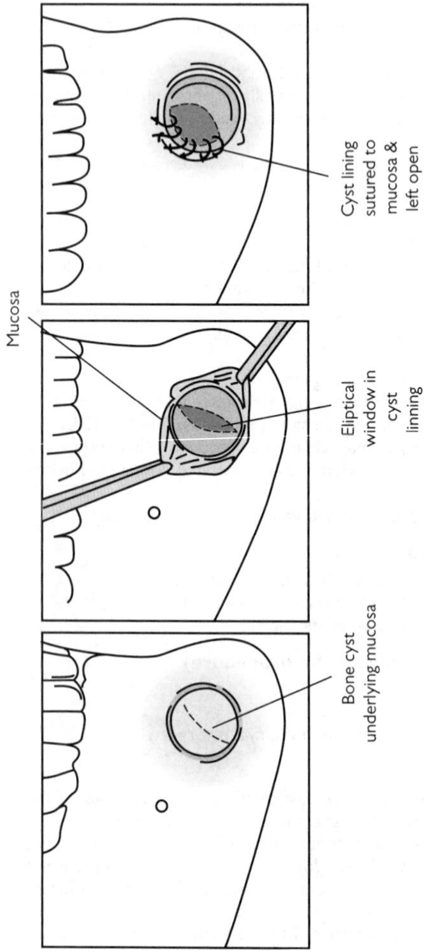
Mucosa
Cyst lining sutured to mucosa & left open
Eliptical window in cyst linning
Bone cyst underlying mucosa

Fig. 15.8 Mucosa sutured to epithelial lining of cyst in marsupialization.

Intra-oral implant insertion

Osseo-integration is the apparent direct connection of live bone to a functioning dental implant without intervening connective tissue. This takes 3–6 months and meticulous surgical technique is critical.

Anatomy

See ➲ 'Maxillary sinus floor elevation' (p. 856) for further relevant anatomy.
- The inferior alveolar canal is 10mm above the inferior border of the mandible, rising upwards and buccally to the mental foramen.
- The floor of the mouth contains, from anterior to posterior, the sublingual artery, submental artery, and mylohyoid branch of the inferior alveolar artery.

Indications (typical)

- To replace an individual tooth with an appropriate abutment.
- To provide implant support for intra-oral prosthetic devices.

Consent

- Bleeding.
- Infection.
- Failure of implant (7–10%).
- Localized gum recession.

Preoperative preparation

- Preoperative imaging: OPG or CBCT.
- A custom-made drill guide/stent.
- 2g amoxicillin PO 1h preoperatively.
- Complete WHO checklist and provide VTE prophylaxis as necessary.
- Chlorhexidine 0.2% mouthwash.
- Regional block with LA and vasoconstrictor.

Position and theatre set-up

Semi-supine.

Procedure

- Create a mucoperiosteal envelope flap over the alveolar crest as previously described (see ➲ 'Surgical tooth extraction', p. 842).
- Assess bone quality, width, and height to determine platform width and length of the implant fixture.
  - Alveolar bone may need reshaping, and unexpected cortical defects may require augmentation and delayed implant placement.
- Mark implant site position with a round bur or precision guide drill; this can be done freehand or by utilizing a drill guide/stent (see Fig. 15.9a).
- Preparation of the implant site (osteotomy) begins using the manufacturer's recommended sequence of bone drills.
- The osteotomy is increased in diameter with sequentially larger twist drills at up to 2,000rpm with copious water cooling.
- Pilot drills are used to enlarge the cortical bone prior to using the next twist drill or to correct the osteotomy direction.

(a)

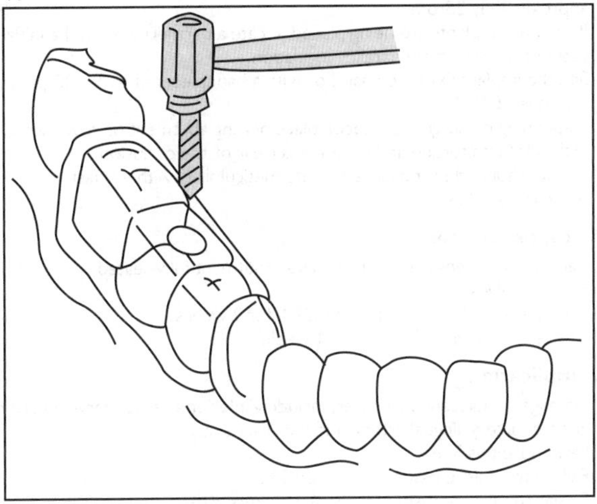

(b)

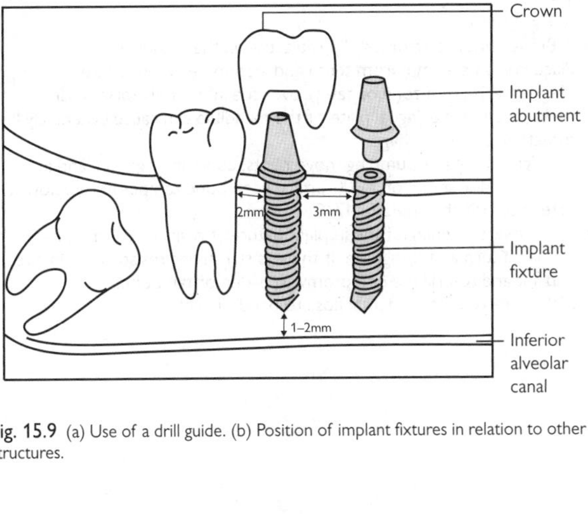
Crown
Implant abutment
2mm
3mm
Implant fixture
1–2mm
Inferior alveolar canal

Fig. 15.9 (a) Use of a drill guide. (b) Position of implant fixtures in relation to other structures.

- Bone taps are used in dense bone to prethread the osteotomy at approximately 25rpm.
- If multiple implants are being placed, locate a paralleling pin in the initial osteotomy to help aid parallel angulation.
- Site the implant fixture by hand or with a handpiece set to 15–20rpm at a torque of 45Ncm.
- Depending on surgical protocol, place healing abutment or cover screw with <15Ncm torque and ensure it is clear of the occlusion.
- Irrigate thoroughly and close the site meticulously with 4-0 fast-resorbing sutures.

Postoperative care

- Radiograph to ensure cover screw or abutment fully seated.
- Simple analgesia.
- Chlorhexidine 0.2% mouthwash QDS for 2 weeks.
- Advise not to wear denture for 1 week.

Complications

- Damage to adjacent structures, including inferior alveolar nerve, inferior alveolar artery, lingual artery, and maxillary sinus.
- Peri-implantitis 5–8%.
- Failure to achieve osseo-integration 2%.
- 5-year survival: non-smokers 93%, smokers 90%.
- Infection <5%.

Tips and tricks

(See Fig. 15.9b)

- A Brånemark retractor aids lip retraction in the mandible.
- Place implants >2mm from teeth and >3mm between fixtures.
- Maintain a 1–2mm zone of safety over the inferior alveolar canal.
- Perforation of the lingual plate of the mandible can cause potentially life-threatening haemorrhage.
- Use light picking or pumping movements, copious irrigation, and a maximum drill speed of 2,000rpm to keep bone temperature below the osteonecrosis threshold of 47°C.
- Avoid overtightening of the implant fixture; if resistance is met, back off half a turn and re-tighten. If there is still strong resistance, remove implant and re-drill the osteotomy to widen or tap bone.
- Make sure you attach dental floss to paralleling pins.

Maxillary sinus floor elevation

Anatomy

- The maxillary sinus floor runs obliquely, lying 6–8mm above the 1st premolar and just 1–2mm above the 2nd molar.
- The lining is called the Schneiderian membrane and is 0.3–0.8mm thick.
- Bony sinus septa are present in 24–31% of patients.

Indications (typical)

- To augment the posterior maxillary sinus prior to implant placement in patients with less than 8mm native bone height.
- A two-stage procedure is required if <4–5mm native bone height.
- A simultaneous procedure can be performed if >5mm native bone height and expected primary stability of implant is >35Ncm.
- Osteotome technique can be used if >6mm of native bone.

Consent

- Infection.
- Bleeding.
- Risk of procedure being abandoned if sinus membrane torn.

Preoperative preparation

- Preoperative radiographs: OPG or cone-beam CT.
- 2g amoxicillin PO 1h preoperatively.
- Complete WHO checklist and provide VTE prophylaxis as necessary.
- Chlorhexidine 0.2% mouthwash.
- Regional block with LA and vasoconstrictor.

Position and theatre set-up

Semi-supine.

Procedure

Lateral antrostomy procedure

(See Fig. 15.10)

- Raise a mucoperiosteal flap as previously described (see ➔ 'Surgical tooth extraction', p. 842) ensuring closure will be over sound bone.
- With a piezo saw or small round bur create a lateral antrostomy around a 15×10mm island of bone in the maxillary wall, below the infraorbital nerve and about 2mm above the estimated sinus floor.
- Reflect the sinus membrane by at least 2mm superiorly, anteriorly, and posteriorly to the antrostomy.
- Reflect the sinus membrane off the floor and up the medial wall.
- Use the bony island as a trapdoor into the sinus, using its superior border as a hinge, and push inwards so it forms the new sinus floor.
- Fill the created defect with particulate xenograft such as Bio-Oss® ensuring the ostium to the nasal passage is not obstructed medially.
- If planned for, place implants (see ➔ 'Intra-oral implant insertion', p. 852).
- A collagen membrane such as Bio-Guide® is then placed over the defect, extending at least 3mm past the borders of the osteotomy.
- Close the mucoperiosteum with 4-0 nylon sutures.

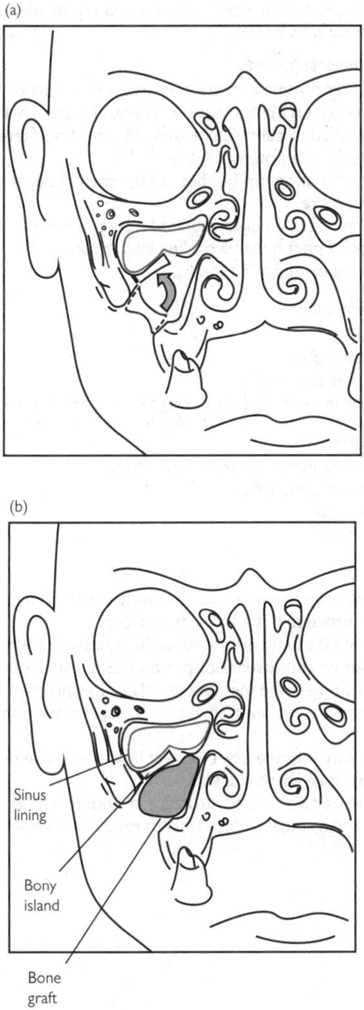
(a)
(b)
Sinus
lining
Bony
island
Bone
graft

Fig. 15.10 (a) Using the bony island as a trapdoor to create the new sinus floor. (b) Particulate bone graft in place.

- If a two-stage procedure is planned, implants can be placed at 9 months and loaded 3 months later.

Osteotome (Summer's) procedure

- Osteotomy sites for implants are prepared 1mm short of sinus floor.
- 3mm of bone graft is placed into the osteotomy and a malleting osteotome is used to gently abfracture the sinus floor, tenting the membrane to form a potential space.
- Membrane perforation can be checked by visual inspection and a Valsalva manoeuvre.
- For each 1mm of bone height required (up to 3–4mm in total), 3mm of particulate bone graft must be packed into the space.
- Implants can be loaded at 3 months.

Postoperative care

- Simple analgesia.
- 5 days oral antibiotics.
- Remove sutures at 1 week.
- Avoid blowing nose or sucking through straws for 2–3 weeks.

Complications

- Perforation of Schneiderian membrane 44%.
- Postoperative sinusitis 10%.
- Graft infection 2%.
- Graft failure <1%.

Tips and tricks

- Small tears of 1–6mm can be patched with a collagen membrane.
    - Abandon procedure if a larger tear occurs.
- The membrane is often perforated whilst creating the window, usually in the anterior or anterosuperior position, as it is thinnest here. Attempting to reflect the membrane only causes propagation of the tear. Instead remove at least 2mm bone around it and continue the dissection.
- Place collagen membrane dry, then wet it with a couple of drops of saline to allow it to adapt and stick.
- Bio-Guide® has a two-layered structure: a smooth surface to abut the soft tissues, and a rough surface to abut regenerated bone.

Removal of a submandibular duct stone

Overview

Submandibular calculi are a common cause of obstructive sialadenitis and can be removed by a transoral technique if distal to the submandibular hilum. Endoscopic or radiological retrieval may be used, but are not usually suitable for impacted, immobile stones or those >4mm. Stones within the hilum or parenchyma are managed by transcervical excision of the submandibular gland (see ➔ 'Submandibular gland excision', p. 790).

Anatomy

(See Fig. 15.11)

- The submandibular duct runs forwards and upwards over the back of mylohyoid and inferomedial to the sublingual gland.
- It opens at the sublingual papilla just adjacent to the midline.
- It is 5–6cm long and normally 2mm in diameter (1mm at papilla).
- The lingual nerve passes under the duct from lateral to medial at the 2nd molar and proceeds anteriorly branching into the tongue.

Indications (typical)

Symptomatic palpable calculi.

Consent

- Infection.
- Bleeding/haematoma.
- Weakness of lip.
- Numbness of tongue.

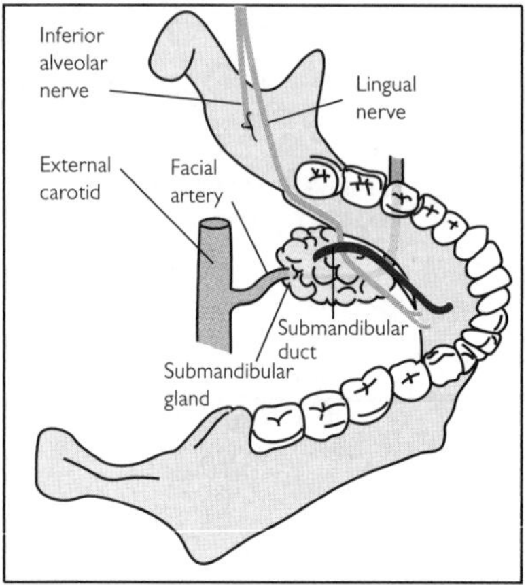
Inferior alveolar nerve
Lingual nerve
External carotid
Facial artery
Submandibular duct
Submandibular gland

Fig. 15.11 Superior oblique view showing relationship between submandibular duct and lingual nerve.

Preoperative preparation

- Antibiotics to treat acute infection prior to surgery.
- Complete WHO checklist and provide VTE prophylaxis as necessary.
- LA with lingual nerve block alone can be used for anterior stones.
- Otherwise GA with nasotracheal intubation + head stabilization ring; infiltration with LA + vasoconstrictor is helpful for haemostasis.

Position and theatre set-up

- Supine with mouth prop between molars of affected side.
- Surgeon stands on unaffected side, assistant on affected side.

Procedure

Stones anterior to the duct crossing the lingual nerve

- Pass a suture into the floor of mouth around the duct behind the stone to prevent it from moving backwards.
- Incise over the palpable stone parallel with the duct.
- If adherent to the duct wall, gently mobilize the stone with a Mitchell trimmer to deliver.
- Irrigate proximally and distally with normal saline.
- Ensure haemostasis and loosely close the mucosa with absorbable sutures; closure of the duct itself increases risk of post-surgical duct stricture.

Stones posterior to the duct crossing the lingual nerve

- Incise the sublingual fold from the 1st molar to just short of the sublingual papilla, staying lateral to the submandibular duct.
    - Stay close to the teeth but leave a cuff of tissue to close.
- Retract the sublingual gland laterally using stay sutures if required.
- Identify the duct anteriorly and place a suture for anterior traction.
- Trace the duct back on its superior medial aspect until the lingual nerve is identified running beneath it at the 2nd molar region.
- Carefully separate the duct and lingual nerve back to the gland.
- Sustained external pressure on the gland upwards elevates it to improve visualization of the stone.
- If required extend the mucosal excision to the 3rd molar keeping the lingual nerve under direct vision.
- Delivery of stone and closure is as described above.

Postoperative care

- Chlorhexidine 0.2% mouthwash 1 week.
- Consider antibiotics if signs of infection.
- Chewing gum can be used to encourage salivary flow.

Complications

- Failure to remove stone requiring sialoadenectomy <2%.
- Lingual nerve damage <1%.
- Submandibular duct stricture.
- Sublingual haematoma.

Sublingual gland excision

Overview

Definitive management of a ranula is transoral sialoadenectomy of the sublingual gland to prevent recurrence. Although a minor oral surgical procedure, difficult access and the fact that it is commonly performed in children usually warrant a general anaesthetic.

Anatomy

(See ➲ 'Removal of submandibular duct stone' (p. 860) for further relevant anatomy.)

- The submandibular duct opens into the mouth at the sublingual papilla, which continues backwards as a ridge called the sublingual fold or *plica sublingualis*.
- The sublingual fold overlies the sublingual gland, which sits on mylohyoid and is bound by the mandible laterally, and submandibular duct and lingual nerve medially.
- 8–20 small ducts of Rivinus drain the gland directly into the floor of mouth along the sublingual fold or into the submandibular duct.

Indications (typical)

- Ranula.
- Salivary gland tumour.

Consent

- Infection.
- Bleeding/haematoma.

Preoperative preparation

- Complete WHO checklist and provide VTE prophylaxis as necessary.
- LA with lingual nerve block and local infiltration.
- Otherwise GA with nasotracheal intubation.

Position and theatre set-up

Supine with head stabilization ring.

Procedure

- Cannulate submandibular duct with a size 00 or 0 lacrimal probe.
- Incise the mucosa of the floor of mouth from the 1st molar to just short of the sublingual papilla, staying lateral to the submandibular duct; stay close to the teeth but leave a cuff of tissue to aid closure (Fig. 15.12).
- Dissect with scissors onto the sublingual gland and ranula, then continue in a submucosal plane medially and identify the submandibular duct; the mucosa is very thin here so be careful not to tear.
- Trace the duct back on its superior medial aspect until the lingual nerve is identified running beneath it at the second molar region.
- Mobilize the duct from the gland and ranula; retract it medially.
- Blunt dissect the gland and ranula free of its attachments.
- Deliver the gland and send for histopathological examination.
- Ensure meticulous haemostasis.
- Loosely close the floor of mouth with resorbable sutures.

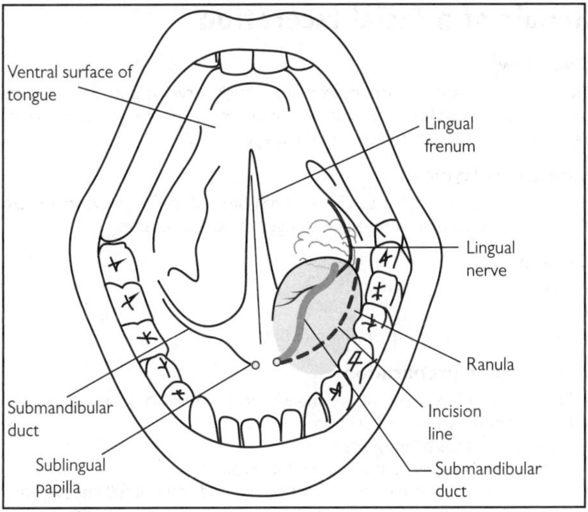
Ventral surface of tongue
Lingual frenum
Lingual nerve
Ranula
Incision line
Submandibular duct
Submandibular duct
Sublingual papilla

Fig. 15.12 Incision marking.

Postoperative care

Simple analgesics.

Complications

- Lingual nerve damage <1%.
- Damage to submandibular duct.
- Haematoma.

Tips and tricks

- Infiltrate local anaesthetic into the floor of the mouth to help haemostasis and provide some hydro-dissection.
- Taking an elipse of overlying mucosa facilitates tissue handling.
- DeBakey tissue forceps are great for handling the fragile tissues.
- Excision of the gland, not the ranula, is the primary aim of surgery; don't hesitate decompressing the ranula if it hinders dissection.
- Peanut swabs are useful adjuncts to blunt dissection, and also dry the field.
- There are always branches of the sublingual artery entering from deep anteriorly so use careful dissection and bipolar diathermy.

Repair of a facial laceration

Overview
Most facial lacerations encountered are straightforward but care must be taken to fully assess for tissue loss, underlying fracture, or injury to the facial nerve, parotid duct, or structures of the eye.

Indications (typical)
Any wound not amenable to closure with Steri-Strips™ or cyanoacrylate skin glue, which require well-aligned edges under no tension.

Consent
- Infection.
- Bleeding.
- Thickened scar (hypertrophic or keloid).

Preoperative preparation
- Mostly LA, unless extensive or underlying structures require repair.
- Document cranial nerve function.
- Consider tetanus prophylaxis.
- Antibiotics if heavily contaminated/bite wound.
- Penetrating neck wounds should *not* be opened without full imaging and facilities to explore fully, in case vascular structures are involved.
- Complete WHO checklist and provide VTE prophylaxis as required.

Position and theatre set-up
- Position is dictated by the position of the laceration.
- Usually semi-supine if under LA, supine with head stabilization ring if under GA.

Procedure
- Apply anaesthesia as a local infiltration or regional block (see ➲ 'Intra-oral nerve blocks', p. 826, and 'Nerve blocks of the face', p. 830).
- Thoroughly toilet the laceration with saline and explore for any foreign bodies.
  - Locating glass can be aided with pre- or perioperative imaging.
- Explore the wound to identify damage to nearby structures.
  - Visual inspection of underlying bone helps exclude bony injuries.
- Debride necrotic areas and trim irregular wound edges.
  - This is usually minimal as the head and neck region has excellent vascularity and wound infections are rare.
- Close skin lacerations in layers to reduce skin edge tension and close dead space using 3-0 undyed absorbable sutures ensuring the knots are buried.
- Close skin using interrupted 5-0 or 6-0 monofilament sutures, with minimal tension on the knots to allow for postoperative swelling.
  - Evert edges to improve the scar.
- Full-thickness lip lacerations require closure in three layers (mucosa, muscle, and skin) and meticulous approximation of the vermillion border to avoid a poor aesthetic result later.

Postoperative care

- Regular barrier dressing with 1% chloramphenicol or Polyfax® ointment.
- Avoid getting the area wet for 24h, then clean twice daily with clean water and careful drying.
- Remove sutures at 5 days to avoid a 'railway track' scar.
- Use sunscreens once the sutures are removed.

Complications

- Wound infection <5%.
- Keloid/hypertrophic scarring 5%.

Tips and tricks

- For oblique wounds, take deeper bites at the thicker edge for better approximation—this shelves the wound.
- Divide a long wound in half with a suture to ensure it is closed symmetrically; repeat process to simplify closure.
- For large flaps of skin keep in mind that tissue elasticity can pull one wound edge far from where it originated; anatomically reapproximate flap and tack into position before beginning definitive closure.
- Thin flaps of skin can be very friable but Steri-Strips™ are useful to hold in correct position; additional suturing through them helps stop sutures pulling through.
- Gravel rash must be thoroughly scrubbed to prevent permanent discoloration.

Facial lacerations: parotid duct repair

Overview

Occasionally facial lacerations result in injury to significant structures, including the parotid duct and facial nerve, in which case intricate repair is required.

Anatomy

- The surface marking of the duct is along the middle-third of a line drawn from the tragus to the midpoint of the upper lip.
- The duct is usually cephalic and deep to the buccal branch of the facial nerve.
- It overlies the superficial surface of the masseter before hooking around its anterior border, piercing the buccinator, to open intraorally at the level of the 2nd maxillary molar.

Indications (typical)

Loss of continuity of the parotid duct.

Consent

- Infection.
- Bleeding.
- Collection or leakage of saliva through wound.
- Weakness of facial muscles.

Preoperative preparation

- Complete WHO checklist and provide VTE prophylaxis as necessary.
- GA to avoid movements being exaggerated under the microscope.

Position and theatre set-up

- Supine with head stabilization ring.
- Operating microscope.

Procedure

- Modify a 16G closed-end epidural catheter by cutting off the closed tip and cannulate the duct intra-orally.
- Advance until visible in the facial wound; if not seen, gently flush with saline or methylene blue to confirm parotid duct injury.
- Identifying the buccal branch of the facial nerve and milking the parotid gland to express saliva help identify the proximal cut end.
- Advance the catheter into the proximal cut end.
- Re-approximate the duct with 6-0 resorbable interrupted sutures.
- The catheter is left in situ as a stent to reduce stricture formation; leave a 2cm length intra-orally and secure to the buccal mucosa with a 4-0 resorbable suture.
- Place size 8 or 10 suction drain to manage residual salivary leakage in the wound and close as previously described (see ➲ 'Repair of a facial laceration', p. 864).

Postoperative care

- Prophylactic antibiotics for 5 days.
- Remove drain when drainage minimal.
- Remove stent at 2/52.

Complications

- Sialocoele.
- Salivary fistula.
- Duct stricture.
- Sialadenitis.
- Facial nerve injury.

Tips and tricks

- If the proximal end is within the substance of the parotid gland, ligate to induce gland atrophy as repair is impossible.
    - Warn the patient of postoperative pain due to obstructive parotitis in this instance.
- Chronic sialocoele and salivary fistula can be treated with intra-parotid injection of botulinum toxin A.

Facial lacerations: facial nerve repair

Overview

Even after successful repair, all patients will have some permanent residual weakness and likely synkinesis. Such moderate dysfunction, however, is still significantly better than the morbidity associated with complete lack of facial nerve function.

Anatomy

(See Fig. 15.13)

- There are five branches of the facial nerve: temporal, zygomatic, buccal, marginal mandibular, and cervical.
- Anterior to a line drawn vertically from the lateral canthus, the branches arborize significantly and cross-innervation between them allows a degree of functional overlap.
- This is greatest in the zygomatic and buccal branches, so damage of these branches is less likely to lead to a permanent facial paralysis.
- The temporal branch crosses the zygomatic arch approximately 1cm in front of the upper anterior attachment of the helix.
- The marginal mandibular branch loosely forms an arc below the inferior border of the mandible, lying up to 1.5cm beneath it.
- See ➔ 'Access: bicoronal flap' (p. 894) for further relevant anatomy.

Indications (typical)

Permanent motor deficit in the distribution of the affected nerve.

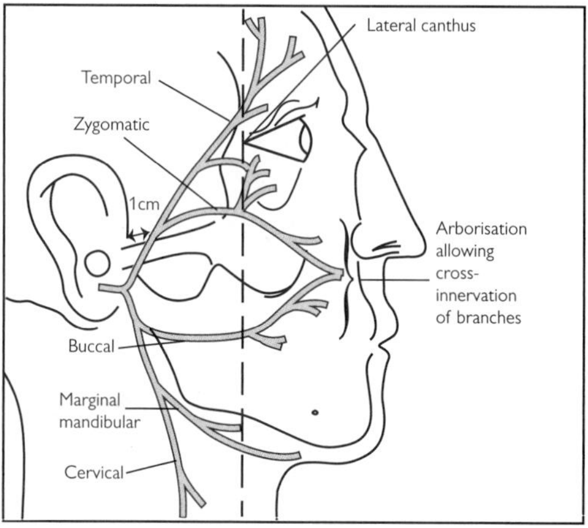
Lateral canthus
Temporal
Zygomatic
1cm
Arborisation allowing cross-innervation of branches
Buccal
Marginal mandibular
Cervical

Fig. 15.13 Anatomy of the facial nerve.

Consent

- Infection.
- Bleeding.
- No improvement in facial movement.

Preoperative preparation

- Preoperative assessment of facial nerve function using House–Brackmann scale.
- Complete WHO checklist and provide VTE prophylaxis as necessary.
- GA to avoid movements being exaggerated under the microscope.

Position and theatre set-up

- Supine with head stabilization ring.
- Operating microscope is required.

Procedure

- Identify and trim the transected nerve ends with microscissors.
- Coaptation is performed by carefully placing two or three interrupted 8-0 nylon sutures through the epineurium to oppose the edges.
  - The first suture should appose the two ends without tension.
- A cable or interpositional nerve graft may be required if tissue has been lost or a tension free repair cannot be obtained.
  - This can be harvested from the great auricular or sural nerve.
- A drain should be sited and meticulous haemostasis achieved to avoid haematoma.
- Closure is in layers as for any other facial laceration.

Postoperative care

- Remove drain at 24h if minimal drainage.
- Antibiotics for 5 days.
- Eye care is necessary if incomplete eye closure is present.
  - Manually blink the eye regularly, especially if it feels dry.
  - Carbomer liquid eye gel (Viscotears®) QDS.
  - Lacrilube® eye ointment +/– eye patch at night.

Complications

- Haematoma.
- Infection.
- Donor-site morbidity if a graft is used (ear or lateral leg numbness depending on whether great auricular or sural nerve is used).

Lateral canthotomy and cantholysis

Overview

This is a sight-preserving emergency procedure that must be familiar to all trainees. The infrequency with which the procedure is required makes this difficult; fortunately, it is simple to conceptualize.

Anatomy

(See Fig. 15.14a)

- The orbital septum is a fibrous sheath arising from the orbital rims that creates a closed orbital space, in which elevated pressures can cause an orbital compartment syndrome leading to ischaemia.
- The lateral canthus overlies the lateral canthal ligament, which anchors the eyelids to the orbit at Whitnall's tubercle.
- The tarsal plates within each eyelid extend laterally, merging to form the lateral canthal ligament; prior to merging, these extensions are called the superior and inferior crura.

Indications (typical)

- Suspected retrobulbar haemorrhage with decreased visual acuity (VA), proptosis, afferent pupillary defect (APD), or elevated intraocular pressure (IOP >40mmHg).

Contraindications

Do not perform in presence of globe rupture.

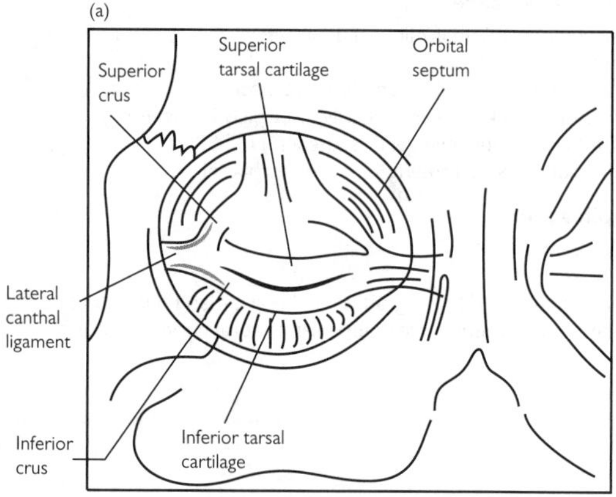
(a)
Superior crus
Superior tarsal cartilage
Orbital septum
Lateral canthal ligament
Inferior crus
Inferior tarsal cartilage

Fig. 15.14 (a) Anatomy of the lateral canthal region. (b) Line of incision. (c) Incision through lateral canthus. (d) Incision through inferior crus.

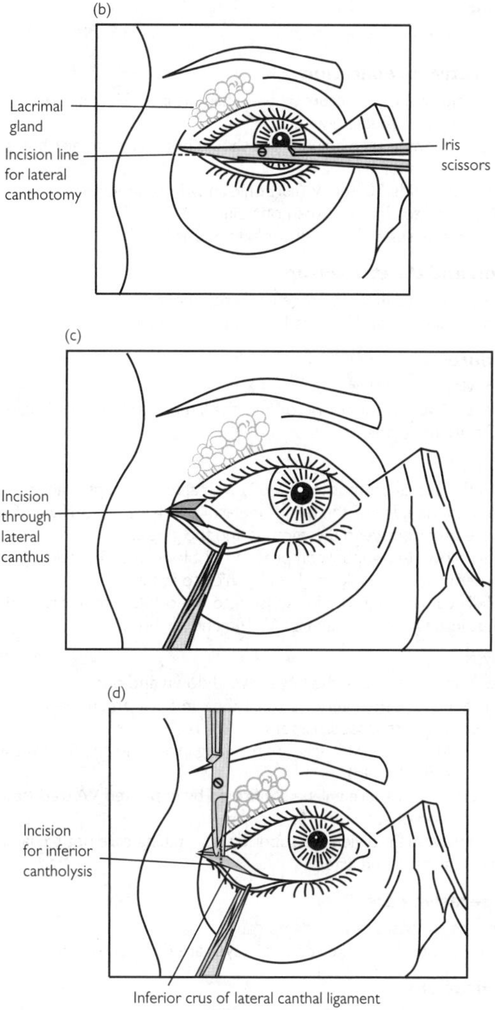
(b)
Lacrimal gland
Incision line for lateral canthotomy
Iris scissors
(c)
Incision through lateral canthus
(d)
Incision for inferior cantholysis
Inferior crus of lateral canthal ligament

Fig. 15.14 (*Contd.*)

Consent

Will require subsequent repair.

Preoperative preparation

- Irreversible visual loss occurs when ischaemia is >120min; surgery must be carried out immediately.
- Medical treatment is an adjunct and should not delay surgery, but is administered as follows:
  - Acetazolamide 500mg IV (carbonic anhydrase inhibitor).
  - 20% mannitol 2g/kg IV (osmotic diuretic).
  - Dexamethasone sodium phosphate 6.6mg IV.

Position and theatre set-up

- Often performed in the emergency department.
- Patient positioned at 30° to reduce venous pressure.

Procedure

- Clean with sterile saline.
- Infiltrate LA and vasoconstrictor into the lateral canthus, taking care not to infiltrate the globe.

Canthotomy

- Clamp the lateral canthus for 30–60s with artery forceps reaching laterally to the edge of the orbit, one arm overlying the surface of the skin, the other between the canthus and the globe.
  - This allows temporary compression of blood vessels, reduction of oedema, and a visible track with which to follow.
- Carefully cut laterally with iris scissors to the orbital rim to divide the canthus into two parts (see Figs 15.14b and 15.14c).

Cantholysis

- Forceps are used to pull the lower eyelid down and out.
- If you cannot see the inferior crus of the canthal ligament try to palpate by strumming with closed scissors.
- Cut the inferior crus with scissors resulting in a loose and floppy lower eye lid (see Fig. 15.14d).
- A successful procedure will be confirmed by improved VA, reduced IOP, and resolution of APD.
- If no improvement divide the superior crus, taking care not to damage the lacrimal gland and artery.

Postoperative care

- Cover the surgical site with damp gauze.
- Closure is considered later once the eyes are deemed stable.

Complications

- Damage to the lacrimal apparatus on cutting the superior crus.
- Damage to the globe or periorbital tissues, especially if the patient is agitated; consider GA.

Tips and tricks

- An APD is demonstrated when the Affected Pupil Dilates on shining a light on it during a swinging flashlight test.
- A crude estimation of IOP can be made by palpating the globe through closed lids and comparing sides.
- Only a small amount of blood is seen with decompression of retrobulbar haemorrhage; improved VA confirms a successful procedure.
- If retrobulbar haemorrhage occurs in the postoperative period of patients who have undergone zygomatic or orbital floor repairs, open the surgical wound to decompress.
- Further management of post-surgical retrobulbar haemorrhage is to remove sutures to open and explore the wound.

Intermaxillary fixation (IMF)

Overview

IMF is used to hold the teeth in the correct functional occlusion by effectively splinting the mandible non-rigidly to the maxilla. There are many forms of IMF, including IMF screws and Ernst ligatures, but the most stable is by application of Erich arch bars, described here.

Indications (typical)

- Prolonged fixation during conservative fracture treatment.
- Facilitation of reduction during open procedures.
- Dentoalveolar fractures.

Consent

Damage to teeth roots.

Preoperative preparation

- Check dentition and occlusion to ensure arch bars can be used; a deep overbite or severe periodontal disease may preclude use.
- Impressions can be taken to fabricate a custom-made arch bar.
- Broad-spectrum antibiotics if open fracture.
- Complete WHO checklist and provide VTE prophylaxis as necessary.
- Nasotracheal intubation; an endotracheal tube placed distal to the last standing molar can be used, but the procedure is made more difficult.
- Warn anaesthetist if fixation is planned to be left in place.

Position and theatre set-up

Supine with head stabilization ring.

Procedure

Attaching the arch bars

- Mobilize and reduce the fracture to align the dental arch.
- Adapt the arch bar to the dental arch with an artery clip.
- Trim the bar so it does not extend past the most distal tooth.
- Ensure cleats face buccally and towards the gingiva.
- A 15cm, 26-gauge stainless steel wire is passed *below* the bar then bucco-palatally through the distal embrasure space of the anchoring tooth.
- Bring the wire back through the mesial embrasure space palato-buccally and *over* the bar (see Fig. 15.15a).
- With an apical pull, artery forceps are used to twist the ligature clockwise until the wire snugly holds the bar against the dental arch.
- Apply individual ligatures on each tooth symmetrically from right to left to ensure even seating.
- Cut each ligature to 1cm and neatly fold into the embrasure space.
- Repeat the process in the opposing jaw, ensuring that the opposing cleats of each bar are positioned symmetrically.
- For very displaced fractures the arch bar is sectioned and one is placed on each fragment; IMF can then be used to reduce the fracture.

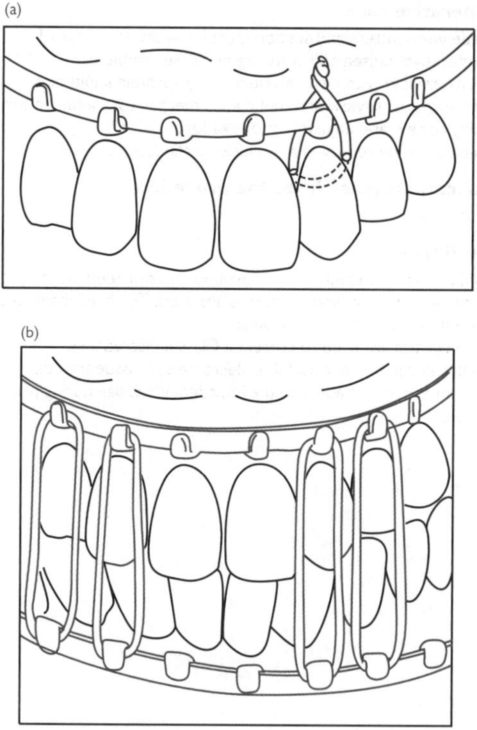

Fig. 15.15 (a) Fixation wire in place around arch bar. (b) IMF using elastics loops.

Applying intermaxillary fixation

- If this is done prior to extubation, ensure any throat packs are removed and the oropharynx is carefully suctioned.
- Place a 26-gauge wire loop around the cleats from the upper and lower arch bars and tighten; place one loop on each side and one loop anteriorly.
- Individual elastic modules or elastic chain can also be used (see Fig. 15.15b).

Postoperative care

- Bedside wire-cutters and suction must be available in case of postoperative nausea and vomiting or airway problems.
- Dietician review with high-calorie and high-protein liquid diet.
- Dental hygienist review and meticulous mechanical plaque control.
- Weekly review and adjustment of fixation.
- Arch bars can be removed at 6 weeks in clinic.

Complications (specific to the procedure)

Malunion 10%.

Tips and tricks

- Individual ligatures can be placed around anterior teeth as long as they are firm and apically-directed forces are used. Teeth adjacent to a fracture line are liable to be avulsed.
- Class II elastics are used to correct a Class II discrepancy.
- Dental wax can be very useful to decrease soft tissue trauma.
- Avoid unnecessary trauma to the interdental papillae during placement of wires.

ORIF mandible

Overview

Occlusal forces and action of the muscles of mastication cause fracture separation at the superior border of the mandible (*tension zone*). The lower border undergoes compression during function (*compression zone*). Ideal placement of plates is therefore as superiorly as possible without damage to the teeth. In the symphysis region there are additional torsional forces requiring an additional plate.

In standard fractures a *load-sharing* (or functionally adequate) technique with a semi-rigid miniplate and two monocortical non-locking screws on each side of the fracture is generally utilized. Rigid buttressing of the fracture fragments by close apposition creates mechanical stability.

Where there are defect fractures or poor bone stock, rigid bony buttressing is not possible, so the plate and screws must create mechanical stability. A *load-bearing* technique with a rigid reconstruction plate and three bi-cortical locking screws each side of the fracture is required. Obviously there are intermediate situations and experience aids choice of hardware.

Anatomy

- The angle is the zone posterior to the 3rd molar and anterior to the posterior inferior attachment of masseter.
- The body is posterior to the canine and anterior to the angle.
- The parasymphysis is the zone between the canines.
- The symphysis is the midline of the mandible.
- The mental foramen is usually apical to the 2nd premolar.

Indications (typical)

Displaced mandibular fractures causing malocclusion of teeth.

Consent

- Infection.
- Bleeding.
- Extractions of teeth that compromise reduction.
- Alteration of bite (malocclusion).
- Failure of bony healing (non-union).
- Bone healing in incorrect position (malunion).
- Permanent numbness of lip and teeth.

Preoperative preparation

- Plain radiographs showing fracture in two planes or CBCT/CT.
- Prophylactic antibiotics ± tetanus prophylaxis.
- Complete WHO checklist and provide VTE prophylaxis as necessary.
- Mostly performed under GA with nasotracheal intubation; simple fractures may be carried out under LA.

Position and theatre set-up

Supine with head stabilization.

Procedure

Access to parasymphysis and body fractures

- Infiltrate with local anaesthetic and vasoconstrictor.
- Incise through the mucosa with a no.15 blade approximately 10mm below the attached gingiva, curving around the arch as needed.
- Posterior to the canines raise the incision to 5mm below the attached gingiva to avoid the mental nerve (see Fig. 15.16a).
- Dissect between the mucosa and mentalis muscle, then incise through mentalis and periosteum near the alveolar ridge.
- Raise a mucoperiosteal flap to the lower border as previously described (see ➲ 'Surgical tooth extraction', p. 842).
- Identify and protect the mental nerve.

Access to angle fractures

- If there is no 3rd molar or it is likely to be left in situ, a vestibular incision as described for BSSO is performed (see ➲ 'Bilateral sagittal split osteotomy', p. 898).
- Otherwise a full-thickness mucoperiosteal envelope flap is raised.

Extra-oral submandibular ± submental approach

- Incision length is dependent on the amount of access required.
- The incision is placed parallel to the lower border of the mandible and approximately 2–3cm below it, often in a skin crease.
- Submandibular (Risdon) incisions can be extended submentally, and even round to the contralateral side if required.
- Incise through the skin with a no.15 blade exposing the surface of platysma (which is thin or absent anteriorly).
- Undermine the skin to reduce traction on platysma.
- Sharply incise through platysma, again 2–3 cm below the lower border of the mandible, and identify the facial artery and vein.
- Ligate these vessels with 3-0 Vicryl® ties and dissect in the plane just beneath them to the lower border of mandible (see Fig. 15.16b).
    - The marginal mandibular branch of the facial nerve is deep to platysma but the vessels overlie it, and it is thus protected.
- Divide the pterygomasseteric sling and carry out subperiosteal dissection to allow excellent access to the ramus and even condyle.
- Anterior subperiosteal dissection exposes the body and symphysis.

Reduction and fixation

- Reduce the fracture to the correct occlusion, either by hand or using intermaxillary fixation (see ➲ 'Intermaxillary fixation', p. 874).
    - IMF may be left in place for fine adjustment of the occlusion postoperatively.
- Pre-contour a miniplate to fit passively around the fracture with at least two screw holes either side of the fracture.
- Depending on bone thickness, drill monocortically perpendicularly through the hole closest to the fracture; 6mm screws are usually sufficient.
- Insert screw at same angle as prepared hole but do not tighten fully.

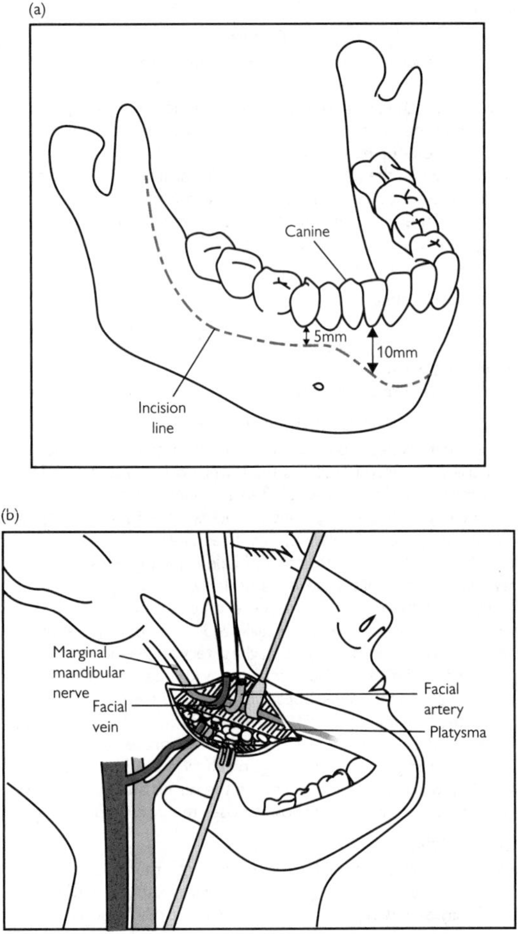
(a)
Canine
5mm
10mm
Incision
line
(b)
Marginal
mandibular
nerve
Facial
vein
Facial
artery
Platysma

Fig. 15.16 (a) Line of incision. (b) Extra-oral approach to mandible with platysma reflected and facial vessels ligated.

- Prepare the hole on the other side of the fracture similarly, but aim for compression of the fracture by drilling eccentrically into the plate hole slightly away from the fracture itself.
- If the occlusion is correct, fully tighten the screws and complete application of screws to the remaining plate holes.
- Attach all necessary plates in this manner.
    - A transbuccal approach with a drill trochar may be required to ensure perpendicular insertion for angle fractures.
- Irrigate thoroughly with saline.

Closure

- Close in layers using 3-0 absorbable sutures, approximating the mentalis muscle first, then the mucosa.
- If access incisions are planned properly the wound should not directly overlie the plate.

Postoperative care

- Prophylactic antibiotics if poor oral hygiene/immunocompromised.
- Chlorhexidine 0.2% mouthwash 1 week.
- Avoid smoking.
- Soft diet 4–6 weeks.
- Meticulous oral hygiene.

Complications (specific to the procedure)

- Damage to inferior alveolar nerve 5–10%.
- Malocclusion due to inadequate reduction 5–10%.
- Infection 10–15%.
- Non-union 1%.
- Long buccal nerve invariably damaged but patients rarely notice.

Tips and tricks

- Blunt dissection to free the mental nerve will allow easier soft tissue retraction.
- Reduce the fracture to the correct occlusion, rather than anatomical reduction—buccal anatomical reduction may result in widening the fracture lingually, with consequent malocclusion.
- Ensure water-cooling is used throughout drilling to prevent early loss of fixation through screw osteolysis.
- If there is lingual widening, pre-plate the fracture, then remove the plate and over-bend it; this will pull the lingual fracture line together when the plate is replaced.
- Bone-holding forceps at the lower border can make the parasymphysis easier to plate.
- Trauma to dental tissues and alveolar bone may accompany mandibular fractures, or may be isolated; whilst specific management is not described here, an excellent up-to-date resource can be found at www.dentaltraumaguide.org.

TMJ: ORIF mandibular condyle

Overview

TMJ fractures may be managed using open, closed, or endoscopically assisted reduction with a 4mm, 30° scope. Closed reduction is described elsewhere (see ➲ 'Intermaxillary fixation', p. 874).

Anatomy

The facial nerve enters the parotid gland almost immediately after leaving the skull and divides within it to supply the facial muscles.

Indications (typical)

Absolute

- Unable to achieve occlusion with closed technique.
- Lateral extracapsular displacement causing cosmetic defect.
- Displacement of fragment into middle cranial fossa.
- Foreign body invasion, such as firearm projectiles.

Relative

- Bony overlap >5mm with resultant loss of ramus height.
- Open fracture as potential for fibrosis.
- Bilateral fractures as ramus height lost.
- Associated midface fracture preventing use of IMF.
- Patient factors such as epilepsy, learning difficulties, or alcohol misuse precluding use of IMF.

Consent

- See ➲ 'ORIF mandible', p. 878.
- Include facial nerve weakness (<1%) and collection or leakage of saliva through wound.

Preoperative preparation

- Complete WHO checklist and provide VTE prophylaxis as necessary.
- Nasotracheal intubation + prophylactic antibiotics at induction.
- Avoid muscle relaxation during parotid dissection to reduce risk of facial nerve injury (although essential during fracture reduction).

Position and theatre set-up

Supine with head stabilization ring.

Procedure

Transparotid retromandibular approach

- Make a 3cm incision parallel to the ramus 1cm behind its posterior border, just under the inferior attachment of the helix (see Fig. 15.17).
- Dissect the superficial layer above the parotid sheath in all directions to allow more retraction.
- Carefully divide the parotid fascia using blunt dissection and continue through the gland parallel to the anticipated facial nerve branches; protect any branches identified.

- Incise masseter in line with its fibres and separate them using blunt dissection.
- Incise the periosteum and dissect subperiosteally to expose the entire lateral ramus, from sigmoid notch to inferior border.
- Reduction of the fracture into the correct anatomical position is facilitated by ensuring the patient is now fully paralysed.
- The proximal fragment is usually medially displaced (medial override) by the action of the lateral pterygoid; manipulate the fragment to make it a lateral override fracture.
- Place two 1mm miniplates in a triangular formation anteriorly and posteriorly, ensuring alignment of the posterior border of the ramus and proximal fragment (see Fig. 15.17).
- A high fracture may preclude two plates due to lack of bone; a single plate can be used but consider a 1.25mm plate to ensure mechanical stability and avoid postoperative plate fracture.
- Check occlusion is satisfactory.
- Close in layers, including masseter and the parotid fascia, with 3-0 absorbable sutures.
- Skin is closed with 5-0 nylon sutures.

Endoscopically-assisted

- Make a vestibular incision 5mm lateral to the attached gingiva from the 1st molar up the external oblique ridge as for a BSSO (see 'Bilateral sagittal split osteotomy', p. 898).
- Dissect subperiosteally to expose the whole lateral surface of the ramus, as described above, thereby creating an optical cavity.
- Insert an optical retractor and engage around the posterior border of the ramus.

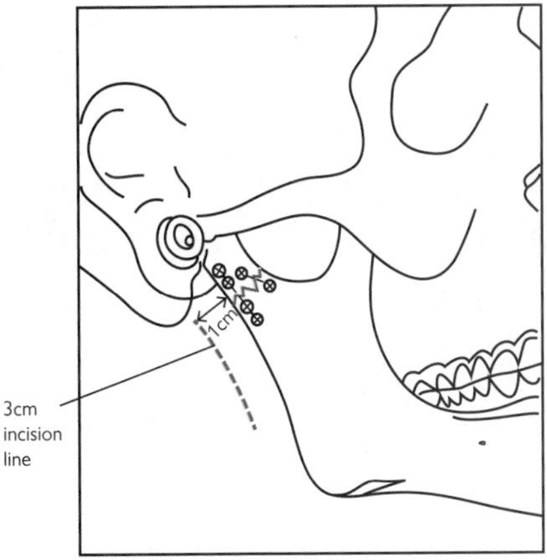
1cm
3cm
incision
line

Fig. 15.17 Position of retromandibular incision and miniplates.

- Insert a 4mm 30° scope and identify the fracture line.
- If medially displaced manipulate the proximal fragment into a lateral override position.
- Subperiosteally dissect the proximal fragment on its lateral side.
- Turn the endoscope 180o to trans-illuminate the cheek and introduce a buccal trocar at this position.
- Plate fragments as described for 'TMJ: ORIF mandibular condyle', p. 882.

Postoperative care

- Postoperative radiographs.
- Review weekly to check occlusion for 4–6 weeks.
- Prophylactic antibiotics for 5 days.
- Skin sutures to be removed at 5–7 days.
- Soft diet 4–6 weeks.

Complications (specific to the procedure)

- Facial nerve damage: 30% temporary, 1% permanent.
- Malunion.
- Condylar necrosis.
- Sialocoele.
- Plate fracture.

Tips and tricks

- Low fractures and lateral override fractures are easiest.
- A coincident mobile mandibular fracture helps with reducing the condyle so fix the condyle first.
- Distraction of the fracture is assisted by using a McKesson mouth prop as a fulcrum whilst pushing up on the patient's chin.

ORIF zygomatic complex

Overview

Fractures of the cheek bones involve both the zygoma and maxilla—the zygomatic (malar) complex. These are referred to as tripod fractures as they displace at three points: the zygomatic arch (ZA), lateral orbital rim, and infraorbital margin. Although stable anatomical reduction can occasionally be achieved by a closed technique, exposure at one or more sites is usually required to confirm reduction or to allow stabilization with miniplate fixation (see Fig. 15.18a). Additionally, orbital reconstruction may be required as the zygomatic complex forms the floor and lateral wall of the orbit (see ➲ 'Repair of orbital floor and wall', p. 890). Isolated ZA fractures may also occur and are treated with a closed approach.

Anatomy

- The zygoma has three processes that terminate at suture lines: the zygomaticomaxillary (ZM), zygomaticofrontal (ZF), and zygomaticotemporal (ZT) sutures.
- If exposure of the ZA is required, a bicoronal approach is used to prevent facial nerve injury (see ➲ 'Access: bicoronal flap', p. 894).

Indications (typical)

- Functional abnormalities—trismus or diplopia.
- Aesthetic abnormalities—facial deformity or abnormal eye position.

Consent

- Infection.
- Bleeding.
- Scar.
- Risk of blindness (1 in 15,000).

Preoperative preparation

- Imaging: plain radiographs in two planes or CT.
- Intraoperative imaging may be useful to confirm fracture reduction.
- GA—fibre-optic nasotracheal intubation may be required if impingement of the ZA on the coronoid process limits mouth opening.
- Complete WHO checklist and provide VTE prophylaxis as necessary.
- Prophylactic antibiotics +/– dexamethasone at induction.
- Orthoptic ± ophthalmic assessment as required.

Position and theatre set-up

Supine with head stabilization ring.

Procedure

Gillies' closed reduction

- With a no.15 blade make a 2cm incision 2.5cm superior and anterior to the upper helical attachment; angle to avoid branches of the superficial temporal artery.

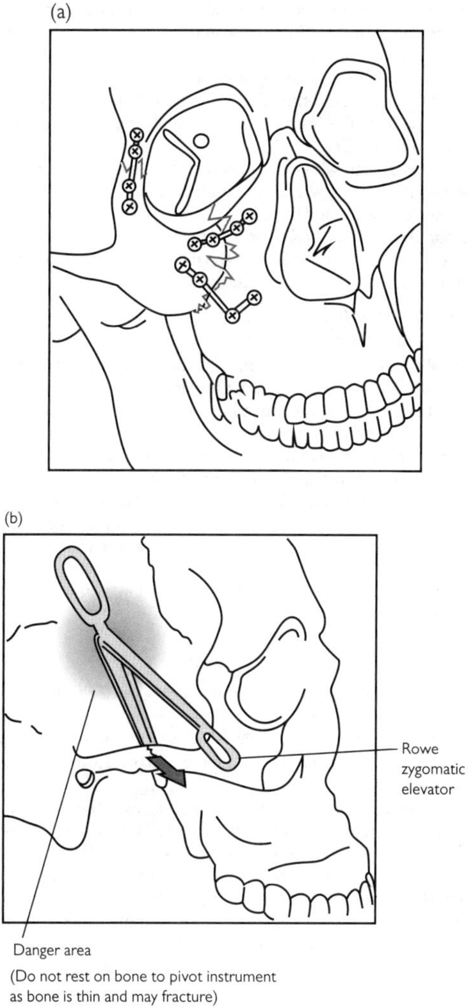
(a)
(b)
Rowe zygomatic elevator
Danger area
(Do not rest on bone to pivot instrument as bone is thin and may fracture)

Fig. 15.18 (a) Miniplate fixation over suture lines and infraorbital rim. (b) Use of Rowe zygomatic elevator.

- Continue dissection through subcutaneous tissue containing temporoparietal fascia (TPF) to expose the white, glistening deep temporal fascia (dTF).
  - Incise through dTF to expose temporalis.
- Use an artery clip to hold the inferior portion of the dTF and introduce a Howarth periosteal elevator with a sweeping motion to reach the deep surface of the ZA.
- Replace the Howarth with a Rowe zygomatic elevator (see Fig. 15.18b).
- Pull the elevator in an upwards and outwards direction to reduce the fracture, which usually audibly clicks.
  - Do not use the temporal bone as a pivot.
- Check reduction is stable and close the incision in a single layer with three interrupted 3-0 black silk sutures.

Open reduction internal fixation

Zygomaticomaxillary (zygomatic) buttress

- Make a full-thickness upper vestibular incision 5mm from the attached gingiva, extending from canine to 1st molar.
- Subperiosteal dissection exposes the anterior and lateral maxilla and the maxillary process of the zygoma.
- Reduce the fracture transorally with a Rowe elevator; keep instruments close to bone to avoid disrupting the buccal fat pad.
- Reduction is checked by confirming the buttress is well aligned.
- Carefully adapt an L-shaped miniplate ensuring it is placed as laterally as possible to make use of the best quality bone; the foot of the plate should run above the roots of the teeth.
- Close in a single layer, ideally including periosteum, with a 3-0 fast-resorbing continuous suture.

Zygomaticofrontal suture

- Lateral eyebrow approach:
  - Apply a corneal shield to protect the globe and infiltrate a vasoconstrictor in the line of incision.
  - Use finger and thumb to stabilize skin over the superolateral orbital ridge and make a 2cm incision within the brow down to periosteum in one stroke.
  - Undermine in a supraperiosteal plane to allow retraction inferiorly with Senn–Miller (cat's paw) retractors to identify the fracture.
  - Incise the periosteum, exposing both sides of the fracture.
  - Subperiosteally dissect medially over the superior orbital rim with a Mitchell trimmer, then slide a Howarth periosteal elevator inferiorly to expose the lateral orbital wall; make sure the elevator is angled away from the globe as dissection proceeds into the orbit.
  - With the fracture fully visualized reduction can be performed by the Gillies' or intraoral method.
  - Correct alignment of the zygoma with the greater wing of the sphenoid along the lateral orbital wall (sphenozygomatic junction) confirms reduction.

- Adapt a five-hole miniplate with an empty hole over the fracture line; screw sequencing is as per ORIF mandible (see ➔ 'ORIF mandible', p. 879).
- Close periosteum with 3-0 absorbable suture and skin with 6-0 nylon interrupted sutures.
- Upper blepharoplasty approach:
  - Place a horizontal incision in the supratarsal skin crease.
  - If there is no crease, or it has been obliterated by swelling, this should be about 10mm above the lashes in the midline and extended laterally to 7mm above the lashes at the lateral canthus.
  - Incise through skin and orbicularis oculi and onto the orbital septum; the skin incision can be extended laterally if required.
  - Blunt dissect with scissors under the muscle towards the superolateral orbital rim and expose periosteum.
  - Reduce, plate, and close as described for 'Lateral eyebrow approach', p. 888.

Infraorbital rim approach

- This can be transcutaneous or transconjunctival (see ➔ 'Repair of orbital floor and wall', p. 892).

Postoperative care

- Eye observations.
- Avoid blowing nose for 10 days.
- If plates are used continue antibiotics for 5 days
- Removal of sutures at 5–7 days.
- Chlorhexidine 0.2% mouthwash if intraoral approach is used.

Complications (specific to the procedure)

- Plate infection <1%.
- Blindness 1 in 15,000.

Tips and tricks

4 mm or 6mm screws are usually used but it is situation-dependent.

- Low-profile 0.5 or 0.7mm plates are used at the ZF and infraorbital margin; 0.7mm or 0.8mm plates at the ZM.
- One-point fixation is usually achieved at the ZF or ZM buttress.
- ZF fixation complements a ZM plate and is the usual configuration for two-point fixation.

Repair of orbital floor and wall

Overview

An orbital blowout fracture is where the orbital rim is intact but a traumatic increase in intra-orbital pressure causes one or more of the walls to fracture, usually the floor or medial wall. The orbital floor must also be explored in zygomatic complex fractures with eye signs.

Anatomy

- The anterior ethmoidal artery is transmitted through the medial wall at 24mm from the anterior lacrimal crest; the posterior ethmoidal artery is 12mm further back and the optic nerve a further 6mm (24/12/6).
- The junction between the floor and medial wall is called the transition zone and is difficult to see intraoperatively.
- The floor forms an S-shape in the sagittal plane creating a post-bulbar constriction that holds the globe forward (see Fig. 15.19a).
- The posterior orbital ledge is just in front of the optic canal and is formed by the orbital process of the palatine bone.

Indications (typical)

- Diplopia and gaze restriction.
- Enophthalmos.
- Large defects that will lead to late enopthalmos.
- Paediatric 'white-eyed' blowout; inferior rectus entrapment causes muscle necrosis and permanent ocular restriction due to fibrosis.

(a)

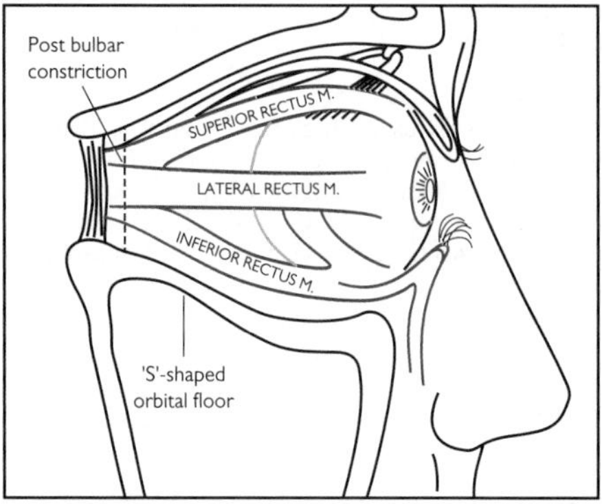
Post bulbar
constriction
SUPERIOR RECTUS M.
LATERAL RECTUS M.
INFERIOR RECTUS M.
'S'-shaped
orbital floor

Fig. 15.19 (a) Saggital view of orbital floor. (b) Transcutaneous approaches. (c) Transconjunctival approach. (d) Preformed mesh secured in place.

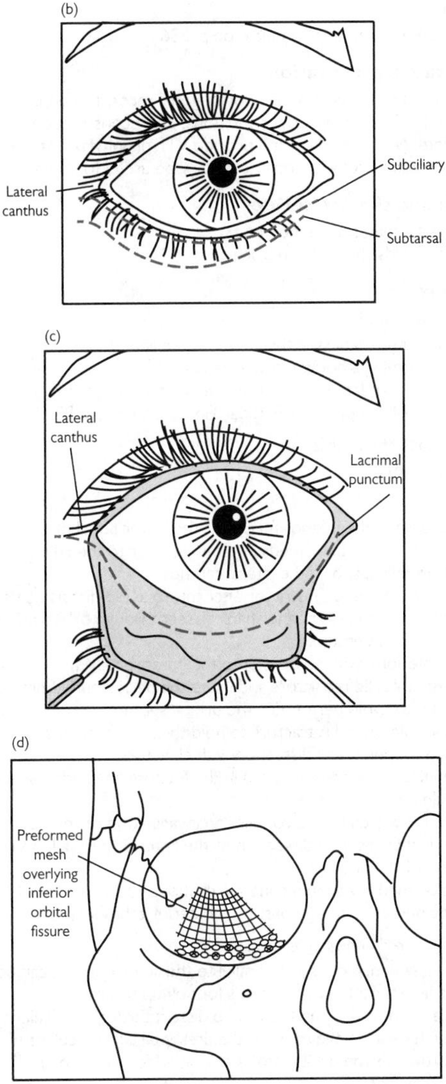
(b)
Lateral canthus
Subciliary
Subtarsal
(c)
Lateral canthus
Lacrimal punctum
(d)
Preformed mesh overlying inferior orbital fissure

Fig. 15.19 (*Contd.*)

Consent

- As for 'ORIF zygomatic complex' on p. 886.

Preoperative preparation

- Fine 1mm-slice CT with 3-plane orthogonal reconstructions and both bone and soft tissue windows; additional 3D reconstructions are great!
- Complete WHO checklist and provide VTE prophylaxis as necessary.
- GA; infiltration with vasoconstrictor may be useful for haemostasis.

Position and theatre set-up

- Supine with head stabilization ring.
- Corneal shields should be in place.

Procedure

Temporary tarsorraphy

- A 6-0 silk suture is passed through the grey line of each lid either side of the pupil forming a horizontal mattress.
- A knot is tied at 2cm so the lid can be opened for a forced duction test at the start of the procedure. (See 'Tips and tricks', p. 893.)

Transcutaneous approaches

(See Fig. 15.19b)

Subtarsal

- A skin crease at the inferior margin of the lower tarsal plate is incised with a no.15 blade. Start medially, 2mm inferior to the lid margin, and extend laterally just past the lateral canthus.
- Infiltrate LA and vasoconstrictor after this to avoid distorting tissues.
- Use skin hooks to retract and sharp dissect through orbicularis oculi onto the orbital septum.
- Dissect inferiorly with scissors onto the infraorbital rim.
- Use Desmarres lid retractors and incise the periosteum 2mm below the orbital rim to avoid perforating the orbital septum.
- Use malleable orbital retractors to hold the periorbital tissues and complete subperiosteal dissection with elevators.
  - The infraorbital nerve is often in the fracture line and dissection should continue above it.
- The inferior orbital fissure contains an invagination of the periosteum; bipolar diathermy, then dissection of the anterior part, allows increased exposure of the floor.
- Dissection medially should continue cautiously to ensure no damage to the optic nerve; do not go past the posterior ethmoidal artery.

Subcilliary (layered Converse technique)

- The initial skin incision is just parallel to the lid margin and can be carried past the lateral canthus in a Crow's foot by up to 2cm.
- Create a 4–6mm skin flap then sharp dissect through orbicularis oculi at the same level as above to enter the preseptal suborbicularis plane.
- Dissect towards the orbital rim as described for the 'Subtarsal' approach, p. 892.

Transconjunctival approach

- Place two 6-0 silk sutures through the lower tarsal plate 4mm below the lid margin to evert the lower lid.
- Perform a lateral canthotomy and cantholysis of the inferior crus (see ➔ 'Lateral canthotomy and cantholysis', p. 872).
- Enter the subconjunctival plane via the canthotomy incision and create a pocket medially extending to the lacrimal punctum.
- Open this pocket by incising the conjunctiva, from the canthotomy laterally to the punctum medially, at a level midway between the lid margin and inferior fornix (see Fig. 15.19c).
- Use a malleable orbital retractor to hold the orbital fat and retract the lid with Desmarres retractors to expose the orbital rim.
- Enter the orbit as described for the 'Transcutaneous approaches', p. 892.

Reconstruction

- A titanium mesh or anatomical titanium plate is adapted to sit passively over the defect and secured with screws over the inferior orbital rim (see Fig. 15.19d).
- It must not be cantilevered from the orbital rim, but sit on a ledge of bone; this invariably means placing it on the posterior orbital ledge.
- The acutely angled medial wall transition zone must be replicated in medial wall defects; anatomical plates help achieve this.
- Check pupil level, correction of enopthalmos, and perform a forced duction test before securing the mesh.

Closure

- Close the periosteum with 4-0 resorbable sutures.
- No muscle sutures are placed in transcutaneous approaches.
- Skin should be closed with interrupted 6-0 nylon sutures.
- Transconjunctival incisions can either be closed with resorbable sutures or left open.
    - Many surgeons leave these open to reduce the risk of entropion.

Postoperative care

- Elevate head (reduces periorbital swelling).
- Hourly eye observations overnight (pain, pupil reflexes, visual acuity, eye movements).
- Remove skin sutures at 5 days.

Complications

- Blindness 1 in 15,000.
- Ectropion.
- Enopthalmos.

Tips and tricks

Forced duction test involves holding the conjunctiva and episclera just shy of the limbus with toothed forceps and checking that the eye moves unhindered in all directions; it is negative in the absence of mechanical restriction.

Access: bicoronal flap

Overview

Access to the facial skeleton is complicated by aesthetic sensitivity and functionally important structures, most notably the facial nerve. The bicoronal flap allows excellent access to much of the facial skeleton and is described here.

Anatomy

(See Fig. 15.20a)

- The scalp has five layers:Skin, subCutaneous tissue, galea Aponeurotica, Loose connective tissue, and Pericranium.
- Inferolaterally the galea becomes the temporoparietal fascia (TPF).
- TPF becomes the superficial muscular aponeurotic system (SMAS) below the zygomatic arch (ZA).
- The deep temporal fascia (dTF) overlies temporalis and is immediately deep to the TPF, attaching to the superior temporal line.
- Inferiorly the dTF becomes the parotidomasseteric fascia and continues in the neck as the deep cervical fascia.
- A superfical fat pad lies between TPF and dTF just above the ZA.
- dTF divides into a superficial and deep portion separated by an intermediate fat pad 2cm above the ZA.
- A deep fat pad lies under the deep portion of dTF and is called the buccal fat pad.
- The deep portion of the dTF inserts into the periosteum of the ZA.
    - The plane just deep to this is used in the Gillies' approach (see ➲ 'ORIF zygomatic complex', p. 886).
    - The plane just superficial to this is used to access the ZA.
- The temporal branch of the facial nerve leaves the parotid gland and traverses within or just deep to the TPF; it crosses the ZA at least 1cm from its root and follows the Pitanguy line (5mm below tragus to 15mm above lateral eyebrow) within the superficial fat pad to enter the frontalis at least 2cm above the zygomaticofrontal suture (see Fig. 15.20b).

Indications (typical)

Access to the frontal bone, upper mid-face, zygomatic arch, orbit, temporal, and infra-temporal fossae.

Consent

- Infection.
- Bleeding.
- Numbness and/or weakness of forehead.
- Loss of muscle bulk in temporal region.
- Hair loss.

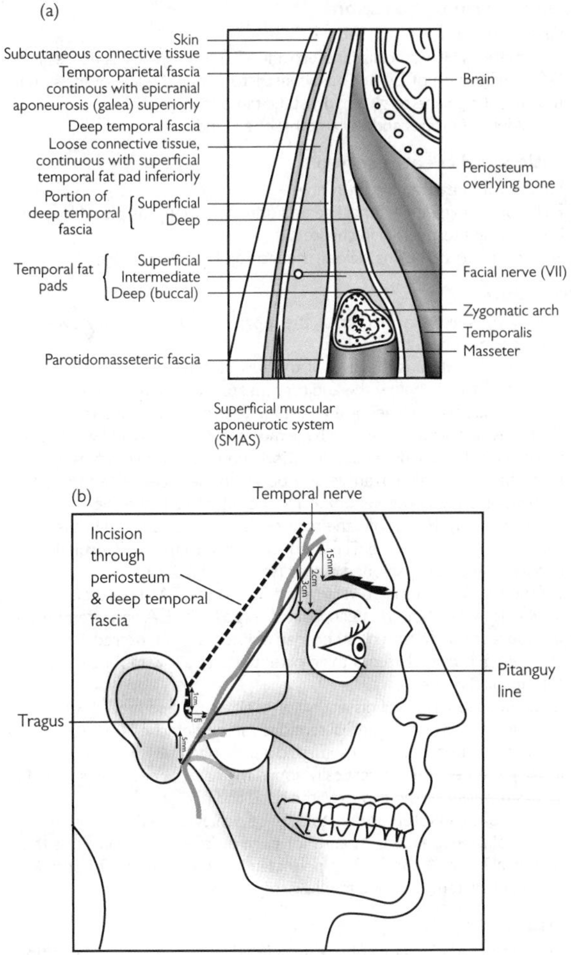
(a)
Skin
Subcutaneous connective tissue
Temporoparietal fascia continous with epicranial aponeurosis (galea) superiorly
Deep temporal fascia
Loose connective tissue, continuous with superficial temporal fat pad inferiorly
Portion of deep temporal fascia
Superficial
Deep
Temporal fat pads
Superficial
Intermediate
Deep (buccal)
Parotidomasseteric fascia
Superficial muscular aponeurotic system (SMAS)
Brain
Periosteum overlying bone
Facial nerve (VII)
Zygomatic arch
Temporalis
Masseter
(b)
Temporal nerve
Incision through periosteum & deep temporal fascia
15mm
2cm
3cm
Pitanguy line
1cm
Tragus
5mm

Fig. 15.20 (a) Coronal section of temporal region. (b) Position of temporal branch of the facial nerve following the Pitanguy line, and position of the incision through periosteum and dTF used to avoid damaging this nerve.

Preoperative preparation

- Group and save.
- Complete WHO checklist and provide VTE prophylaxis as necessary.
- GA + infiltration of LA and vasoconstrictor along the line of incision in the subgaleal plane to give hydrostatic tamponade.
- Consider antibiotics and dexamethasone at induction.

Position and theatre set-up

- Supine with head stabilization ring.
- Full monitoring with arterial line and urinary catheter as blood loss can be significant, especially in children.
- Shaving a corridor of hair along the incision line aids closure.

Procedure

- Make a bow-like skin incision to the subgaleal plane coronally over the vertex 5cm behind the hairline.
- The inferior extent is the level of the auricular helix.
  - Extend to just below the auditory meatus to access the ZA.
  - Continue to the level of the earlobe to access the condyles.
- Compress the wound edges with haemostatic Raney clips and wet gauze.
- Continue subgaleal dissection anteriorly until 3cm above orbital rim.
- Incise the pericranium transversely between the superior temporal lines at this point and continue forward in the subperiosteal plane.
- Approximately 1cm above the root of the ZA, incise through the superficial portion of the dTF, then connect with the supraorbital periosteal incision fashioned earlier (see Fig. 15.20).
- Extend this fascial incision vertically down to the ZA and dissect forwards in the subperiosteal plane to expose the ZA and lateral orbit.
- If a supraorbital foramen rather than a notch is encountered it is converted into the latter with an osteotome to allow mobilization of the supraorbital nerve.
- Continue subperiosteal dissection of orbital roof and medial wall.
- The medial and lateral canthal tendons can be detached if further access is required but mark with a suture to aid reattachment.
- Incising the periosteum vertically above the nasal bones as it is raised allows mobility of the flap over the nose and mid-face.
- Access to the infratemporal fossa can be achieved by dissecting the temporalis muscle along its anterior edge or its entire origin along the temporal bone. A 1cm cuff of periosteum and muscle is left just below the superior temporal line to allow resuspension.

Closure

- The canthal tendons must be resuspended in their anatomical position within the orbit and not to the orbital rim.
  - Use miniplates if attachments have been lost traumatically.
- Resuspend temporalis if elevated; the anterior portion of the muscle is attached via drill holes in the lateral orbital rim.
- Resuspend the incised superficial portion of the dTF.
- Remove Raney clips stepwise and perform meticulous haemostasis.

- Place size 12 suction drains bilaterally.
- The galea should be closed with 2-0 resorbing sutures.
- The scalp is closed with skin staples and skin with 5-0 non-resorbing sutures.

Postoperative care

- Remove drains when <30ml/day.
- Sutures to be removed at 5–7 days, staples at 10 days.

Complications

- Numbness (supraorbital and ZT nerve) 17%.
- Partial unilateral frontal motor deficit 11%.
- Varying degrees of alopecia 18%.
- Haematoma 5%.
- Temporal hollowing 45–76%.

Tips and tricks

- Bevel the incision to avoid hair follicles, thereby minimizing peri-incisional alopecia.
- The standard straight incision leaves a noticeable scar causing hair to part away from it, especially when wet. A stealth incision with geometric zig-zags is used to allow a less conspicuous scar.
- For balding patients, the incision can be extended as far posteriorly as the upper part of the occiput.
- If a pericranial flap is required, incise transversely through pericranium further from the supraorbital rim with lateral incisions along the superior temporal lines to create an apron of tissue.
    - Its blood supply is anterior so keep periosteum attached to the galea/frontalis muscle layer anteriorly as far as possible.
- Prevent temporal hollowing by keeping the intermediate fat pad attached to the deep portion of the dTF.

Bilateral sagittal split osteotomy

Overview

This versatile technique to correct prognathia and retrognathia has been extensively modified and improved upon but has changed little since first described by Hugo Obwegeser in 1953.

Anatomy

- The IAN branches from the posterior division of the mandibular nerve before entering the mandibular canal at the lingula, and exiting at the mental foramen as the mental nerve.
- The facial vessels lie near the inferomedial surface of the mandible before curving round the inferior border at the anterior border of masseter to ascend towards the angle of the mouth.

Indications (typical)

- Significant malocclusion of mandibular origin causing masticatory difficulty, facial deformity or airway problems.
- As part of a bimaxillary procedure for facial rejuvenation or obstructive sleep apnoea.

Consent

- Infection.
- Bleeding.
- Relapse.
- Numbness to lip and teeth.
- May require teeth to be wired shut for up to a month postoperatively.

Preoperative preparation

- Accurate pre-assessment of new mandibular position is mandatory.
    - Position is predicted by simulation of intended osteotomies on study models.
    - Acrylic occlusal wafers are fabricated to facilitate final repositioning.
- Group and save.
- Complete WHO checklist and provide VTE prophylaxis as necessary.
- GA with nasotracheal intubation.
- Hypotensive anaesthesia (less bleeding and postoperative swelling).
- Antibiotics and dexamethasone at induction.

Position and theatre set-up

Supine with head stabilization ring.

Procedure

- Insert a large McKesson mouth prop.
- Infiltrate local anaesthetic with vasoconstrictor.
- Incise to bone over the external oblique ridge on the anterior surface of the ramus half way between the dental arches.
- Extend anteriorly to the first molar tooth 3mm below the level of the attached gingiva (see Fig. 15.21a).
- Raise a buccal mucoperiosteal flap down to the inferior border.

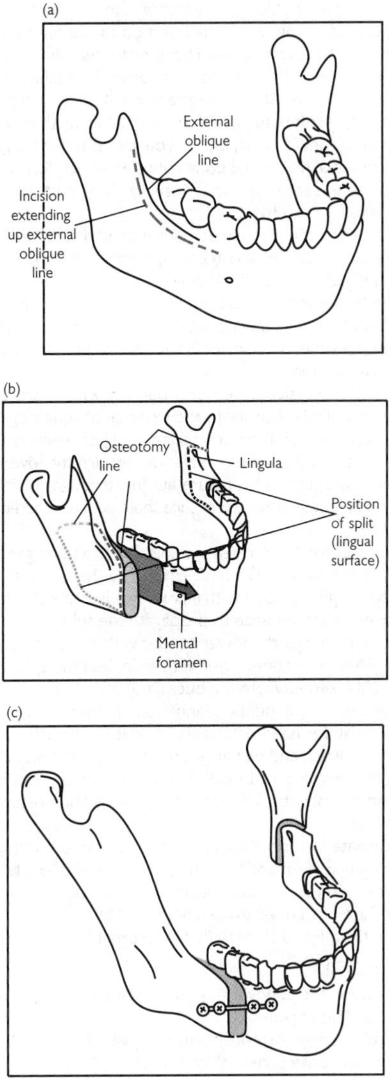
(a)
External
oblique
line
Incision
extending
up external
oblique
line
(b)
Osteotomy
line
Lingula
Position
of split
(lingual
surface)
Mental
foramen
(c)

Fig. 15.21 (a) Incision. (b) Bone cuts. (c) Bone fragments fixed in intended position.

- Elevate the periosteum along the anterior ramus up to the base of the coronoid process, stripping off the insertion of the temporalis.
  - Retract using a curved Kocher clamp or forked ramus retractor.
- Continue on the lingual surface to 2cm above the occlusal plane.
- Identify the lingula and IAN, then raise periosteum to the posterior border, retracting soft tissues medially with a Howarth elevator.
  - Seeing the coronoid notch means you are above the lingula.
- Begin with a medial horizontal bone cut using an acrylic finishing bur to remove part of the anterior ramus lingually giving better visualization of the lingula (see Fig. 15.21b).
- With a long side-cutting Lindemann bur extend this cut to make a unicortical medial horizontal osteotomy parallel with the occlusal plane just above and *just* distal to the lingula.
- Remove the McKesson mouth prop and ramus retraction.
- Place an Obwegeser channel retractor in the 2nd molar region buccally so it fully engages the lower mandibular border, protecting the soft tissues and facial artery.
- Make a vertical unicortical osteotomy buccally with a fissure bur from the inferior mandibular border to the external oblique ridge.
  - Gently paint through the buccal plate until just reaching cancellous bone (bleeds), and ensure completion through the lower border.
- Join the two bone cuts with a fissure bur just through cortical bone.
- Use fine flexible osteotomes to ensure the unicortical osteotomies are complete.
- Use wedge osteotomes to open the split 2–3mm using gentle malleting.
- Introduce a Smith bone spreader 2–3mm into the split with the two prongs buccally; gently open with incrementally increasing force, pausing briefly between each squeeze to propagate the split.
- If it fails to 'pop', mallet the lower border with a fine osteotome, keeping the IAN under direct vision, to complete the split.
- Ensure the IAN is freed from the buccal cortical plate.
- Ensure fragments move independently to confirm split is complete.
- Site a tonsil swab for haemostasis and repeat on the other side.
  - Remove all swabs and throat packs once haemostasis achieved.
- Place into IMF using a prefabricated occlusal wafer if required.
  - The condyles must be fully seated superiorly and posteriorly in the glenoid fossa.
- Internal miniplate fixation is applied in the corrected position using the same technique as for mandibular fractures (see Fig. 15.21c).
  - Alternatively three titanium bicortical screws can be used, ensuring that they are positioned away from the IAN.
- Remove elastic IMF and close with 3-0 resorbable sutures.

Bad split (up to 23%)

- This occurs when the condyle stays on the anterior fragment.
- Complete the split as planned.
- Perform a subcondylar osteotomy to readjust.
- Plate the condyle onto proximal fragment.

Postoperative care

- Postoperative imaging the following day.
- Dexamethasone for 24h.
- Antibiotics 5 days.
- Chlorhexidine 0.2% mouthwash for 1 week.

Complications

- Damage to the IAN: temporary 100%, permanent 30%.
- Relapse advancement 8%.
- Relapse setback 22%.
- Damage to the facial vessels; extra-oral ligation is rarely required.
- Bad split 23%—patient may require prolonged IMF.

Maxillary osteotomy

Overview

Osteotomies can be performed at the Le Fort I, II, or III level, depending on the underlying skeletal abnormality. Once the tooth-bearing portion of the maxilla is mobilized, it can be repositioned within its soft tissue envelope anteriorly, superiorly, or inferiorly. The Le Fort I osteotomy is the most common and is described here. Dramatic changes in facial profile can be obtained, especially when used as a bimaxillary procedure

Anatomy

- The maxilla is supplied by a rich mucosal anastomotic vascular network derived from the:
  - Descending palatine branch of the maxillary artery.
  - Alveolar branches of the maxillary artery.
  - Ascending palatine branch of the facial artery.
  - Anterior branch of ascending pharyngeal artery.
- A mobilized maxilla may therefore be safely reliant on branches of the facial and pharyngeal arteries via the soft palate.
- The thick pterygoid plates are attached to the posterior maxilla by a thin bridge of bone.

Indications (typical)

Significant malocclusion of maxillary origin causing masticatory difficulty or facial deformity.

Consent

- Infection.
- Bleeding.
- Relapse.
- Numbness of face.

Preoperative preparation

- Accurate pre-assessment of new maxillary position is mandatory.
  - Position is predicted by simulation of intended osteotomies on study models.
  - Acrylic occlusal wafers are fabricated to facilitate final repositioning.
- Group and save.
- Complete WHO checklist and provide VTE prophylaxis as necessary.
- GA (nasotracheal intubation) + infiltration of LA and vasoconstrictor.
- Antibiotics and dexamethasone at induction.

Position and theatre set-up

Supine with head stabilization ring.

Procedure

- A fixed reference position is created by placing a temporary IMF screw in the glabella region
- A horseshoe mucoperiosteal vestibular incision 4mm from the attached gingiva is made between the first molar teeth.

- Bring the incision out towards the parotid duct laterally to give a broad soft tissue pedicle.
- Elevate the periosteum with Obwegeser periosteal elevators in a superior direction to just below the infraorbital rims, preserving the infraorbital neurovascular bundles.
- Continue medially to expose the piriform aperture.
- Use a Mitchell trimmer and Howarth periosteal elevator to free the mucosa of the floor and walls of the nose to the level of the inferior turbinates superiorly, extending to a depth of approximately 30mm.
- Elevate periosteum laterally past the ZM buttresses creating a mucosal tunnel that exposes the maxillary tuberosities; ensure the pterygoid plates can be located with elevators.
- Use a Langenbeck retractor to fully visualize the maxilla and mark the intended osteotomy.
    - This mark should start from the lateral part of the piriform aperture, between the floor and inferior turbinate, and extend laterally, a few mm above the root apices, angled towards the inferior extent of the pterygoid plate.
- Locate a small Lack tongue depressor on the pterygoid plate in the mucosal tunnel overlying the tuberosity.
- Use a reciprocating saw to cut towards the piriform aperture.
    - Start near the ZM buttress.
    - The bone is thick here and it can take a few seconds to get going.
- On nearing the piriform aperture, angle the saw parallel to the lateral nasal wall, protecting nasal mucosa with a Howarth elevator.
- Remove the saw, then cut back towards the tongue depressor through the ZM buttress under direct vision to ensure the cut has reached (but not involved) the pterygoid plate.
- Use curved, guarded osteotomes to complete the lateral nasal wall cuts and a forked osteotome for the septum; 30mm depth is safe.
- Use curved pterygoid chisels to cause dysjunction from the maxilla.
- Down-fracture the maxillary segment with light digital pressure.
    - Smith spreaders, Rowes' disimpaction forceps, and Tessier retromaxillary levers are all used to aid down-fracture.
- Locate and mobilize the vascular pedicles by gentle dissection with a Mitchell trimmer to allow tension-free repositioning.
- Bone removal using rongeurs and an acrylic trimming bur is undertaken in a stepwise fashion to allow impaction as required.
- Position the maxilla in the intended occlusion with the mandible, ensuring the mandibular condyles are seated correctly in the glenoid fossae then apply elastic or wire IMF (see ➔ 'IMF', p. 874).
- Check the intended movements have been performed using the temporary IMF screw placed at the beginning as a reference point
- Secure with miniplates at the nasomaxillary and ZM buttresses (see Fig. 15.22a).
- Remove IMF and the temporary IMF screw and check the occlusion.

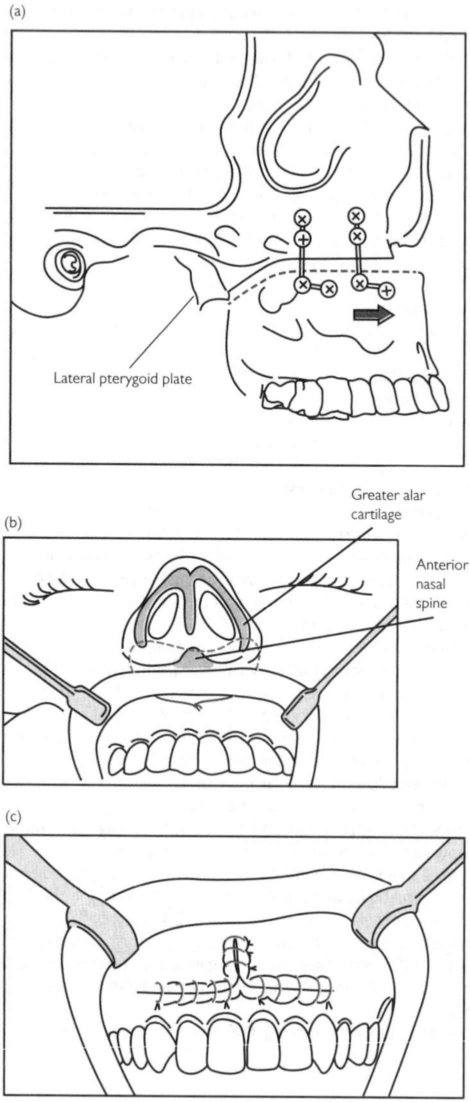
(a)
Lateral pterygoid plate
(b)
Greater alar cartilage
Anterior nasal spine
(c)

Fig. 15.22 (a) Maxilla fixed in planned position. (b) Alar cinch suture. (c) V-Y closure of soft tissues.

Closure

- Close with a continuous 3-0 fast-resorbing suture.
- Control alar width with an alar cinch suture, passing first through the mucosa of one ala, and then the other; narrow the alar base by tightening the suture and tie at the correct width (see Fig. 15.22b).
- Use V-Y closure if lip lengthening is required (see Fig. 15.22c).
  - Pull the midline of the upper wound margin upwards with a skin hook such that it approximates with itself for 1cm either side.
  - Suture this approximated 1cm to shorten the upper wound.
  - Thereafter, close the remaining horizontal wound as normal.

Postoperative care

- Continue antibiotics and dexamethasone for at least 24h.
- Postoperative radiographs the following day.
- Meticulous oral hygiene (dental hygienist instruction required).
- Chlorhexidine 0.2% mouthwash for 1 week.

Complications

- Paraesthesia: temporary 30%, permanent 6%.
- Infection of plates.
- Non-union.
- Relapse 3–28%.

Tips and tricks

- Reduce nasal septum to prevent buckling when impacting maxilla.
- A 4–5mm vertical step downwards at the zygomatic buttress can be helpful as curving below the zygoma here can make controlled horizontal manoeuvring of the maxilla more difficult.
- Avoid disrupting the buccal fat pad as herniation into the operative field reduces visibility.

TMJ arthrocentesis

Overview

TMJ lysis and lavage is a straightforward, minimally invasive treatment of temporomandibular dysfunction (TMD) that gives symptomatic improvement for 70% of patients.

Anatomy

- The TMJ is a synovial joint surrounded by a dense fibrous capsule.
- The joint space is divided into upper and lower spaces by a fibrocartilaginous articular disc called the meniscus (see Fig. 15.23a).
- The mandibular condyle is circumferentially supplied by the superficial temporal artery (STA) and the maxillary artery.
  - Anterior surface: posterior deep temporal branch of the maxillary artery.
  - Posterior surface: STA.
  - Superficial surface: transverse facial branch of the STA.
  - Deep surface: anterior tympanic, middle meningeal and inferior alveolar branches of the maxillary artery.
- It is primarily innervated by the auriculotemporal branch of V3.
- Point A (see Fig. 15.23b) represents the maximum concavity of the glenoid fossa.
- Point B represents the articular eminence.

Indications (typical)

- Myogenous TMD refractory to non-surgical management.
- Arthrogenous TMD with disc derangement; especially a closed lock of the TMJ.
- Arthrogenous TMD with degenerative joint disease.

Consent

- Infection.
- Bleeding.
- No improvement of symptoms.

Preoperative preparation

- Complete WHO checklist and provide VTE prophylaxis as necessary.
- GA or IV sedation with infiltration of LA and vasoconstrictor.

Position and theatre set-up

Supine with head stabilization ring.

Procedure

- Mark out points A and B on a line from the lateral canthus to the most posterior and central point of the tragus (Holmlund–Hellsing line) (see Fig. 15.23b).
- Infiltrate local anaesthetic at planned entry points.
- With the mouth open, insert a 19G needle at point A and angle anterosuperiorly to enter the posterior recess.

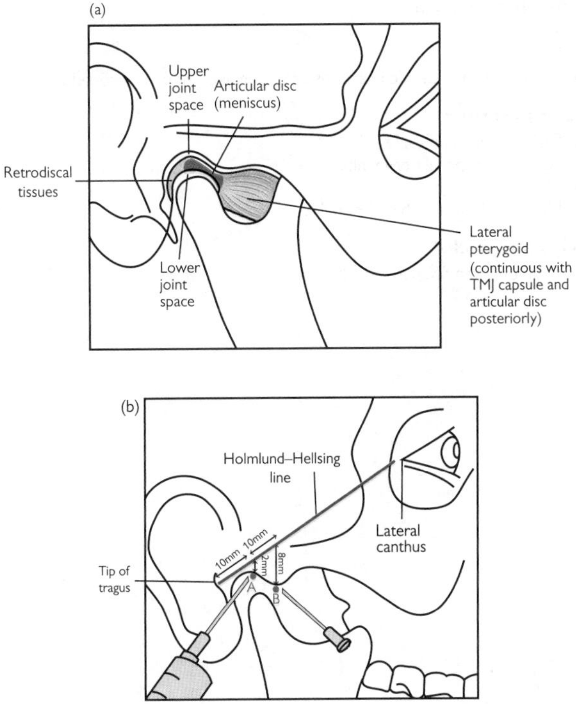
(a)
Upper joint space
Articular disc (meniscus)
Retrodiscal tissues
Lower joint space
Lateral pterygoid (continuous with TMJ capsule and articular disc posteriorly)
(b)
Holmlund–Hellsing line
Lateral canthus
Tip of tragus
10mm
10mm
2mm
8mm
A
B

Fig. 15.23 (a) TMJ structure. (b) Surface markings: point A is 10mm along the Holmlund–Hellsing line and 2mm below; point B is 20mm along and 8mm below.

- Distend the upper joint space with up to 5ml of Hartmann's solution to break down adhesions.
  - Mandibular movement should be felt.
- Insert a second 19G needle at point B and angle posterosuperiorly to enter the anterior recess; correct positioning is confirmed by drainage when closing the mouth.
- Connect a three-way stopcock on an extension tube to the first needle.
- Support both needles and ask the assistant to flush at least 100ml of solution under pressure to lavage the joint space.
- Remove the first needle then introduce 1ml triamcinolone acetonide 40 mg/ml intra-articularly.
- Place a small fabric plaster over the entry points and apply pressure.

Postoperative care

- Simple analgesia.
- Soft diet.
- Self-physiotherapeutic exercises as undertaken prior to procedure.

Complications

- Facial nerve injury 0.7%.
- Auriculotemporal nerve injury 2.4%.
- TMJ haemarthrosis.
- Needle fracture within joint 0.1%.

Tips and tricks

A double-lumen Shepard needle can be used but it is quite large.

TMJ eminoplasty and condyloplasty

Overview

The articular eminence is a tubercle projecting inferiorly from the zygomatic arch. It forms the anterior border of the glenoid fossa and contributes to joint stability.

Anatomy

- The STA divides into an anterior and posterior branch 2cm above the ZA.
- The middle meningeal branch of the maxillary artery is closely associated with the auriculotemporal branch of V3; both structures are deep to the condyle approximately 10mm from its articular surface.
- The auriculotemporal nerve passes in an anteroposterior direction and emerges 1–2 mm posterior to the condyle, turning superiorly to follow the STA.
- The ZA is formed by the zygomatic process of the temporal bone and temporal process of the zygoma.
- The middle cranial fossa can be <1mm deep to the glenoid fossa.
- See ➲ 'Access: bicoronal flap' (p. 894), 'TMJ: ORIF mandibular condyle' (p. 882), 'TMJ arthrocentesis' (p. 906) for further relevant anatomy pertaining to the temporal fascia, facial nerve, and superficial temporal vessels.

Indications (typical)

- Recurrent TMJ dislocation.
- Reshaping the mandibular fossa to accommodate TMJ replacement.

Consent

- Infection.
- Bleeding.
- No improvement of symptoms.
- Weakness of facial muscles.

Preoperative preparation

- Complete WHO checklist and provide VTE prophylaxis as necessary.
- GA.

Position and theatre set-up

Supine with head turned to the contralateral side.

Procedure

Access to the condyle

- Make a skin incision in the crease anterior to the attachment of the helix, extending no further than the inferior portion of the tragus; a 1–2cm hockey-stick extension in hair-bearing temporal skin angled 45° above the ZA aids exposure (see Fig. 15.24a).
- At the superior part of the incision continue through the subcutaneous tissue and TPF to expose the dTF.

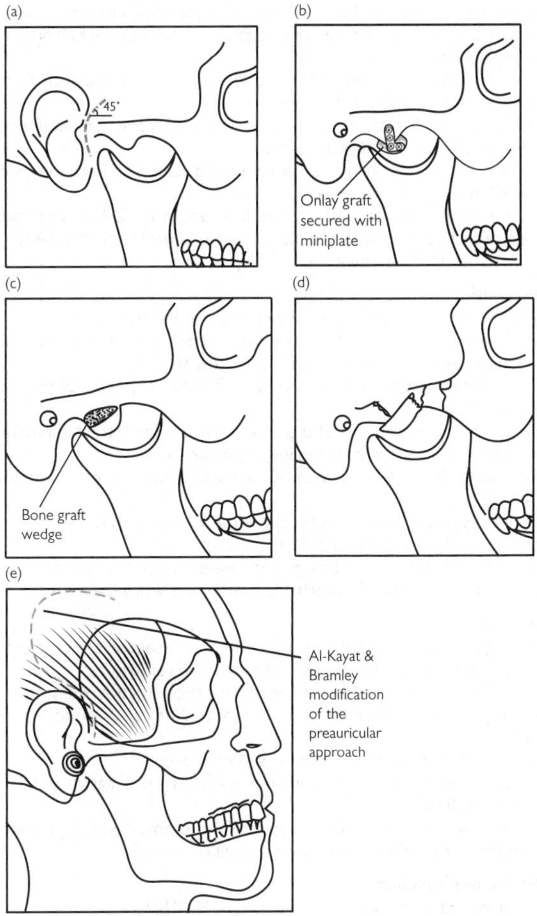
(a)
45°
(b)
Onlay graft
secured with
miniplate
(c)
Bone graft
wedge
(d)
(e)
Al-Kayat &
Bramley
modification
of the
preauricular
approach

Fig. 15.24 (a) Preauricular incision with hockey-stick extension. (b) Eminence augmentation using onlay graft, (c) interpositional graft, and (d) Dautrey procedure. (e) Al-Kayat and Bramley incision.

- At the inferior part of the incision sharp dissect down the anterior wall of the cartilaginous meatus to a similar depth, staying behind the parotid gland.
- Blunt dissect the avascular plane over the dTF 10–15mm anteriorly and continue over the ZA at this depth.
  - Retract this flap carefully as it contains the STA and auriculotemporal nerve, as well as the facial nerve.
- Make a 15mm incision in an anterior superior direction from the root of the ZA through the superficial layer of the dTF.
- Complete this incision vertically over the root of the ZA down to bone, then raise a subperiosteal flap along the lateral surface of the ZA to expose the articular eminence and TMJ capsule.

High condylar shave

- The lower joint space is opened with a horizontal incision.
  - Opening and closing the mouth helps to demonstrate the articular space, which is usually about 5mm below the ZA.
  - A further vertical incision to create a T allows exposure of the condylar neck.
- Place retractors each side of the condylar head and distract it inferiorly with a Howarth elevator in the lower joint space.
- Remove 2–4mm of the articular surface with a water-cooled tungsten carbide fissure bur.
- Deliver resected bone by dissecting it free with a Mitchell trimmer.
- Smooth with a tungsten carbide acrylic trimmer.
- Inspect the meniscus for damage and carefully close the capsule.
- Close in layers with 3-0 absorbable sutures and skin with 5-0 nylon.

Eminectomy

- Staying extra-capsular continue subperiosteal dissection to completely expose the articular eminence, and retract the soft tissues.
- Use a fissure bur to perform a horizontal glenotemporal osteotomy, keeping parallel to the base of skull to reduce the risk of perforating the middle cranial fossa.
  - The osteotomy should be at least 15mm deep.
  - Use a fine osteotome to complete it at the medial margin and deliver resected bone.
- Alternatively, the eminence can be carefully removed with an acrylic trimmer using the glenoid fossa as a guide to depth.

Eminence augmentation

- A number of techniques are possible (see Fig. 15.24b–d):
  - Onlay graft: cortical bone graft is shaped then secured on the eminence using miniplate fixation.
  - Inter-positional graft: a lateral glenotemporal osteotomy is performed and a wedge of bone is secured between the osteotomized fragment and ZA with a miniplate.
  - Dautrey procedure: an oblique osteotomy is performed through the ZA, then greenstick-fractured anteriorly, and rotated downwards.

Postoperative care

- Simple analgesia.
- Suture removal at 5 days.
- Postoperative physiotherapy should be arranged.

Complications

- Failure of resolution of symptoms.
- Temporary facial nerve injury 9% (18% if had previous surgery).
- Permanent facial nerve injury <1%.
- Auriculotemporal nerve injury: paraesthesia, Frey's syndrome.
- Infection <1%.

Tips and tricks

- The temporal extension of the incision should try to avoid the STA so modify the angle if required.
- An Al-Kayat and Bramley question mark incision gives even greater exposure and reduces facial nerve traction injuries (see Fig. 15.24e).
- Avoid catching the parotid fascia as it tends to bleed.

TMJ disc procedures

Overview

Displacement of the articular disc of the TMJ or *meniscus* can cause pain, trismus, and joint clicking. Disc procedures aim to either reposition (meniscopexy) or replace (meniscectomy) the articular disc.

Anatomy

Relevant anatomy pertaining to the temporoparietal fascia, relationship of the facial nerve to the TMJ, superficial temporal vessels, and articular eminence is given elsewhere: see ➲ 'Access: bicoronal flap' (p. 894), 'TMJ: ORIF mandibular condyle' (p. 882), 'TMJ arthrocentesis' (p. 906), 'TMJ eminoplasty and condyloplasty' (p. 910).

Indications (typical)

Severe cases of internal joint derangement refractory to conservative treatments.

Consent

As for 'TMJ eminoplasty and condyloplasty' (p. 910).

Preoperative preparation

- Preoperative MRI to diagnose internal disc derangement.
- Complete WHO checklist and provide VTE prophylaxis as necessary.
- GA with nasotracheal intubation.

Position and theatre set-up

- Supine with head turned to the contralateral side.
- Surgical magnification with loupes.

Procedure

- Approach to the joint capsule is as previously described (see ➲ 'TMJ eminoplasty and condyloplasty', p. 910).
- Infiltrate LA with vasoconstrictor into retrodiscal tissues for haemostasis.
- Distract the joint inferiorly and maintain in this position to exaggerate the articular space.
- The upper joint space is opened with a horizontal incision through the capsule just below the ZA leaving a cuff of tissue to aid closure.
- Retract the capsule and dissect it from the lateral border of the disc.
- The lower joint space is entered by a horizontal incision through the collateral ligament at the lateral margin of the disc.

Meniscopexy

- Use toothed Adson forceps to manipulate the disc and reposition it backwards to a near-anatomical position.
- Further mobilization can be achieved by using a Freer periosteal elevator to carefully buttonhole the anterior disc attachments; this is the same principle as meshing skin grafts for more length.
- Excise a strip of avascular posterior disc tissue, then plicate the disc posteriorly to the retrodiscal tissues with interrupted 4-0 absorbable sutures on an 8mm half-circle reverse cutting needle (see Fig. 15.25).

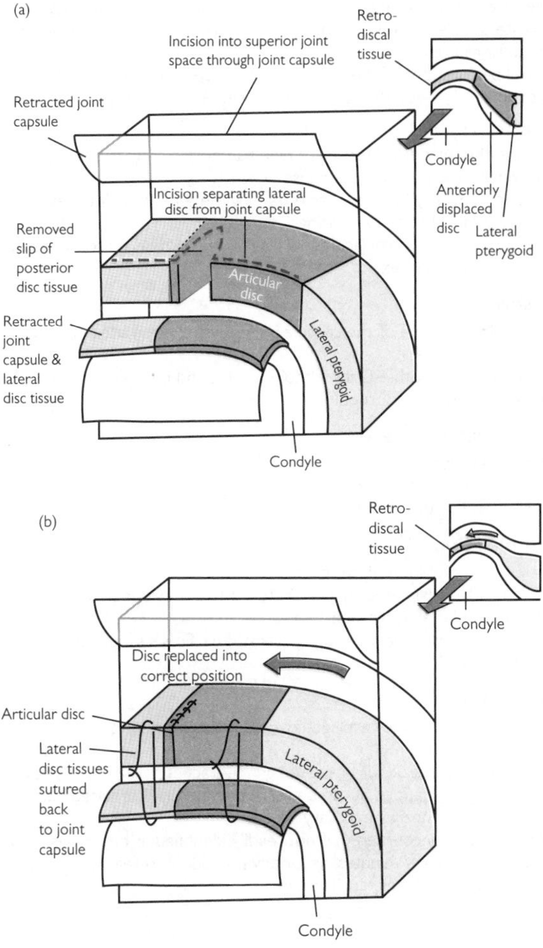
(a)
Retro-
discal
tissue
Incision into superior joint
space through joint capsule
Retracted joint
capsule
Condyle
Anteriorly
displaced
disc
Lateral
pterygoid
Incision separating lateral
disc from joint capsule
Removed
slip of
posterior
disc tissue
Articular
disc
Retracted
joint
capsule &
lateral
disc tissue
Lateral pterygoid
Condyle
(b)
Retro-
discal
tissue
Condyle
Disc replaced into
correct position
Articular disc
Lateral
disc tissues
sutured
back
to joint
capsule
Lateral pterygoid
Condyle

Fig. 15.25 (a) Conceptual diagram of meniscopexy, demonstrating incision into superior joint space, separation of lateral disc from joint capsule, and removal of wedge of posterior disc tissue. (b) Position of disc after plication.

- Release distraction and allow condyle to seat in the glenoid fossa.
- Plicate the disc laterally to the lateral collateral ligament to reinforce the posterior plication.
- Small perforations of the disc are incorporated into the resection if possible; otherwise they are repaired with 4-0 absorbable sutures.

Meniscectomy

- Clamp the retrodiscal tissues to help haemostasis and excise the posterolateral portion of the disc.
- Allis forceps may be useful for retracting the remaining disc tissue into the surgical field before excising.
- An autologous disc replacement is fashioned with dermis or a pedicled temporalis fascia flap.

Closure

- Meticulous closure of the capsule is required to promote healing of the synovial membrane.
- Close in layers with 4-0 absorbable sutures and 6-0 nylon for skin.
- A suction drain is not required.

Postoperative care

- Simple analgesia.
- Suture removal in 5 days.
- Postoperative physiotherapy.

Complications

- Failure of resolution of symptoms.
- Temporary facial nerve injury 9% (18% if had previous surgery).
- Permanent facial nerve injury <1%.
- Auriculotemporal nerve injury: paraesthesia, Frey's syndrome.
- Infection <1%.

Tips and tricks

- Avoid damage to the cartilage-covered articulating surfaces of the condyle.
- If the disc cannot be fully released gentle traction will give an idea on where it is trapped; it can be released medially if required but be mindful of the nearby maxillary artery.
- Any bleeding encountered, if not readily identified, is best managed with pressure for a few minutes, as for any procedure; reseating the condyle into the fossa will help achieve this.

Pectoralis major myocutaneous flap

Overview

This axial pattern pedicled flap allows reconstruction of cutaneous and mucosal defects in the head and neck as far superiorly as the ZA externally and the superior tonsillar pole intraorally. Although superseded in the main by free flaps for primary reconstruction, it is still a valuable tool in the reconstructive surgeon's armament.

Anatomy

- The pectoral branch of the thoracoacromial artery runs in a fascial plane deep to pectoralis major to supply the muscle.
- The lateral thoracic artery, a branch of the axillary artery, gives a variable secondary supply laterally.
- Internal mammary artery perforators supply the medial portion.
- A random pattern blood supply allows extension of the skin paddle beyond the inferior border of pectoralis major at the 6th rib.
- Innervation is from the lateral pectoral nerve within the pedicle.
- Innervation is also provided by the medial pectoral nerve, which has two to three branches; these pass through pectoralis minor to supply pectoralis major from its deep surface.

Indications (typical)

- Free flap salvage.
- Previously irradiated patients with no free flap recipient vessels.
- Myofascial flaps can be used to provide additional coverage over neck vessels; especially important in previously irradiated patients.
- Infected recipient sites (due to rich vascularity of the flap).

Consent

- Infection.
- Bleeding.
- Failure of flap.
- Scar.
- Alteration of breast position.

Preoperative preparation

- Group and save.
- Complete WHO checklist and provide VTE prophylaxis as necessary.
- GA—usually nasotracheal, depending on the site of the defect.
- Broad-spectrum antibiotics at induction.

Position and theatre set-up

Supine with head stabilized and arm abducted at 90°.

Procedure

- Mark a line from the acromion to xiphisternum and intersect it with a second line dropped vertically from the midpoint of the clavicle.
  - This approximates the thoracoacromial vascular pedicle.
- Mark out a skin paddle over the inferomedial chest wall, corresponding with the lateral border of the sternum and the 6th to 2nd ribs; size and shape depends on the defect (see Fig. 15.26).
- Incise circumferentially around the skin paddle down to the pectoralis major; bevel the incision radially through subcutaneous tissue to maximize the number of perforating vessels.
  - Shearing injury to perforators is reduced by suturing the skin paddle to underlying muscle.
- Incise along the anterior axillary fold towards the axilla, exposing the lateral border of pectoralis major; widely elevate skin and subcutaneous tissue off the pectoralis muscle up to the clavicle.
- Divide the muscle medially and inferiorly to the skin paddle, then start to elevate off the chest wall.
- Continue to release the muscle up the lateral edge of the sternum, controlling internal mammary perforators prior to transecting them.
- Raise the muscle along its lateral border to identify pectoralis minor.
  - Pectoralis major and the deep fascia containing the pedicle are easily freed by finger dissection.
- With the pedicle under direct vision, divide the branches of the medial pectoral nerve, the lateral thoracic artery, and the lateral border of the pectoralis major, which inserts into the humerus.

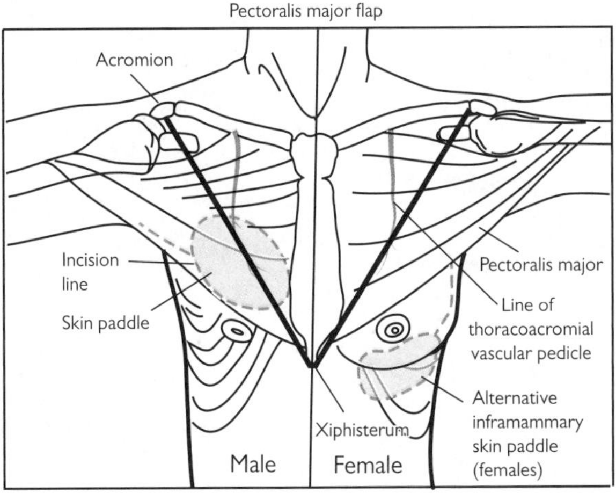
Pectoralis major flap
Acromion
Incision line
Skin paddle
Pectoralis major
Line of thoracoacromial vascular pedicle
Alternative inframammary skin paddle (females)
Xiphisterum
Male
Female

Fig. 15.26 Position of skin paddles, incisions and vascular pedicles in male and female patients.

- A sub-dermal tunnel is made over the clavicle by blunt dissection; it should be a width of four fingers to prevent vascular compression.
- Pass the flap through this tunnel, ensuring it does not twist.
- The donor site is closed primarily with a size 14 closed suction drain in situ; undermining skin aids closure, though a split skin graft may also be required.

Postoperative care

- Monitor flap at least twice per day.
- Continue antibiotics for at least 24h.
- Drains out when bleeding is minimal.

Complications

- Complete flap necrosis 1%.
- Partial flap necrosis 10%.
- Haematoma.
- Seroma.

Tips and tricks

- An infra-mammary skin paddle avoids excess bulk and distortion of the female breast by medial displacement on closure (see Fig. 15.26).
- The distance from inferior border of clavicle to recipient site should not exceed that between inferior border of clavicle and top of flap.
- Placing the flap under the clavicle can increase length.
- Avoid transecting the internal mammary perforating vessels by taking the medial border lateral to these; this allows salvage if required with a deltopectoral flap.

Radial forearm free-flap harvest

Overview

The forearm flap is extremely versatile and can be used in almost every situation in head and neck reconstruction if required. Donor site morbidity has seen other flaps become more fashionable over recent years but the reliable, long pedicle, coupled with a thin, pliable skin paddle, still make this flap relevant.

Anatomy

(See Fig. 15.27a)

- The pedicle consists of paired venae comitantes (VC) and the radial artery; it lies superficially in an intermuscular septum between the tendons of brachioradialis and flexor carpi radialis (FCR).
- The radial artery supplies the hand via the deep palmar arch.
- The ulnar artery forms a collateral supply via the superficial palmar arch; it is *complete* if it supplies every digit itself, or may be *completed* by communications with the deep palmar arch.
- The superficial venous system is drained by the cephalic vein and the deep venous system by the VC; the systems anastomose via a communicating vein between the medial cubital vein and VC in the antecubital fossa.
- The cephalic vein lies lateral to the pedicle in subcutaneous tissue.
- The lateral antebrachial cutaneous (LABC) branch of the musculocutaneous nerve lies lateral and superficial to the cephalic vein.
- The superficial branch of the radial nerve accompanies the radial artery proximally, passing underneath brachioradialis to approach the wrist lateral to the cephalic vein, supplying sensation to the dorsum of the hand.

Indications (typical)

- Almost any soft tissue defect; can be tubed for pharyngeal reconstruction.
- An osteocutaneous flap can be used to reconstruct small bony defects with a 13 × 120mm maximal dimension.

Consent

- Infection.
- Bleeding.
- Failure of flap.
- Scar.
- Numbness over thumb.

Preoperative preparation

- Allen's test *must* be performed:
  - A normal test with adequate ulnar blood flow is negative.
  - Occlude ulnar and radial arteries and ask patient to pump hand.
  - Open hand avoiding hyperextension.
  - Release ulnar artery; refill should be within 6s.
  - Repeat with the radial artery.

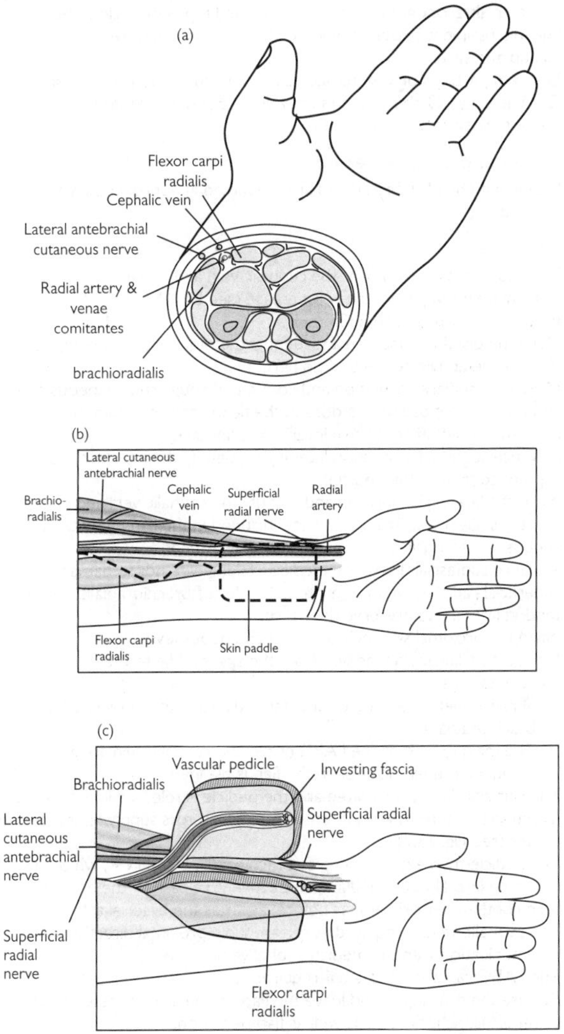
(a)
Flexor carpi radialis
Cephalic vein
Lateral antebrachial cutaneous nerve
Radial artery & venae comitantes
brachioradialis
(b)
Lateral cutaneous antebrachial nerve
Brachio-radialis
Cephalic vein
Superficial radial nerve
Radial artery
Flexor carpi radialis
Skin paddle
(c)
Vascular pedicle
Investing fascia
Brachioradialis
Superficial radial nerve
Lateral cutaneous antebrachial nerve
Superficial radial nerve
Flexor carpi radialis

Fig. 15.27 (a) Cross-sectional anatomy of the distal forearm. (b) Incision markings. (c) Flap just prior to division of the pedicle proximally.

- Doppler ultrasonography can be performed if positive Allen's test.
- Suitable recipient vessels should be identified preoperatively.
- Group and save.
- Ensure no arterial or venous access is obtained from the donor side.
- Complete WHO checklist and provide VTE prophylaxis as necessary.
- GA with nasotracheal intubation.

Position and theatre set-up

- Supine with head stabilized and arm abducted at approximately 90°.
- Tourniquet.

Procedure

- The flap axis is centred over the cephalic vein and radial artery with the distal margin away from the wrist crease (see Fig. 15.27b).
- Inflate the tourniquet to 250mmHg.
- Make the distal skin incision and identify the radial artery and adjacent VCs; divide and ligate the pedicle here.
- Make the medial skin incision and continue through subcutaneous tissue and fascia to expose the tendons in the flexor compartment; the thin paratenon is left intact to maximize skin graft take.
- Advance subfascial dissection laterally to identify the intermuscular septum containing the pedicle.
- Make the lateral skin incision and identify the cephalic vein and LABC nerve distally; these are divided and included in the flap if additional venous anastomosis or nerve coaptation is planned.
- Advance subfascial dissection medially, taking care not to damage the superficial radial nerve on the lateral border of brachioradialis; retract its tendon laterally to preserve the nerve.
- Make the proximal skin incision to subcutaneous level.
- Make a curvilinear skin incision from the skin paddle to the antecubital fossa.
    - Skin is undermined in the subcutaneous plane to expose FCR and brachioradialis.
    - The main branch of the LABC nerve and cephalic vein are also identified if their inclusion in the flap is planned.
- The skin paddle is gently lifted and the pedicle is released in a proximal direction by cauterizing and transecting perforators supplying the deeper tissues (see Fig. 15.27c).
- The pedicle then extends deep to brachioradialis and FCR, which are retracted laterally and medially, respectively; release of the pedicle is then continued proximally, as before, as far as the brachial artery.
- The cephalic vein, if required, is released in a proximal direction to its communication with the median cubital vein.
- The LABC can also be taken if required.
- Release the tourniquet and leave the flap on the arm for at least 20min to reperfuse; check hand as well as flap perfusion.
- Fully define the venous anatomy to locate the communication of the VC with the median cubital vein if required.

- Once the recipient site is prepared, clamp the pedicle with curved artery forceps and harvest the flap.
- A 3-0 transfixion suture is applied for haemostasis.
- A suction drain can be placed at the donor site and a skin graft, preferably full-thickness, is used to close it (see ➲ 'Harvesting a full-thickness skin graft (FTSG)', p. 534).

Postoperative care

- As for fibula free flap (see ➲ 'Fibula free-flap harvest', p. 933).
- Assess donor site skin graft at 10 days and weekly thereafter.

Complications

- Flap failure <4%.
- Radial fracture after composite flaps including bone used 17%.
- Damage to superficial branch of radial nerve (base of thumb) 75%.
- Infection with total graft failure and tendon exposure <1%.

Tips and tricks

- Placing the skin paddle more lateral makes picking up the cephalic vein easier.
- Placing the skin paddle more medial avoids a hairy skin paddle.

Osteocutaneous iliac crest flap harvest

Overview

This versatile flap can be used for complex composite reconstructions in the head and neck region. The muscle flap can be wrapped around the cut bone margin on the opposite side to the skin paddle and be left to mucosalize, allowing a tripartite reconstruction of skin, bone, and oral mucosa. The bone height and volume lends itself to dental implant placement, especially in the dentate patient.

Anatomy

(See Fig. 15.28)

- The pedicle consists of the deep circumflex iliac artery (DCIA) and the deep circumflex iliac vein.
- The pedicle runs behind and parallel to the inguinal ligament in a sheath formed by condensation of the transversalis and iliacus fasciae; at the ASIS it enters a groove medial to the iliac crest.
- An ascending branch supplies the internal oblique and is found 1cm medial to the ASIS.
- The lateral femoral cutaneous nerve lies variably near the ASIS and should be preserved if possible.

Indications (typical)

- Reconstruction of bony defects of the mandible and maxilla 6–16cm in length.
- A myocutaneous element can be included for simultaneous soft tissue reconstruction.

Consent

- Infection.
- Bleeding.
- Failure of flap.
- Scar.
- Pain and prolonged limp.
- Numbness over thigh.
- Hernia.

Preoperative preparation

- Suitable recipient vessels should be identified preoperatively.
- Group and save.
- Complete WHO checklist and provide VTE prophylaxis as necessary.
- GA.
- Broad-spectrum antibiotics at induction.
- Stool softeners may be started 1 week prior to surgery to avoid excessive straining postoperatively.

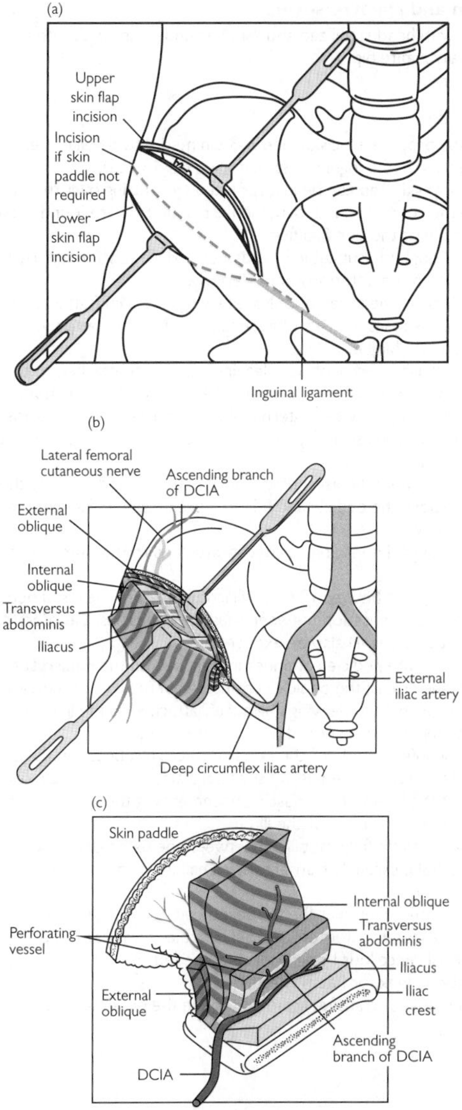
(a)
Upper skin flap incision
Incision if skin paddle not required
Lower skin flap incision
Inguinal ligament
(b)
Lateral femoral cutaneous nerve
Ascending branch of DCIA
External oblique
Internal oblique
Transversus abdominis
Iliacus
External iliac artery
Deep circumflex iliac artery
(c)
Skin paddle
Internal oblique
Transversus abdominis
Perforating vessel
Iliacus
Iliac crest
External oblique
Ascending branch of DCIA
DCIA

Fig. 15.28 (a) Incision markings. (b) Anatomy of the DCIA. (c) Layers of an osteocutaneous iliac crest flap.

Position and theatre set-up

- Supine with head stabilized and sandbag under hip to elevate and externally rotate hip.
- Catheter.

Procedure

- Mark the proposed incision line 2–3 cm medial to the iliac crest parallel and just above the inguinal ligament (see Fig. 15.28a).
- A fusiform skin flap can be incorporated by centring over the iliac crest, where the zone of musculocutaneous perforators are found; dissect the upper pole of the skin flap first.
- Incise through the subcutaneous tissues and identify the external oblique fibres, which run anteriorly and inferiorly.
- Incise through the external oblique leaving a 2cm cuff attached to the ilium; this exposes internal oblique fibres, which run perpendicularly to the external oblique.
- Incise through internal oblique leaving a 2cm cuff attached to the ilium; this exposes transversus abdominis (TA) fibres, which run horizontally.
- Open the plane between internal oblique and TA; this will expose tributaries of the ascending branch of DCIA on the under-surface of internal oblique.
- Dissect following the ascending branch inferiorly and medially through TA to expose the pedicle and follow it proximally to the external iliac artery and vein.
- Incise through TA leaving a 2cm cuff attached to the ilium; this exposes iliacus.
- Open the plane between TA and iliacus to expose the distal pedicle in the fascial condensation between these two muscles; the lateral femoral cutaneous nerve will also be exposed.
- At the ASIS the pedicle continues in a groove on the iliac crest between the TA and iliacus; the pedicle runs hidden in the cuff of muscles.
- Incise through iliacus leaving a 2cm cuff attached to the ilium; the inner table of the ilium is exposed.
- Incise the inferior pole of the skin flap through subcutaneous tissue to expose the gluteus medius, tensor fascia lata, and sartorius muscles.
- Transect the lateral thigh muscle attachments at the iliac crest and expose the outer table of the ilium.
- With the pedicle fully mobilized between the external iliac vessels and the ASIS, carefully transect the remaining portion of iliacus and sartorius.
- Incise the periosteum at the proposed osteotomy sites and use an oscillating saw or osteotome to define a bicortical iliac bone flap.
- Additional cancellous bone is taken if needed.
- Apply bone wax for haemostasis.
- When ready for transfer, ligate and divide the proximal pedicle.

Closure

- A drain is placed to avoid haematoma and an epidural catheter is sited to allow infiltration with levobupivicaine for postoperative analgesia.
- The inner abdominal wall is reconstructed by approximating the TA and the internal oblique to iliacus.
    - Sutures can be passed through oblique drill holes placed in the cut ilium bone edge to reinforce closure.
- The outer abdominal wall is reconstructed by approximating external oblique to the gluteus medius.
- If internal oblique is taken a polypropylene mesh repair of the inner abdominal wall is fashioned to prevent a hernia.
- Subcutaneous 3-0 resorbable and 4-0 nylon skin sutures are used to close the wound.

Modifications

- An osteomusculocutaneous flap can be designed by harvesting a substantial portion of internal oblique.
- A bicortical or unicortical bone flap can be harvested as necessary.

Postoperative care

- As for 'Fibula free-flap harvest' (p. 933).

Complications

- Flap failure 2–5%.
- Hernia avoided if mesh repair used.
- Haematoma.
- Paraesthesia lateral thigh (lateral femoral cutaneous nerve).

Fibula free-flap harvest

Overview

This versatile flap is a workhorse in head and neck reconstruction due to the length of bone that can be harvested and consistency of the pedicle.

Anatomy

(See Fig. 15.29a)

- The fibula articulates with the tibia above and talus below.
- 22–25cm of bone can be harvested maintaining at least 6cm proximally and distally; this preserves ankle joint stability and avoids the peroneal nerve, which courses anteriorly around the fibular head.
- The popliteal artery bifurcates at the knee into the anterior and posterior tibial artery (PTA), which travel down the leg in their respective compartments either side of the interosseous membrane.
- The PTA then divides after 2–3cm giving off the peroneal artery.
- The peroneal artery and its paired VCs form the pedicle; it runs between tibialis posterior and flexor hallucis longus (FHL), and has one endosteal and multiple periosteal branches.
- Multiple perforators supply the skin; these can be septocutaneous, through the posterior crural intermuscular septum, or musculocutaneous, through FHL and soleus.

Indications (typical)

- Reconstruction of bony defects of the mandible and maxilla.
- Composite osteocutaneous flaps for simultaneous soft tissue reconstruction.

Consent

- Infection.
- Bleeding.
- Failure of flap.
- Scar.
- Foot drop.

Preoperative preparation

- Vascular supply to the lower limb must be assessed clinically.
  - CT or MR angiography is advised to confirm presence of the peroneal artery and exclude peronea arteria magna (dominant blood supply to lower limb from large peroneal artery).
- Suitable recipient vessels should be identified preoperatively.
- Group and save.
- Complete WHO checklist and provide VTE prophylaxis as necessary.
- GA—usually nasotracheal depending on the site of the defect
- Broad-spectrum antibiotics at induction.

(a)

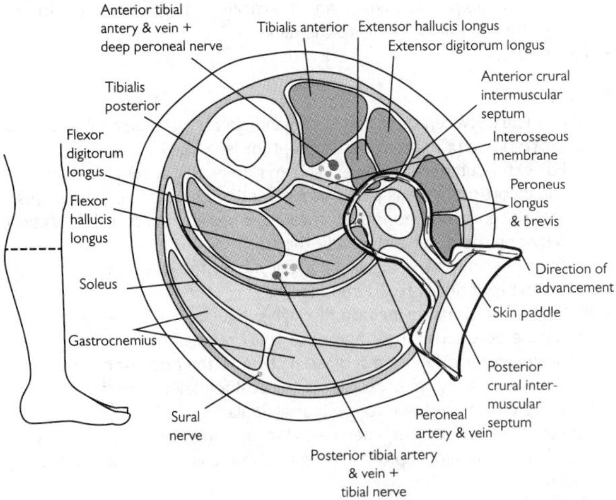
Anterior tibial antery & vein + deep peroneal nerve
Tibialis anterior
Extensor hallucis longus
Extensor digitorum longus
Anterior crural intermuscular septum
Interosseous membrane
Peroneus longus & brevis
Direction of advancement
Skin paddle
Posterior crural inter-muscular septum
Peroneal artery & vein
Posterior tibial artery & vein + tibial nerve
Sural nerve
Gastrocnemius
Soleus
Flexor hallucis longus
Flexor digitorum longus
Tibialis posterior

(b)

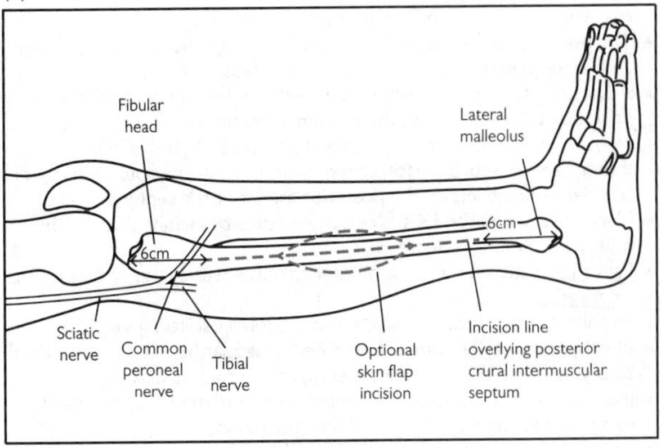
Fibular head
Lateral malleolus
6cm
6cm
Sciatic nerve
Common peroneal nerve
Tibial nerve
Optional skin flap incision
Incision line overlying posterior crural intermuscular septum

Fig. 15.29 (a) Cross-sectional anatomy of the leg demonstrating direction of advancement during dissection of the flap. (b) Incision markings.

Position and theatre set-up

- Supine with hip partially flexed and internally rotated; the knee is bent to expose the lateral leg at 40° to the table.
- Tourniquet.

Procedure

- Mark a line between the fibular head and lateral malleolus; this outlines the posterior crural intermuscular septum (see Fig. 15.29b).
  - For osteocutaneous flaps a fusiform skin paddle is centred over this line incorporating any perforators identified by Doppler; the largest calibre septocutaneous perforators are usually found at the junction between the distal and middle-thirds.
  - For bone-only flaps, a straight incision over the line is used.
- Inflate the tourniquet to 300mmHg.
- Make the anterior skin incision through subcutaneous tissues and fascia to expose peroneus longus and peroneus brevis.
- Advance posteriorly in the subfascial plane to the posterior crural intermuscular septum; preserve any musculocutaneous perforators.
- Follow the septum down to the lateral fibula.
- Transect medially through peroneus longus and brevis to the anterior crural intermuscular septum leaving a <1mm cuff of muscle on the fibula.
- Divide the anterior crural intermuscular septum longitudinally and continue transecting medially through extensor hallucis longus until reaching the interosseous membrane.
- The posterior skin incision is then made through subcutaneous tissues and fascia to expose gastrocnemius and soleus.
- Advance anteriorly in the subfascial plane to the previously identified posterior crural intermuscular septum; if septal perforators were identified musculocutaneous perforators may be ligated.
- If there are no septal perforators dissect down to the fibula with a cuff of soleus muscle left on the posterior aspect of the septum.
- Mark the proximal and distal osteotomy sites by incising through the muscular cuff and periosteum.
- Pass a periosteal retractor around the fibula ensuring the pedicle is not captured.
- Perform the osteotomies with a water-cooled oscillating saw.
- Identify the anterior compartment neurovascular bundle (anterior tibial artery, vein and deep peroneal nerve) and retract medially.
- Incise through the interosseous membrane 1cm medial to the fibula exposing the chevron fibres of tibialis posterior.
- Access is now improved by applying bone clamps and distracting the fibula laterally; the distal pedicle is transected and controlled with a 2-0 ligature.
- Expose the whole length of the pedicle by carefully dividing tibialis posterior.
- With the pedicle safe, under direct vision dissect through flexor hallucis longus leaving a cuff to free the fibula.

- Release the tourniquet and leave the flap on the leg for at least 30 minutes to reperfuse; haemostasis and vessel preparation can then be performed.
- Closure is in layers with 3-0 non resorbable sutures loosely approximating the muscle; muscle closure is over a drain if used.
- Close skin with 4-0 nylon sutures; if a skin paddle >5cm wide is used a split-skin graft is used to avoid excess tension contributing to compartment syndrome (see ➲ 'Taking a split skin graft', p. 518).
- A wool and crepe dressing is placed for comfort.

Postoperative care

- Monitor the flap if there is a skin paddle.
- Maintain normothermia.
- MAP up to 65mmHg; avoid vasoconstricting vasopressors.
- Urine output 1ml/kg/h.
- Haematocrit >27%.
- Transfuse if Hb <80 g/l.
- Nurse at 45° to enhance venous drainage.
- Start NG feeding when bowel sounds are heard.
- Appropriate analgesia.
- Drains out when bleeding is <30ml/day.

Complications

- Haematoma 25%.
- Flap failure <5%.
- Loss of skin paddle 5–10%.
- Instability of ankle joint.
- Foot drop.
- Postoperative compartment syndrome.

Tips and tricks

- A longer pedicle is created by harvesting a longer portion of fibula, then discarding the excess bone.
- Due to lateral distraction of the bone the pedicle appears to run medially near its origin at the PTA.

Chapter 16

Orthopaedics

Application of a secondary cast to forearm or leg

Overview

When applying a cast, whether in the A&E department, theatre or the plaster room, the following steps should always be followed.

Consent

- Verbal informed consent is usually obtained in A&E or clinic settings. If in theatre under general anaesthetic, a formal signed consent should be obtained.
- An explanation of the procedure and its implications should be given, i.e. the length of immobilization, need for regular follow-up, and imaging to check maintenance of reduction, weight-bearing status.
- Risks: skin irritation, plaster sores, nerve compression (commonly superficial radial at the wrist and common peroneal at fibular neck), loss of reduction, re-application of cast, compartment syndrome.
- Ensure the correct 'surgical' site is clearly marked.

Preparation

- Having an assistant is essential to apply an effective cast.
- Gather required equipment:
  - Cast type ('plaster of Paris'/Gypsona or soft cast).
  - Select the appropriate width (1in up to 8in).
  - Continuous roll or sheet from a box.
  - Measure the length required and cut beforehand.
  - Under cast padding.
  - Bucket of warm water (tepid not cold speeds up the setting process).
  - Appropriate setting (plaster room in clinic or A&E, theatre).
  - Couch or chair for patient.

Procedure

Assuming the fracture has been reduced/alignment restored:

- Attend to any wounds appropriately and ensure they are properly covered.
- Ask your assistant to stabilize limb whilst a double layer of padding is added.
- Ensure prominent areas have extra protection (e.g. malleoli, heel, olecranon, tibial spine).
- Dip cast in water; if using a roll, wait until the bubbles have stopped.
- Do not wring out cast as this makes application more difficult.
- Mould cast appropriately to stabilize fracture avoiding deep ridges, as these will produce pressure sores. Moulding should be done with the palms of the hand.
- Different fracture patterns will require different casting techniques.

- Rotationally unstable fracture requires immobilization of the joint above and below. For example, a both bone forearm fracture (radius and ulna) requires the cast to extend from just proximal to the metacarpophalangeal joints to the proximal upper arm, thus immobilizing the wrist and elbow and minimizing rotation.
- When applying the cast, the joints proximal and distal to the cast ends need to have adequate clearance in order to preserve function. For example, a below-knee cast for a stable ankle fracture will include the ankle joint but stop a hand's breadth distal to the knee crease to allow unhindered knee flexion.

Post-procedure

Clear documentation of the procedure and follow-up plan must be recorded in the operation or patient's notes, this should include:

- When the patient can be discharged, if relevant.
- When to return for follow-up.
- Whether further X-rays are needed and when.
- What complications to be aware of and the need to return to the plaster room if they have any concerns.

Ideally a printed leaflet including all this information should be provided.

Further reading

Charnley J. *The Closed Treatment of Common Fractures*. Cambridge: Colt Books, 1999.

Manipulation under anaesthetic (MUA) of a distal radius fracture +/– insertion of Kirschner (K) wires

Anatomy

- Sound knowledge of the osteology and its ligamentous attachments is essential.
- The dorsal aspect of the distal radius is covered by the compartments of the extensor tendons (Fig. 16.1). The volar aspect is covered with the flexor compartment, median, and ulnar nerves. The radial artery runs along the radial aspect.
- The superficial radial nerve is at risk on the radial border during insertion of the styloid wire.

Indications

- Displaced and unstable distal radius fractures
- The vast majority of these fractures are dorsally displaced or angulated (Colles' fractures).
- Volar angulated and displaced articular fractures may require plating and may not be suitable for MUA and K wiring.
- Assess the AP and lateral X-rays for (Fig. 16.2).
    - Radial height/ulnar variance.
    - Volar inclination.
    - Degree of dorsal comminution.
    - Co-existing ulnar styloid fractures.
    - The greater the alteration to these factors the more unstable the fracture pattern.
- The aim of reduction is to restore the above parameters.

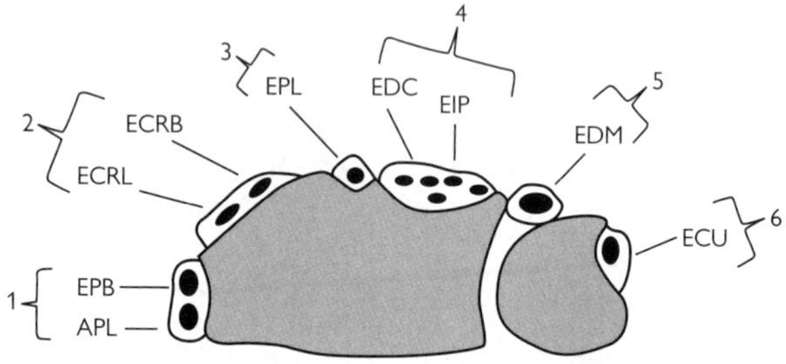
4
3
EPL
EDC
EIP
5
2
ECRB
EDM
ECRL
ECU
6
1
EPB
APL

Fig. 16.1 The dorsal compartments of the wrist. 1. APL (abductor pollicis longus), EPB (extensor pollicis brevis). 2. ECRL (extensor carpi radialis longus), ECRB (extensor carpi radialis brevis). 3. EPL (extensor pollicis longus). 4. EDC (extensor digitorum communis), EIP (extensor indicis proprius). 5. EDM extensor digiti minimi). 6. ECU (extensor carpi ulnaris).

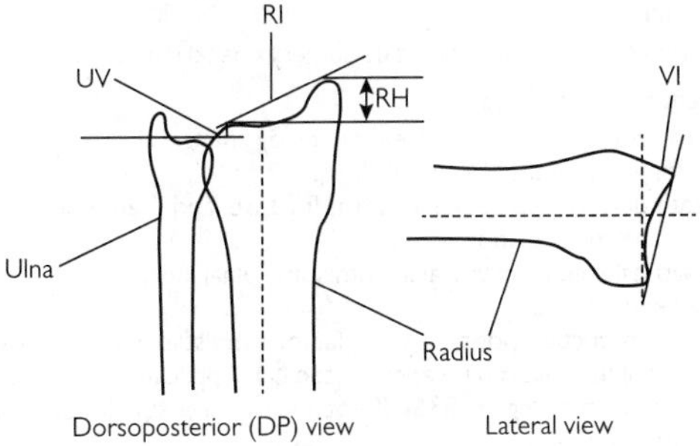
RI
UV
RH
VI
Ulna
Radius
Dorsoposterior (DP) view
Lateral view

Fig. 16.2 Anatomical relationships to observe around the distal radius. UV (ulnar variance), RH (radial height), RI (radial inclination), VI (volar inclination).

Preoperative preparation

History and examination

- Mechanism of injury, neurological symptoms, PMH (previous medical history), DH (drug history), occupation.
- Document neurovascular status and degree of deformity.
- Assess for open wounds.

X-rays

- Posteroanterior (PA) and lateral images centred on the distal radius required.

Obtain informed consent

- Explain procedure to patient
- Risks: infection, nerve injury (superficial radial, median), stiffness of wrist, malunion, removal of metal work, compartment syndrome.
- Ensure the correct surgical site is clearly marked.

Liaise with anaesthetist

- GA most common, can be performed under nerve block.
- Antibiotics on induction (follow local hospital protocol).

Liaise with the scrub team and ensure equipment is available

- Wiring set essential, including 1.6mm and 2.0mm K-wires.
- Have a small fragment set available or distal radius plating set if need to undertake internal fixation arises.
- Radiographer and image intensifier (II) available.
- Fracture table with radiolucent arm table attachment.
- An assistant is useful to help obtain and hold reduction.

Position and theatre set-up

- Table running perpendicular to anaesthetic machine, arm on an arm board.
- Operating seat in axilla, scrub nurse and trolley at end of arm board with II screen in clearly visible position, II coming in from head end.
- Place a high arm tourniquet but only inflate if performing internal fixation.

Procedure

The World Health Organization safe surgery checklist must be completed.

Closed reduction of fracture

- Prior to arm prep as plan of treatment may change.
- Apply longitudinal traction for 1–2min.
- Recreate deformity by dorsiflexion at fracture, and then reduce using traction and manipulation.
- Keep wrist flexed palmar-wards with some ulnar deviation.
- Check reduction using II.
- If fracture reduction position is satisfactory and stable, a full below-elbow moulded cast can be applied (see ➲ 'Application of a secondary cast to forearm or leg', p. 936). If not and requires stabilization, prepare for K-wire fixation.

K-wire fixation

- Preparation of the arm to tourniquet, in line with local policy (iodine-based aqueous or alcoholic, or chlorhexidine). Drape using a specific adhesive isolation drape or arm extremity drape.
- Reduce fracture again and check position with II.
- Generally three wires are use: two dorsally and one oblique via the radial styloid.
- Use II to locate the optimum position for wire placement.
- Make longitudinal stab incisions at the optimum points and bluntly dissect to bone using an artery clip or dissecting scissors to ensure no tendons or neurovascular structures are penetrated by the wires (dorsal tendons and superficial radial nerve).

Intrafocal wiring

- Start dorsally to correct dorsal translation and angulation.
- Insert two 1.6mm K-wires, by hand, into fracture site dorsally at the previously prepared incisions, until the far cortex (palmar) is felt.
- Lever the wires until the distal fragment is in the desired position, evaluate with II, and drive the wires into palmar cortex.
- Next correct radial inclination.
- Insert one 1.6mm K-wire into the radial fracture site and repeat as above, but this time lever in an ulnar direction and then drive into ulnar cortex of radius.
- Check position on II.

Interfragmentary wiring

- Start on the radial side.
- The assistant holds the fracture reduced.
- Using the premade incision, insert a 1.6mm K-wire, using the wire driver, into the tip of the radial styloid and drive in an ulnar direction to engage and fix in the ulnar cortex of the radius, proximal to the fracture site.
- Now insert the dorsal wires.
- Via the dorsal incisions, place two 1.6mm K-wires into the dorsal cortex of the distal fracture fragment.
- Drive the wire proximally at an angle that allows the wire to engage and fix into the palmar cortex of the radius, proximal to the fracture.
- Check position on II.

Closure

- Close the wounds only if too long using a monofilament absorbable or non-absorbable suture (3.0).
- Bend the wires using wire-bending pliers, approximately 1cm above skin edge.
- Cut the ends of the wire leaving 1cm length after the bend.
- Use sterile dressings (jelonet and dressing gauze or a simple dry dressing).
- Apply a back slab (see ➲ 'Application of a secondary cast to forearm or leg', p. 936), this allows for swelling, which a complete cast does not.

Postoperative care

- Elevate limb.
- Check neurovascular status.
- Plan for discharge either same day or next day when safe to do so.
- Review in clinic at 1 week:
  - X-ray the distal radius (AP and lateral) to ensure reduction is maintained.
  - Complete the cast in the plaster room.
- Review again in 1 week and check position of fracture with an X-ray (AP and lateral).
- At 4 weeks postoperatively, X-ray again and if suitable remove the K-wires in clinic (see ➲ 'Removal of K-wire', p. 941).
- Following removal place back into a cast for 2 more weeks.
- At 6 weeks remove cast and begin physiotherapy for movement and strengthening.

Complications

- Infection (superficial and deep) of pin sites.
- Pressure sore under cast.
- Loss of reduction leading to malunion.
- Stiffness and weakness.

Removal of K-wire

- Once the decision to remove wires has been made and the position of the wires checked on X-rays.
- Obtain verbal consent from the patient and explain procedure.

Preparation

Suitable room, plaster saw, skin preparation (iodine-based or chlorhexadine), sterile wire-holder or pliers, dressings.

Procedure

- Seat or lay the patient down with arm supported.
- Remove the plaster, padding, and dressings.
- Clean the area around the wire and skin, remove scabs.
- Warn the patient when you are beginning.
- Rotate the wires first to loosen, then expeditiously pull the wires in a longitudinal direction.
- Repeat for the other wires.
- Apply a compressive gauze to control bleeding.
- Apply sterile dressing and further cast if required.

Tips and tricks

- When reducing the fracture, make sure the volar cortex is reduced and not overlapping, as this will help to maintain length and reduction.
- When placing interfragmentary wires, place the dorsal wire close to the subchondral bone of the radius articular surface, this is the strongest bone and will lead to less risk of collapse and loss of position.

Further reading

(http://www.aofoundation.org).
Charnley J. *The Closed Treatment of Common Fractures*. Cambridge: Colt Books, 1999.

Operative fixation of Weber B fracture of ankle

Overview

Successful fixation of ankle fractures requires sound knowledge of the surgical approach to distal fibula and fracture site, and application of a lateral plate to distal fibula fracture.

Anatomy

- The ankle mortise forms an intimate housing for the body of Talus (Fig. 16.3), failure to restore this relationship and stability alters the contact pressures across the ankle joint leading to early degeneration. It comprises:
  - Laterally, the distal fibula.
  - Medially, the medial malleolus (projection of distal tibia).
  - Superiorly, the distal tibia.
- Ligaments support the osseous structures:
  - Laterally, the anterior and posterior tibiofibular ligaments (syndesmosis), anterior and posterior talofibular ligaments, and the calcaneofibular ligament.
  - Interosseous membrane running the length of fibula attached to the tibia.
  - Medially, the two-layered deltoid ligament; superficial, fan-shaped, tibiocalcaneal ligament, and the deep anterior and posterior talotibial ligaments.

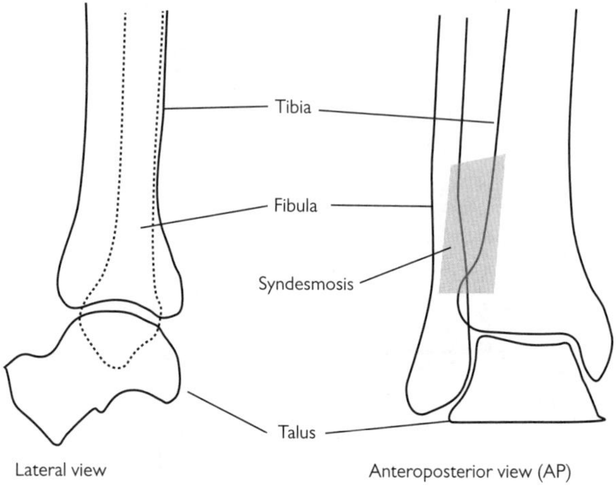
Tibia
Fibula
Syndesmosis
Talus
Lateral view
Anteroposterior view (AP)

Fig. 16.3 Showing lateral and anteroposterior depictions of the tibia–fibula–talus complex.

- The peroneal tendons (brevis and longus) run behind the lateral malleolus.
- The superficial peroneal nerve runs anteriorly and the sural nerve runs posteriorly to the distal fibula.

Indications

Fixation is indicated for unstable fractures/fracture-dislocations of the ankle joint such as:

- Bimalleolar fractures (medial and lateral malleolus).
- Displaced isolated medial malleolar fractures.
- Lateral malleolar fractures with associated talar shift (widening of the gap between the medial malleolus and talus).
- Open fractures (see ➔ 'Surgical debridement of traumatic wounds', p. 971).
- Isolated fibula fractures above the syndesmosis (representing a syndesmotic disruption).

Preoperative preparation

- Adequate preoperative work-up (history, examination, investigations, as required).
- Ensure soft swelling is not excessive as this will not allow wound closure.
  - If swelling is from fracture haematoma, early fixation is feasible to decompress the haematoma and allow wound closure.
  - If the soft tissues around the ankle swell, delay in fixation may be required to allow swelling to subside (up to 7 days).
  - A reduced fracture immobilized in cast, foot pumps, elevation, and ice will help reduce swelling.
  - If swelling is severe or if skin fracture blisters develop and reduction cannot be held in a cast, consider the application of a temporary external fixator.
- Ensure the correct surgical site is clearly marked.
- Obtain informed consent:
  - Explain procedure.
  - Risks: infection, damage to nerves and vessels, stiffness, compartment syndrome, degenerative changes in ankle joint, malunion, metalwork prominence and removal, DVT, and PE.
- Liaise with anaesthetist:
  - General anaesthetic (fast 6h) or spinal anaesthetic
  - Antibiotics on induction (follow local hospital protocol).
- Liaise with the scrub team and ensure equipment is available:
  - Small fragment set (3.5mm fully threaded cortical, 4.0mm fully and partially threaded cancellous screws, washers).
  - 1.6mm and 2mm AO wires/K-wires
  - Standard fracture fixation set (as per local policy).
  - Radiographer and image intensifier (II) available.
  - Radiolucent table.

Position and theatre set-up

- Radiolucent table, patient supine, feet away from anaesthetic machine.
  - Sand bag under ipsilateral buttock and the leg raised on a radiolucent block helps with surgical access and ability to take X-rays.
- Apply high-thigh tourniquet.
- Image intensifier (II) to be positioned from opposite side of table perpendicular to leg.
- An assistant is useful but not essential.

Procedure

- The World Health Organization safe surgery checklist must be completed.
- Preparation of the lower leg and toes, in line with local policy (iodine-based aqueous or alcoholic or chlorhexidine). Drape allowing adequate access to the whole lower leg. Cover the toes (glove, drape tape).
- Mark out incision with a sterile skin marker.
- Longitudinal incision over lateral malleolus, the length dictated by fracture pattern.
- Incise anterior to the peroneal tendons, working distal to proximal helps with delineation.
  - Avoid the superficial peroneal nerve anteriorly and the sural nerve posteriorly. Staying directly lateral over the fibula helps avoid nerve injury.
- Clear the fracture site of periosteum, clot and any other soft tissues that may hinder reduction.
  - Use saline wash and suction.
  - Ensure you can see the apices of the fracture to ensure direct visualisation of fracture reduction.
- Reduce the fracture and hold with pointed bone reduction clamp, perpendicular to fracture line.
- If the fracture pattern allows and bone quality adequate, insert a lag screw (provides absolute stability).
  - Usually easiest in an anterior to posterior direction.
  - Use a 3.5mm drill and drill the near cortex of fibula at central point of fracture, perpendicular to fracture line.
  - Insert the reduction sleeve or a 3.5mm drill guide (for the 2.5mm drill) into the hole and drill the far cortex with a 2.5mm drill.
  - Measure the screw length using a depth gauge.
  - Tap the far cortex for a 3.5mm cortical screw. Countersink the near cortex (spreads load of screw head and reduces screw head prominence).
  - Insert appropriate length 3.5mm fully threaded cortical screw until tight (finger tight only as over tightening can strip threads and it will fail).
  - Check reduction with II.
- Next apply a lateral plate to fibula (neutralization plate if used in conjunction with a lag screw).
  - Select an appropriate length 1/3 tubular plate. Aim for three screws each, distal and proximal to the fracture.

  - Pre-contour plate minimally to shape of fibula and apply to fibula using a clamp, check position with II.
  - Drill proximal screws first; 2.5mm drill and guide. Drill both cortices. Measure using a depth gauge, tap both cortices (3.5mm cortical screw tap), insert appropriate length fully threaded 3.5mm cortical screw (usually 2mm longer than measured). Repeat this step for all diaphyseal screws (proximal).
  - Drill unicortically in the distal segment so as to avoid entering the ankle joint. Measure screw length and use either fully threaded 3.5mm cortical or 4.0mm fully threaded cancellous screws (no difference in pullout strength) without tapping. The three screw tips tend to converge towards distal joint line.
  - Check reduction and implant position with II.
- Washout wound thoroughly and ensure haemostasis.

Closure

- Leave deep fascia open.
- Close subcutaneous fascia using an appropriate suture (2.0 Vicryl® or PDS).
- Close skin with either a subcutaneous suture method (3.0 absorbable monofilament) or interrupted mattress sutures (3.0 non-absorbable monofilament).
  - Do not use clips, as this will be under a cast.
- Infiltrate local anaesthetic if appropriate.
- Apply dressing (local protocol).
- Cover lower leg with layer of padding.
- Apply a posterior plaster splint (back-slab) below knee (distal to popliteal fossa ending at the metatarsal heads) with the foot plantigrade and ankle at 90°.

Postoperative care

- Elevate leg.
- Check neurovascular status.
- Allow toe movement.
- Mobilize non-weight bearing on operative leg.
- VTE prophylaxis as per local policy.
- Review in clinic at 2 weeks to remove sutures, check wound, and obtain an X-ray.
- Re-apply a below-knee cast and remain non-weight bearing.
- Review in clinic at 6 weeks, remove cast, and X-ray.
- Start full weight-bearing if appropriate.
- Discharge to physiotherapy if this service is in place, if not review for final time at 12 weeks.

Complications

- Infection (superficial or deep).
- Nonunion or malunion.
- Prominence of metal work and need for removal.
- Stiffness of ankle.
- Degenerative changes in ankle joint.
- Numbness or painful neuroma from nerve injury.

Tips and tricks

- Ensure you can clearly see the apices of the fracture when reducing the lateral fracture, as anatomical restoration of length and rotational alignment is crucial.
- Make sure the talus is reduced in the mortise. Occasionally, when fixing an isolated lateral malleolar fracture, the deltoid ligament can be trapped between the medial malleolus and talus preventing reduction. If so this needs to be removed.
- 3.5 DCP (dynamic compression plate) without contouring should be used for more proximal fibular fractures.
- Pre-contoured plates for the fibula may be used if available.

Further reading

(http://www.aofoundation.org).

Hoppenfeld S, deBoer P, Buckley R. *Surgical Exposures in Orthopaedics: The Anatomic Approach*, 4th edn. Lippincott Williams & Wilkins, 2009.

Dynamic hip screw (DHS) fixation for extra-capsular neck of femur fracture

Overview

- Extra-capsular fractures of the neck of the proximal femur are unstable, painful, and prevent mobilization. They all require surgical stabilization to:
  - Allow early mobilization.
  - Avoid the complications of decubitus (chest infections, bed sores, and often death).
  - Reduce pain.
- Surgical management of intertrochanteric fractures of the proximal femur requires excellent knowledge of the:
  - Reduction of intertrochanteric fractures on fracture table.
  - Approach and technique of insertion of guide wire for intertrochanteric fracture.
- DHS fixation of proximal femur for intertrochanteric fracture.

Anatomy

See ➲ 'Surgical anatomy and approaches to the hip joint', p. 1000.

Indications

- Any intertrochanteric fractured neck of femur (see Fig. 16.18).
- Undisplaced intracapsular fractured neck of femur.

Contraindications

- It is less suitable for reverse oblique or subtrochanteric configurations.
- Pathological fractures which require IM nailing.

Preoperative preparation

- Consider the National Institute of Health and Care Excellence (NICE) guidelines on fractured neck of femur management (1).
- In the United Kingdom, a tariff is offered for best clinical practice related to hip fractures (2). Six criteria are measured.
- All patients aged 60 and above:
  - Time to theatre (all cases) <36h.
  - 36h from arrival in Emergency Department (or time of diagnosis if an inpatient) to the start of anaesthesia.
  - Admitted under the joint care of a consultant geriatrician and a consultant orthopaedic surgeon.
  - Admitted using an assessment tool agreed by geriatric medicine, orthopaedic surgery, and anaesthesia.
  - Assessed by geriatrician in perioperative period (defined as 72h of admission) (geriatrician defined as consultant, SAS or ST3+)
  - Postoperative geriatrician-directed:
    —Multi-professional rehabilitation team.
    —Fracture-prevention assessments (falls and bone health).
  - Pre- and postoperative abbreviated mental test score (AMTS).

- Adequate preoperative work-up (history, examination, investigations, as required). Essential information:
  - Mechanism of injury (trip or medical cause for fall, e.g. blackout, cardiac disease, etc.).
  - Pre-injury level of function (e.g. walks with two sticks or is a keen walker and swims).
  - Previous medical history.
  - Thorough drug history, including allergies.
  - Social situation (living accommodation, any regular help, house modifications, who does the shopping).
  - CXR.
  - ECG.
  - Blood tests, including FBC, U and E, coagulation, group and save.
  - Ensure the correct surgical site is clearly marked.
- Obtain informed consent:
- The treating doctor, in the patient's best interest, should sign consent if the patient lacks mental capacity to consent (e.g. longstanding dementia or confusion).
- Always consult the patient's family prior to consent and procedure.
  - Explain procedure if patient able to comprehend.
  - Risks: infection, bleeding, damage to nerves, poor mobility, failure of fixation, DVT, and PE.
- Liaise with anaesthetist:
  - General anaesthetic (fast 6h) or spinal anaesthetic.
  - Antibiotics on induction (follow local hospital protocol).
- Liaise with the scrub team and ensure equipment is available:
  - DHS fracture fixation set (as per local policy), ensure all implant sizes are available.
  - Radiographer and image intensifier (II) available.
  - Radiolucent fracture table that will allow leg positioning and traction.

Position and theatre set-up

- The head is by the anaesthetic machine. Table runs down the centre of the theatre.
- Instruments and scrub nurse on the operative side.
- II from opposite side, ensure II monitor can be clearly seen at the foot of the table.

Position and fracture reduction

- Patient is positioned supine.
- A radiolucent, well-padded pudendal post is placed on the correct side of the traction table and the patient is gently moved down the table to engage post between legs (ensure, where appropriate, catheter, scrotum, and penis are moved and protected).
- Padding is placed around the foot and ankle of the fractured side.
- The foot is secured into the boot or footplate at the distal end of the leg extension of the traction table.
- The contralateral leg is placed into leg holder with the hip and knee flexed up (a Lloyd–Davies support works well—ensure well-padded to avoid injury to peroneal nerve).

- The distal table ends are removed and the table height is set.
- Ensure the patient is securely held on the table, a chest strap can help.
- The II is positioned to provide an anterior-posterior (AP) image of the hip.
- Gentle longitudinal traction and internal rotation is applied to the limb to reduce the fracture.
- Check reduction with II both AP and lateral images.
- Unstable fractures may not reduce with these methods and require open reduction.
- Securely lock the traction table to ensure reduction is maintained.

Procedure

- The World Health Organization safe surgery checklist must be completed.
- Preparation of the lower leg, in line with local policy (iodine-based aqueous or alcoholic or chlorhexidine). Drape using a specific adhesive isolation drape.

The direct lateral approach to the proximal femur

- Mark out proximal femur and incision, longitudinally from level of greater trochanter to a point 10–15cm distal in line with femur.
- Make incision in skin and subcutaneous fat to level of fascia lata.
- Check position of femur under fascia lata and make incision centrally in fascia lata and extend using heavy curved scissors proximally and distally, revealing underlying vastus lateralis muscle.
- Check position of femur and either incise muscle fascia centrally and split muscle fibres longitudinally down to the bone or lift the vastus lateralis anteriorly, releasing it from the lateral intermuscular septum.
- Watch for perforating vessels running posterior to anterior, control bleeding from these.
- Hold the muscle apart using a deep self-retainer (Norfolk and Norwich).
- Clear the muscle from lateral aspect of the proximal femur.

Insertion of guide wire

- Use a 3.2mm threaded guide wire through a 135° fixed guide.
- The starting point is usually at the level of the lesser trochanter.
- Use II to accurately place guide wire in both AP and lateral planes.
- Place the footprint of the guide parallel to the longitudinal axis of the femur.
- The wire must be inserted with the tip ending in the subchondral bone at the apex of the femoral head.
- It should be central in the femoral head on the AP and lateral views.
- Measure the remaining length of guide wire using the measuring device. This length dictates your sliding hip screw (SHS) length and what to set the triple reamer to.
- If tip in subchondral bone subtract 5mm from the measurement. This is the length of SHS and the depth setting of the triple reamer.

Insertion of the SHS and plate

- Ream over the guide wire using the triple step reamer.
- Drip wash fluid on to tip to keep it cool and avoid thermal damage to bone.
- Use II to ensure wire not driven into pelvis and is still in situ on removal of reamer.
- Tap the reamed canal over the wire (not essential in very osteoporotic bone).
- Insert the selected SHS using the centralizing sleeve.
- Check position with II. This should be central in the head on the AP and lateral X-rays and the tip in the subchondral bone.
- The tip–apex distance dictates the ideal position of the SHS tip. This is calculated by the sum of distance from tip of SHS to apex of femoral head on both AP and lateral views. This sum should be less than 25mm.[3]
- Ensure the final position of the T-handle SHS driver is parallel to the shaft of the femur. This will allow the barrel of the plate to sit in the appropriate position.
- Slide the barrel of the plate over the SHS and tap this until it is flush on the femur.
- Remove the SHS retaining rod and guide wire.
- Ensure the plate is central on the bone and fix in situ using four cortical 4.5mm fully threaded screws.
- Use the drill (3.5mm), measure (depth gauge), tap (4.5mm), screw insertion sequence.
- Reduce the traction on the affected limb. Obtain final II images (AP and lateral).
- A compression screw can be placed into the end of the SHS if required.
- Ensure haemostasis and lavage thoroughly.

Closure

- Close the muscle fascia (no. 1 Vicryl®).
- Close the fascia lata (no. 1 Vicryl®).
- Close the subcutaneous fascia (2.0 Vicryl®).
- Close the skin.
- Dress the wound.

Postoperative care

- Antibiotics and VTE prophylaxis as per local policy.
- Check FBC and U&E next day.
- Allow weight bearing as tolerated.
- Ensure rehabilitation and a discharge plan is established with multidisciplinary team input (surgeons, orthogeriatricians, physiotherapists, occupational therapists, family, social services).
- Follow-up as per local protocol.

Complications

- Superficial and deep infection.
- Failure of fixation (cut out).
- DVT and PE.
- Chest infection.
- Poor mobility.

Tips and tricks

- A lateral wall must be present in the distal segment to provide support to the medial/proximal fracture segment during compressive loading. If this is not present a intramedullary device should be considered.
- Ensuring the guide wire, and thus the SHS, is in the centre of the head on the AP and lateral X-rays will reduce the risk of cut out and failure.

Further reading

Baumgaertner MR, Curtin SL, Lindskog DM, Keggi JM. The value of the tip-apex distance in predicting failure of fixation of peritrochanteric fractures of the hip. *J Bone Joint Surg Am*. 1995 Jul; 77(7):1058–64. (http://www.aofoundation.org).

References

1 NICE Guidelines Hip Fractures: (http://guidance.nice.org.uk/CG124Hip fracture tariff).
2 Best Practice Tariff: (http://www.nhfd.co.uk/003/hipfractureR.nsf/vwContent/BestPracticeTariff).
3 Baumgaertner MR, Curtin SL, Lindskog DM, Keggi JM. The value of the tip-apex distance in predicting failure of fixation of peritrochanteric fractures of the hip. *J Bone Joint Surg Am*. 1995 Jul; 77(7):1058–64. (http://www.aofoundation.org).

Hemiarthroplasty for intra-capsular fracture neck of femur

Displaced intra-capsular fractures of the neck of femur need replacing as the blood supply to the head is disrupted (see ➲ 'Surgical anatomy and approaches to the hip join', p. 1000). This predisposes to avascular necrosis and a higher rate of non-union if fixation is not undertaken. It also avoids complications of decubitus for the patient.

Anatomy

See ➲ 'Surgical anatomy and approaches to the hip join', p. 1000, and Fig. 16.19.

Indications

- Displaced intra-capsular fractures of the neck of femur.
- Consider total hip replacement in high demand patients.
- For NICE Guidelines see ➲ 'Dynamic hip screw (DHS) fixation for extra-capsular neck or femur fracture', p. 950.

Preoperative preparation

Assessment and preparation of the patient for surgery is the same as for intertrochanteric fractures (see ➲ 'Dynamic hip screw (DHS) fixation for extra-capsular neck or femur fracture', p. 950).

- Mark the affected limb.
- Informed consent is required.
  - Always consult the patient's family prior to consent and procedure.
  - Risks: infection, bleeding, damage to nerves (sciatic and superior gluteal), poor mobility, fracture during stem insertion, dislocation, revision surgery, DVT, and PE.
- Liaise with anaesthetist:
  - General anaesthetic (fast 6h) or spinal anaesthetic.
  - Antibiotics on induction (follow local hospital protocol).
  - Ensure thromboprophylaxis is commenced in line with Trust policy.
- Liaise with the scrub team and ensure equipment is available:
  - Hip instrument tray and retractors.
  - Double mix of cement.
  - Ensure all hemiarthroplasty implant sizes are available (see local Trust policy on brand of implant).
  - Standard operating table.
  - Anterior and posterior supports (if lateral positioning) and sandbags (if supine).

Position and theatre set-up

- The head end is by the anaesthetic machine. Table runs down the centre of theatre.
- Positioning is surgeon-dependent:
  - Supine with sandbag under buttock of operative side.
  - Lateral decubitus (more common)—operative side up, maintained with rigid side supports front and back (anteriorly at level of ASIS and posteriorly on sacrum).
- Surgeon on posterior side and assistant anteriorly. Scrub nurse is at foot of bed.

Procedure

- The World Health Organization safe surgery checklist must be completed.
- Preparation of the lower leg in line with local policy (iodine-based aqueous or alcoholic or chlorhexadine). Drape using a specific hip draping pack, stockinette over lower leg.
- Mark out surface anatomy:
  - Femoral shaft.
  - Greater trochanter.
  - Wing of ilium.
  - ASIS.

Approach

Commonly the Hardinge approach is used (see ➔ 'Surgical anatomy and approaches to the hip joint', p. 1002).

Neck cut and canal preparation

- Maintain the hip position and allow the tibia to rest perpendicular to the floor.
- Make a neck cut, using an oscillating saw, from the level of the superior edge of the lesser trochanter, along the base of the neck to exit in the piriform fossa of the superior neck.
- Using a trial implant or broach can help to mark out the neck cut.
- This cut is for a Thompson's prosthesis, where the collar sits on the lesser trochanter. If using a different prosthesis, ensure the appropriate neck cut is made.
- Remove the femoral head by inserting a 'corkscrew' in to the centre of the neck. Rotate until the head rotates, indicating no soft tissue remains attached (capsule or ligamentum teres).
- Size the removed head using the measures provided.
- This corresponds to the size of the Thompson's monobloc prosthesis that will be used.
- If in between sizes, always choose 1mm smaller.
- Externally rotate the leg, keeping hip flexed to 90° to reveal the neck cut.
- Prepare the canal by opening it proximally with a straight pencil reamer or Trethowan spike.
- Broach the canal with the specific Thompson's broach.
- If not fitting, clear out the posterolateral part of the canal and trochanter using a curette.
- Insert a Charnley cement restrictor into the prepared canal, measure how far to insert the restrictor against the stem of the implant.
- Thoroughly wash and dry the canal with pulsed lavage, suction and a clean swab.

Cementation of the prosthesis

- Open the prosthesis, ensuring it is the correct size and not out of date.
- Having an old prosthesis on the set is useful to ensure the stem will fit in the canal prior to cementation, if not use the new prosthesis but clean after.
- Be aware of what cement is being used, e.g. a 'normal' viscosity cement gives 10min before it is set but only about 6min of working time!

- Ensure you are ready for cementation—implant ready, new gloves, instrument to remove excess cement, and implant impactor.
- Instruct the scrub nurse to mix cement and inform the anaesthetist. A timer will be started when mixing commences.
- Take the cement at 2min and fill canal.
- Retrograde fill the canal, by allowing the cement to push the tip of the cement gun out of the canal.
- Pressurization with thumb pressure is adequate. Excessive pressurization can be dangerous if there is diminished cardiopulmonary reserve.
- Between 3 and 4min insert the prosthesis by hand, ensure the point of the collar is slightly anterior to the lesser trochanter, which will recreate some of the anteversion of the femoral neck.
- Clear excess cement and pressurise until 8–10min.
- Once the cement has cured, thoroughly wash the acetabulum and remove any debris.
- Reduce the hip with longitudinal traction and internal rotation.
- Wash and ensure haemostasis.

Closure

- Close the capsule first with a heavy braided suture (no. 2 Vicryl®).
- Repair the abductors back to the cuff of tendon left on the trochanter using a heavy braided suture (no. 2 Vicryl®).
- Repair the fascia lata (no. 1 Vicryl®).
- Close subcutaneous fascia (2.0 Vicryl®) and skin using an absorbable monofilament (3.0 Monocryl®).
- Apply a dry dressing.

Postoperative care

- Prescribe further antibiotics and VTE prophylaxis as per local protocol.
- Obtain a set of bloods (FBC and U&E) and X-ray of the hip the next morning.
- The patient can mobilize full weight-bearing.
- Rehabilitation and follow-up arrangements should be made as per local hospital policy.
- Review by an orthogeriatrician is essential and multidisciplinary team assessment is required to ensure safe discharge is achieved.

Further reading

Hardinge K. The direct lateral approach to the hip. *J Bone Joint Surg Br* 1982; 64(1): 17–19.

Hoppenfeld S, deBoer P, Buckley R. *Surgical Exposures in Orthopaedics: The Anatomic Approach*, 4th edn. Lippincott Williams & Wilkins, 2009.

Fixation of patella fracture by tension band wiring

Anatomy

See ➲ 'Diagnostic arthroscopy and simple arthroscopic procedures', p. 986, and Figs 16.3 and 16.13.

- The patella is a large sesamoid, which sits anteriorly at the knee joint. It is suspended between the patellar tendon inferiorly via its inferior pole, which inserts into the tibial tuberosity, and superiorly into the distal conjoint tendon of the quadriceps (rectus femoris centrally, vastus lateralis, medius, and intermedius). The medial and lateral insertions to the patella are the retinaculae and medially the medial patellofemoral ligament.
- It forms a joint between the posterior articular surface of the patella and the anterior articular surface of the distal femur, the trochlear groove.
- A displaced fracture of the patella disrupts the extensor mechanism of the leg at the knee.

Indications

- Transverse fractures of the patella.
- Multi-fragmentary patellar fractures, used in combination with other fixation techniques (lag screws, circlage wires).

Preoperative preparation

- History and examination, mechanism of injury, neurological symptoms, PMH, DH, occupation.
- Document neurovascular status.
- Assess for open wounds.

X-rays

- AP and lateral radiographs of the knee required.
- If concerns over associated injury to the patellar tendon or quadriceps tendon an ultrasound or MRI scan can be useful.

Obtain informed consent

- Explain procedure to patient.
- Risks: infection, nerve injury (infrapatellar branch of saphenous nerve), stiffness of knee, malunion, removal of metalwork, development of arthritis, compartment syndrome.
- Ensure the correct surgical site is clearly marked.

Liaise with anaesthetist

- GA most common, can be performed under nerve block.
- Antibiotics on induction (follow local hospital protocol).

Liaise with the scrub team and ensure equipment is available

- Wiring set essential, including 1.6mm and 2.0mm K-wires, 1.25mm circlage wire.
- Have a small fragment set available (3.5mm cortical and 4.0mm partially threaded cancellous screws) if need to undertake internal fixation arises.

- Radiographer and image intensifier (II) available.
- Radiolucent fracture table.
- Tourniquet and padding.
- An assistant is useful to help obtain and hold reduction.

Position and theatre set-up

- Head end of table next to anaesthetist.
- Nurse and instrument trolley on operative side, image intensifier on opposite side.
- Patient supine with a small bolster under the operative leg.
- Apply a high-thigh tourniquet (inflate to 300mmHg) and inflate after preparation and draping to reduce bleeding.

Procedure

- The World Health Organization safe surgery checklist must be completed.
- Preparation of the leg to the level of the tourniquet, in line with local policy (iodine-based aqueous or alcoholic or chlorhexadine).
- Drape using a specific adhesive isolation drape or leg extremity drape.
- Place the foot in a stockinette and wrap in a crepe bandage.
- Incise the skin longitudinally starting up to 5cm proximal and extending 5cm distal to the patellar poles.
- Incise the superficial fascia in line with the skin incision.
- This will bring you onto the disrupted fascia and periosteum overlying the patella.
- If an open wound is present, debride this thoroughly and lavage with up to 9l of sterile warmed saline.
- Clear the ends of the fracture of soft tissue and debris only, leaving as much soft tissue attached to the patellar fragments.
- Wash thoroughly.
- Reduce the fracture fragments together and hold with a large, pointed reduction clamp.
- Leg extension by assistant can help with reduction.
- Check reduction by palpation of the articular surface via rents in the retinaculum and with II.
- Using a wire driver, pass two parallel 2mm K-wires from proximal to distal (antegrade), spaced ~1–2cm apart, in the anterior half of the patella.
- Leave 3cm of K-wire protruding distally.
- Take a 20–30cm length of 1.25mm circlage wire, push under the proximal K-wires, close to the proximal pole of the patella, through the substance of the quadriceps tendon, from lateral to medial.
- Using a large-bore cannula can help, by leaving the plastic sheath in situ and passing the circlage wire through this.
- Make a single twist in the circlage wire (medially), pass obliquely across the patella, and repeat the above step but this time through the patella tendon, under the distal wires, medial to lateral.
- Cross the circlage wire centrally and make a second twist with the other free end of the circlage wire, creating a 'figure of 8 circlage' with two twisted loops on either side for tightening.

- Tighten the loops simultaneously with wire holders, checking reduction as above.
- Cut and bend the K-wires, rotate the bent ends posterior to cause the least soft tissue irritation (see Fig. 16.4).
- Final II AP and lateral radiographs.
- Wash out wound.

Closure

- Close the retinaculum with a strong braided suture (no.1 Vicryl®).
- Close the superficial fascia (2.0 Vicryl®) and the skin (3.0 absorbable monofilament).
- Adhesive dressing, padding and crepe bandage, straight-leg rigid splint.

Postoperative care

- Allow partial weight-bearing for 6 weeks in the splint.
- Start passive range of movement of the knee with physiotherapy (0–90° flexion).
- Review wound at 2 weeks.
- Review in clinic at 6 weeks with AP and lateral radiographs of the knee.
- Once the fracture has united start active range of movement, full weight-bearing and strengthening exercises.

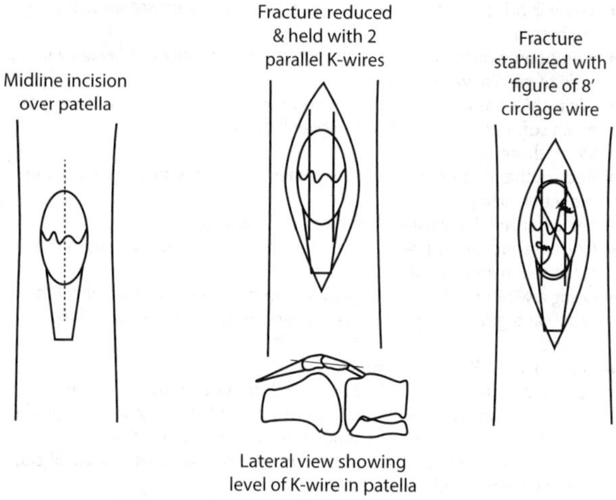
Midline incision over patella
Fracture reduced & held with 2 parallel K-wires
Fracture stabilized with 'figure of 8' circlage wire
Lateral view showing level of K-wire in patella

Fig. 16.4 Diagrams showing incision, reduction of patella fracture with K-wires, and completed tension band wire construct.

Complications

- Early and late infection.
- Prominence of the metalwork and need for removal (usually after 6 months if fracture united.)
- Arthritis of the patellofemoral joint.

Tips and tricks

- Keeping the knee slightly flexed during insertion of the K-wire will allow the correct trajectory across the patella, but will also keep the ends of the K-wire visible distal and proximal to the patella and quadriceps tendons.
- Always take a longer length of circlage wire than you think you will need, then, you will not run out and have to start again.

Further reading

(http://www.aofoundation.org).

Insertion of traction pins

Anatomy

Distal femur

- Distal femur traction pins are used for pelvic and acetabular fractures, proximal femoral fractures.
  - Use for longer than 2–3 weeks can result in knee stiffness.
- The lateral knee joint capsule reaches 1.25–2cm above knee joint line, avoid entering the joint as this predisposes to septic arthritis.
- Avoid too proximal pin insertion as this risks injury to femoral artery in Hunter's canal.
- If using in children, do not forget to avoid the distal femoral physis.

Proximal tibia

- Proximal tibial traction pins are used for femoral shaft, hip, pelvic and acetabular fractures.
- Contraindicated if a ligament injury to ipsilateral knee exists.
- Never used in children as recurvatum can occur due to injury of proximal tibial physis.
- Remember pins are inserted from the lateral side to avoid damaging the common peroneal nerve.

Calcaneal

- Calcaneal traction pins are used for tibial fractures.
- The pin should be inserted as far posterior as possible while still engaging sound bone, in order to avoid the tendons and neurovascular bundle passing behind the malleoli and the subtalar joint.
- The posterior tibial nerve branches after it passes behind the medial malleolus:
  - Medial plantar nerve (motor branches to: abductor hallucis, flexor digitorum brevis, flexor hallucis brevis, 1st lumbrical; sensory branches to: plantar medial 3.5 digits and medial 3.5 dorsal nailbeds).
  - Lateral plantar nerve (motor branches to: quadratus plantae, flexor digiti minimi, adductor hallucis, interossei, three lateral lumbricals, abductor digiti minimi; sensory branches to: lateral plantar surface, lateral 1.5 toes and lateral 1.5 dorsal nailbeds).
  - Medial calcaneal nerve (sensory to the plantar medial aspect of the heel).

Indications

- Traction is a useful technique for aiding in the maintenance of fracture reduction. These can be used temporarily or for the duration of fracture healing in combination with a traction-pulley system.
- Traction pins are also used intraoperatively in combination with a fracture operative table to maintain reduction.
- The lower limb is the commonest site for traction pin insertion; either at the distal femur, proximal tibia, or calcaneum.

Preoperative preparation

- History and examination, supported by investigations.
- Appropriate radiological imaging.
- Select appropriate form of traction required depending on location and configuration of fracture.
- Discussion with senior colleague important.

Obtain informed consent

- Explain procedure to patient.
- Risks: infection (superficial, septic arthritis, osteomyelitis), nerve injury, vessel injury, joint stiffness.

Liaise with anaesthetist

- General anaesthetic (fast 6h) or spinal anaesthetic.
- Antibiotics on induction (follow local hospital protocol).

Liaise with the scrub team and ensure equipment is available

- Traction pins: Steimann pins (3.6mm diameter, variable lengths), Denham pins (4.0mm and 5.0mm diameter, lengths 20 or 23cm, centrally threaded).
- Bohler stirrup.
- Thomas pin mount or Steimann pin screw caps.
- Universal chuck with T-handle.
- Radiolucent operating table.
- Image intensifier with sterile covers and radiographer.

Position and theatre set-up

- For all the following, set up is supine.
- Table running down centre of the theatre, head at anaesthetic machine.
- A sandbag under the ipsilateral buttock can help with leg rotational control.
- A sterile bolster for under the knee or raise the heel.
- II coming from the opposite side to surgery, screens at foot of table.

Procedure

- The World Health Organization safe surgery checklist to be completed.
- Preparation of the limb, in line with local policy (iodine-based aqueous or alcoholic or chlorhexidine).
- Drape using a specific adhesive isolation drape or leg extremity drape.

Distal femur traction pin

- Bring in II and obtain a lateral image of the knee in extension.
    - Mark on the medial side of the leg, the level of the proximal pole of the patella (at this level, the pin will be just proximal to the adductor tubercle and will avoid injury to the collateral ligaments) and the midpoint of the femur at that level (Fig. 16.5).
    - Then mark a line on the anterior surface of the distal thigh a line that is parallel to the knee joint, running medial to lateral.
- Place the bolster under the knee to allow slight flexion:
    - Pin insertion from the opposite side of the table (medial to lateral).
    - Obtain a lateral X-ray.
    - Places the periarticular soft tissues in the position they will occupy while the limb is in traction, reducing pressure necrosis of the skin.

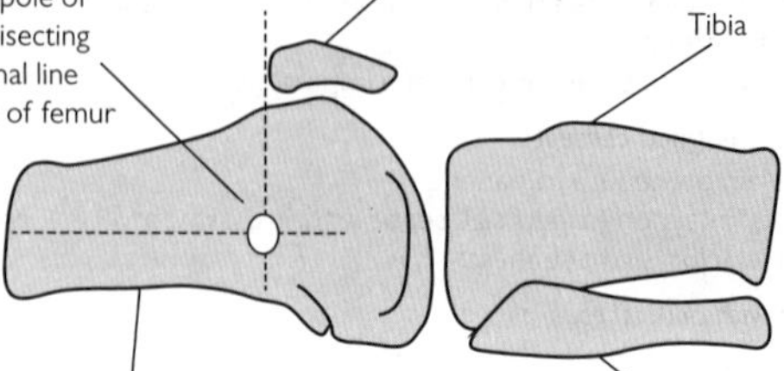
Entry point of traction pin: Line at level of superior pole of patella, bisecting longitudinal line midpoint of femur
Patella
Tibia
Femur
Fibula

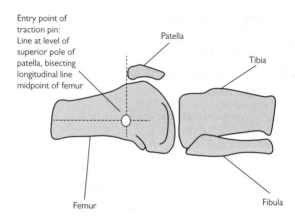

Fig. 16.5 Placement of the distal femoral traction pin.

- Make a 0.5cm incision on the medial side of the distal femur at the marked point.
- Take a 5.0mm Denham pin and load this into the universal chuck and T-handle.
- Gently pass the point of the pin through the soft tissues to engage the medial femoral cortex.
    - Obtain an X-ray to confirm entry point (proximal pole of patella and just posterior to midline in lateral image).
- Drive the pin through the femur parallel to the knee joint line (an AP X-ray can help).
- As the pin exits laterally, make a further incision to accommodate the pin.
    - A small cut in the iliotibial band around the pin will help with free movement of the pin during traction.
    - Ensure the skin is not under tension at the entry or exit points.
- Ensure equal lengths of the pins protrude from either side and the central thread is within bone (to avoid sliding of pin).

Proximal tibial traction pin

- Place the bolster under the knee to allow flexion, this will facilitate obtaining a lateral X-ray.
- Bring in II and obtain a lateral image of the knee.
- Mark on the lateral side a point 2.5cm posterior and 2.5cm distal to tibial tubercle (Fig. 16.6).
- Mark a line on the anterior surface of the lower leg, a line that is parallel to the knee joint, running lateral to medial.
- Remember too proximal pin placement, places it through much weaker cancellous bone, running the risk of cut out.

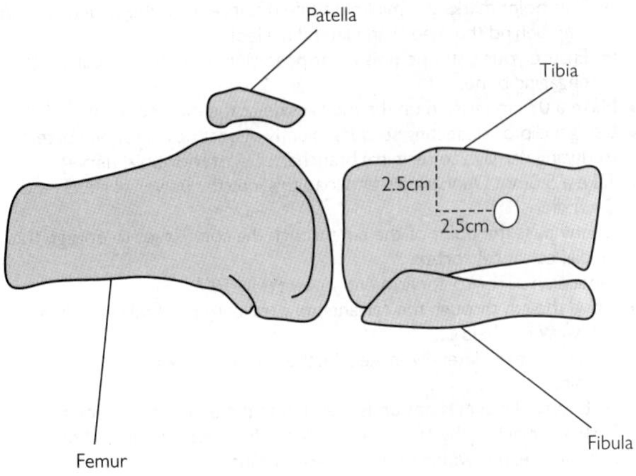
Patella
Tibia
2.5cm
2.5cm
Fibula
Femur

Fig. 16.6 Placement of proximal tibial traction pin.

- Too distal pin placement will be in stronger cortical bone, but puts the peroneal nerve at risk as it passes anteriorly after it passes around the fibular neck.
- Make a 0.5cm incision on the lateral side of the proximal tibia at the marked point.
- Take a 5.0mm Denham pin and load this into the universal chuck and T-handle
- Gently pass the point of the pin through the soft tissues to engage the lateral tibial cortex.
- Obtain an X-ray to confirm entry point.
- Drive the pin through the tibia parallel to the knee joint line (an AP X-ray can help).
- Ensure not to drift anterior.
- As the pin exits medially make a further incision to accommodate the pin.
  - Ensure the skin is not under tension at the entry or exit points.
- Ensure equal lengths of the pins stick out from either side and the central thread is within bone (to avoid sliding of pin).

Calcaneal traction pin

- Place the bolster under the heel in order to obtain an unobstructed lateral X-ray.
- Bring in II and obtain a lateral image of the ankle and calcaneum. Mark on the medial side a point 2.5cm inferior and 2.5cm posterior to the medial malleolus (or on the lateral side a point 2cm inferior and posterior to the lateral malleolus, these should coincide).

- This point marks the minimum safe distance from the structures running behind the medial and lateral malleoli.
- Ensure your entry point is as far posterior as possible yet still engaging bone.
- Make a 0.5cm incision on the medial side at the marked point.
- Using a clip or dissecting scissors, bluntly dissect down to the cortex (reducing damage to terminal branches of posterior tibial nerve).
- Take a 5.0mm Denham pin and load this into the universal chuck and T-handle.
- Gently pass the point of the pin through the soft tissues to engage the medial calcaneal cortex.
- Obtain an X-ray to confirm entry point (Fig. 16.7).
- Drive the pin through the calcaneum, parallel to the ankle joint line (an AP X-ray can help).
- As the pin exits laterally make a further incision to accommodate the pin.
    - Ensure the skin is not under tension at the entry or exit points.
- Ensure equal lengths of the pins stick out from either side and the central thread is within bone (to avoid sliding of pin).

For all pin types

- Attach an appropriate-sized Bohler stirrup and secure this in place by tightening the locking screws.
- Cut the sharp ends of the pins using pin or bolt-cutters.
- Cover the cut ends to avoid injury (short segments of oxygen tubing used for masks, can be useful here).

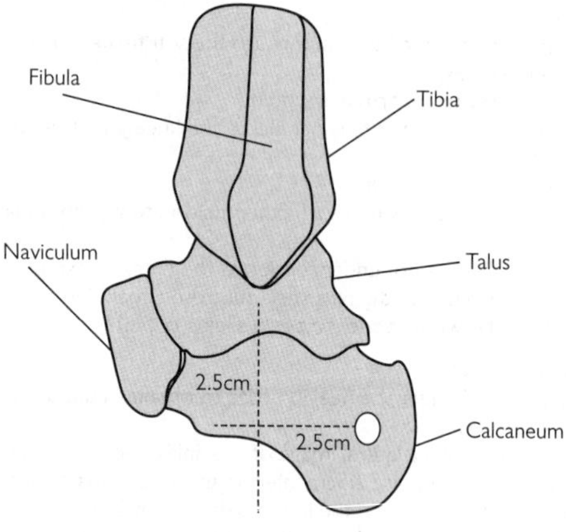
Fibula
Tibia
Naviculum
Talus
2.5cm
2.5cm
Calcaneum

Fig. 16.7 Placement of calcaneal traction pin.

Pin site care

- Apply a slit gauze swab around the pin and do not remove the crust that develops around the pin on the skin.
- The gauze swab should only be changed infrequently.
- No closure is required.

Postoperative care

- Appropriate traction needs to be constructed on an orthopaedic traction bed (beyond the scope of this book).
- The traction should be used for shortest time necessary.
- Regular pressure area care is essential.
- VTE prophylaxis as per local protocol.

Complications

- Pin site infection.
- Pin loosening.
- DVT/PE.
- Pressure sores.
- Stiff joints.

Tips and tricks

- The use of bolsters is essential for a successful procedure, keeping the opposite leg out of the operative field as well as allowing the image intensifier in for a clear view.
- Remember to have your spare hand well out of the way of the exiting pin—it is very easy to impale yourself or your assistant!

Surgical debridement of traumatic wound

Indications

- Any upper or lower limb trauma with associated soft tissue injury.
- Often wounds overlie fractures.

Classification of open wounds associated with fractures

Gustillo and Anderson (1)

- Type I: wound <1cm.
- Type II: wound 1–10cm.
- Type III: wound >10 cm or high-energy injury (comminuted/segmental fractures).
  - A—adequate tissue remaining for closure/coverage.
  - B—extensive periosteal stripping and soft tissue loss—requires flap coverage.
  - C—vascular injury requiring vascular repair.

The true extent of the soft tissue injury cannot be correctly classified until debridement is complete.

Preoperative preparation

- ATLS approach (2)—ensure primary survey (ABCDE) is complete before assessing the affected limb.
- Thorough history and examination (information from paramedics and resuscitation team essential).
- Assess the wound and level of contamination (farmyard/marine).
- Assess neurological status.
  - Sensation and motor to affected limb distal to injury.
- Assess vascular status.
  - White and cold; capillary refill; peripheral pulses if weak use a hand held Doppler.

Guidelines on management of open fractures

British Orthopaedic Association/British Association of Plastic, Reconstructive and Aesthetic Surgeons combined guidelines.

- IV antibiotics (co-amoxiclav 1.2g or cefuroxime 1.5g) within 3h of injury, until time of debridement.
- Regular assessment of neurovascular status, especially if the limb is moved or splints applied.
- Any vascular injury treated surgically within maximum 6h warm ischaemia time.
- Compartment syndrome treated immediately with complete fasciotomy of all compartments of affected limb.
- Remove gross contamination from wound, photograph, and dress with saline soaked gauze.
- Apply appropriate splint and reassess neurovascular status.
- Always have a multidisciplinary team approach to management—early involvement of plastic and vascular surgeons essential.

- Consider early transfer to Major Trauma Centre if safe to do so.
- Surgery can take place on next planned trauma operating list (unless immediate surgery required as above).

Obtain informed consent if possible

- Explain procedure to patient.
- Risks: infection, damage to nerves and vessels, further debridement, soft tissue coverage (skin grafts, flaps), compartment syndrome, amputation.
- Ensure the correct surgical site is clearly marked.

Liaise with theatre staff and anaesthetic team as soon as possible if planning surgery

- Equipment requirements will depend on injury severity and site.
- Open fractures may require IM nailing, external fixation or plating.
- Standard orthopaedic set required for debridement.
- Have 9l of warmed normal saline for irrigation available (an arthroscopic giving set is a controlled mode of delivery to the wound).
- Image intensifier and radiographer required.
- Alert other speciality teams if required.

Position and theatre set-up

- This will depend on the site of wound and associated injuries.
- In principle, a radiolucent table required if associated fractures.
- Tourniquet application can be useful in some cases if applicable.
- II from the opposite side, scrub nurse on the same side as surgeon.

Procedure

- The World Health Organization safe surgery checklist must be completed.
- Preparation of the limb, in line with local policy (iodine-based aqueous or alcoholic or chlorhexidine).
- Drape using a specific adhesive isolation drape or arm extremity drape.
- Clear gross contamination from wounds.
- Extend wounds longitudinally as less likely to compromise subsequent flaps.
- Remove all devitalized soft tissue, including skin, fascia, muscle, periosteum, and bone devoid of any soft tissue attachment.
- Aggressive debridement is essential to reduce the risk of subsequent infection.
- Assessing muscle viability is difficult—pinching with forceps to see if it contracts can help.
- Once appropriate debridement is achieved, lavage with 9l of warmed normal saline.
- Stabilize fractures as appropriate.
- Leave wounds open and dress with non-adhesive dressings.

Postoperative care

- Continue antibiotics until definitive soft tissue coverage is achieved.
- Prepare for a second debridement with or without coverage at 48h.
- Involve the plastic surgery team, if they are not already.

Complications

- Infection (acute or chronic).
- Breakdown of closure/coverage (split skin graft or flap).
- Amputation.

Tips and tricks

- The key to a successful outcome is a calm, stepwise, multidisciplinary initial management of these injuries.
- Antibiotics are crucial early.
- Remember there is no need to do this in the middle of the night, the next safe operation list is the safest option for both patient and surgical team.

Further reading

BOAST 4: The Management of Severe Open Lower Limb Fractures. ☞ (www.boa.ac.uk)

References

1 Gustilo RB, Anderson JT. Prevention of infection in the treatment of one thousand and twenty-five open fractures of long bones: retrospective and prospective analyses. *J Bone Joint Surg Am.* 1976. 58(4):453–8.

2 ATLS: ☞ (http://www.facs.org/trauma/atls/).

Fasciotomy for compartment syndrome of the lower leg

Fasciotomy for compartment syndrome of the lower leg

Overview

The diagnosis and management of compartment syndrome is an essential requirement for all surgical trainees. Compartment syndrome can occur in the upper limbs, lower limbs, hands, feet, and abdomen. This chapter focuses on the leg.

It is a surgical emergency and, as such, prompt diagnosis and management are mandatory. Inform senior colleagues as soon as the diagnosis is suspected.

Anatomy

The leg contains four fascial compartments and each of these contains several important structures (Table 16.1 and Fig. 16.8).

Indications

Clinically diagnosed compartment syndrome.

Preoperative preparation

- Ensure thorough history and examination are undertaken.
- Key features in diagnosis include:
  - Severe pain out of proportion to injury.
  - Pain failing to improve as expected.
  - Pain aggravated by passive muscle stretch.
  - Sensory loss can be useful early sign.

Table 16.1 Summary of the contents of the four compartments of the leg

Compartment	Muscles	NV structures
Anterior	Tibialis anterior Extensor hallucis longus Extensor digitorum longus Peroneus tertius	Anterior tibial artery Anterior tibial vein Deep peroneal nerve
Lateral	Peroneus brevis Peroneus longus	Superficial peroneal nerve
Superficial Posterior	Gastrocnemius Soleus	Long saphenous nerve and vein (run superficial to compartment)
Deep Posterior	Flexor digitiorum longus Flexor hallucis longus Tibialis posterior	Peroneal artery Peroneal vein Posterior tibial artery Posterior tibial vein Tibial nerve

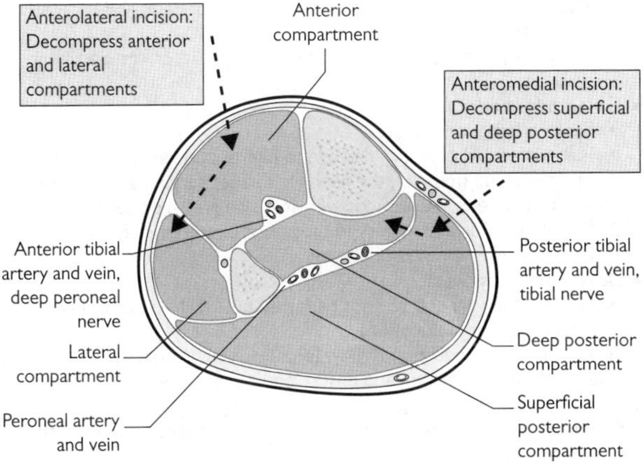
Anterolateral incision: Decompress anterior and lateral compartments
Anterior compartment
Anteromedial incision: Decompress superficial and deep posterior compartments
Anterior tibial artery and vein, deep peroneal nerve
Posterior tibial artery and vein, tibial nerve
Deep posterior compartment
Lateral compartment
Superficial posterior compartment
Peroneal artery and vein

Fig. 16.8 Diagram showing the compartments of the leg (mid-calf level), the relevant neurovascular structures, and direction of incision through the fascia to decompress all four compartments.

- Common factors involved in development of compartment syndrome:
  - High-energy injuries (open fractures, road traffic accidents).
  - Young men with large calf muscles and tibial fracture.
  - Post IM nailing of tibia.
  - Tight casts/backslab post-surgery.
- Initial management:
  - Ensure an ATLS approach to management has been undertaken.
  - A low threshold of suspicion is required for diagnosis.
  - Assess limb as described above.
  - Ensure all casts, backslabs, and bandages are split to skin on affected side.
  - Inform senior colleagues immediately if compartment syndrome is suspected.
  - Order and have available appropriate radiographs and scans of associated injuries that may require simultaneous management.
  - Contact theatres and on-call anaesthetist to make them aware of plan for surgery in the form of fasciotomy.
  - If present in your institution, contact the on-call plastic surgery team.
- Diagnosis in patients with impaired consciousness, children (under sedation), or those with regional nerve blocks:
  - The use of intra-compartmental pressure (ICP) monitors is advocated.
  - Most theatres have ICP monitoring devices, otherwise a manometer can be set up (this will require anaesthetic help to set up device).

    - The difference between diastolic blood pressure and ICP is calculated.
    - A value equal or less than 30mmHg is suggestive of compartment syndrome.
- Obtain informed consent.
    - Explanation of procedure.
    - Risks: infection, bleeding, damage to nerves and vessels, debridement of dead tissue (muscle), the need for further surgery and debridement, closure of the wounds with split skin grafts, possibility of amputation, further surgery for cosmesis or to return function.
    - Mark the level and side of surgery.
- Liaise with anaesthetist:
    - GA—explain patient may not be fasted but will have to proceed (rapid sequence intubation).
    - Antibiotics on induction (follow local hospital protocol).
- Liaise with the scrub team and ensure equipment is available including:
    - Image intensifier is required.
    - Ensure all procedure-specific equipment (if fracture fixation or stabilization is required) is available.
    - Tourniquet.

Position and theatre set-up

- Head at anaesthetic machine end.
- Table running down centre of theatre.

Procedure

(See Figs 16.8 and 16.9)

- The World Health Organization safe surgery checklist must be completed.
- Preparation of the leg to the level of the tourniquet, in line with local policy (iodine-based aqueous or alcoholic, or chlorhexidine).
- Drape using a specific adhesive isolation drape or leg extremity drape.
- Marking out (see Fig. 16.9):
    - Mark out the subcutaneous border of the tibia, then mark points 2cm medial and 2cm lateral to the subcutaneous borders.
    - Draw longitudinal lines either side of tibia, full length, for line of incision.
    - Placing the leg on a radiolucent block, will give better access for incisions, fixation, and II if required
- Start medially, incise the full length of the marked out incision, down through skin and fat to the level of the muscle fascia.
- Skin incision length should be approximately 16cm, depending on the size of leg, but it does need to be generous as this plays a role in the compression.
- Be aware that the long saphenous nerve and vein are close by and could be transected.
- Incise the fascia just behind the tibia, which will open the superficial posterior compartment, using scissors.

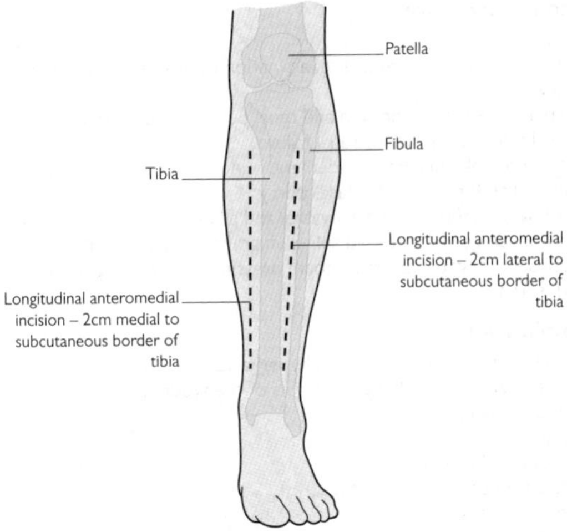
Patella
Fibula
Tibia
Longitudinal anteromedial incision – 2cm lateral to subcutaneous border of tibia
Longitudinal anteromedial incision – 2cm medial to subcutaneous border of tibia

Fig. 16.9 Frontal view of the leg showing marking out of subcutaneous border of tibia and optimal lines of incision (2cm medial and lateral).

- This is the full length of the incision—muscle will bulge through the incision.
- It is recommended that the approach is not too posterior as this risks damaging the perforator branches of the posterior tibial artery.
- Sticking close to the posterior tibia, incise the fascia between superficial and deep compartments longitudinally, taking care not to injure the posterior tibial artery and vein.
- Ensure compartments adequately released.
- Now make the incision on the anterolateral side as before.
- Incise the fascia over the anterior compartment longitudinally.
- Proceed through the fascia into the lateral compartment.
- Be careful not to injure the superficial peroneal nerve.
- Once all four compartments are released, inspect the muscles for viability.
- Assess colour (pink, grey, or black).
- Squeezing muscle between forceps will result in contraction if viable.
- If unsure, make a small cut in the muscle and wait for bleeding—this will give an idea of present blood supply.
- Any non-viable tissue must be excised.
- Ensure haemostasis and thorough washout with normal saline.
- Dress with jelonet (roll) directly onto exposed muscle, dressing gauze.
- A waterproof, adhesive dressing will retain moisture and prevent ooze all over dressings and bedding.
- Wrap loosely in wool and crepe bandages.

Postoperative care

- Analgesia.
- Full neurological and vascular examination to ensure no iatrogenic nerve injury.
- Maintain adequate hydration and renal perfusion. Be watchful of hyperkalaemia and risk of renal failure.
- A second look, further debridement, and closure of wounds are required at 48h after initial fasciotomy.
- If primary closure is not achievable, and all devitalized tissue is removed, early coverage with meshed split-skin grafts is the best option.
- The use of negative pressure foam dressings is becoming more widespread.

Complications

- Myoglobinuria and renal failure; hyperkalaemia.
- Altered sensation within the margins of the wound.
- Dry, scaly skin.
- Pruritus.
- Discoloured wounds.
- Swollen limbs.
- Tethered scars.
- Recurrent ulceration.
- Muscle herniation.
- Pain related to the wound.
- Tethered tendons.
- Volkmann's contracture.
- Weak dorsiflexors.
- Claw toes.
- Sensory loss.
- Chronic pain.
- Amputation.

Tips and tricks

- This is predominantly a clinical diagnosis—pain out of proportion to injury and passive stretch aggravating symptoms.
- Do not delay surgery (irreversible damage by 6h).
- Inform a senior early.
- A two-incision technique is recommended, ensuring all four compartments are decompressed.

Further reading

British Orthopaedic Association and British Association of Plastic, Reconstructive and Aesthetic Surgeons clinical guidelines on open fractures of the lower limb. (www.bapras.org.uk).

Fitzgerald AM, Gaston P, Wilson Y, Quaba A, McQueen MM. Long-term sequelae of fasciotomy wounds. *Br J Plas Surg* 2000; 53: 690–93.

McQueen MM, Court-Brown CM. Compartment monitoring in tibial fractures. The pressure threshold for decompression. *J Bone J Surg Br* 1996; 78: 99–104.

Intra-articular injections and joint aspiration

Indications

- Therapeutic injections of joints with local anaesthetic and steroid.
- Aspiration of effusions to diagnose septic arthritis, crystal or inflammatory arthropathy, or pain relieving (haemarthrosis/sterile effusion).
- The joints most commonly injected or aspirated are the knee, shoulder, wrist, and ankle. The hip, or small joints of the hand and foot are often performed in theatre under radiological image guidance.

Anatomy

For the knee and shoulder see ➲ 'Diagnostic arthroscopy and simple arthroscopic procedures' (p. 986); for the wrist see ➲ 'Carpal tunnel decompression' (p. 994).
(See Fig. 16.3)
The anterior structures of the ankle from medial malleolus to lateral malleolus include:

- Tibialis anterior.
- Extensor hallucis longus.
- Anterior neurovascular bundle (anterior tibial artery and deep peroneal nerve).
- Extensor digitorum longus.
- Peroneus tertius.

Preoperative preparation

- An explanation of procedure and consent is required (ideally written informed).
- Risks: infection (very low ~1:15000), allergy, damage to local structures. If steroid used, steroid flare (acute pain lasting up to 48h), fat necrosis, skin depigmentation.
- A suitable treatment room with an assistant.
- Sterile dressing pack, with gauze swabs, galley pot (for preparation), sterile disposable drape.
- Skin preparation product (iodine-based aqueous or alcoholic, or chlorhexadine).
- Sterile needles (wide bore for aspiration, 18-gauge, white; or 21-gauge, green) and sterile syringes (5, 10, and 20ml).
- Have local anaesthetic available (1% lignocaine).
- Sterile gloves.
- Receptacle for aspirate (sterile microbiology or biochemistry pots).
- Appropriate drugs for administration (check dose and expiry date).
- Sterile dressing.

Position and theatre set-up

- Ensure patient comfy and well supported prior to commencing (in case of a vasovagal episode).
- An examination couch is often useful.
- Set up all equipment on a clean trolley, open all required equipment onto the sterile dressing pack prior to commencing. Having an assistant is useful here.

Procedure

Aseptic technique should be observed for all aspirations:

- Thorough hand washing.
- Sterile gloves.
- Appropriate skin cleansing (iodine-based aqueous or alcoholic, or chlorhexidine) of the affected joint.
- Draping ensuring entry site exposed.
- Use of single use sterile needles and syringes.
- New needle for administering after drawing up drugs.

Knee

- Prepare a wide-bore needle (18-gauge, white) and 20 ml syringe if aspirating; green needle (21-gauge) and appropriate syringe for drugs if injecting.
- The commonest approach is the lateral retropatellar (Fig. 16.10).
    - The patient is supine, lower limb fully exposed, and knee fully extended.
    - Prepare knee using aseptic technique. A 5–10ml of 1% lignocaine can be injected as a field block if pain may be a problem.
    - Palpate the superolateral corner of the patella.
    - Any effusion will be easy to palpate proximal to this in the suprapatellar pouch.

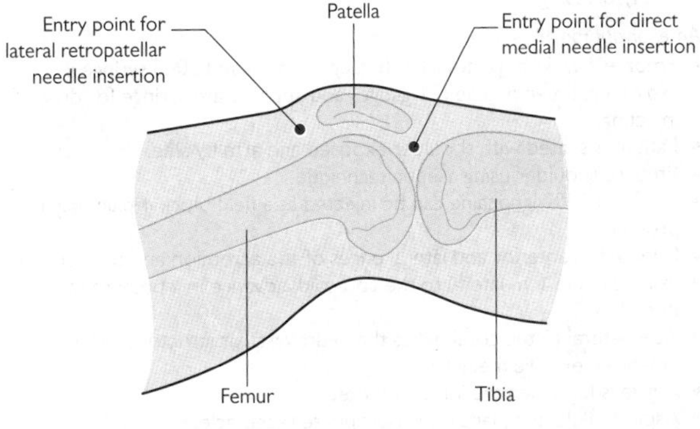
Entry point for lateral retropatellar needle insertion
Patella
Entry point for direct medial needle insertion
Femur
Tibia

Fig. 16.10 Showing the common sites for needle insertion around the knee—the lateral retropatellar and direct medial.

- Insert the needle 5mm posterior to the superolateral corner aiming perpendicular to the leg into the suprapatellar pouch.
- A give should be felt on entering the joint, between the patella and femoral condyles.
- Aspirate as much fluid as possible and place into appropriate receptacle.
- If injecting drugs into the knee, aspirate first to confirm needle is correctly placed in the joint, then inject drugs.
- Apply a dressing.

Shoulder

The shoulder can be accessed posteriorly, anteriorly, and laterally; this is very similar to the portals used in shoulder arthroscopy (see Fig. 16.14). The safest of is the posterior approach, but this can be difficult in a patient with large body habitus.

Posterior approach

- Prepare a wide-bore needle (18-gauge, white) and 20ml syringe if aspirating; green needle (21-gauge) and appropriate syringe for drugs if injecting.
- Patient is seated with shoulder exposed and arm by side.
- Prepare shoulder using aseptic technique.
- 5–10ml of 1% lignocaine can be injected as a field block if pain may be a problem.
- Palpate the posterolateral corner of the acromion.
- Insert the needle 2cm inferior and 2cm medial to this point, directing the needle towards the tip of coracoid. This can be palpated with the index finger of your opposite hand to guide direction.
- Ensure the needle is not directed superiorly as this will enter the subacromial space.
- A give is felt when the joint is entered.
- Aspirate fluid and place into appropriate receptacle.
- Apply dressing.

Anterior approach

- Prepare a wide-bore needle (18-gauge, white) and 20ml syringe if aspirating; green needle (21-gauge) and appropriate syringe for drugs if injecting.
- Patient is seated with shoulder exposed and arm by side.
- Prepare shoulder using aseptic technique.
- 5–10ml of 1% lignocaine can be injected as a field block if pain may be a problem.
- Palpate the anterior and lateral edges of the acromion and the coracoid.
- Insert needle 1cm lateral to the coracoid, advance in a posteroinferior direction.
- Keep lateral to the coracoid as the neurovascular structures of the brachial plexus lie medially.
- A give is felt when the joint is entered.
- Aspirate fluid and place into appropriate receptacle.
- Apply dressing.

Ankle

- Prepare a wide-bore needle (18-gauge, white) and 20-ml syringe if aspirating; green needle (21-gauge) and appropriate syringe for drugs if injecting.
- The most common and safest approach is anterolateral, if this fails an anteromedial approach is helpful (Fig. 16.11). If administering a therapeutic injection, image control can help to safely access the joint.
- The patient is supine, lower limb fully exposed, and leg extended, allowing the foot to naturally plantar-flex.
- Prepare ankle using aseptic technique.
- 5–10ml of 1% lignocaine can be injected as a field block if pain may be a problem.

Anterolateral

- Palpate the distal tip and anterior border of the fibula.
- Insert the needle approximately 5mm medial to the anterior fibula, 2–3cm proximal to the tip (a soft spot is usually felt).
- Proceed in a posteromedial direction, with a slight proximal inclination.

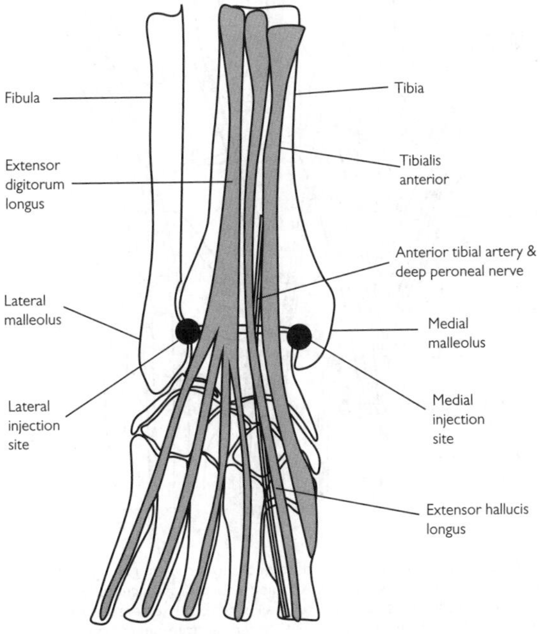
Fibula
Tibia
Extensor digitorum longus
Tibialis anterior
Anterior tibial artery & deep peroneal nerve
Lateral malleolus
Medial malleolus
Lateral injection site
Medial injection site
Extensor hallucis longus

Fig. 16.11 Ankle joint and relationship of anterior tendons and anterolateral and anteromedial injection or aspiration sites.

- A give is felt as the joint is entered.
- Aspirate fluid and place into appropriate receptacle.
- Apply dressing.

Anteromedial

- Palpate the soft spot just medial to the tibialis anterior tendon and lateral to the medial malleolus, 2–3cm proximal to the tip.
- Insert the needle into this space, proceeding in a posterolateral direction, with a slight proximal inclination.
- A give is felt as the joint is entered.
- Aspirate fluid and place into appropriate receptacle.
- Apply dressing.

Wrist

- The wrist is one of the more difficult joints to access. Remember the intercarpal joints tend to drain to the radiocarpal joint.
- The radiocarpal joint is entered via a dorsal approach (Fig. 16.12).

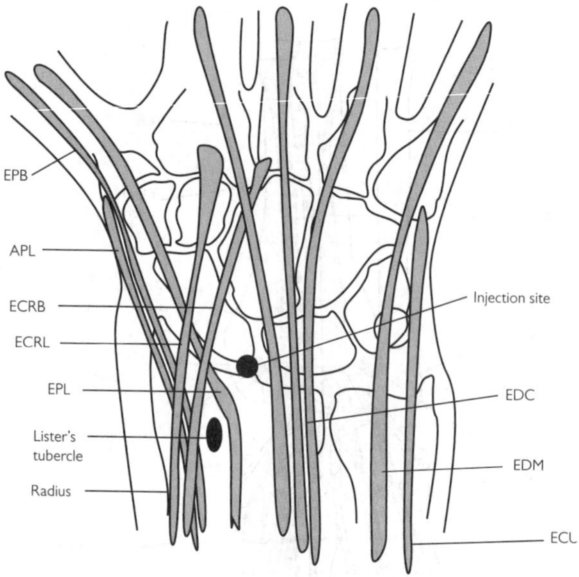
EPB
APL
ECRB
ECRL
EPL
Lister's tubercle
Radius
Injection site
EDC
EDM
ECU

Fig. 16.12 Relationship of dorsal wrist tendons to carpus and appropriate site for injection or aspiration of wrist joint: APL, abductor pollicis longus; EPB, extensor pollicis brevis; ECRL, extensor carpi radialis longus; ECRB, extensor carpi radialis brevis; EPL, extensor pollicis longus; EDC, extensor digitorum communis; EIP, extensor indicis proprius; EDM, extensor digiti minim; ECU, extensor carpi ulnaris.

- The patient is positioned seated or semi-recumbent, the wrist and hand supported and slight palmar-flexion helps.
- Prepare wrist using aseptic technique.
- 5–10ml of 1% lignocaine can be injected as a field block if pain may be a problem.
- Prepare a wide-bore needle (18-gauge, white) and 5ml syringe if aspirating; green needle (21-gauge) and appropriate syringe for drugs if injecting.
- Larger syringes cause too great a vacuum on aspiration and collapse the joint, thus, less effective for aspiration.
- Palpate the soft spot 1cm distal to Lister's tubercle on the dorsum of the wrist, between the tendons of extensor carpi radialis brevis and extensor pollicis longus radially, and extensor digitorum communis on the ulnar side.
- Insert the needle at this point in a dorsal to volar direction, with a 10° proximal inclination to allow for the volar inclination of the radius.
- A give is felt as the joint is entered.
- Aspirate fluid and place into appropriate receptacle.
- Apply dressing.

Postoperative care

- If administered therapeutic injections, review the patient 15min post-procedure to assess effect and ensure patient has had no adverse reaction.
- If aspiration for diagnostic purposes, await the results of either urgent Gram staining in the case of infection, or crystallography if suspecting gout or pseudogout.
- Treatment ongoing is dependent on the outcome of the tests.

Tips and tricks

- Always prepare all the equipment you need prior to commencing the procedure, as it is very frustrating if you have to stop halfway through to fetch something you have forgotten.
- Have an assistant if possible—this makes the whole procedure much smoother.

Diagnostic arthroscopy and simple arthroscopic procedures

Overview

Arthroscopy is widely used in the knee, shoulder, ankle, wrist, and elbow. The technique of arthroscope insertion and a diagnostic examination of the knee and shoulder are valuable skills to assess and treat common intra-articular pathology or washout an infected joint.

Knee arthroscopy

Anatomy

Surface anatomy is key, mark out:

- Patella.
- Patellar tendon.
- Tibial plateau.
- Femoral condyles.
- Medial and lateral collateral ligaments (Fig. 16.13).

The medial and lateral femoral condyles articulate with the corresponding condyles of the proximal tibia. They are stabilized primarily via the concavity created by the mensici and the ligaments of the knee joint; medial and lateral collateral ligaments (MCL and PCL) and the anterior and posterior cruciate ligaments (ACL and PCL).

The medial and lateral menisci are crescent-shaped fibrocartilaginous structures. They are concave on their superior surface, which articulates with the condyles of the femur, and are flat on their inferior surfaces. The inferior surface is attached to the condyles of the tibia via strong circumferential coronary ligaments. They have poor blood supply, which feeds via the periphery.

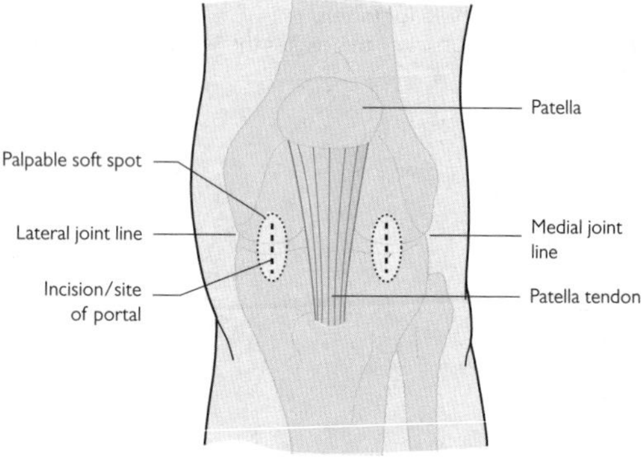
Patella
Palpable soft spot
Lateral joint line
Medial joint line
Incision/site of portal
Patella tendon

Fig. 16.13 Surface anatomy of knee showing patella, patellar tendon, medial and lateral joint lines, and entry points for portals marked.

The cruciate ligaments provide resistance to anterior (ACL) and posterior (PCL) translation of the tibia upon the femur. The ACL originates from the anteromedial aspect of the tibial intercondylar eminence. It has two bundles: the anteromedial and posterolateral. They insert in to the posterolateral aspect of the femoral intercondylar notch. The PCL arises from the central portion of the posterior tibia proximally, just below the articular surface, and inserts onto the lateral edge of the medial femoral condyle and the roof of the intercondylar notch.

The patella is suspended between the patellar tendon inferiorly and the insertion of the quadriceps conjoint tendon superiorly. The patellar tendon runs from the inferior pole of the patella, inserting onto the tibial tuberosity of the anterior proximal tibia.

Indications

Washout of sepsis, mensical tears, chondral defects, and removal of loose bodies, cruciate ligament reconstruction, synovectomy, excision of soft tissue lesions, assessment of intra-articular fractures and their reduction.

Preoperative preparation

- History and examination to obtain likely diagnosis.
- Imaging:
  - AP and lateral X-rays of the knee should be performed.
  - MRI to diagnose soft tissue pathology as indicated by clinical assessment.
- Obtain informed consent.
  - Explain procedure to patient
  - Risks: infection (superficial wound and septic arthritis), nerve injury (infrapatellar branch of long saphenous nerve), neuropraxia due to tourniquet, effusion, DVT, and PE.
- Ensure the correct surgical site is marked.
- Liaise with anaesthetist.
  - GA most common.
  - Antibiotics on induction if any implants are used.
- Liaise with the scrub team and ensure equipment is available:
  - Appropriate table to allow required positioning.
  - A side support or post.
  - Tourniquet and padding.
  - 'Arthroscopy stack' to include: monitor, light source, camera with imaging and recording capability, fluid management system.
  - High-flow arthroscope cannula.
  - 4 mm arthroscope (30° viewing angle).
  - Shaver, radio-frequency ablator, arthroscopic instrument tray.
  - An assistant is useful but not essential.

Position and theatre set-up

- Head end of table next to anaesthetist.
- Nurse and instrument trolley on operative side, stack and drivers for equipment on opposite side.

- Patient supine.
  - A well-secured and padded post at the level of the upper mid-thigh on the operative side can be useful to lever open the medial compartment.
- Apply a high-thigh tourniquet (inflate to 300mmHg) and inflate after preparation and draping to reduce intra-articular bleeding.

Procedure

- The World Health Organization safe surgery checklist must be completed.
- Examination under anaesthetic:
  - Range of motion (in degrees)—flexion and extension (hyperextension).
  - Any instability: ACL, PCL, MCL, LCL.
  - Patellar tracking and instability.
  - Document this clearly.
- Preparation of the leg to the level of the tourniquet, in line with local policy (iodine-based aqueous or alcoholic or chlorhexidine).
- Drape using a specific adhesive isolation drape or extremity drape.

Insertion of arthroscope

- Marking out surface anatomy is useful.
- Flex knee to 70–90° helps palpate the joint lines and surface anatomy.
- Remember that routinely used arthroscope has a viewing angle of 30°; direction of view is away from where the light source attaches to the arthroscopic cannula. A 70° viewing angle arthroscope may be used in special circumstances where steeper angle of viewing is required.
- Anterolateral portal (see Fig. 16.13):
  - Usually created first. Palpate the soft spot 1cm above and lateral to the angle formed by lateral aspect of the patellar tendon and the anterolateral aspect of lateral tibial condyle.
  - Make a stab incision here, either horizontal or vertical, but ensure the capsulotomy is horizontal, to reduce the risk of injury to lateral meniscus.
  - Take the trochar and cannula (ensure they are secured together), keeping the knee flexed, pass through the incision.
  - Aiming towards the intercondylar notch, apply gentle pressure until resistance decreases and the capsule is breached.
  - Extend the leg and pass through the patellofemoral joint into the supra-patellar pouch. Remember this is a blind manoeuvre, thus care must be taken not to drive into and damage the articular surface.
  - Moving the cannula side to side freely confirms position.
  - Remove the trochar and insert the arthroscope attached to the camera (ensure white balancing has taken place prior to insertion).
  - Attach the inflow tube to the tap on the cannula and turn on, distending the joint.
  - Washout of the joint may be required to clear blood and synovial fluid to provide a clear picture.
  - Focus camera.

- Anteromedial portal (see Fig. 16.13):
  - This is created under direct vision once the diagnostic investigation of the knee joint has reached the medial compartment.
  - Allow the knee to flex over the edge of the table, this allows easier access to the medial compartment.
  - Insert a needle into the medial compartment, watching for its entry on the monitor. The entry point is similar to the lateral side: 1cm medial to patellar tendon and 1cm superior to the medial tibial condyle. The needle should pass just superior to the medial meniscus.
  - Remove the needle and make a stab incision as for the lateral portal in the same orientation, avoiding damage to the medial meniscus.
  - A probe can now be passed to aid with the assessment of the knee joint.
- Inspection of the knee joint:
  - Navigate around the joint in a systematic fashion to ensure all anatomy is seen and no pathology is missed:
    - —Suprapatellar pouch (knee extended).
    - —Lateral gutter (knee extended).
    - —Patellofemoral joint (under surface of patella, trochlea groove of femoral condyle).
    - —Medial gutter (knee extended).
    - —Medial compartment (knee flexed over side of bed, slight extension is helpful to view posterior horn of mensici; assess medial meniscus, medial tibial and femoral condyles).
    - —Intercondylar notch (knee flexed; ACL, PCL, and horns of mensici).
    - —Lateral compartment ('figure of 4' position; assess lateral meniscus, lateral tibial, and femoral condyles).
  - Remember to move the light lead of the scope around to change the viewing angle.
  - Take photographs of the anatomy as seen for documentation purposes.
  - Once diagnostic assessment is complete, management of the pathology can be undertaken.
  - Safely pass the scope and instruments to senior surgeon and explain findings.

Closure
- Some surgeons leave portals unsutured and just apply an adhesive paper strips and dressing.
- If closing, use a non-absorbable monofilament (3.0 nylon) and dry adhesive dressing.
- Apply a layer of padding and a crepe bandage for 24h.
- Deflate tourniquet.

Postoperative care
- Construct a detailed operation note and annotate the photographs that have been taken.
- Follow-up as per local protocol, depending on procedure performed.
- Weight bear and begin range of movement early.
- Physiotherapy is essential to reduce the risk of postoperative stiffness.
- Remove sutures at 10–14 days.

Shoulder arthroscopy

Anatomy

Surface anatomy is key (Fig. 16.14). Mark out:

- Acromion.
- Spine of scapula.
- Clavicle.
- Acromioclavicular joint.
- Coracoid.

The glenohumeral joint consists of the articulating surfaces of the head of the humerus and the glenoid.

The glenoid is pear shaped and shallow in its concavity, making it quite unstable but affords a large range of motion.

The thick rim of labrum attached circumferentially deepens the glenoid and creates a 'suction cup' effect on the humeral head.

The joint capsule is attached between the glenoid and the humerus (neck) and within it has thickenings known as the glenohumeral ligaments (GHL):

- Superior (SGHL).
- Middle (MGHL).
- Inferior (IGHL).

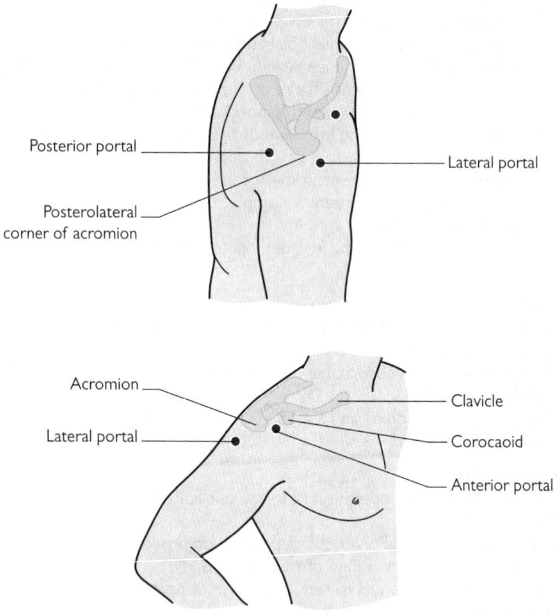
Posterior portal
Lateral portal
Posterolateral corner of acromion
Acromion
Clavicle
Lateral portal
Corocaoid
Anterior portal

Fig. 16.14 Surface anatomy of shoulder, with coracoid, acromion, and clavicle marked out, and entry points of common portals.

The rotator cuff can be visualized intra-articularly and from the bursal space of the subacromial joint:

- Subscapularis runs anteriorly from the anterior scapular body and inserts onto the lesser tuberosity.
- Supraspinatus runs superiorly from the supraspinatus fossa of the scapula posteriorly and inserts into the greater tuberosity.
- Infraspinatus runs postero-superiorly from the infraspinatus fossa of the posterior scapular body and inserts onto the greater tuberosity.
- Teres minor runs postero-inferiorly from the medial border of the inferior tip of the posterior scapula and inserts again into the greater tuberosity.

The long head of biceps (LHB) tendon runs in the bicipital groove into the GHJ, and inserts into the superior aspect of the glenoid and amalgamates with the superior labrum.

Indications

Washout of sepsis, diagnosis of joint pathology, labral tears, SLAP lesions, long head of biceps' pathology, adhesive capsulitis, rotator cuff tears, impingement, excision lateral end of clavicle, chondral defects, and removal of loose bodies.

Preoperative preparation

- History and examination to obtain likely diagnosis.
- Choice of imaging to be guided by clinical assessment:
  - AP of the glenohumeral joint, axillary view and scapula Y X-rays of the shoulder should be undertaken.
  - Ultrasound scan to assess rotator cuff.
  - MRI to aid diagnose soft tissue pathology as indicated by clinical assessment (SLAP lesion, labral injury, cuff tear).
  - CT scan to assess bony pathology (bony bankart lesion, Hill Sachs' lesion).
- Obtain informed consent.
  - Explain procedure to patient.
  - Risks: infection (superficial wound and septic arthritis), nerve injury (supra clavicular branches of nerve, musculocutaneous nerve, axillary nerve, suprascapular nerve), stiffness, DVT, and PE. Procedure-specific complications.
- Liaise with anaesthetist.
  - GA most common, can be performed under nerve block (interscalene, axillary, and suprascapular nerve).
  - Antibiotics on induction if any implants are used.
- Liaise with the scrub team and ensure equipment is available:
  - Appropriate table to allow required positioning.
  - Arm traction set if appropriate.
  - 'Arthroscope stack' to include: monitor, light source, camera with imaging and recording capability, fluid management system.
  - High-flow arthroscope cannula
  - 5mm arthroscope (30/70°).
  - Shaver, burr, radio-frequency ablator, arthroscopic instrument tray, cannulae of varying size.
  - An assistant is useful but not essential.

Position and theatre set-up

- Head end of table away from anaesthetist.
- Nurse and instrument trolley on operative side, stack and drivers for equipment on opposite side.
- 'Beach chair' position:
  - Semi-seated, ensure pillow under legs to prevent slippage, head well secured, and lateral corner of table can be removed (for operative shoulder). Traction can be added if required.
- Lateral position:
  - Back towards the edge of the table, patient secured with front and back supports, head supported (gel ring). Longitudinal traction is applied with arm in approximately 45° abduction and 30° flexion, apply 4–5 kg of weight.
- Remember to perform examination under anaesthetic prior to setting traction.

Procedure

The World Health Organization safe surgery checklist must be completed.

- Examination under anaesthetic:
  - Range of motion (degrees)—flexion, abduction, internal, external rotation.
  - Instability: sulcus sign, dislocatable shoulder, anterior, posterior, or inferior laxity.
- Preparation of the arm and shoulder, in line with local policy (iodine-based aqueous or alcoholic, or chlorhexidine).
- Drape using a specific adhesive isolation drape or arm extremity drape.

Insertion of arthroscope

Some surgeons like to distend the GHJ capsule with saline prior to scope insertion. If this is desired, pass a needle as if inserting the scope and distend the joint—look for back-filling of syringe to conform the capsule is intact. This usually requires about 40ml.

- Palpate the soft spot between infraspinatus and teres minor; 2cm medial, and 2 cm inferior to the posterolateral corner of the acromion. Make a stab incision here.
- Ensure the trochar is securely fastened within the metal high-flow cannula. Place opposite hand on shoulder to palpate the tip of the coracoid.
- Push the trochar in an inferomedial direction to the tip of the coracoid (aiming for palpating finger).
- Once through the deltoid muscle, the lip of the glenoid and the humeral head can be felt with the tip.
- Push between these two structures, through the posterior capsule and into joint. A pop is felt.
- Remove trochar, attach the fluid inlet tube to the tap on the scope. Insert the scope attached to the camera (ensure white balance has been completed), lock the scope into the cannula, and turn on the fluid tap.
- Distend the joint, with a pressure setting on the pump of between 40 and 60 mmHg.
- Washout out joint if image is poor.
- Focus camera.

- Navigate around the joint in a systematic fashion to ensure all anatomy is seen and no pathology is missed:
  - LHB tendon (SGHL).
  - Subscaspularis tendon (rotator interval).
  - Rotator cuff (supraspinatus, infraspinatus and teres minor).
  - Inferior capsule and arcade of IGHL.
  - Posterior and anterior labrum and MGHL.
  - SLAP region (superior glenoid insertion of LHB).
  - Articular surface of glenoid and humeral head.

Once glenohumeral arthroscopy is completed, remove the arthroscope, re-insert the trocar into the arthroscope cannula and redirect it to the subacromial space and bursa. Withdraw from joint, stay under the deltoid but superficial to the rotator cuff, and direct the tip of the trocar to the undersurface of anterolateral corner of acromion.

Navigate in subacromial space to view:

- Subacromial bursa.
- Coraco-acromial arch and ligament.
- Bursal surface of rotator cuff.
- Inferior surface of acromioclavicular joint.

Take photographs of the anatomy as seen for documentation purposes.

Other portals can be created to pass instruments, but description of this is beyond the scope of this chapter.

Ensure safe handover of instruments to senior colleague.

Closure

- Some surgeons leave portals unsutured and just apply an adhesive dry dressing.
- If closing, use a non-absorbable monofilament (3.0 nylon).
- Dress as for the knee and apply an absorbable dressing over the top to absorb any fluid that may leak out (for 24h only).
- A sling is often used and if no soft tissue repairs have been undertaken, it can be discarded as pain allows.

Postoperative care

- Construct a detailed operation note and annotate the photographs that have been taken.
- Follow-up as per local protocol, depending on procedure performed.
- Physiotherapy is essential to reduce the risk of postoperative stiffness.
- Remove sutures 10–14 days.

Tips and tricks

- Having a logical sequence to your diagnostic investigation of the shoulder or knee will help to avoid missing intra-articular pathology.
- Using the light lead to change viewing angle will improve the efficiency and ease of the arthroscopy.

Further reading

Hoppenfeld S, deBoer P, Buckley R. *Surgical Exposures in Orthopaedics: The Anatomic Approach*, 4th edn. Lippincott Williams & Wilkins, 2009.

Carpal tunnel decompression

Anatomy

The carpal tunnel is a fibro-osseous tunnel on the palmar aspect of the wrist, defined by the carpal bones and flexor retinaculum (also known as the transverse carpal ligament (TCL)).

The carpal bones are (anticlockwise from scaphoid) (Fig 16.15):

- Scaphoid.
- Lunate.
- Triquetrum.
- Pisiform (volar to triquetrum in flexor carpi ulnaris).
- Hamate.
- Capitate.
- Trapezoid.
- Trapezium.

The carpal bones form an arch dorsally, with the prominences of the:

- Scaphoid tubercle (radial) and pisiform (ulnar) attaching the retinaculum proximally.
- Tubercle of trapezium (radial) and hook of hamate (ulnar) attaching the retinaculum distally.

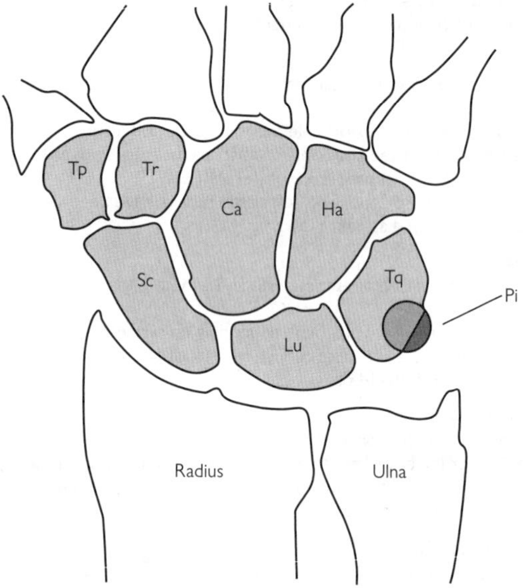
Tp
Tr
Ca
Ha
Sc
Tq
Pi
Lu
Radius
Ulna

Fig. 16.15 The bones of the carpus. Sc =scaphoid, Lu= lunate, Tq = Triquetrum, Pi = Pisiform, Ha = Hamate, Ca = Capitate, Tr = Trapezoid, Tp = Trapezium.

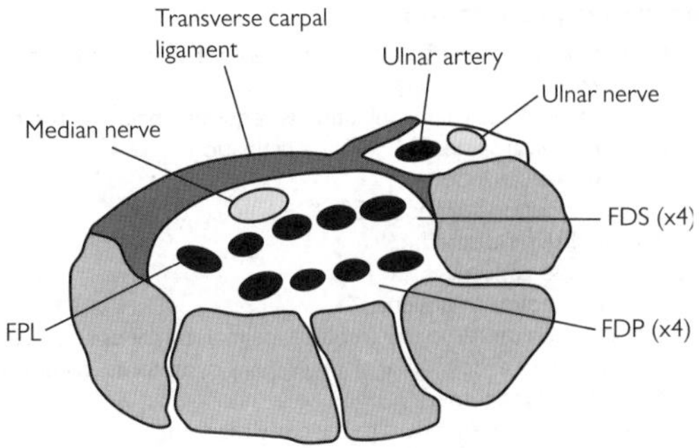
Transverse carpal ligament
Ulnar artery
Ulnar nerve
Median nerve
FDS (x4)
FPL
FDP (x4)

Fig. 16.16 Carpal tunnel cross-sectional anatomy.

Within the carpal tunnel run 11 structures (Fig. 16.16):

- Most volar the four tendons of flexor digitorum superficialis (FDS) and the median nerve.
- Dorsal and radial is flexor pollicis longus (FPL); and the four tendons of the flexor digitorum profundus (FDP).
- The flexor carpi radialis (FCR) tendon lies in a separate compartment on the radial aspect of the tunnel.
- The ulnar nerve and artery lie superficial to the ulnar aspect of the flexor retinaculum and are not within the carpal tunnel.
- The palmar cutaneous branch of the median nerve arises 5cm proximal to the flexor retinaculum and courses distally and on the radial side of the median nerve, staying superficial to the retinaculum, to supply the proximal palmar skin.
- It is in danger if the incision is too radial.
- The recurrent motor branch of the median nerve supplies the muscle of the thenar eminence. The point where this branch arises from the median nerve and its course are variable and thus place it at risk during release of the retinaculum.
- Most often (50%) it arises distal to the TCL and proceeds retrograde to supply the thenar eminence.
- It can arise within the carpal tunnel itself and either pass out beneath the TCL distally and curve back (30%)
- or pass directly through the TCL to the thenar muscles (20%).

Indications

- Compression of the median nerve at the carpal tunnel, as it passes beneath the transverse carpal ligament.
- Release of sepsis.
- Part of a fasciotomy of the forearm for compartment syndrome.
- Compression of the median nerve at the wrist following distal radius fracture.

Preoperative preparation

- History and examination usually are sufficient for diagnosis of carpal tunnel syndrome.
  - Thorough neurological examination is required, including the entire limb and cervical spine. PMH, DH, occupation.
- Investigations may include:
  - Nerve conduction studies (NCS).
  - Cervical MRI if indicated.
- Obtain informed consent:
  - Explain procedure to patient.
  - Risks: infection, nerve injury (median, palmar cutaneous), radial artery, scar tenderness, pillar pain, ongoing symptoms, complex regional pain syndrome.
  - Ensure the correct surgical site is clearly marked.
- LA commonly used.
  - General or regional anaesthesia used in revision surgery or those unable to tolerate a local procedure.
- Liaise with the scrub team and ensure equipment is available:
  - A basic soft tissue tray.
  - Bipolar diathermy.
  - Standard operating table with arm table attachment.
  - Antibiotics not required.

Position and theatre set-up

- Table running perpendicular to anaesthetic machine.
- Patient positioned supine with operative arm on arm table.
- Operating seat in axilla, scrub nurse and trolley at end of arm board.
- Place a high-arm tourniquet.
- Loupe magnification is useful if neurolysis required.

Procedure

- The World Health Organization safe surgery checklist must be completed.
- Apply high-arm tourniquet and set to 250mmHg.
- Prepare operative hand with iodine-based aqueous or alcoholic, or chlorhexadine.
- Infiltrate LA (10ml 1% lignocaine or 10ml 1% lignocaine and 0.5% bupivacaine 1:1 mixture) as a field block in the area of the likely wound.
- Usually from the distal wrist crease to the proximal palmar crease, in line with the radial border of the ring finger.
- Now scrub.
- Prepare the arm to the level of the tourniquet, in line with local policy (iodine-based aqueous or alcoholic, or chlorhexidine). Drape using a specific adhesive isolation drape or arm extremity drape.
- Elevate arm or use crepe to exsanguinate the limb and inflate tourniquet.
- Make incision in line with the radial border of the ring finger (2–3mm ulnar to the thenar skin crease), running from Kaplan's cardinal line distally (thumb extended to 90°, parallel line drawn across palm from distal border of thumb, marks the level of deep palmar arch) (Fig. 16.17) to the distal wrist crease.

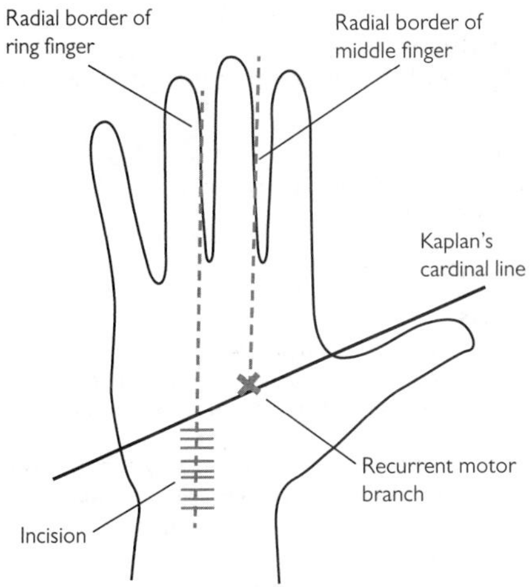
Radial border of
ring finger
Radial border of
middle finger
Kaplan's
cardinal line
Recurrent motor
branch
Incision

Fig. 16.17 Surface anatomy of the palm of the hand and landmarks used for surgery of the carpal tunnel.

- If proximal extension is required, curve incision ulnarwards so not to cross wrist joint at 90°.
- Keeping incision slightly ulnar reduces risk of injuring the palmar cutaneous nerve and the deep motor branch of the median nerve.
- Continue with sharp dissection in line with incision, proceeding through fat, occasionally the belly of flexor pollicis brevis (divide), to the superficial palmar fascia.
- The palmaris longus tendon (present in 90%) inserts here.
- Divide the flexor retinaculum carefully in line with incision.
- Once the carpal tunnel is entered, the median nerve will be seen.
- Insert a McDonald dissector between the median nerve and retinaculum distally, elevating the retinaculum away from the nerve, cut down onto the McDonalds, thus protecting the nerve.
- Repeat proximally.
- Ensure complete release of the retinaculum is obtained.
- Distally the perivascular fat often marks the extent and may need retraction to fully achieve release
- Proximally retraction is useful to complete release under direct vision.
- Reduce tourniquet and ensure haemostasis.
- Observe 'blush' of nerve on tourniquet release to confirm healthy nerve and absence of constricting bands around the nerve itself, which may need release/neurolysis.

Closure

- Close with 4.0 interrupted nylon monofilament suture.
- Adhesive dressing and compressive hand bandage, ensuring fingers free to move.

Postoperative care

- Encourage elevation and finger movement.
- Reduce bandage at 48h.
- Remove sutures at 10–12 days.
- 6–8 week clinical review and discharge.

Tips and tricks

- When making your incision, and progressing through the subsequent layers of the transverse carpal ligament, ensure you remain perpendicular to the palm, otherwise you can easily stray into Guyon's canal.
- Keep the hand fully supinated on the table, using either an assistant or lead hand. The hand had a natural tendency to pronate.

Surgical anatomy and approaches to the hip joint

Overview

An understanding of the key anatomy of the hip joint is vital for planning operative management of hip fractures and understanding the approaches to the hip for both trauma and elective surgeries.

Anatomy

The intertrochanteric region runs from the greater trochanter to the lesser trochanter of the proximal femur (Fig. 16.18). It marks the insertion of the joint capsule, and with it the basis of the classification of proximal femoral fractures as intra-capsular or extra-capsular.

- The distinction between intra- and extra-capsular fractures is made in relation to the blood supply to the femoral head.
- Displaced intra-capsular fractures have a disrupted blood supply and are prone to non-union and avascular necrosis, thus requiring replacement.
- Extra-capsular fractures have a maintained blood supply and will heal.
- The blood supply is threefold (Fig. 16.19):
    - Superiorly from the ligamentum teres.
    - Distally via the interosseous vessels.
    - The extra-capsular circumflex arterial anastomosis, made up of the medial and lateral circumflex arteries, which are branches of the profunda femoris. These in turn give rise to the ascending capsular vessels, which supply the head.
- The hip abductors (gluteus medius and minimus) insert onto the greater trochanter.
- The hip flexor iliopsoas inserts onto the lesser trochanter.

Approaches to the hip joint

The posterior (Moore or southern) approach

- Commonly used for total hip arthroplasty. It has no true inter-nervous plane. This involves splitting the fascia lata in a posterior fashion proximally into the gluteus maximus. The short external rotator of the hip (piriformis, superior and inferior gemelli, obturator internus, and pronator quatdratus) are exposed and lifted from the posterior aspect of the trochanter to reveal the hip capsule. The sciatic nerve is at risk here as this passes through the greater sciatic notch, usually inferior to the piriformis and lies on the short external rotators.

The anterior (Smith–Petersen) approach

- Commonly used in paediatric surgery or for washing out a septic hip joint. It reduces the risk of damaging the blood supply to the head of the femur. It has a true inter-nervous plane between the femoral nerve and superior gluteal nerve. This involves an incision from the ASIS vertically down over the interval of the sartorius and tensor fascia lata. Superficially, develop the interval between sartorius (femoral nerve) and tensor fascia muscle (superior gluteal nerve), identifying the lateral cutaneous nerve of thigh and retracting it medially with sartorius. The

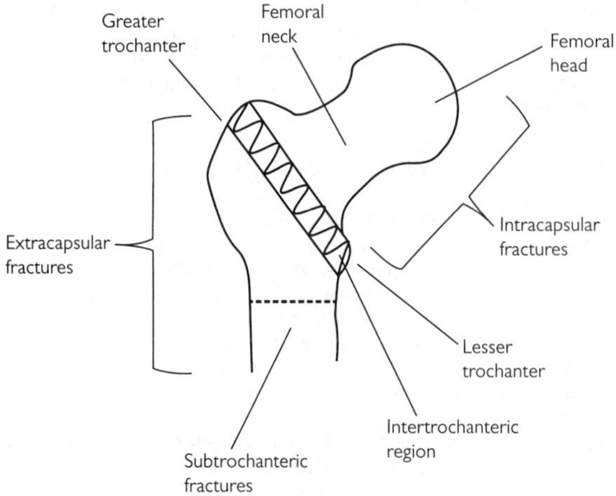
Greater
trochanter
Femoral
neck
Femoral
head
Extracapsular
fractures
Intracapsular
fractures
Lesser
trochanter
Intertrochanteric
region
Subtrochanteric
fractures

Fig. 16.18 Classification of hip fracture—intra-capsular or extra-capsular.

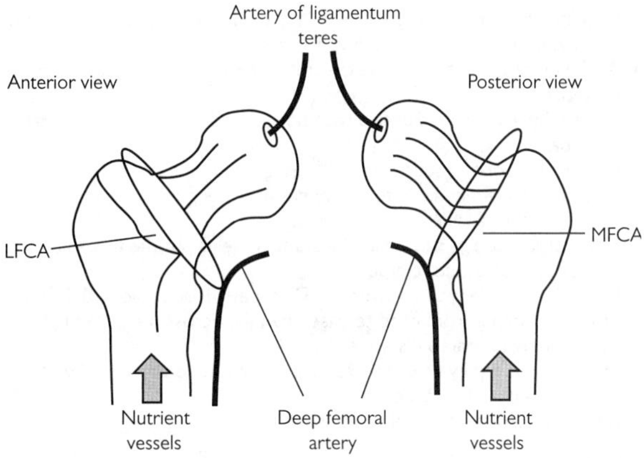
Artery of ligamentum
teres
Anterior view
Posterior view
LFCA
MFCA
Nutrient
vessels
Deep femoral
artery
Nutrient
vessels

Fig. 16.19 The blood supply to the femoral head: MFCA (medial femoral circumflex artery), LFCA (lateral femoral circumflex artery).

ascending branch of the lateral femoral circumflex artery crosses the gap between sartorius and tensor fascia lata and often requires ligation. Deep to this, the interval between the rectus femoris (femoral nerve) and gluteus medius (superior gluteal nerve) is exploited to gain access to the joint capsule.

The lateral (Hardinge) approach

- Often used for hip hemiarthroplasty and THA. It has no true inter-nervous plane (1).
- Incision runs longitudinally 10cm superior to, and over, the centre of the greater trochanter, and 10cm distal, in line with shaft of femur.
- Incise fat to the level of the fascia lata maintaining haemostasis, incise fascia lata in line with skin incision, with a gentle posterior curve proximally to allow easier delivery of the proximal femur at dislocation.
- Insert a Charnley Bow self-retaining retractor with the 'D' side facing distally.
- Be aware of the sciatic nerve posteriorly as this can be trapped under the lip of the retractor.
- Incise the bursa and clear from the greater trochanter by sweeping away with a swab, revealing the muscle of the gluteus medius.
- Split the gluteus medius muscle in line with its fibres, leaving the posterior 1/3 to 1/2 attached to the greater trochanter (for later reattachment).
- Do not stray more than 5cm proximal with the split as this puts the superior gluteal nerve at risk.
- Continue the incision to the level of the greater trochanter tip, along the trochanter and distally into the vastus lateralis muscle.
- At the distal end there are the circumflex vessels, which need to be cauterized.
- Ensure the gluteus medius flap has enough tendon left on the trochanter for repair.
- Lift the anterior flap subperiosteally using a cutting diathermy, subsequently lifting the gluteus minimus lying deep to the medius. This will reveal the capsule of the hip joint.
- External rotation of the leg by the assistant helps put the tissues under tension and eases the release.
- Incise the capsule with an inverted 'T'-shaped incision, along the centre of neck of femur from head to base, then the across the base of the neck from proximal to distal.
- Dislocate the hip by flexing to 90° and externally rotating, this will bring the fractured neck into view.
- Re-adjust retractors to hold soft tissue.

Further reading

Hoppenfeld S, deBoer P, Buckley R. *Surgical Exposures in Orthopaedics: The Anatomic Approach*, 4th edn. Lippincott Williams & Wilkins. 2009.

Reference

1 Hardinge K. The direct lateral approach to the hip. *J Bone Joint Surg Br*. 1982. 64(1): 17–19. 1982.

Surgical approach to great toe metatarsophalangeal joint (MTPJ)

Anatomy

The first MTPJ is formed between the articular surfaces of the base of the proximal phalanx and head of the metatarsal, surrounded by a fibrous capsule. The sesamoids (medial and lateral) sit beneath the metatarsal head, within the tendons of the flexor hallucis brevis. The flexor hallucis longus (FHL) runs between the sesamoids, inserting on to the plantar surface of the distal phalanx. The extensor halluces longus (EHL) tendon runs on the dorsal aspect of the joint and inserts onto the base of the distal phalanx, dorsal surface; the extensor hallucis brevis inserts onto the dorsal aspect of the proximal phalanx. The adductor hallucis muscle inserts onto the lateral aspect of the proximal phalanx, blending with the joint capsule. The abductor hallucis muscle inserts onto the medial aspect of the proximal phalanx, blending with the joint capsule (Fig. 16.20).

The dorsomedial digital nerve runs along the dorsal aspect of the great toe, medial to the EHL tendon. On the plantar aspect, medially, runs the medial plantar hallucal artery and nerve. Both these structures can be injured during dissection, if the incision is placed too dorsal or plantar.

Indications

Commonly used for cheilectomy, arthrodesis, and replacement of the osteoarthritic MTPJ (hallux rigidus); correction of hallux valgus. Useful for fracture surgery of the 1st ray of the foot.

Preoperative preparation

- Ensure thorough history and examination is undertaken.
- Order and have available appropriate radiographs.
- Obtain informed consent:

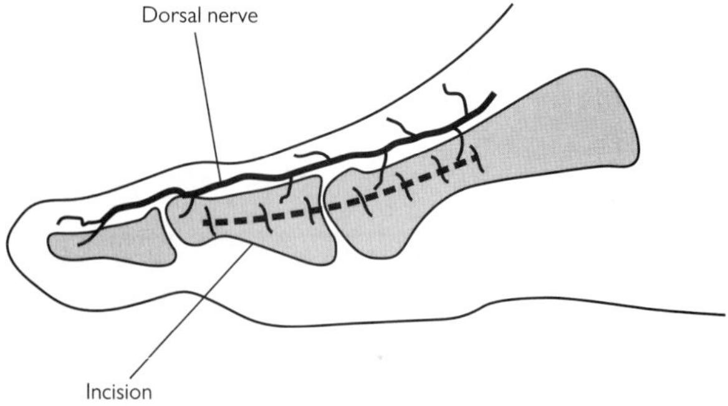
Dorsal nerve
Incision

Fig. 16.20 Anatomy and medial incision for approach to 1st MTPJ.

- Explanation of procedure.
- Risks: infection (superficial, septic arthritis), nerve injury (dorsomedial nerve), vessel injury, DVT/PE.
- Correct limb and toe marked.

- Liaise with anaesthetist:
  - GA (need 6h fast).
  - Antibiotics on induction (follow local hospital protocol).
- Liaise with the scrub team and ensure equipment is available including:
  - Image intensifier if required.

Position and theatre set-up

- Position patient supine, with head at anaesthetic end, table running down centre of theatre.
- High-thigh or ankle tourniquet for bloodless field.
- A raised block can be useful to place foot on, or cross patient's leg over for an unrestricted operative field.
- Scrub nurse positioned at foot of bed on the operative side.
- Image intensifier (II) from the opposite side if required.

Procedure

- The World Health Organization safe surgery checklist must be completed.
- Preparation of the limb, in line with local policy (iodine-based aqueous or alcoholic, or chlorhexidine).
- Drape using a specific adhesive isolation drape or leg extremity drape.
- Elevate limb and inflate tourniquet.
- The incision is on the medial side, longitudinal, centred over the metatarsal head, extending from the distal metatarsal shaft to the shaft of the proximal phalanx.
- Carefully dissect down to the joint capsule.
- Raise a dorsal flap, allowing visualisation of the dorsomedial nerve of the great toe.
- Raise a similar flap on the plantar side to expose the capsule.
- Make a longitudinal incision in the capsule in line with skin incision.
- Free off any adhesions and, sticking to bone, lift off the capsule on the dorsal and plantar side of the metatarsal and proximal phalanx.
- This will allow visualization of the joint and any further bony work can be undertaken.

Closure

- Capsule closed with absorbable suture (braided no. 1 Vicryl® suitable).
- Skin closure interrupted non-absorbable monofilament (3.0 nylon) or a subcuticular absorbable monofilament (3.0 Monocryl®).
- Local dressing and forefoot dressing of padding and crepe bandage.

Postoperative care

- Elevation to reduce swelling.
- Analgesia.
- Heel-bearing shoe commonly used to avoid loading forefoot.
- Removal of sutures if required at 12–14 days.
- Specific instruction will depend on the procedure undertaken.

Complications

- Infection, nerve injury (dorsomedial nerve), bleeding.
- Specific complications depending on procedure.

Tips and tricks

- The use of a square bolster to lift the foot off the table will help with easy access to the first ray. This will also allow unrestricted access for the image intensifier.
- When lifting the thick capsule sharply off the metatarsal and phalanx, placing a mini-Homman retractor inside to place the tissues under tension is useful.

Surgical approach to the lumbar spine

The commonest approach is the posterior approach.

Anatomy

- The lumbar spine consists of five vertebrae, which are continuous with the thoracic spine caudally and sacrum rostrally. Each vertebra has a body, two pedicles posteriorly (which form a ring posteriorly completed by the laminae and spinous process). This posterior ring surrounds the spinal cord.
- Lateral projections from the pedicle/laminae complex, the transverse processes, serve as attachment for the strong posterior spinal musculature (Fig. 16.21).
- The vertebral bodies are separated by the intervertebral discs, to which they are strongly adherent.
- Running along the anterior aspect of the vertebral column is the anterior longitudinal ligament, attached to the anterior vertebral bodies, similarly the posterior longitudinal ligament attaches to the posterior aspect of the vertebral bodies.
- A thick ligament, the ligmentum flavum runs between the laminae at each level.
- The opening created posteriorly between the pedicles and laminae, on each side, allow exit of the nerve roots.
- The spinous processes are connected by the interspinous ligament and supraspinous ligament.
- Beneath the lumbodorsal fascia lie the posterior paraspinal muscles, from central to lateral, the multifidus, longissimus and iliocostalis. The quadratus lumborum extends from the tip of the transverse processes. Anteriorly lies the psoas muscle.

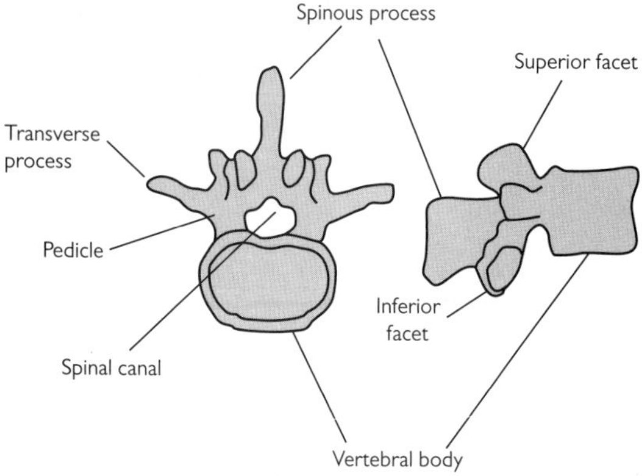
Spinous process
Superior facet
Transverse process
Pedicle
Inferior facet
Spinal canal
Vertebral body

Fig. 16.21 Bony anatomy of a lumbar vertebra.

Indications

- The posterior approach allows access to the posterior elements of the vertebrae, including the spinous process, laminae, facet joints, and pedicles.
- It subsequently provides access to the spinal cord itself and intervertebral discs.
- Uses include discectomy, interbody fusion, nerve root decompression, and excision of tumours.

Preoperative preparation

- Ensure thorough history and examination is undertaken.
- Order and have available appropriate radiographs and MRI scans.
- Obtain informed consent.
  - Explanation of procedure.
  - Risks: nerve root injury, damage to the spinal cord and coverings (dural tear), infection, thromboembolic event. Other risks are procedure-dependent.
  - Mark the level and side of surgery.
- Liaise with anaesthetist:
  - GA (need 6h fast).
  - Antibiotics on induction (follow local hospital protocol).
- Liaise with the scrub team and ensure equipment is available including:
  - Image intensifier is required.
  - Ensure all procedure specific equipment is available.
  - Montreal mattress or Jackson frame required to allow patient to be positioned prone.

Position and theatre set-up

- Head at anaesthetic machine end. Table running down centre of theatre.
- Position prone on Montreal mattress or Jackson frame.
  - Abdominal cut out leaves the abdomen free. This reduces the venous plexus filling around the spinal cord.
- The arms on arm boards, with shoulders flexed and abducted to 90°, ensure no pressure over the ulnar nerves at the elbow. Ensure a well-padded head support is used and there is no pressure on the orbits.
- Setup II with full c-arm sterile cover.

Procedure

- The World Health Organization safe surgery checklist must be completed.
- Preparation of the back, in line with local policy (iodine-based aqueous or alcoholic, or chlorhexidine).
- Drape using a specific adhesive isolation drapes, square draping the operative area.
- Use the Image Intensifier (II) to mark the correct spinal operative level.
- This is done by placing a metal implement or a needle on the tip of the correct spinous process for the operative level; once the correct level is found, mark this with a sterile marker pen.
- Make a longitudinal midline incision, centred over the operative level extending at least one level caudal and rostral.

- Superficially, incise fat and the lumbodorsal fascia in line with incision, to the level of the spinous process.
- Preserving the interspinous ligament, detach paraspinal muscles, on both sides if required using a periosteal elevator. Lift off the muscle, down the spinous process and lamina to reveal the facet joint.
- If complete exposure of the facet joint or transverse process is required, continue to lift the muscles off the superior and inferior facets, care should be taken to spare the capsule if the facets joints are to be preserved. Continue anterior to the transverse process as necessary.
- At this level, the segmental vessels and nerves, that supply the paraspinal muscles, will be encountered as they cross between the transverse process and facet joint. Cautery will be required.
- Deeper dissection involves removing ligamentum flavum by cutting the attachment to superior edge of the inferior lamina. Continue to the under-surface of the inferior edge of the superior lamina. An up-cutting spinal punch is useful to safely achieve this.
- Below the ligamentum lies the epidural fat and bluish coloured dura.
- Using blunt dissection stay lateral to dura, retract the dura and nerve roots medially, continuing to the floor of spinal canal, giving access to the pathology.

Closure

- Close the lumbodorsal fascia using an absorbable braided suture (no. 1 Vicryl®).
- 2.0 Vicryl® for the subcutaneous layer.
- 3.0 Monocryl® for skin.

Postoperative care

- Analgesia.
- Full neurological examination to ensure no iatrogenic nerve injury.
- Mobilization with physiotherapists should begin the next day.
- Full rehabilitation protocol will depend on the procedure undertaken.
- Follow-up in clinic 8 weeks post-procedure.

Complications

- Bleeding, haematoma causing neural compression, dural tear and escape of cerebrospinal fluid, neurological injury, infection.
- Specific complications dependent on procedure undertaken.

Tips and tricks

- Ensure you carefully mark out the operative level before you commence, it is very easy to be a level too high or too low!
- A Cobb periosteal elevator is excellent for the dissection of the paraspinal muscles.

Index

D

E

F

G

H